AF556792

Vascular Diseases

A Concise Guide to Diagnosis, Management, Pathogenesis, and Prevention

Edited by
Sandor A. Friedman

John Wright • PSG Inc
Boston Bristol London
1982

Library of Congress Cataloging in Publication Data
Main entry under title:

Vascular diseases.

Bibliography: p.
Includes index.
1. Blood-vessels--Diseases. I. Friedman, Sandor A. [DNLM: 1. Vascular diseases. WG 500 V3313]
RC691.V37 616.1'3 81-16105
ISBN 0-7236-7000-5 AACR2

Published by:
John Wright • PSG Inc, 545 Great Road, Littleton, Massachusetts 01460, U.S.A.
John Wright & Sons Ltd, 42–44 Triangle West, Bristol BS8 1EX, England

Medicine is an ever-changing science. As new research and clinical experience broaden our knowledge, changes in treatment and drug therapy are required. The editor and the publisher of this work have made every effort to ensure that the treatment and drug dosage schedules herein are accurate and in accord with the standards accepted at the time of publication. Readers are advised, however, to check the product information sheet included in the package of each drug they plan to administer to be certain that changes have not been made in the recommended dose or in the indications and contraindications for administration. This recommendation is of particular importance in regard to new or infrequently used drugs.

Printed in Great Britain by
John Wright & Sons (Printing) Ltd. at The Stonebridge Press, Bristol.

International Standard Book Number: 0-7236-7000-5

Library of Congress Catalog Card Number: 81-16105

Joel M. Schwartz, MD
Chief, Division of Hematology
Coney Island Hospital
Associate Professor of Medicine
State University of New York
Downstate Medical Center
Brooklyn, New York

Edward H. Smith, MD
Professor and Chairman
Department of Radiology
University of Massachusetts
Medical Center
Worcester, Massachusetts

Francis U. Steinheber, MD
Chief, Division of Gastroenterology
Coney Island Hospital
Assistant Professor of
Clinical Medicine
New York University School
of Medicine
New York, New York

CONTRIBUTORS

Harry Bienenstock, MD
Chief, Division of Rheumatology
Coney Island Hospital
Brooklyn, New York
Director, Division of Rheumatology
Long Island College Hospital
Associate Attending Physician
Hospital for Special Surgery
Clinical Assistant Professor of Medicine
Cornell University Medical College
New York, New York

Sandor A. Friedman, MD
Chief, Department of Medicine
Coney Island Hospital
Professor of Medicine
State University of New York
Downstate Medical Center
Brooklyn, New York

Shafkat Hussain, MD
Associate Chief, Division of Hematology
Coney Island Hospital
Assistant Professor of Medicine
State University of New York
Downstate Medical Center
Brooklyn, New York

Anthony M. Imparato, MD
Professor of Surgery
New York University Medical School
Director, Division of Vascular Surgery
New York University Medical Center
New York, New York

David A. Phillips, MD
Associate Professor of Radiology
Director, Vascular Radiology
University of Massachusetts Medical Center
Worcester, Massachusetts

Robert B. Rakow, DPM, FACFS
Chief, Division of Podiatry
Coney Island Hospital
Attending-in-Charge, Division of Podiatry
Caledonian Hospital
Brooklyn, New York

Herman Rosen, MD
Chief, Nephrology Division
Coney Island Hospital
Associate Professor of Clinical Medicine
State University of New York
Downstate Medical Center
Brooklyn, New York

Marvin L. Sachs, MD
Assistant Professor of Medicine
School of Medicine
University of Pennsylvania
Director of Vascular Laboratories
Department of Medicine
Hospital of the University of Pennsylvania
Philadelphia, Pennsylvania

Gary S. Saphire, DPM
Associate Attending, Division of Podiatry
Coney Island Hospital
Associate Attending Podiatrist
Maimonides Medical Center
Caledonian Hospital
Brooklyn, New York

DEDICATION

To our patients and students from whom we continue to learn.

CONTENTS

ACKNOWLEDGMENTS

The editor wishes to express his gratitude to Ms Rebecca Edison for her tireless and dedicated aid in preparing the manuscript of this book. Mr Robert Schwartz, Coney Island Hospital medical photographer, also deserves recognition for his prompt and careful preparation of illustrative material.

INTRODUCTION

Traditionally, the peripheral circulation has not been the focus of much attention in medical education. Medical students generally receive little formal instruction concerning circulatory diseases distal to the aortic valve and this situation prevails through most medical residency programs and, to a lesser extent, throughout most surgical training programs.

As a result of this limited clinical exposure, many practicing physicians do not feel competent to manage peripheral vascular problems. Numerous surveys, for example, have demonstrated physicians' widespread inability to palpate peripheral pulses properly. Even well-trained cardiologists, who are capable of eliciting the most subtle cardiac signs, admit to much difficulty in palpating popliteal pulses. In the training of a cardiologist, there is much emphasis on arteriosclerotic heart disease and coronary bypass procedures but relatively little attention is paid to the same disease process in the cerebral, mesenteric or extremity vessels. The importance of detecting abdominal aortic aneurysms is not stressed in undergraduate medical education, or even in public health courses, even though this lesion is a major cause of death in older people. These are just a few examples in a long list of deficiencies. Certainly medical education has not kept pace with the rapid advances in diagnosis and treatment of vascular diseases.

This book represents an attempt to review the management of the major circulatory diseases and to summarize newer concepts in pathogenesis, diagnosis, and therapy. The text is organized into chapters dealing with the circulation of specific organ systems and others concerned with specific kinds of lesions, such as aneurysms, dissections, and arterial emboli. A chapter on diabetic neuropathy is included because it is so often a complicating factor in patients with occlusive arterial disease.

In the last decade, there have been rapid advances in diagnostic radiology, sonography, and nuclear medicine, which make possible complicated diagnoses with noninvasive tools. The purpose of the chapter on noninvasive diagnosis is to acquaint the clinician with the availability, scope, and accuracy of these new techniques in assessing the vascular system. A chapter on invasive vascular procedures also describes some new techniques and provides an angiographic atlas of vascular lesions.

The chapter on thrombosis is concerned with current concepts of vascular thrombus formation and prevention. It summarizes what is known and what is still speculative about the roles of platelets, fibrinogen, and a host of clot-promoting and inhibiting factors in the pathogenesis of venous and arterial thrombi. This is a rapidly changing field, and the purpose of the chapter is to provide a background for following new developments.

The intention throughout the book is to present a comprehensive, but not exhaustive, review of clinical vascular disorders. The approach is pragmatic and clinically oriented. References were chosen to illustrate and amplify rather than to document each point. Much controversy remains about the diagnostic and therapeutic approach to a number of vascular problems. We have tried to present a balanced account of often conflicting data before offering our own points of view. We hope that this book will have educative value to medical students and will function as a helpful guide to practicing physicians.

1 Arteriosclerosis Obliterans of the Lower Extremities

Sandor A. Friedman

Although often overlooked in routine screening of patients, peripheral arteriosclerosis is a major clinical problem. The true incidence of this disease in various population groups is not precisely known because standards of diagnosis have varied widely.

The Framingham study found the annual incidence of intermittent claudication to be 2.6 and 1.1 per thousand for men and women, respectively.[1] The incidence rises sharply with age, most new cases arising between the ages of 50 and 70. A radiologic study reported aortic calcification in 10% of 40-year-old individuals, and a rising incidence with age.[2] Obviously, these studies grossly underestimate the true incidence of the disease.

CRITERIA FOR DIAGNOSIS

We now know that the posterior tibial pulse is always present in normal individuals. This fact was well established by examining a large group of small children.[3] The normal absence of the dorsalis pedis pulse has been a matter of debate for many years. Surveys on this issue have found that from 5% to 20% of the normal population lack one or more dorsalis pedis pulses. More recent studies have narrowed the range from 5% to 12%.[3] There are major problems in performing what may seem to be a simple study. First, there is great variability among examiners in their abilities to palpate peripheral pulses. Second, one must define the normal population studied. It should be a young, nondiabetic group. Third, the dorsalis pedis pulse is subject to vasoconstriction, and thus subjects must be examined in a relaxed state and in a warm environment. Since these conditions are difficult to meet, we believe that the true incidence of missing dorsalis pedis pulses in a young, normal population is under 5%. With the advent of the portable Doppler machine, it may now be possible to obtain more objective data.

Since the peripheral arterial system is so accessible to physical examination, it is surprising how often the diagnosis is missed unless symptoms occur. Most patients with missing or absent peripheral pulses are asymptomatic. Even the asymptomatic patients represent a small minority of those afflicted with widespread arteriosclerosis. Before one can measure even a slight drop in pressure across an arterial segment, at least two thirds of the lumen must be occluded. Thus, the clinical expression of disease is the last stage of a pathologic process that began many years before.

The purpose of this chapter is to explore the clinical manifestations, risk factors, and treatment of occlusive arterial disease of the lower extremities.

RISK FACTORS

Diabetes Mellitus

Diabetes mellitus is certainly the most prominent of the associated findings in patients with peripheral arteriosclerosis. Clinical evidence of arterial insufficiency has been found 11 times more frequently in the diabetic than the normal population.[4] This is also a difficult statistic to corroborate because the definition of diabetes mellitus is not well established for people over the age of 60. Standards of glucose tolerance were developed by studying normal subjects in the third decade. We know that glucose tolerance decreases with age, but there is no definite agreement on normal glucose standards for older people. It is clear, however, that a very large percentage of patients with peripheral arteriosclerosis are diabetic, at least 15% to 20% of patients with femoropopliteal disease.[5,6] In fact, the majority of femoropopliteal patients under the age of 55 probably have diabetes mellitus. Aortoiliac disease is associated with a somewhat lower incidence of diabetes. Certainly, these statements are correct if we take one of the following criteria as sufficient evidence for the presence of diabetes mellitus:

1. A long-standing documented history of treatment for diabetes mellitus,
2. Persistent elevation of blood sugar levels over 180 mg/100 ml, with intermittent glucosuria,
3. Two-hour postprandial blood sugar level over 200 mg/100ml, or
4. Two-hour postprandial blood sugar level over 180 mg/100ml, with a history of diabetes mellitus in a parent.

The relationship between diabetes and peripheral arteriosclerosis is epidemiologically difficult to study for still another reason. Within the group of diabetics, there is no correlation between the extent of glucose intolerance and the likelihood or severity of peripheral arterial disease. Thus, a graph plotting the level of blood sugar against the presence of peripheral arterial disease would grossly underestimate the importance of diabetes as an etiologic factor because the mildest diabetic has the same risk as the most severe.

Of those patients with peripheral arteriosclerosis, those with the most severe arterial insufficiency tend to be diabetics. The incidence of missing pulses rises sharply in the general population over the age of 60, but relatively few nondiabetics ever develop gangrene. An autopsy study found gangrene to be 40 times more common in diabetics than nondiabetics over the age of 50.[7] Almost all patients who develop gangrene in the presence of a palpable pedal pulse are diabetic. Thus, it is fair to state that diabetes mellitus is the most important etiologic and prognostic factor in peripheral arteriosclerosis. Rarely does a nondiabetic lose a limb secondary to arteriosclerosis. Unfortunately, we do not understand why diabetes accelerates arteriosclerosis.

Hyperlipidemia

The second major etiologic factor is hyperlipidemia. Many patients under the age of 50 with peripheral arterial disease have some form of hyperlipidemia. Although there is a great deal of overlap and confusion about the kinds of hyperlipidemia, the classification of congenital hyperlipidemias by Fredrickson et al[8] is still clinically useful in assessing patients. Briefly, they divided inherited abnormalities into five categories as follows:

Type I:	Hyperchilomicronemia–elevation of low molecular weight triglycerides
Type II:	Betahyperlipoproteinemia
Type III:	Broad-beta hyperlipoproteinemia
Type IV:	Pre-beta hyperlipoproteinemia
Type V:	Type I and Type IV

The most common form of hyperlipidemia seen in patients with peripheral arterial disease is Type IV, although sometimes it is difficult to categorize the problem precisely. In Type IV hyperlipidemia, the fasting triglyceride level is disproportionately high, while serum cholesterol concentration is either normal or elevated to a much lesser degree. It tends to be induced by a high carbohydrate intake and, in some people, is associated with alcohol. Many patients with this lipid abnormality are overweight, and serum triglyceride levels may fall to normal with weight loss. These people can then be maintained in a normal state by preventing weight gain and restricting carbohydrates.

People of normal weight and Type IV hyperlipidemia usually require drug therapy as well as carbohydrate restriction. Clofibrate is very effective in lowering triglyceride levels. Once they have been lowered to normal, it is reasonable to stop this drug and determine whether carbohydrate restriction alone can keep triglyceride levels in the normal range. Long-term, continuous use of clofibrate is associated with an increased incidence of gallstones.

Even when an individual with Type IV hyperlipidemia does not appear to be overweight for his height and bone structure, it is useful to inquire about his weight when he first reached full maturity (about age 25). There is statistical evidence to suggest that weight gain after age 25 can be well correlated with elevation of serum triglyceride levels. Thus, a rather thin individual may gain 20 pounds over the course of 20 years and develop hyperlipidemia even though he is still not obese. Loss of this 20 pounds may be quite beneficial for his triglyceride level.

Types III and V, which are rather rare, are sometimes confused with Type IV hyperlipidemia on lipoprotein electrophoresis. These types are also carbohydrate-dependent and related to premature atherosclerosis. All three are also strongly associated with diabetes mellitus. Although often subclinical, diabetes mellitus or a prediabetic state is present in the majority of patients with Type IV hyperlipidemia. Careful glucose-tolerance testing after cortiscosteroid administration may be necessary to uncover the defect in carbohydrate metabolism. The relative importance of diabetes mellitus and hypertriglyceridemia in the pathogenesis of arterial lesions is not clear. It is interesting that glucose intolerance and hypertriglyceridemia are also linked in chronic renal failure, a condition known to predispose to premature arteriosclerosis.

Type II, betahyperlipoproteinemia, is the second most common hyperlipidemia and is recognized by a disproportionate elevation of serum cholesterol with relatively normal triglyceride levels. These patients also develop premature atherosclerosis and can sometimes be recognized by the presence of xanthelasma and tendinous xanthomas. A common location for xanthoma is over the Achilles tendon where it produces a hard subcutaneous mass. Type II hyperlipidemia is often associated with enhanced platelet aggregation, which may contribute to arterial thrombosis. It is basically a fat-induced defect, which is more difficult to treat than the carbohydrate-induced hyperlipidemias. A low-fat diet, particularly low in saturated fat, must be combined with drug therapy. Since the main route of cholesterol excretion is in the bile, the most effective agent is one that interferes with the enterohepatic circulation of bile and binds cholesterol in the gut. Thus, drugs such as cholestyramine and colestipol are quite effective in lowering serum cholesterol levels. Although they are quite safe and rarely cause malabsorption of other substances, one must be certain that these agents do not interfere with bioavailability of other medications. It may be important to check blood levels of concomitantly taken drugs such as digitalis. Unfortunately, abdominal discomfort, nausea, and bloating severely limit the ability of many patients to continue taking cholesterol-binding agents.

Another facet of lipid metabolism that has taken on importance recently is the serum concentration of high density lipoproteins (HDL). HDL appear to offer a protective effect against the development of arterial disease.[9] Since HDL contain cholesterol, a serum cholesterol level reflects both arteriosclerosis-promoting and -inhibiting factors. A complete lipid profile should include lipoprotein electrophoresis and cholesterol, triglyceride, and HDL levels determined from blood drawn after a 12-hour fast. The development of methods to raise HDL would be an effective approach to the lipid problem. There is preliminary evidence to suggest that regular, strenuous exercise may be one way of accomplishing this goal.[10] Cigarette smoking appears to lower HDL.

Cigarette Smoking

Cigarette smoking is another important risk factor. Numerous epidemiologic studies have confirmed a statistical relationship between smoking and arteriosclerosis in the coronary, cerebral, and peripheral vessels. In one study, only 2.5% of patients with peripheral arterial disease were nonsmokers as compared to 25% of controls.[11] Patients who stopped smoking had a lower rate of amputation than those who continued.

The effects of smoking on the peripheral circulation are multiple. First, tobacco accelerates the arteriosclerotic process through mechanisms that are totally unknown. There is a dearth of information about products of smoking that may affect the arterial wall. There is some evidence, however, to suggest that increased blood levels of carboxyhemoglobin may injure the arterial intima.[12] Second, nicotine in cigarettes acts as a peripheral vasoconstrictor. This further compromises cutaneous blood flow in an ischemic limb. Third, smoking may accelerate platelet aggregation and cause an increased tendency to thrombosis.[13]

Hypertension

Hypertension can be correlated with peripheral arterial disease, although the relationship is not nearly as strong as its association with cerebrovascular disease. In fact, hypertension is probably not a completely independent factor. Many hypertensive patients are also diabetic and often have lipid abnormalities. Hypertension seems to potentiate the harmful effects of these other factors. There is epidemiologic evidence to support this view. In certain parts of Africa, for example, severe hypertension is present in endemic proportions and yet the incidence of coronary and peripheral arteriosclerosis is quite low.

Menopause

In women, early castration seems to be an important risk factor. Bilateral ovariectomy, particularly before the age of 45, is associated with an increased incidence of coronary and peripheral arteriosclerosis. This probably accounts for a high proportion of the aortoiliac disease encountered in female patients.[14] Use of replacement estrogen does not prevent this process.

Recent evidence suggests that even hysterectomy without ovariectomy predisposes women to early arteriosclerosis.[15] The mechanism is unknown. The epidemiologic data, taken as a whole, indicate that removal of female organs is potentially atherogenic and that we have no way of counteracting this effect. It behooves the clinician, therefore, to be very conservative in recommending hysterectomy in patients without uterine cancer.

Polycythemia

Another risk factor is polycythemia. The relative red cell mass (hematocrit) is the major determinant of whole blood viscosity. As viscosity rises, it produces an increased shearing force against the intimal lining of blood vessels, leading to multiple sites of injury. Whenever there is intimal injury, atherosclerosis gains an easier foothold. This probably accounts for the propensity of atheromas to form at sharply angulated branching points in the arterial tree such as the terminal aorta. The rise in viscosity begins as the hematocrit exceeds 45%, but is of minimal importance below 50% to 55%. Blood generally becomes quite viscous when the hematocrit exceeds 55%. This effect is independent of true red cell mass, and even a chronically low plasma volume is a risk factor for arteriosclerosis. The most common cause of low plasma volume is iatrogenic overuse of diuretic agents. It is wise to use these agents sparingly in the therapy of congestive heart failure and hypertension, and to check the hematocrit periodically. In hypertension, the goal of diuretic use should be to eliminate hypervolemia but not to produce hypovolemia. Similarly, in congestive heart failure, therapy should not depend solely on diuresis.

Heavy cigarette smoking may cause mild polycythemia even in the absence of lung disease. Smoking produces carbon monoxide, which combines with and inactivates hemoglobin, leading to tissue hypoxia. This chronic hypoxia is a stimulus to erythropoietin secretion. In obese individuals, smoking may produce a rather striking rise in hematocrit. Basal atelectasis during sleep in these individuals is a further stimulus to erythropoietin production.

Maintenance of a slightly lower hematocrit may be one reason for the low incidence of arteriosclerosis in premenopausal women. Slight iron deficiency may keep their blood viscosity at a lower level than their male counterparts'. It may not always be wise to treat the iron deficiency in an asymptomatic woman.

In patients under the age of 60 with arterial occlusion, who have none of the above risk factors, one must search for other systemic disease before assuming that they have atherosclerosis.

PHYSIOLOGY

In studying the peripheral circulation, one must consider separately the physiology of muscle and cutaneous blood flow. Because of vastly different blood flow requirements and patterns of autonomic innervation, they are often affected quite differently by occlusive arterial disease. The arteriolar network of the skin is under strong autonomic control and is subject to marked extremes of vasoconstriction and vasodilatation. Blood flow to the skin can vary from unmeasurable levels up to 100 ml of tissue/min. An average flow of only a few ml/mg of tissue/min is adequate to maintain its nutrition and integrity.

Blood flow to resting muscle is always quite low. This circulation is under relatively little autonomic control. Local ischemia during exercise induces vasodilatation which, combined with an increase in cardiac output, increases blood flow to leg muscles five- to tenfold during normal walking.

Since the foot is composed mostly of skin and subcutaneous tissue, significant ischemia does not occur until arterial insufficiency is quite advanced. Muscle has adequate blood flow in the resting state even when the foot has become gangrenous. In fact, blood flow to resting muscle is normal or near normal in most people with peripheral arterial disease.[16] Exercise, however, demonstrates quite quickly the deficit in blood flow to the extremity. Even with maximal vasodilatation, arteries supplying the muscle cannot effect the enormous increase in blood flow that is necessary for walking or lifting an arm. It is not surprising, then, that intermittent claudication is usually the first symptom of arterial insufficiency in active individuals. On the other hand, if arterial occlusion is confined predominantly to the distal tibial arteries, beyond the branching of most of the muscle blood supply, rest pain in the foot may be the first symptom. This is also true of sedentary individuals who rarely walk more than a few hundred feet at a time.

SYMPTOMS OF ARTERIAL INSUFFICIENCY IN THE LOWER EXTREMITIES

Intermittent claudication is the only specific symptom of peripheral arterial disease. Like its counterpart, angina pectoris, claudication is a result or inadequate oxygenation of exercising muscle. Unlike angina, which may have many variants and atypical features, claudication in the lower extremities is quite constant. Pain occurs only during walking and is promptly relieved by rest. Standing still for a few minutes should be sufficient to give relief. Most important is the compelling nature of claudication, which forces the patient to stop completely. The pain becomes intolerable and is not relieved by merely slowing the pace. If an occasional patient attempts to continue walking with pain, he will eventually fall down as his hypoxic leg muscles suddenly fail to function.

The distance that a patient can walk depends on the extent of arterial insufficiency in the muscle circulation. Claudication distance varies from less than 50 feet with severe disease up to about six city blocks. Obviously, any factor that increases the work of the leg muscles will shorten the distance. Claudication distance may vary with the speed of walking, inclination of the course, meteorological conditions, and type of surface. The effect of walking surface can be surprisingly important. Some patients with arterial insufficiency may be able to walk long distances on a springy surface such as a boardwalk, and yet are limited to two blocks or less when walking on concrete. Treadmill studies have shown that, under standardized conditions, claudication distance varies very little from day to day. The patient who can walk a half mile one day and only two blocks the next day probably does not have intermittent claudication. With the passing of time, claudication distance may increase or decrease significantly. Each time after pausing to rest for a few minutes, the patient with claudication can generally walk about the same distance again and, in this way, can manage to travel long distances on foot. One encounters an occasional patient whose claudication distance progressively decreases during a walk, so that his total trip is limited. Conversely, a few patients with arterial insufficiency can walk much farther after stopping the first few times—so called second-wind phenomenon. The gait of claudicators is always normal since there is no intrinsic musculoskeletal disease. Once muscle ischemia develops, the patient must stop rather than limp. Any patient who obtains relief or can significantly extend his ambulatory capacity with canes or crutches is not suffering from intermittent claudication.

The nature of pain in claudicators is variable. Most commonly, patients describe a tightening or pressing pain in their calves or buttocks, not unlike the classical description of angina. Others complain of sharp, crampy calf pain which may be excruciating. Finally, some patients feel only a sense of achiness or weakness in their legs and stop walking because they do not have the strength to continue. Some of this latter group probably have a high pain threshold and do not experience any problem until muscular function begins to fail.

In summary, intermittent claudication is a discomfort in a lower extremity, usually in the calf or buttock, which occurs only during walking, disappears quickly with rest, and is relatively constant in its appearance from day to day. If the clinician adheres to this strict definition, he will generally not overdiagnose the condition. Unfortunately, there is a tendency within the medical community to ascribe unexplained chronic complaints about the lower extremities to intermittent claudication. Misdiagnosis can be a very serious matter because it can lead to inappropriate therapy. Most patients with arterial disease of the lower extremities are asymptomatic. If they develop a nonvascular cause of leg discomfort that is mistaken for intermittent claudication, they may be subjected to unnecessary arteriography and arterial bypass surgery.

Radicular pain from arthritis or herniated intervertebral discs of the lumbosacral spine is frequently confused with intermittent claudication. This pain is worsened by walking, but it also appears at rest and is aggravated by coughing and straining. The presence of diabetic peripheral neuropathy sometimes can confuse the issue. Since this complication is very common in diabetics (and many patients with peripheral arterial disease are diabetic), the two disorders frequently coexist. A small percentage of neuropathic patients have shooting pains in the lower extremities, which are often aggravated by walking. However, this pain is also severe at rest and often awakens the patient at night. A few patients may have both neuropathic pain and intermittent claudication, and it may be difficult to assess the relative role of each disorder in the patient's symptomatology.

There is a widespread misconception that nocturnal cramps may be related to peripheral arterial disease. In fact, these cramps have nothing to do with vascular disease. They are very common, particularly in people over the age of 50, and often coexist with peripheral arterial disease. Again, serious consequences may result if they are mistaken for intermittent claudication. These cramps occur during sleep and are relieved by walking.

A rare disease that may simulate intermittent claudication very closely is glycogen storage disease of skeletal muscle (McArdle's disease). This inherited disorder may first become clinically apparent in young adults; the first symptom is often crampy pains in the leg muscles on walking. In this condition, the patient's muscles are hypoxic because of insufficient glucose rather than lack of oxygen. Lactate and pyruvate levels in femoral vein blood do not rise significantly during exercise because muscle cells cannot break down glycogen to glucose.

The other symptoms of peripheral arterial disease relate to the cutaneous circulation and are nonspecific. When they are caused by arterial insufficiency, they indicate rather advanced disease because skin and subcutaneous tissue require very little blood flow to maintain normal nutrition.

Coldness and Paresthesias

The most frequent, but least reliable, symptom is coldness of a foot. Many people have cold feet a good deal of the time because they have an intrinsically high vasomotor tone. However, if a patient complains of unilateral coldness or coldness of recent onset, one must suspect the possibility of arterial insufficiency. Many people have cold feet when they first go to bed, but usually experience vasodilatation during the night. If a patient awakens each morning with cold feet, he is likely to have arterial insufficiency.

Numbness or paresthesias often occur with peripheral arterial disease, but also with many neurologic disorders. In particular, one must consider diabetic peripheral neuropathy. In fact, bilateral foot numbness is more often caused by diabetic neuropathy than ischemia in patients with arterial insufficiency. One must be wary of assessing the degree of arterial insufficiency on the basis of paresthesias. Paresthesias (or numbness) that occur on walking are an entirely different matter. Some patients with arterial disease develop paresthesias of their toes rather than calf pain when they walk. This symptom is a clinical equivalent of intermittent claudication and occurs because of ischemia to peripheral nerves. With a decreased proximal arterial pressure, maximally vasodilated muscle arterioles "steal" blood from the cutaneous arterioles.

Rest Pain

Pain in a foot at rest is a dire symptom if caused by arterial insufficiency. It indicates failure of collateral vessels to supply adequate blood flow to peripheral nerves and skin. The resulting ischemic neuritis produces severe pain, usually described by the patient as burning, numbing, pricking, or a combination of all three. Pain is usually more prominent at night and gradually becomes more severe until the patient may have to sit up to obtain relief. Perfusion pressure is often so low that the relative effect of gravity on total blood flow to the foot is considerable.

It is extremely important to distiguish between ischemic rest pain and other causes of foot pain. Ischemic foot pain indicates a total blood flow capacity to the foot of less than 10% of normal. Prognosis for the foot is poor unless blood flow can be increased. On the other hand, many people with mild peripheral arterial disease may have foot pain related to arthritis, bony spurs, or neurologic disorders.

CLINICAL SIGNS

Careful pulse palpation is the key to accurate diagnosis of peripheral arterial disease. The femoral pulse is relatively easy to palpate in the inguinal area, but proper evaluation of the popliteal, posterior tibial, and dorsalis pedis pulses may cause difficulty for the inexperienced examiner. The Doppler flowmeter has achieved wide popularity as a substitute for pulse palpation. This portable machine is a combination of transmitter and recorder of ultrahigh frequency sound waves. When the transmitter is placed on the skin over an artery, the sound waves are beamed into the artery. If there is a moving plane (blood flow), these waves are deflected back and recorded as a noise. The Doppler flowmeter is unquestionably useful, but a word of caution is necessary. It is extremely sensitive and will register a noise even in the presence of severe stenosis as long as there is a little blood flow. It may also register sounds from large collateral vessels. Thus, a Doppler sound is a reliable sign of patency only if it is used to measure the blood pressure of an extremity. With a sphygmomanometer, one can determine the systolic pressure above which no sound is received. By comparing the blood pressure obtained in this way with the blood pressure in the other extremities, one can make a diagnosis of peripheral arterial disease and also assess in hemodynamic terms how severe it is. The blood pressure in one leg should not be lower than in the other, and leg pressure should never be lower than arm pressure.

Examination of the foot is very important in assessing the adequacy of the cutaneous circulation. With mild to moderate decreases in cutaneous blood flow capacity, the foot or a portion of the foot tends to blanch on elevation above heart level. This may require 20 to 30 seconds of elevation and is often best seen on the plantar surface of the foot. Generally, cutaneous ischemia is most marked in the most distal portion of the extremity, so that the toes may be the only area to blanch. The next maneuver is to place the foot in a dependent position and time the return of normal color. The rapidity of color return is inversely proportional to the degree of ischemia. Pallor that persists for more than 30 seconds indicates moderately severe ischemia, and its persistence beyond 60 seconds is an ominous sign.

Another useful observation involves the peripheral veins. The rate of filling of the dorsal foot veins when the leg is lowered below heart level is proportional to cutaneous blood flow, provided that the patient does not have varicose veins. Since the latter fill in retrograde fashion, they render venous filling time useless in the evaluation of blood flow. Under normal conditions, the dorsal foot veins fill within 10 to 15 seconds when the leg is placed in a dependent position. Vasoconstriction as well as arterial insufficiency can slow venous filling but, in the case of the former, this abnormality is generally bilateral. A difference between the two legs usually indicates decreased skin blood flow capacity.

Rubor on dependency is a sign of severe ischemia. In a foot with ischemic rest pain, one should always find either dependent rubor or prolonged pallor (beyond 60 seconds) in the dependent position. This rubor is a homogeneous, violaceous color on the dorsum of the foot (Figure 1-1). It is most marked on the toes and extends proximally a variable distance. Rubor begins after the pallor has disappeared and reaches its maximum between 30 and 120 seconds after the leg has been placed in a dependent position. This rubor is a reflection of tissue hypoxia, and reactive arteriolar and capillary dilatation. Ischemic tissue extracts more oxygen from arteriolar blood. The resulting deoxygenated blood remains in dilated capillaries because of the low perfusion pressure. Dependent rubor must be distinguished from the violaceous hue seen in chronic venous insufficiency. With venous disease, cyanosis appears as soon as the leg becomes dependent, and is scattered throughout the foot rather than homogeneous and concentrated. Some feet develop digital, homogeneous erythema rather than a violaceous color on assumption of the dependent position. This represents a reactive hyperemia secondary to less severe ischemia.

Temperature of the foot is of limited usefulness as a clinical sign of ischemia. Foot temperature depends to a large extent on environmental temperature and its state of vasomotor tone. One can sometimes recognize the effect of vasoconstriction if the foot is sweaty as well as cold. Unilateral coldness without sweating usually indicates arterial insufficiency. An experienced examiner can learn to distinguish a difference of 1 °C with careful palpation.

With advanced ischemia, skin ulcers and gangrene may develop.

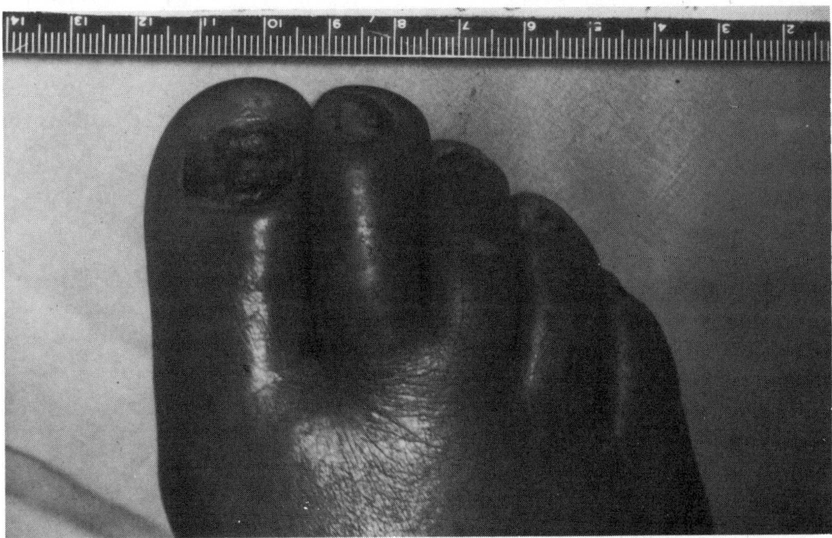

Figure 1-1 An ischemic foot with severe dependent rubor. Small areas of subungual gangrene can be seen.

Ischemic ulcers are most often located on a toe, the lateral malleolus, or the heel, but they can occur almost anywhere on the foot. They tend to be pale with a poorly granulated base and may have a cyanotic border. Very often, the ulcer is secondary to trauma but perpetuated by arterial insufficiency. These ulcers are better vascularized and slow to heal only because of a relative lack of blood flow. Many patients with diabetic neuropathy are subject to frequent inapparent trauma, and the resulting ulcers heal slowly because of arterial disease. Arterial ulcers must be distinguished from venous ulcers, which are hyperemic and associated with other signs of venous insufficiency.

The so-called trophic changes—hair loss, callus formation, and dystrophy of the toenails—are not well correlated with the presence or severity of arterial insufficiency. They are not useful in assessing the circulatory status.

GENERAL MEASURES FOR THE TREATMENT OF PERIPHERAL ARTERIAL DISEASE

Most patients with peripheral arterial disease are asymptomatic and have no signs of cutaneous ischemia. The diagnosis can be made only by careful palpation of peripheral pulses on routine examination. The finding of a pulseless foot is extremely important. Blood flow capacity may appear quite adequate for ordinary circumstances, but still be insufficient to meet extraordinary demands. Any trauma to the foot may increase tissue metabolism and consequent need for blood flow beyond what the collateral vessel can supply. For this reason, every patient in this category should receive detailed foot care instructions. We give our patients the following advice verbally and in the form of a printed handout:

Instructions for Care of the Feet for Patients with Poor Circulation of the Legs

1. Tobacco: Do not smoke.
2. Cold: Avoid extreme cold. Dress very warmly in winter. Do not bathe or swim in cold water.
3. Heat: Never apply heat or ice to the feet. Avoid exposure of feet or legs to the sun.
4. Position: Sleep with your legs on the level with the bed. Never sit with legs crossed.
5. Cleanliness: Wash your feet with a mild soap in lukewarm water only. Dry feet carefully, especially between toes.

6. Dry scaly skin: You may apply lanolin or cold cream to your feet—gently massage into the dry, scaly areas.
7. Toenails: Should be cut by a podiatrist or a member of your family. Cut the toenails straight across; never cut in at the corners or too close to the skin.
8. Corns and calluses: Should be taken care of by a podiatrist.
9. Shoes and socks: Never walk in your bare feet. Wear only comfortable, properly fitting shoes and socks. Square- or round-toed shoes preferred. Clean pair of socks each day. Do not wear circular garters or hose with elastic tops.
10. Local medication: Never use strong antiseptic; no tincture of iodine. No corn remedies or corn plasters on your feet. Use only medications ordered by your physician.
11. Exercise: Walking is a good way to improve your circulation.
12. Injuries: Try to avoid even minor injuries to your feet by following the above rules. Consult your physician at the first sign of discomfort in your legs or any injury to your legs or feet.
13. Self-inspection: You may not be able to feel pain in your feet as well as you should. Therefore, examine your feet every week. If there are cracks or cuts in the skin or new color changes, consult your physician even if you have no pain.

It is particularly important to emphasize the danger of applying direct heat to a foot. Heat causes local vasodilatation and also increases the metabolic rate of tissue and local oxygen demand. In the normal limb, the increase in blood flow is more than adequate to meet increased oxygen requirements up to about 45°C. With occlusive arterial disease, delivery of blood to the foot is outstripped by oxygen demand at lower temperatures. Thus, the foot may suffer burns at temperatures only slightly above body temperature. Thermal injury is particularly common in diabetic patients with peripheral neuropathy, since they may not perceive the heat of bath water or electric blankets. Diabetic patients should be instructed to check their bath water with their elbows. For the same reason, all diabetics should inspect their feet periodically, using a hand mirror to see the plantar surfaces.

Vasodilating drugs have long been advocated for improving blood flow. These agents include alpha-adrenergic antagonists and a variety of agents that act directly on arteriolar walls. There has never been any convincing evidence that they increase muscle blood flow as much as normal walking, and their effects on cutaneous blood are questionable.[17] They probably cause more vasodilatation in areas of normal blood flow than in areas of occlusion. They are of very limited use in the treatment of peripheral arterial disease.

Anticoagulants have not been proven effective in the long-term treatment of chronic arterial disease. They are probably indicated in patients who have episodes of acute arterial thrombosis in situ. Recently, much attention has been focused on the possible benefits of antiplatelet drugs, but long-term studies of their effect have not yet been completed.

It is extremely important for patients with peripheral arterial disease to stop smoking. The likelihood of serious complications such as amputation is certainly higher if smoking continues.[11] This observation is analogous to the increased incidence of sudden death in patients with coronary heart disease who continue to smoke. Patients who already have impaired cutaneous flow are at double risk. The vasoconstrictive effect of smoking further limits blood flow, while tobacco accelerates the atherosclerotic process.

Many patients with peripheral arterial disease have coronary artery disease and/or hypertension for which beta-blocking agents may be prescribed. These agents have a variable effect on the peripheral circulation. Although they cause generalized vasodilatation indirectly by inhibiting the production of renin, they also block the action of beta-adrenergic (vasodilating) sympathetic fibers. In some patients, the latter action may result in significant vasoconstriction of both muscle and cutaneous arterioles, increasing the severity of ischemia and intermittent claudication. Beta blockers should be used with caution in patients with peripheral arterial disease. Cautious tapering of the dosage is often advisable for patients who develop claudication while taking beta-blocking agents.

AORTOILIAC DISEASE

Occlusive disease of the terminal aorta and common iliac artery is one of the earliest atherosclerotic lesions. The mean age of patients presenting with isolated aortoiliac occlusion was 49 years in one series.[14] Surgically-induced, early menopause is a significant factor in women with aortoiliac disease. Diabetes mellitus, although a very definite risk factor, appears to be less important in the genesis of this proximal lesion than femoropopliteal and tibial artery disease.

The classic presentation of patients with aortoiliac disease is Leriche's syndrome, consisting of bilateral intermittent claudication and, in males, impotence. The claudication is usually in the area of the hips and buttocks, but this is not invariable. For unknown reasons, some patients with pure aortoiliac occlusion have only calf claudication. However, one must always suspect the concomitant presence of femoropopliteal disease in these patients.

Hip claudication can be easily missed or confused with musculoskeletal problems. The patient's complaint of fatigue in the hips or lower back on walking may be dismissed as a manifestation of poor physical conditioning. At times, the pain can be rather intense and extend almost to the lower back. If the pain occurs after very short distances, it may be mistakenly ascribed to a herniated lumbar disc or osteoporosis of the lower spine. If only one common or external iliac artery is involved, claudication will be unilateral and may be confused with osteoarthritis of the hip.

Impotence

Aortoiliac disease is one of the very few causes of true failure of penile erection. Impotence sometimes dominates the clinical picture since claudication can be extremely mild in the beginning, especially in patients who tend to be sedentary. Impotence, like claudication, may develop gradually over a period of months as proximal perfusion pressure decreases. The patient may first notice gradual increased difficulty during sexual intercourse and occasional inability to have an erection. Both he and his mate may attribute this problem to emotional problems or physical exhaustion. It is not uncommon for such a patient to seek marriage counseling or psychiatric consultation without realizing the organic nature of his problem.

The mechanism of impotence in aortoiliac disease is a decreased perfusion pressure in the pudendal artery. Since this vessel is supplied by both internal iliac (hypogastric) arteries, bilateral occlusion is necessary to produce impotence. The lesions may be in the terminal aorta, common iliac, or hypogastric arteries. In the rare individual with isolated, bilateral hypogastric artery occlusion, there is generally no claudication. The vascular nature of impotence in a patient with normal femoral pulses can be discovered by penile plethysmography.

Clinical Signs

Because of the proximal location of aortoiliac disease, there is great potential for collateral circulation bypassing the obstruction. Aortography often demonstrates anastomoses of branches of the superior mesenteric and renal arteries with branches of the hypogastric arteries. These, in turn, connect with the deep femoral system. In unilateral iliac stenosis or occlusion, there is usually collateralization between the two hypogastric systems.

As a result of this extensive collateral circulation, serious cutaneous ischemia is unusual in isolated aortoiliac occlusion. Mild to moderate pallor on elevation is generally the only finding other than pulse deficits. Gangrene rarely occurs, and the prognosis for limb survival is excellent. Gangrene or dependent rubor strongly suggests the presence of more distal disease.

In well-established aortoiliac disease, the femoral pulses are absent or clearly weak, but in milder cases this may not be so. In fact, patients may have definite intermittent claudication with femoral pulses that appear normal on palpation. It may be necessary to measure the blood pressure in the lower extremities in order to make the diagnosis. Systolic pressure can be measured by inflating a cuff over the lower calf to the point of extinction of the dorsalis pedis or posterior tibial artery. The pulse can be monitored by finger palpation or, more accurately, with a Doppler flowmeter. Systolic pressure is determined in the supine position and compared with arm pressure. If there is no occlusive disease, leg blood pressure should not be lower than arm pressure.

Occasionally, arm and leg blood pressures may appear approximately equal in a patient whose history is strongly suggestive of aortoiliac disease. In this case, exercising the leg is crucial for correct diagnosis. Blood pressure tends to fall distal to an arterial obstruction during exercise, perhaps because of the large run-off of blood into muscle vessels. The decline in blood pressure and duration of this decline after exercise are proportional to the insufficiency of muscle blood flow.[18]

By checking postexercise blood pressure, one may discover an aortoiliac obstruction with a systolic pressure gradient as small as 20 to 30 mm Hg. It has been shown in in vitro experiments with isolated arterial segments that this small pressure loss can account for a 33% decrease in blood flow.[14] Thus, a patient with seemingly normal femoral pulses may have very significant claudication. Listening for a bruit over the femoral artery after exercise is another way of detecting the presence of mild aortoiliac obstruction.

Therapy

Therapy for aortoiliac disease hinges on the symptoms and their severity. Patients with mild symptoms can be given foot care instructions and examined periodically. They should be encouraged to stop smoking, lose weight, and continue walking. Walking is a good stimulus to collateral circulation, and the patient should be encouraged to walk long distances, stopping to pause each time claudication begins. A significant number of newly-diagnosed patients report improvement in their claudication symptoms during the first three to four months. If there is no improvement within six months, the patient is not likely to improve further.

If, after four to six months, the patient still has very severe claudication that seriously interferes with his lifestyle, bypass surgery can be contemplated. The factors determining this decision are complex and include the general health of the patient. If he has significant coronary artery or cerebrovascular disease, the risk of a three-hour operation under general anesthesia is considerable. Furthermore, a patient's apparently mild angina before surgery may turn out to be more severe postoperatively. If the patient's walking distance is still severely limited even when he no longer has claudication, not much has been accomplished. If surgery is contemplated, aortography must be performed first. If there is a patent arterial segment beyond the obstruction, surgery is possible. The better the distal run-off, the better are the chances of long-term surgical success. Aortography should not be performed unless surgery is contemplated. It is an invasive procedure with potential for occasional complications. These include traumatic dissection of an artery, perforation, intimal tears, and traumatic thrombosis.

The results of aortoiliac or aortofemoral bypass surgery for claudication, if obstruction is confined to the aortoiliac area, are excellent. Almost all patients receive partial or total relief of the symptom. Five-year graft patency rates for pure aortoiliac disease are over 85% in several series. The results are not as good if there is also femoropopliteal disease. In a Mayo Clinic series of 401 patients undergoing aortoiliac repair, 75% of the survivors were free of symptoms five years after aortoiliac repair.[19] In localized aortoiliac disease, endarterectomy is as effective as bypass grafting.[20]

The treatment of impotence is much more complicated. In general, the results of aortoiliac surgery for this symptom have been very poor, probably for a variety of reasons. First, aortofemoral bypass performed for relief of claudication does not increase hypogastric blood flow. The surgeon must perform an aorto-common-iliac bypass if the lesion is confined to the aorta, or an aortohypogastric bypass if the common iliac arteries are occluded. The latter is not always possible because the run-off in the distal hypogastric arteries may not be adequate. Second, some of these patients are diabetic, and diabetes mellitus is associated with impotence, perhaps due to peripheral neuropathy and/or small vessel disease. The aortoiliac disease may be only a contributing factor in these patients. Third, autonomic ganglia responsible for erection may be destroyed during surgery. In fact, impotence is sometimes a complication of aortoiliac surgery.

Recent reports have suggested that well-planned bypass surgery with particular attention to autonomic ganglia in carefully selected patients may relieve impotence. In fact, iliopudendal bypass has been successfully performed in cases of impotence due purely to hypogastric artery occlusion. However, one must warn the impotent patient in advance that his chances of gaining normal penile function are poor. It is very important to realize that many patients who complain a great deal about claudication are really more concerned with their impotence. Physician and patient must understand each other and plan realistic goals before embarking on aortoiliac surgery.

Evaluation and Treatment of Impotence

Patients with impotence and normal blood pressures in the lower extremities must be carefully evaluated. Psychological, endocrine, and neurologic causes as well as vascular disease should be considered. Nocturnal tumescence studies are useful in distinguishing between psychological and organic impotence. If nocturnal erections are absent, further evaluation should include a search for diabetic neuropathy and microadenoma of the pituitary gland. The latter can be detected by measuring serum prolactin levels. An elevated prolactin level is an indication for polytomography of the sella turcica.

Penile plethysmography is easily employed to detect arterial insufficiency beyond the common iliac arteries.[21] A combination of penile blood pressure measurement with a Doppler flowmeter and impedance plethysmography can detect and partially localize arterial obstruction. A low blood pressure suggests large artery obstruction, whereas a constellation of normal blood pressure and decreased penile blood flow as measured by impedance plethysmography indicates small vessel disease. Arteriography is indicated only if the blood pressure is low and the patient is willing to undergo surgery.

Other Procedures

Alternative procedures for the relief of limb ischemia in aortoiliac disease include axillofemoral[22] and cross-over femorofemoral bypass grafting. Axillofemoral grafts have a low, long-term patency rate[23] and should be reserved for patients with severe ischemia who are poor risks for general anesthesia and abdominal surgery, or have intraabdominal infections. The procedure involves tunnelling a graft subcutaneously from the axillary to the ipsilateral femoral artery, and can be performed with local anesthesia. Femorofemoral grafting can be performed only in the presence of unilateral iliac disease. Results of this procedure in selected cases are almost as good as those of aortoiliac bypass.[24,25]

FEMOROPOPLITEAL DISEASE

Femoropopliteal occlusion tends to develop later than aortoiliac disease. Symptoms do not usually appear before the seventh decade. Diabetes mellitus is the major risk factor, and almost all patients with femoropopliteal disease under the age of 55 have diabetes and/or hyperlipidemia. Most patients present with calf claudication, but cutaneous ischemia is quite common in contradistinction to aortoiliac disease. Older, more sedentary individuals may never have claudication. These patients are asymptomatic until they have serious deficits in blood flow to the foot. The diagnosis of femoropopliteal occlusive disease depends on the demonstration of a normal femoral pulse and an absent or weak popliteal pulse. Posterior tibial and dorsalis pedis pulses are also weak or absent. The popliteal pulse is difficult to palpate, and inexperienced examiners often overdiagnose femoropopliteal disease. With practice, however, one can learn to evaluate this pulse quite accurately in all but very obese individuals. The popliteal pulse is best examined with the patient in a relaxed, supine position and the examiner on the same side as the pulse in question. Using both hands, the examiner should palpate carefully under the knee. The popliteal pulse may be located laterally or medially in the popliteal space and generally requires deep palpation.

The posterior tibial pulse may also be difficult to palpate. It may be quite deep within the subcutaneous tissue and hidden by the protruding medial malleolus. Dorsiflexion and eversion of the foot may sometimes be helpful as one palpates under the medial malleolus. The examiner should be on the same side as the pulse with the examining hand in a comfortable position.

Treatment

Treatment of femoropopliteal disease depends largely on the degree of foot ischemia. In most cases, the patient can usually be followed conservatively with detailed foot care instructions. The indications for femoropopliteal bypass surgery are:

1. Severe ischemia of the foot.
2. Disabling intermittent claudication.
3. Nonhealing ischemic ulcers.

Definite dependent rubor, marked pallor in the horizontal position, or a cold cyanotic foot with or without ischemic rest pain may be a good reason for bypass surgery. One must recognize that many patients, especially those with diabetic neuropathy, may have severe, limb-threatening ischemia without pain. If these individuals are in good general condition and able to withstand surgery, a bypass is appropriate even if they are asymptomatic. However, in the case of high-risk patients, such as those with frequent angina, congestive heart failure, and cerebrovascular disease, it may be advisable to refrain from surgery unless skin breakdown begins. If this decision is made, these asymptomatic individuals must be followed very closely and instructed to inspect their feet daily for signs of ulceration or gangrene. This conservative approach is particularly hazardous in patients with severe diabetic neuropathy, who are subject to frequent inapparent trauma.

Surgical Approach If ischemic rest pain begins, the physician is generally forced to consider more aggressive therapy within a few months. The pain gradually becomes more constant and severe, and the patient may beg for an amputation. He may eventually require narcotic analgesics, become anorectic, and lose weight. At this point, bypass surgery or amputation becomes necessary.

Femoropopliteal bypass for intermittent claudication alone was quite common 15 years ago, but subsequent experience has tempered enthusiasm for this approach. In the first place, femoropopliteal atherosclerosis is usually bilateral. Careful blood pressure measurements in an asymptomatic limb will often reveal some pressure gradient when the other leg develops claudication. The patient may have unilateral claudication only because he cannot walk far enough to develop pain in the other leg. Successful bypass grafting, by eliminating claudication in one leg, may bring out claudication in the other leg. Thus, patient and physician have to be prepared for the possibility of a second operation.

Second, unsuccessful bypass surgery may actually aggravate arterial insufficiency. In order to insert a graft from the upper femoral to the popliteal artery, the surgeon must transect many collateral vessels. A foot with previously good blood flow capacity may now show pallor on elevation or even develop gangrene. The patient must be made aware of this risk before he agrees to surgery.

Third, the long-term results of femoropopliteal bypass surgery are very variable. They depend largely on the progression of atherosclerosis distal to the graft. As the distal run-off decreases, blood flow through the graft also diminishes and the probability of graft thrombosis and occlusion increases. Therefore, the results of surgery vary widely with the patient population served by each surgical group. Patients with mild claudication have, on the average, more slowly progressive disease than those with severe disease and, therefore, are likely to enjoy better five-year patency rates. However, the ultimate rate of progression in an individual patient is impossible to predict.

The best results are obtained with autogenous saphenous vein grafts, but other techniques such as the use of freeze-dried hemografts must be employed if the patient does not have a healthy saphenous vein of at least 4 to 5 mm caliber throughout its length. With autogenous vein grafts, long-term patency rates of 70% to 90% have been reported.[26,27] Even in a series of patients with severe ischemia, patency rates of 96% at one year, 83% at three years, and 72% at five years have been reported.[28] Similar results have been obtained with grafts fròm the femoral to the proximal tibial artery.[27] However, in diabetic patients, the reported long-term success rate is much lower (probably below 50%).[19]

If surgery is contemplated, arteriography of the entire arterial tree from the terminal aorta to the foot should be performed. This is generally performed through a catheter inserted into the lower aorta in retorgrade fashion through a femoral artery. Not uncommonly, a patient may have major occlusions in both the iliac and femoropopliteal areas. As previously pointed out, a mild to moderate stenosis of an iliac artery may not be appreciated by palpation of the femoral pulse. Proximal stenosis must always be surgically corrected before the distal lesion, if the graft is to remain patent. It is not advisable to perform simultaneous aortoiliac and femoropopliteal grafts because the proximal graft is usually sufficient.[29]

The major reason for arteriography is to assess both the proximal and distal arterial run-off beyond the occlusion. There must be a major patent vessel beyond the obstruction in which to insert the distal end of the graft. The likelihood of prolonged patency of this graft depends on the flow of blood into the foot. (Figure 1-2 A, B, C). The decision to operate depends on the condition of the limb and number, caliber and distal extent of patent vessels beyond the insertion of the graft. If the limb is threatened with ischemic necrosis, femoropopliteal bypass may be indicated even with poor distal run-off. On the other hand, surgery for claudication should require excellent proximal and distal run-off.

TIBIAL ARTERY DISEASE

Tibial artery disease increases sharply after the age of 60, and a significant portion of the elderly population has some degree of obstructive disease. The posterior tibial artery is more commonly occluded than the dorsalis pedis. Most patients with this lesion are asymptomatic, but proximal posterior tibial occlusion may produce calf or instep claudication. Tibial artery occlusion is one of the earliest

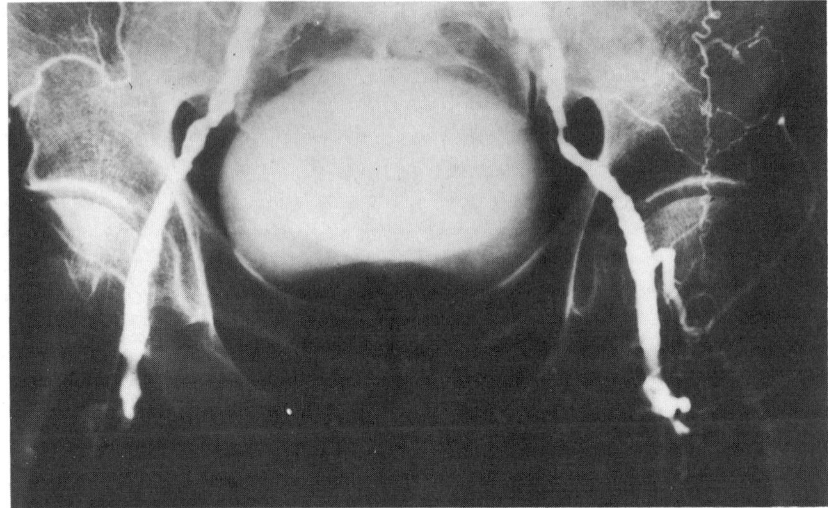

A

B

Figure 1-2A & B An aortogram demonstrates occlusion of both superficial femoral and profunda femoral arteries. Patient is inoperable because of poor distal run-off. **C** A femoral arteriogram shows occlusion of a superficial femoral artery with reconstitution of the popliteal artery through collateral vessels. A bypass procedure is feasible.

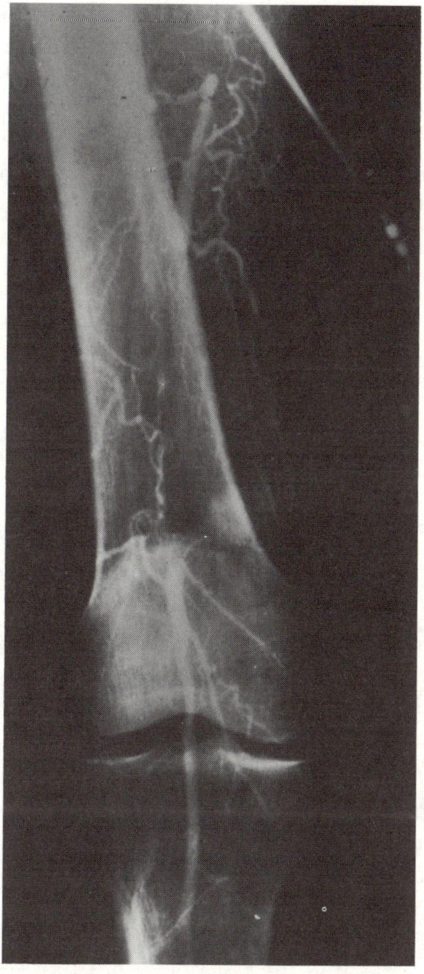

C

clinical signs of atherosclerosis. Narrowing or occlusion of these arteries is a definite risk factor for atherosclerosis elsewhere. In one study, 50% of patients entering a coronary care unit for the first time already had evidence of tibial artery disease.[30]

When the foot is pulseless, blood flow capacity may be reduced. In most cases, it is adequate under normal circumstances, but may not suffice if a strain is placed upon it. Thus, palpation of foot pulses is one of the most important items in the routine examination of older people. A very significant percentage of patients over the age of 60 should receive detailed foot care instruction.

With severe tibial artery disease or combined popliteal and tibial occlusion, severe ischemia may occur. In most cases, arterial bypass surgery is not feasible because the vessels tend to be too small to accept a graft. In selected cases, femoro-distal tibial bypass is possible. If ischemia is limb-threatening and arteriography shows adequate run-off, this kind of surgery can be attempted with the aid of an operating microscope. In selected cases the procedure may be initially successful in about 50%. Nevertheless, the presence of a good popliteal pulse usually indicates that bypass surgery is not feasible.

ALTERNATIVE PROCEDURES FOR TREATING LOWER LIMB ISCHEMIA

Profundaplasty is another reconstructive arterial procedure advocated for the treatment of femoropopliteal occlusive disease. With stenosis and occlusion of the superficial femoral artery, the major source of collateral vessels for the lower leg is the profunda branch of the common femoral artery. Branches of the profunda femoral artery anastamose with geniculate arteries around the knee. Thus, occlusion of the femoropopliteal axis is much more serious if there is also stenosis of the profunda. Endarterectomy and widening of the profunda, in this situation, may improve collateralization and blood flow to the lower leg and foot if there is distal run-off. This operation is sometimes performed in an attempt to salvage an ischemic limb when bypass is not feasible. The results are generally poor.

Lumbar sympathectomy as a means of increasing blood flow remains a very controversial procedure. It certainly has little or no effect on the muscle circulation and should never be employed for intermittent claudication. It is also clear that severely ischemic feet with dependent rubor or gangrene do not benefit from sympathectomy. Some surgeons believe that sympathectomy, by causing total vasodilatation and perhaps allowing collateral vessels to open, may make a difference in the moderately ischemic foot. They contend that patients with recurrent arterial ulcers may benefit from this procedure. There are no controlled studies to confirm any efficacy from lumbar sympathectomy.

ATHEROSCLEROSIS OF THE UPPER EXTREMITIES

Although much less common than in the lower extremities, asymptomatic arterial occlusion can be found with careful examination in a significant number of older individuals, especially patients with diabetes mellitus. Studies of normal individuals have indicated that the radial pulse is never normally absent, and all but about 3% of the normal population also have ulnar pulses.[31] When the ulnar pulse is congenitally absent, this is generally a bilateral phenomenon. The ulnar pulse is usually not checked during routine examination, but a significant number of older people lack one or both ulnar pulses. It is often buried under tendons and difficult to palpate, but one can generally feel it by shaking hands with the patient and palpating with the other hand. Less commonly but not rarely, there may be an absent or weak brachial pulse in the antecubital fossa, which may not be appreciated by measuring blood pressure in the upper arm. Palpation of radial pulses with the cuff over the forearm will reveal a blood pressure difference. In a thin arm, the diseased brachial artery can often be palpated throughout its entire course in the upper arm, and the point of occlusion precisely delineated.

A pulseless hand may be paler than the uninvolved side, and slightly cooler. However, the capacity for collateral circulation is much greater in the upper extremity, and rarely will occlusive lesions of the subclavian axillary-brachial axis lead to serious cutaneous ischemia of the hand. Ischemic tissue necrosis in the upper extremities almost always indicates the presence of a nonatherosclerotic disease. If there is no history of frostbite, one must search extensively for a systemic problem leading to small vessel disease in the hands. This evaluation must include a search for collagen-vascular disease and various coagulopathies, which will be considered in other chapters.

The reactive hyperemia (Allen test) is a useful clinical procedure for assessing the adequacy of cutaneous circulation in the hand. The wrist pulses are obliterated by pressure from the examiner's hand while the patient opens and closes the fist vigorously until pallor is produced. With release of pressure, the normal hand quickly becomes erythematous. This exercise-induced hyperemia is probably mediated through local metabolites. Any area of decreased blood flow remains pale or shows delayed return of color. If this test is positive bilaterally and uniformly, it probably indicates arteriospasm. Unilateral or focal abnormalities suggest occlusive disease. The test can also be performed differentially for the radial and ulnar arteries. Most people have a complete palmar arterial arch feeding the digital arteries and fed, in turn, by both radial and ulnar arteries. Failure to achieve hyperemia when pressure is released from one pulse indicates either occlusion of that artery or an incomplete arterial arch. With the advent of indwelling arterial lines to monitor blood pressure, the Allen test has assumed increased importance. One should not place an arterial line in a wrist artery unless the other wrist artery can be shown by the Allen test to perfuse the entire hand.

Patients with subclavian, axillary, or brachial artery occlusion may have upper extremity claudication. Since exercise in the arms is not standardized as it is in the lower extremities, the diagnosis of claudication becomes more difficult. The patient may complain of pain or aching in the upper arm, but usually he describes fatigue and weakness that limit his ability to perform simple acts. For example, he may have difficulty in brushing his hair or carrying a bag of groceries. One must always think of the possibility of intermittent claudication in any patient who complains of weakness in an upper arm. The presence of a weak subclavian or axillary pulse, or a subclavian bruit at rest or on exercise points to the possibility of subclavian-axillary disease. This can be objectively confirmed by finding a consistent difference in systolic blood pressure of more than 20 mm Hg between the two arms. Exercising the arms is the key to confirming the presence of claudication. The arm generally has normal strength on formal testing, but will fatigue more quickly with exercise.

Whenever the proximal subclavian artery is involved, the patient may also have symptoms and signs of basilar artery insufficiency such as dizziness, diplopia, and even syncope. This can occur through three major mechanisms:

1. Unilateral subclavian artery stenosis with a rudimentary or absent contralateral vertebral artery,
2. Bilateral subclavian artery stenosis, or
3. Unilateral subclavian artery stenosis with a subclavian steal syndrome.

The subclavian steal syndrome will be discussed in detail in another chapter.

Subclavian artery disease without neurologic symptoms is a common complication of a thoracic outlet syndrome which involves the artery distal to the origin of the vertebral artery. This will also be considered in another chapter.

Bypass surgery in the upper extremity is rarely warranted. An occasional patient with subclavian artery occlusion may require this procedure if his lifestyle involves vigorgous exercise of the upper extremity. Professional athletes, for example, may fall into this category. For example, subclavian stenosis or occlusion with resulting claudication is one of the many arm problems that may end the career of a baseball pitcher.

REFERENCES

1. Kannel WB, Skinner JJ Jr, Schwartz MJ, et al. Intermittent claudication: Incidence in the Framingham study. *Circulation* 41:875, 1970.

2. Schilling FJ, Christakis G, Hempel HH, et al. The natural history of abdominal aortic and iliac atherosclerosis as detected by lateral abdominal roentgenograms in 2663 males. *J Chronic Dis* 27:37, 1974.

3. Barnhorst DA, Barner HB. Prevalence of congenitally absent pedal pulses. *N Eng J Med* 278:264, 1968.

4. Dry TJ, Hines EA Jr. The role of diabetes in the development of degenerative vascular disease: With special reference to the incidence of retinitis and peripheral neuritis. *Ann Intern Med* 14:1893, 1941.

5. Schadt DC, Hines EA Jr, Juergens JL, et al. Chronic atherosclerotic occlusion of the femoral artery. *JAMA* 175:937, 1961.

6. Bartels CC, Rullo FR. Unsuspected diabetes mellitus in peripheral vascular disease. *N Engl J Med* 259:633, 1958.

7. Bell ET. Incidence of gangrene of extremities in nondiabetic and in diabetic persons. *Arch Pathol* 49:469, 1950.

8. Fredrickson DS, Goldstein JL, Brown MS. The familial hyperlipoproteinemias. In Stanbury JB, Wyngaarden JB, Fredrickson DS (eds). *The Metabolic Basis of Inherited Disease,* Fourth Edition. New York, McGraw-Hill Book Company, 1977, pp 604.

9. Gordon T, Castelli WP, Hjortland MC, et al. High density lipoprotein as a protective factor against coronary heart disease: The Framingham study. *Am J Med* 62:707, 1977.

10. Hartung GH, Foreyt JP, Mitchell RE, et al. Relation of diet to high-density lipoprotein cholesterol in middle-aged, marathon runners, joggers and inactive men. *N Eng J Med* 302:357, 1980.

11. Juergens JL, Barker NW, Hines EA Jr. Arteriosclerosis obliterans: Review of 520 cases with special reference to pathologic and prognostic factors. *Circulation* 21:188, 1960.

12. Wald N, Howard S, Smith PG, et al. Association between atherosclerotic diseases and carboxyhaemoglobin levels in tobacco smokers. *Br Med J* 1:761, 1973.

13. Levine PH. An acute effect of cigarette smoking on platelet function: A possible link between smoking and arterial thrombosis. *Circulation* 48:619, 1973.

14. Friedman SA, Holling HE, Robert B. Etiologic factors in aortoiliac and femoropopliteal vascular disease: The Leriche syndrome. *N Eng J Med* 271:1382, 1964.

15. Gordon T, Kannel WB, Hjortland MC, et al. Menopause and coronary heart disease. The Framingham Study. *Ann Intern Med* 89:157, 1978.

16. Holling HE, Boland HC, Russ E. Investigation of arterial obstruction using mercury-in-rubber strain gauge. *Am Heart J* 62:194, 1961.

17. Coffman JD. Vasodilator drugs in peripheral vascular disease. *N Engl J Med* 300:713, 1979.

18. Skinner JS, Strandness DE Jr. Exercise and intermittent claudication. II. Effect of physical training. *Circulation* 36:23, 1967.

19. Gomes MR, Bernatz PE, Juergens JL. Aortoiliac surgery: Influence of clinical factors on results. *Arch Surg* 95:387, 1967.

20. Butcher HR Jr, Jaffe BM. Treatment of aortoiliac arterial occlusive disease by endarterectomy. *Ann Surg* 173:925, 1971.

21. Gaskell P. The importance of penile blood pressure in cases of impotence. *Can Med Assoc J* 105:1047, 1971.

22. Blaisdell FW, Hall AD. Axillary-femoral artery bypass for lower extremity ischemia. *Surgery* 54:563, 1963.

23. Mannick, JA. Are there practical alternatives to aortoiliac reconstruction? *Am J Surg* 122:344, 1971.

24. Plecha FR, Pories WJ. Extra-anatomic bypasses for aortoiliac disease in high-risk patients. *Surgery* 80:480, 1976.

25. Brief DK, Alpert J, Parsonnet V. Crossover femoro-femoral grafts. *Arch Surg* 105:889, 1972.

26. Vollmar J, Trede M, Laubach K. Reconstructive procedures for chronic femoropopliteal occlusions: A report on 546 operations. *J Cardiovasc Surg (Torino)* 9:297, 1969.

27. Darling RC, Linton RR, Razzuk MA. Saphenous vein bypass grafts for femoropopliteal occlusive disease: A reappraisal. *Surgery* 61:31, 1967.

28. Wheelock FC Jr, Filtzer HS. Femoral grafts in diabetics: Resulting conservative amputations. *Arch Surg* 90:776, 1969.

29. Szilagyi DE, Smith RF, Elmquist JG, et al. Angioplasty in the treatment of peripheral occlusive arteriopathy: A summary of 12 year's experience. *Arch Surg* 90:617, 1965.

30. Noon GP, Diethrich EB, Richardson WP, et al. Distal tibial arterial bypass. *Arch Surg* 99:770, 1969.

31. Friedman SA. Prevalence of palpable wrist pulses. *Br Heart J* 32:316, 1970.

2 Acute Arterial Obstruction

Sandor A. Friedman

The development of sudden ischemia in a limb is always a matter of urgent concern. Often the symptoms and signs are sufficiently dramatic to lead the patient to seek immediate medical attention, and the physician to make an obvious diagnosis. On other occasions, the symptoms may be subtle and the diagnosis overlooked. Prompt recognition is important not only to preserve the limb but also to establish the cause of the ischemia. In most cases, limb ischemia is a result of arterial embolism which may be a prelude to even more disastrous emboli in vital areas such as the cerebral, mesenteric, and renal arteries. However, there are other important causes of acute limb ischemia which must not be overlooked. This chapter will explore the diagnosis, causes, and treatment of sudden ischemia in an arm or leg.

ACUTE ARTERIAL INSUFFICIENCY

When blood flow through an artery is abruptly cut off, the effect on an extremity is much different from the situation in chronic arterial insufficiency, where perfusing pressure decreases gradually over months or years. Time is required for the development of adequate collateral flow as dormant arterial branches proximal to the obstruction gradually widen and anastomose with small vessels distal to the obstruction. It is for this reason that the maximum effect of an aortoiliac or femoropopliteal bypass is often not seen in the first week after surgery if there is obstructive disease distal to the graft. Blood flow must literally work its way through dormant collateral vessels, propelled by the newly achieved proximal perfusion pressure.

Some collateral vessels open immediately. A femoral arteriogram taken 24 hours after a traumatic occlusion of the popliteal artery often shows numerous collateral branches from the profunda femoral clustered around the hip, but these vessels are not delivering much blood to vessels beyond the obstruction. In contrast, a femoral arteriogram of a patient with chronic femoropopliteal disease usually shows a wide profunda femoral artery extending halfway down the thigh with ramifications that meet elongated geniculate arteries or collaterals from the tibial arteries. In such cases, extensive blood flow through these alternate channels effectively nourishes the limb.

Because of the collateral supply, the patient with chronic disease does not have symptoms at rest until arterial obstruction is very advanced and extensive. On the other hand, in the patient with sudden occlusion of an artery, there may be insufficient blood flow to meet the relatively small requirements of the foot or even resting muscle.

Not all acute arterial occlusions are catastrophic. The severity of the insult depends to a large extent on the patient's ability to summon immediate collateral circulation. The speed of opening of collateral vessels is quite variable and is governed by several factors. The length of the occluded arterial segment, the prior status of the peripheral circulation, and the location of the occlusion affect the outcome. A long thrombus developing in a patient with previous peripheral arterial disease produces much more ischemia than a small embolus entering a healthy artery. A more proximally located occlusion allows more capacity for collateral flow than distal obstruction. Thus, an aortoiliac or subclavian artery occlusion is less likely to threaten limb survival than a popliteal or brachial artery occlusion. There must also be other factors which we do not understand because clinical signs vary a great deal from patient to patient with similar arteriographic findings.

Symptoms

Symptoms of acute arterial obstruction are quite unpredictable. In the classic situation, the patient notices the abrupt onset of excruciating pain, most marked in the distal portion of the extremity.

This pain may be knife-like or have a burning, paresthetic quality. After a few hours, pain may abate as numbness supervenes. The other major symptom is a feeling of coldness in the extremity. Some patients complain of an icy numbness in the foot or hand.

Many patients have less prominent symptoms, and some may have no symptoms at all. Pain may be fleeting and mild. Numbness and coldness may be the only symptoms. Some patients may report that a foot or hand felt unusually cold for a few hours and then warmed up. Others may have noticed transient numbness followed by "pins and needles" or electric feeling in a foot for several days.

Occasionally, an acute arterial obstruction causes virtually no immediate symptoms. However, the patient may begin to have intermittent claudication in the affected limb a few days later when he walks a considerable distance. In taking a history of intermittent claudication of recent onset, one should attempt to determine exactly when and how abruptly this symptom began. If the patient can remember the very first time he had any claudication, and if his walking distance was less than one block on that first occasion, it is quite possible that he has suffered an acute occlusion. He may be able to recall transient numbness, coldness, or pain shortly before the onset of claudication. It is important to evaluate him for possible causes of acute arterial occlusion.

Several factors account for the marked variability of symptoms. First, severity of the ischemic insult affects the clinical picture in unpredictable ways. Up to a certain point, increasing ischemia creates more pain, but when ischemia is very marked, there may actually be less pain. When peripheral nerves become very ischemic, axonal degeneration occurs and the extremity becomes numb. In severe cases of acute arterial obstruction, this numbness may be the initial symptom. In general, it implies a worse prognosis than pain. Sense of coldness also depends on the sensory threshold.

Another factor is the presence of chronic neurologic disorders that may blunt pain perception. Many of the diseases that lead to acute arterial occlusion are closely associated with diabetes mellitus. Patients with diabetic peripheral neuropathy may have acute arterial embolism and gangrene without symptoms. Other patients have sensory deficits secondary to cerebrovascular disease. Finally, there are marked individual variations in pain threshold, and many people may pay little attention to feelings of coldness or "pins and needles" unless they are persistent.

Findings

Clinical findings in acute arterial obstruction also vary. If the patient is examined soon after the onset of symptoms, there are always abnormalities, but it may be difficult to distinguish acute from chronic arterial insufficiency. If the patient gives a clear history of an abrupt nature and has no prior history of peripheral arterial disease, the diagnosis is quite simple to make.

The distal portion of the acutely affected extremity is colder than its counterpart, and there is generally a rather abrupt border between the cold area and the more proximal warmer area. The segment of occluded artery is always more proximal than the upper border of coldness, at least by several inches.

Distal pallor and/or cyanosis is generally seen with the limb at heart level. The foot or hand usually becomes extremely pale when it is elevated above this level. Loss of distal peripheral pulses is the general rule except for a small subset of patients with small-vessel occlusions located in branches beyond the wrist or pedal pulses. This group of patients with the "small-vessel syndrome" will be considered in a separate section. If only one pedal or wrist pulse becomes acutely occluded, the patient will usually be asymptomatic and lack clinical signs of ischemia. The anastomotic connections between the radial and ulnar arteries at the palmar arch and the branches of the dorsalis pedis and posterior tibial arteries are well established before ischemia occurs.

There are occasional patients who develop ischemia of half a hand or foot with occlusion of one of these vessels, because anastomoses are congenitally absent. This problem can be iatrogenically induced. Patients with arterial lines placed in a radial artery for blood pressure monitoring or with arteriovenous fistulas for hemodialysis may develop pallor, cyanosis, and gangrene of several fingers. In order to avoid this complication, an Allen test should be performed on a hand before these procedures are carried out. Both the radial and ulnar pulses are occluded with digital pressure and the hand is allowed to become pale. Then, each pulse is released separately and watched for the speed and degree of reactive hyperemia throughout the hand. Neither wrist artery should be used for invasive procedures of any kind unless flow from each produces prompt hyperemia to the entire hand.

Neurologic abnormalities are generally seen within the first few hours. Distal pin sensation is decreased or absent, and the patient may also lose proprioceptive sense. The proximal extension of sensory loss is variable, but it never extends above the area of coldness. Motor weakness or even paralysis of the hand or foot may also occur. Severe sensory or motor loss is a prognostic sign and suggests that gangrene may soon ensue.

Acute arterial occlusion does not cause generalized edema of the ankle or leg, but a tender area of swelling may appear in the mid-calf area. This represents infarction of skeletal muscle in the gastrocnemius sheath and is associated with a poor prognosis for the viability of the limb. Initially, there is local calf tenderness and only mild subcutaneous induration, but the area of circumscribed swelling increases during the first 24 hours. In severe cases, the entire gastrocnemius area may become boggy and indurated due to necrosis.

If one does not see the patient on the first day of the insult, clinical signs may be quite misleading. Provided that the occluded vessel has recanalized, there may be no signs of cutaneous ischemia. Even with good collateral circulation, there will be at least a mild temperature difference between the extremities, and some pallor on elevation of the limb. If the occlusion is bilateral, this slight temperature difference will be absent. Distal sensory deficits may persist for weeks or months, even after the circulatory status has improved.

If a patient has a history of peripheral arterial disease including intermittent claudication and a feeling of coldness in his foot, it may be very difficult to evaluate the limb should he suddenly develop new symptoms. It is for this reason that documentation of the pulse is so important. Loss of pulse proximal to the area of old disease clearly indicates the presence of a new occlusion. Without this information, it may be impossible to determine clinically whether the patient has a superimposed new arterial obstruction or progressive ischemia because of his chronic arterial insufficiency.

Occasionally, an obtunded or immobilized patient is seen with an ischemic limb. With an unclear history, it is very difficult to determine whether the arterial disease is chronic or acute. There are some clinical signs that may be useful in making this differentiation, but it is usually difficult to be certain of the diagnosis. Arteriography and/or exploration of the occluded artery may be necessary. Muscle enzyme studies may be helpful in such cases. In particular, the creatine phosphokinase (CPK) level tends to rise to high levels in acute arterial occlusion. A small elevation is not helpful because even slight trauma such as an intramuscular injection can elevate the CPK. Cardiac causes of CPK elevation can be eliminated by measuring isozymes and demonstrating an elevation predominantly of the M-M fraction. Differences between acute and chronic arterial insufficiency are summarized in Table 2-1. It should be remembered that there is a great deal of overlap in individual cases.

CAUSES OF ACUTE ARTERIAL OCCLUSION

Once the diagnosis of acute arterial occlusion has been made or suspected, it is imperative to look for the causes. Systemic therapy and local care of the limb often depend on accurate location of the source of

Table 2-1
Differential Diagnosis of Acute Arterial Occlusion and Chronic Arterial Insufficiency

	Acute Arterial Occlusion	Chronic Arterial Insufficiency
Temperature of limb	usually very cold	variable
Demarcation of temperature	usually sharp drop in temperature	more gradual decrease in temperature
Total loss of digital sensation	common	rare, unless associated with diabetic neuropathy
Dependent rubor	often absent	usually present
Mottled cyanosis and pallor	usually present	usually absent
Pallor on dependency	usually present	usually absent
Calf muscle induration	often present	absent
Arteriogram	smooth arteries with circumscribed obstruction	beaded and ragged vessels with long and/or multiple stenoses and occlusion
Muscle enzyme elevation	common	unusual

the problem. In fact, recognition of a potential source often leads to the suspicion that acute ischemia has occurred. For example, if a young woman with no history of atherosclerosis suddenly develops intermittent claudication and is found on examination to have mitral stenosis, arterial embolism should be strongly suspected. The major causes of acute, large- and medium-artery occlusion can be categorized as follows:

1. Arterial embolism,
2. Dissection of the aorta and its branches,
3. Acute arterial thrombosis, or
4. Intense arteriospasm.

ARTERIAL EMBOLISM

Arterial embolism is by far the most common cause of acute arterial occlusion of the extremities. There are many causes of embolism, most of them involving the heart. One logical classification of arterial emboli, according to their source, is shown in Table 2-2.

Table 2-2
Causes of Arterial Embolism

I Cardiac
- A. Valvular
  1. Mitral stenosis and regurgitation
  2. Infective endocarditis
  3. Prosthetic heart valves
  4. Marantic endocarditis
  5. Mitral prolapse syndrome
  6. Atrial myxoma
- B. Arrhythmias
  1. Atrial fibrillation
  2. Sick sinus syndrome
- C. Mural thrombus
  1. Ventricular aneurysm
  2. Acute myocardial infarction
  3. Cardiomyopathies
- D. Paradoxical emboli

II Arterial
- A. Aneurysms
  1. Popliteal aneurysms
  2. Femoral aneurysms
  3. Subclavian aneurysms
  4. Abdominal aortic aneurysms
- B. Atheromas
  1. Carotid artery
  2. Aorta

Mitral Stenosis

Mitral valve disease, particularly mitral stenosis, may be totally silent until arterial embolism occurs. It has been estimated that 20% or more of patients with this disorder have at least one embolus in a lifetime.[1] A clot in the left atrium develops over a period of months to years because of stagnation of blood within the left atrium. This stagnation is based both on obstruction to flow across the mitral valve and lack of atrial contraction. A patient with mitral stenosis will only rarely develop an embolus before atrial fibrillation has occurred. This fibrillation need not be constant, and the patient may even be more prone to embolism if the cardiac rhythm changes intermittently from atrial fibrillation to sinus rhythm.

The likelihood of embolization is not well correlated with the degree of stenosis. Many patients with hemodynamically insignificant stenosis have large multiple emboli. At first glance, this may seem somewhat paradoxical because a tightening of the stenosis raises the left atrial pressure, dilates the left atrium, decreases forward flow, and should lead to further thrombus formation within the left atrium. On the other hand, a wider mitral orifice allows large clots to pass into the left ventricle more easily. Thus, there are factors that make mitral stenosis of any degree extremely dangerous.

It is obvious that mitral stenosis is an important disorder to recognize during routine examination of apparently normal people. One must look especially carefully at patients with atrial fibrillation. Many cases of fibrillation ascribed to arteriosclerotic or hypertensive heart disease represent occult mitral stenosis, even in older individuals. The mid-diastolic rumbling murmur is often difficult to hear and may be easily missed if cardiac auscultation is not performed carefully in a quiet room. Since this murmur is of low pitch, it is much better heard with the bell of the stethoscope than the diaphragm. One should listen with the patient in the left lateral decubitus position and the stethoscope directly over the point of maximal impulse. Occasionally, exercising the patient may amplify the murmur. Despite these steps, the murmur may be intermittently or continuously inaudible in a significant number of patients.

There are other helpful signs in patients with inaudible murmurs. Many individuals with mitral stenosis, especially women, have a slight malar erythema or flush that may be noticeable only in a well-lit area. Auscultation may reveal a loud first sound and an opening snap, which is pathognomonic for mitral stenosis, even in the absence of a murmur. A very loud and palpable first heart sound in association with atrial fibrillation should make one suspect the presence of mitral stenosis.

With simple laboratory tools, an unequivocal diagnosis of mitral stenosis can be made in almost every case. If the patient does not have atrial fibrillation, a deep biphasic P wave in leads V1 to V2 strongly suggests mitral valve disease. A plain chest roentgenogram often shows evidence of left atrial enlargement. On the posteroanterior view, one sees straightening or convexity of the lower left heart border and, with marked left atrial enlargement, there is a double density over the heart shadow and a lifting up of the left mainstem bronchus. If these signs are present in the absence of hypertension or obvious mitral regurgitation, they point strongly to the diagnosis of mitral stenosis.

The most useful diagnostic procedure is echocardiography.[2,3] If this is performed correctly, it will establish the presence or absence of mitral stenosis with almost 100% accuracy. Every patient with unexplained atrial fibrillation or even atrial fibrillation in the presence of coronary heart disease should have an echocardiogram, provided the first sound is loud.

The echocardiographic diagnosis of mitral stenosis depends on an understanding of the physiology of the normal motion of the mitral valve. The normal mitral valve closes in early diastole after rapid filling of the left ventricle, opens again during atrial systole, and closes again as a result of ventricular systole and atrial relaxation (Figure 2-1). The anterior mitral leaflet (AML) and posterior mitral leaflet (PML) move as mirror images in opposite directions during early diastole, and come together when the valve closes. In mitral stenosis, early diastolic closure is absent or slow (decreased E to F slope), and the posterior mitral leaflet moves in the same direction (upward) as the anterior mitral leaflet when the valve opens in early diastole (Figure 2-2).

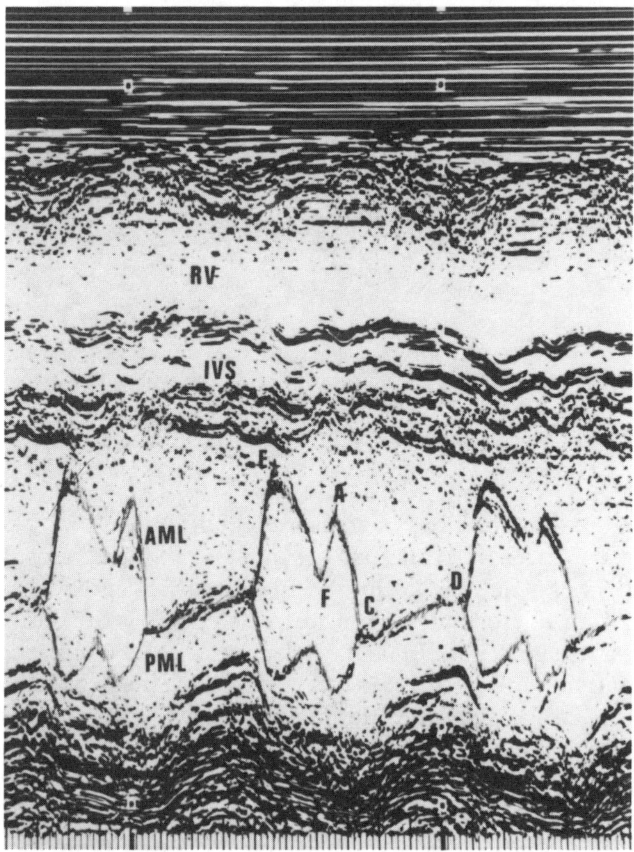

Figure 2-1 Echocardiogram showing a normal mitral valve. Note the sharp E-F slope.

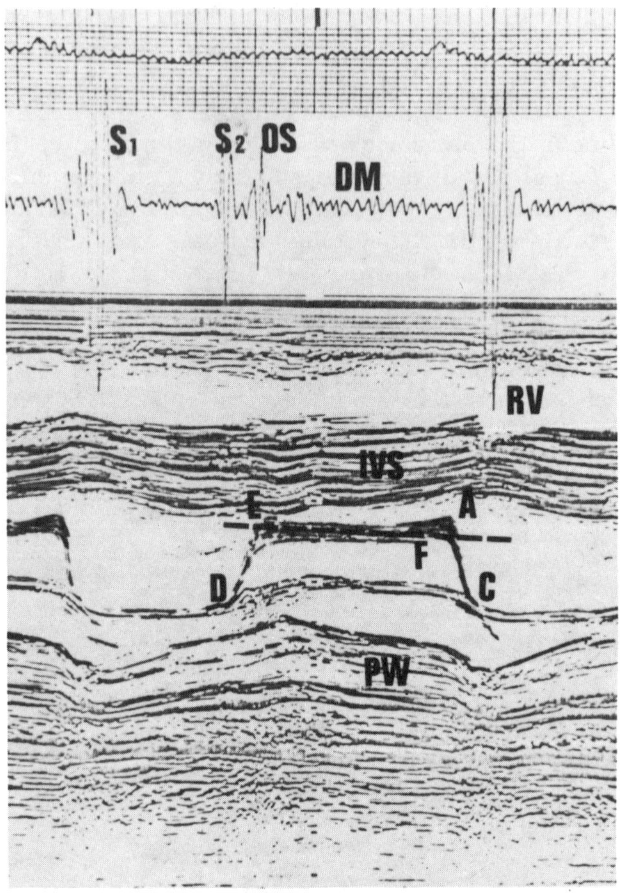

Figure 2-2 Echocardiogram of a patient with mitral stenosis. Note the flat E-F slope.

When the diagnosis has been established, precautions against embolization are necessary. The patient must be followed closely for the development of atrial fibrillation. Most authorities agree that the combination of atrial fibrillation and mitral stenosis is an indication for lifelong anticoagulation. In fact, it is reasonable to instruct an intelligent patient with mitral stenosis to check his pulse on a daily basis. If he notices irregularity, he should seek medical attention as soon as possible. Ambulatory, 24-hour electrocardiographic recording may then be required to determine that he has intermittent atrial fibrillation and, therefore, is a candidate for anticoagulation.

For elderly patients or those with definite contraindications to anticoagulation, antiplatelet therapy may be an alternative. Platelet kinetic studies have shown an increased platelet turnover in patients with mitral stenosis who have had an embolism.[4] A recent clinical report provided preliminary evidence that sulfinpyrazone has a protective effect against arterial embolism in mitral stenosis.[5] This drug is virtually free of hemorrhagic complications. The overall efficacy of antiplatelet drugs in preventing emboli in patients with mitral stenosis is still unknown, and conventional anticoagulation remains the first therapeutic choice in the absence of contraindications.

Mitral Prolapse

The mitral prolapse syndrome has received a great deal of attention in recent years. This disorder is very common, particularly in women, and is usually of no consequence. It has been reported in 21% of normal young women[6] and 6% of young adults.[7] A minority of patients may have nonspecific chest pain, premature ventricular contractions, and, rarely, congestive heart failure. The mitral prolapse syndrome may also be a source of arterial emboli. It has been implicated as a possible cause of transient attacks of cerebral ischemia.[8] Diagnosis depends on hearing a mid- or late-systolic click and/or murmur or on the echocardiographic demonstration of posterior displacement of the posterior mitral leaflet in mid-systole[9] (Figure 2-3). The murmur and click are best heard when the patient is standing and can be accentuated with the Valsalva maneuver.

Even when mitral prolapse has been discovered in a patient with arterial embolism, an exhaustive search should be made for other sources of thrombus since the prolapse may be merely an incidental finding, and its causal relationship to embolism is still somewhat speculative. In particular, one should look for subacute bacterial endocarditis, which may be a complication of mitral valve prolapse. In fact, the recognition of this disorder behooves the physician to advise the patient of the need for prophylactic antiobiotic therapy at the time of surgery or dental work. There is certainly no justification for anticoagulation unless arterial embolism has already occurred.

Endocarditis

Infectious endocarditis must always be considered in the differential diagnosis of arterial embolism. The natural history of endocarditis has been altered by the appearance of valvular infection in drug addicts and older people. The increased incidence of bacterial endocarditis in elderly patients may be partially a result of an increased longevity. Older people develop papillary muscle dysfunction secondary

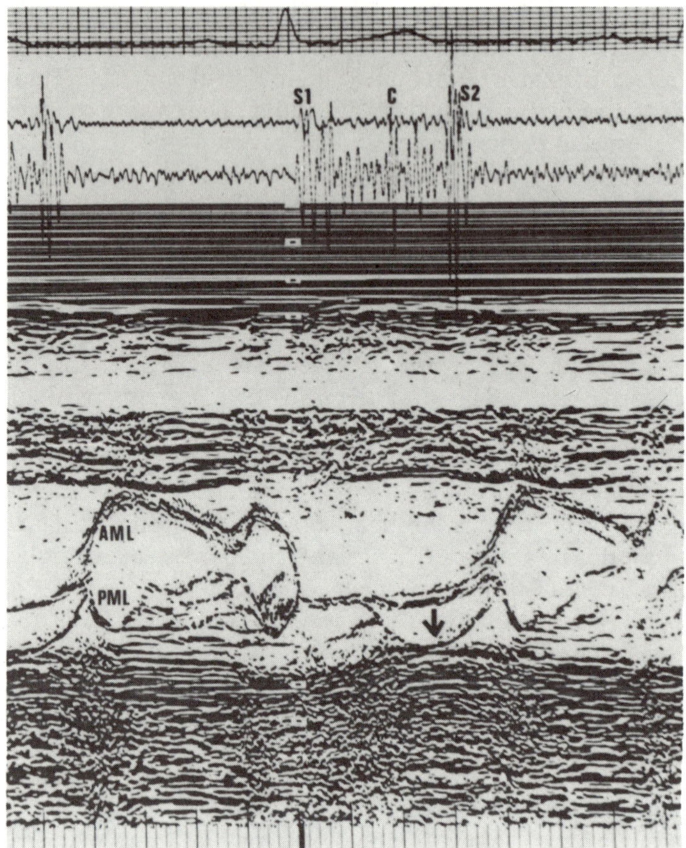

Figure 2-3 Echocardiogram of a patient with mitral valve prolapse. Note the billowing of the posterior mitral leaflet (PML) in late systole (↓).

to coronary heart disease and degenerative changes in the vicinity of the aortic valve and the root of the aorta, lesions that predispose to bacterial implantation. As many as 15% of patients may have no audible murmurs early in the course of the illness.[10]

In many cases of bacterial and, especially, fungal endocarditis, systemic embolization is the first manifestation. Systemic emboli occur in 15% to 35% of cases of endocarditis.[11] Since neurologic sequelae often herald the onset of the disease, endocarditis must be a primary consideration in an individual without hypertension or diabetes mellitus, who presents with a stroke. Embolic petechiae are often a clue to the diagnosis; but other peripheral signs are rarely present.

Fungal endocarditis, once a rare disorder, occurs more frequently in immunosuppressed patients and drug addicts. *Candida,* the usual etiologic agent, has a tendency to form large fungal balls on a valve with little or no inflammatory reaction.[12] These large vegetations embolize quite easily to major arteries in patients who may have no signs of toxicity or leukocytosis and little or no fever. Successful treatment requires a combination of valvular surgery and chemotherapy with amphotericin B and 5-fluorocytosine.

Acute staphylococcal endocarditis often presents with toxicity, fever, and embolization. Heart murmurs are often absent. This syndrome occurs in normal individuals but is more likely seen in drug addicts and patients with poor defense mechanisms. The source of the staphylococcus is often the skin, so that careful examination for open ulcers or pustules is a worthwhile endeavor in any patient with unexplained arterial embolism to an extremity, or neurologic symptoms compatible with a cerebrovascular accident. Pneumococcal infection may occasionally cause an endocarditis. If a patient with pneumonia develops a positive blood culture for pneumococcus, one must watch carefully for the appearance of murmurs. Both staphylococcal and pneumococcal endocarditis are quite lethal, and one must treat the patient vigorously, even if its presence is only suspected.

Because of the reversibility and lethality of infective endocarditis, blood cultures are recommended in all patients with arterial embolism, particularly if they have prior valvular disease. A portion of thrombus recovered from embolectomy should always be placed in culture broth rather than fixed in formalin. More attention should be paid to the aortic systolic murmurs often heard in middle-aged and elderly individuals. Patients with loud murmurs should be considered candidates for antibiotic prophylaxis before surgery, even if they do not have hemodynamically significant aortic stenosis.

Echocardiography may confirm the diagnosis of infective endocarditis if the vegetations are large enough to be seen as multiple echoes in the area of the involved valve[13,14] (Figure 2-4). However, a blood culture is a more sensitive test for the disease. In cases of acute fulminant endocarditis, the echocardiogram may suggest the diagnosis before blood culture results are available. In subacute bacterial endocarditis, tests for rheumatoid factor are often positive.

Marantic Endocarditis

Marantic endocarditis is seen in debilitated patients, especially those with advanced neoplastic disease. This disorder is characterized by sterile, thrombotic valvular vegetations. Although rarely diagnosed antemortem, marantic endocarditis accounts for a very significant proportion of emboli in chronically ill patients.[15]

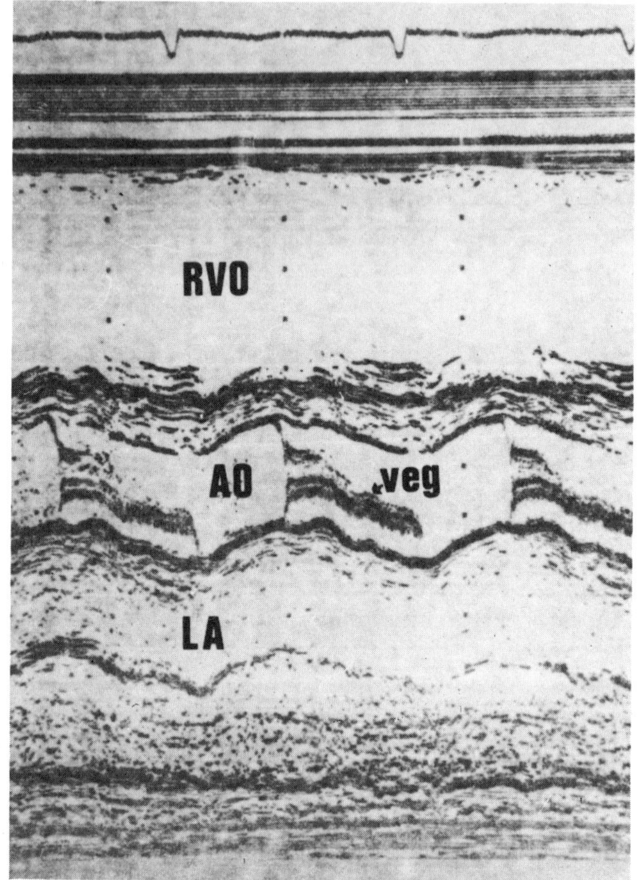

Figure 2-4 Echocardiogram of a patient with bacterial endocarditis. Note the dense echo representing a vegetation on the aortic valve.

Prosthetic Heart Valves

Prosthetic heart valves, whether of disc or ball-valve construction, are associated with a high incidence of arterial emboli, especially in cerebral vessels, in non-anticoagulated patients.[16] Even the recently introduced porcine valve is subject to this complication. At the present time, long-term prophylactic anticoagulation is recommended for all patients who undergo valve replacement.

The formation of a thrombus on these valves also compromises proper valve functioning, slowing and delaying the motion of the ball or disk. Massive thrombosis has resulted in sudden death due to failure of valve opening. Careful auscultation may offer a clue to the presence of significant valvular thrombus before symptoms occur. Failure to hear the opening snap of the mitral or ejection click of the aortic prosthetic valve is an indication for further evaluation, including echocardiography and often cardiac catheterization.

Left Atrial Myxoma

A rare cause of arterial embolism is a left atrial myxoma, which usually occurs as a pedunculated tumor near the foramen ovale. Patients may present with any or all of the following findings: 1) tumor emboli, 2) fever of unknown origin, 3) weight loss and anemia, 4) symptoms and signs suggestive of a collagen disease, 5) mitral murmurs that may change with position, 6) blood pressure changes with position, 7) signs of mitral stenosis without an opening snap, and 8) atrial arrhythmias.

One should seriously consider the diagnosis of atrial myxoma in patients with emboli of unknown cause or fever and murmurs in association with negative blood cultures. The diagnosis can generally be made through histologic examination of an embolus removed at surgery, or by echocardiography (Figures 2-5A, B). Treatment is surgical removal of the tumor, and results have generally been excellent.

Atrial Arrhythmias

Atrial arrhythmias that result in left atrial stasis may lead to thrombus formation and subsequent embolization. Theoretically, every patient with chronic atrial fibrillation is a candidate for arterial embolism, but relatively few ever have this problem. However, since atrial fibrillation is a very common arrhythmia, it is probably the most frequent cause of embolism to all but very small arteries. The incidence of arterial embolism in atrial fibrillation depends largely on the associated findings. Paroxysmal atrial fibrillation in a patient without intrinsic heart disease, or atrial fibrillation related to thyrotoxicosis, almost never leads to thromboembolism. With increasingly severe heart disease, the risk of embolism rises. As the left atrium progressively distends, the tendency to stasis of blood and consequent thrombosis becomes more extensive. The presence of mitral valve disease greatly increases the chance of thromboembolism. Patients with coronary and hypertensive heart disease who are in chronic atrial fibrillation may have emboli after they develop papillary muscle dysfunction.

There are, of course, exceptions to the rule. Occasionally, one sees a fibrillating patient with repeated emboli and little or no cardiac symptomatology. Echocardiography is advisable in such a patient to rule out occult mitral stenosis. Some patients develop thrombus in the

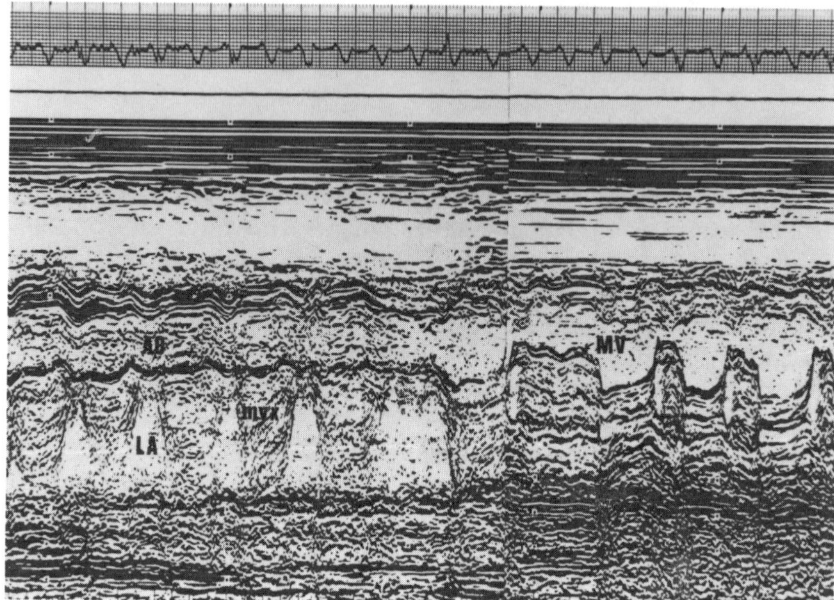

Figure 2-5A M-mode echocardiogram shows a mass of echoes arising from a myxoma within the left atrium. These echoes are seen appearing between the leaflets of the mitral valve in diastole, indicating that the tumor is prolapsing into the mitral orifice. AO: aorta, LA: left atrium, MV: mitral valve, myx: myxoma.

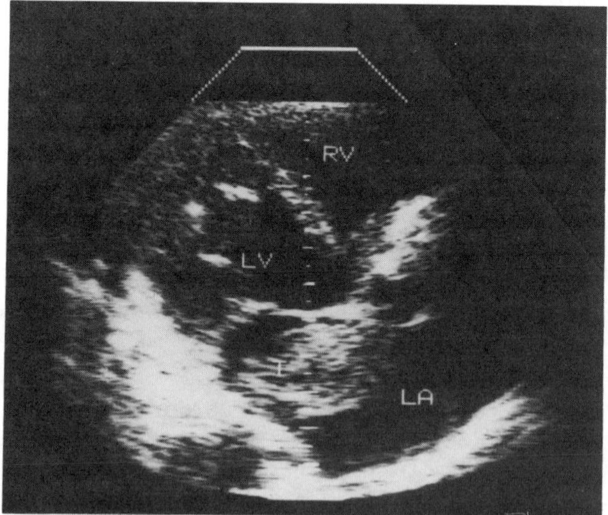

Figure 2-5B Sector scan of the heart shows an oval mass of echoes originating from a myxoma within the left atrium. The tumor was attached to the atrial septum by a peduncle and was noted to prolapse into the mitral valve orifice in diastole. LA: left atrium, T: tumor, LV: left ventricle, RV: right ventricle.

left atrium while fibrillating and tend to embolize with resumption of atrial contraction as their rhythm switches to sinus rhythm. Treatment with digitalis and an antiarrhythmic drug may be useful in these cases in an attempt to keep the patient in normal sinus rhythm.

Another rhythm disorder that may lead to emboli is the sick sinus syndrome.[17] Patients with sinus node disease may have runs of sinus arrest, sinoatrial block, and sinus bradycardia interspersed with episodes of supraventricular tachycardia and atrial fibrillation. Any or all of these rhythms may occur asymptomatically or produce spells of weakness, dizziness, or syncope.

If there is frequent sinus arrest, a thrombus can form in the static left atrium, and the return of atrial contraction may result in systemic embolization. This explanation should be accepted only after all other causes of emboli have been excluded. Since the arrhythmias of sick sinus syndrome are often paroxysmal and asymptomatic, 24-hour electrocardiographic monitoring is indicated whenever there is no obvious explanation for arterial emboli.

Patients with emboli secondary to atrial arrhythmias should be anticoagulated for long periods of time. There is no general agreement on how long anticoagulation should be continued, but lifelong therapy may be advisable. An attempt at cardioversion should be considered for patients with chronic atrial fibrillation who embolize while receiving anticoagulation. The incidence of embolism in atrial arrhythmias is not high enough to justify the risks of prophylactic anticoagulation in patients who have never suffered an arterial embolus.

Ventricular Thrombus

Stasis of blood may also lead to mural thrombosis within the cavity of the left ventricle. Arterial embolus is one of the dread and, fortunately, infrequent late complications of transmural myocardial infarction, generally occurring in the second to third week. The damaged akinetic area of myocardium serves as a substrate for thrombus accumulation during the first two weeks after infarction. Occasionally, patients may have silent myocardial infarcts and develop an arterial embolus a few weeks later. This is particularly true in patients with diabetes mellitus. Careful interrogation of the patient may extract a history of mild dyspnea or atypical pain consistent with an infarct. The electrocardiogram will almost always be abnormal in this situation. In some cases, the thrombus does not embolize until several months after an infarct.

Chronic heart disease with marked dilatation of the left ventricle is another predisposing factor for mural thrombosis. The cardiomyopathies have great potential for ventricular dilatation and are, therefore, a frequent source of systemic emboli. Alcoholism is probably the most frequent cause for this kind of heart disease. Physical examination often reveals a flabby point of maximum impulse to the left of the midclavicular line, with prominent gallops. There is a disproportion between the electrocardiogram and the chest roentgenogram. The former tends to show normal or low voltage in most leads, while the latter demonstrates a large, dilated heart. Some patients with cardiomyopathy have emboli early in the course of the disease, but they usually first develop congestive heart failure. Recurrent pulmonary emboli from the right ventricle are also quite common. Treatment of cardiomyopathy is that of congestive heart failure. Anticoagulation is usually employed only for patients who have had systemic or pulmonary embolism.

The most insidious cause of a mural thrombus is dyskinesia of the left ventricular muscle.[18] As a result of extensive coronary artery disease, focal areas of fibrosis, which are akinetic, and ischemic areas of muscle, which contract poorly, may be found in the left ventricle. A large fibrotic area may become a so-called ventricular aneurysm, which bulges out during cardiac systole. Blood stagnates and clots inside this area.

In its extreme form, a ventricular aneurysm can represent more than 25% of the left ventricular cavity, collecting large thrombi that readily embolize on repeated occasions. Such a large aneurysm is usually easy to recognize for several reasons. First, on physical examination one may palpate a diffuse point of maximum impulse over a wide area and notice a rocking motion. There is a lack of synchrony among different points in the area of this wide impulse. With coins placed at different points over this impulse, one can often see the asynchrony. Most of these patients have rather marked congestive heart failure, and many have premature ventricular contractions. Electrocardiography will often show an area with peristent S-T elevations as well as evidence of an old transmural infarct. The left ventricle will appear to be bulging on chest roentgenogram. Such a large, obvious ventricular aneurysm is a frequent source of emboli and justifies the use of prophylactic anticoagulation. Large ventricular aneurysms can often be diagnosed with conventional M-mode echocardiography.[19,20]

More often, patients with coronary heart disease have smaller aneurysms that may not even cause overt congestive heart failure, although ventricular function is certainly impaired, and the ejection fraction is significantly decreased. Physical examination may reveal a flabby, diffuse point of maximum impulse. Electrocardiography may show nothing more than ischemic changes, and the chest roentgenogram may indicate only a slight enlarged heart shadow. In the case of small aneurysms, conventional echocardiography is often not sufficiently sensitive for diagnosis, but two-dimensional echocardiography is very helpful.

An alternative to two-dimensional echocardiography is real-time radionuclide cineangiography.[21] With this technique, a direct view of ventricular contraction is obtained after intravenous injection of radioactive technetium, during rest and exercise. Small areas of dyskinesia can be seen with this method. Cineangiocardiography with radiopaque dye can also be utilized, but this is a more invasive procedure.

There is no doubt that arterial thromboembolism can result from relatively small aneurysms even in the absence of overt congestive heart failure. However, a careful search for other sources of thrombus is advisable before ascribing arterial emboli to abnormal ventricular motion. Long-term anticoagulation is indicated when embolism has occured or ventricular clot is noted on angiography or echocardiography. In patients with absolute contraindications to anticoagulation, surgical resection of the aneurysm may be indicated. Antiplatelet drugs may be given, but their efficacy has not yet been fully established.

Paradoxical Emboli

Paradoxical arterial embolism represents the least common cause of acute arterial embolism, but it is not as rare as was once believed.[22] It probably accounts for less than 1% of all systemic emboli. A paradoxical embolus is defined as a thrombus originating in a vein and traveling to a systemic artery. The route, except in patients with congenital septal defects, is through an anatomically open foramen ovale. Many normal people have an open foramen ovale, which is functionally closed because of the difference in arterial pressure between the systemic and pulmonary circulations. With the development of pulmonary hypertension, this difference decreases. When pulmonary artery pressure approaches aortic pressure, particulate matter suspended in blood can find its way through the foramen ovale after entering the right atrium. Patients with right-sided heart failure have an increased incidence of venous thromboembolic disease. One of the unusual complications of severe cor pulmonale, therefore, is paradoxical embolization.

As might be expected, patients with paradoxical emboli generally have pulmonary emboli at the same time. In fact, the pulmonary embolism often establishes the acute cor pulmonale necessary for reversed flow across the foramen ovale. It is difficult to estimate the true incidence of paradoxical embolism because it is often overlooked in the differential diagnosis. It is possible that some of the neurologic sequelae of patients with respiratory failure, generally ascribed to hypoxia, hypercapnia, and cerebrovascular accidents, may be manifestations of paradoxical embolism.

This diagnosis should always be considered in patients with known pulmonary hypertension or acute dyspnea who develop strokes or other manifestations of acute arterial occlusion. One should measure the width of the lower extremities and examine carefully for clinical signs of deep vein thrombosis. As in the case of pulmonary embolism, the majority of patients with paradoxical embolism will not have manifest clinical signs of venous thrombosis, but presence of unilateral leg swelling certainly supports the diagnosis. The diagnosis is almost impossible to prove and ultimately depends on exclusion of all other causes of arterial embolism and the presence of severe pulmonary hypertension. Laboratory evidence of pulmonary embolism or venographic proof of deep vein thrombosis should be sought as confirmatory evidence. If the pulmonary hypertension is chronic, long-term anticoagulation may be indicated. Interruption of the inferior vena cava is advisable for patients who cannot be anticoagulated.

Occasionally, the diagnosis can be supported with a nuclear flow scan or echocardiogram. Early detection of radioactive technetium in the left ventricle on scan indicates the presence of a functioning right-to-left shunt. Similarly, echocardiography after intravenous injection of indocyanine green produces early echoes in the left ventricle[23,24] (Figure 2-6).

Aneurysms

Arterial aneurysms usually acquire at least some mural thrombus and are always a potential source of arterial embolization. The distally located aneurysms are more likely to produce emboli, probably because they have a smaller surface area to which the thrombus can adhere. Aneurysms of the popliteal artery are notorious in this regard.[25] The vulnerable position of the artery behind the knee makes it the second most frequent site of arteriosclerotic aneurysm formation.

Recurrent acute episodes of distal ischemia in one leg should always suggest the presence of a popliteal aneurysm, which can usually be palpated as a pulsatile mass behind the knee. If it is occluded, one feels a firm or cystic mass. Ultrasound can identify it as a clotted aneurysm. Femoral and subclavian artery aneurysms also cause a great deal of thromboembolism.

The most common arteriosclerotic aneurysm, located at the terminal aorta, is an infrequent source of acute arterial embolism although it tends to develop a significant amount of mural thrombus.

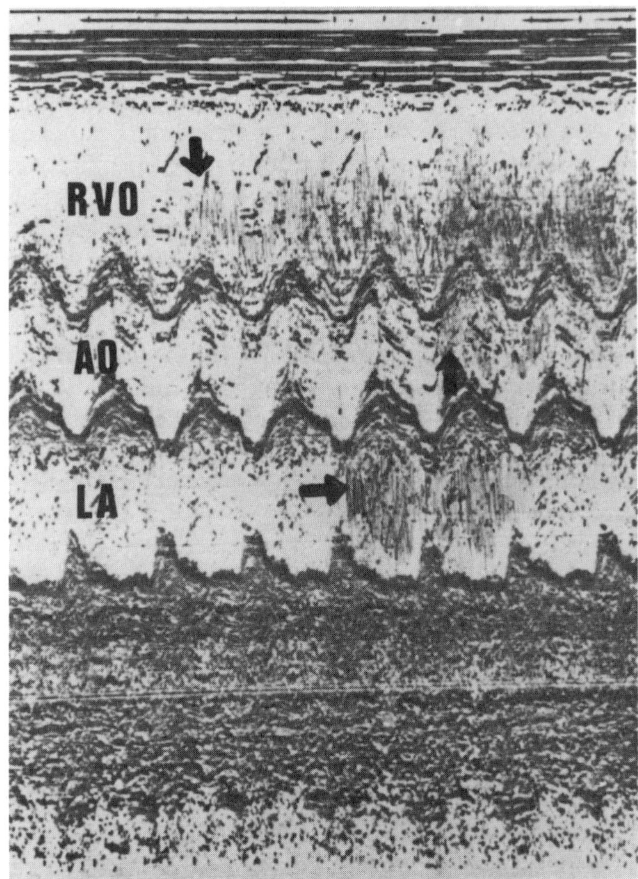

Figure 2-6 Echocardiogram of a patient with pulmonary hypertension and a patent foramen ovale. A dense shadow of saline is seen in the left atrium just as it reaches the right ventricular outflow tract.

On occasion, however, it can produce major emboli to the femoral or popliteal arteries, or microemboli to the feet. It is possible that the incidence of embolization from aortic aneurysms has been grossly underestimated. Small thrombi may repeatedly break away from the aorta and accumulate in the femoral and popliteal arteries, leading to gradual occlusion of these vessels. In support of this thesis is the observation that femoropopliteal occlusive disease is more common than aortoiliac occlusion in patients with aortic aneurysms.[26]

Anticoagulation is best avoided in patients with arterial aneurysms, especially aortic aneurysms. A decrease in hemostasis increases the chances of a catastrophic hemorrhage if a small leak develops. The aneurysm must be surgically repaired.

Atheromas

Probably the most frequent sources of emboli are atherosclerotic arteries. Atheromas are friable, and the shearing force of blood often ruptures them, liberating cholesterol crystals and complexes of fibrin and platelets. The resulting emboli usually lodge in small vessels, but occasionally large arteries can be occluded. Athermatous emboli originate most commonly from the abdominal aorta and carotid arteries. In the case of the abdominal aorta, there may be a syndrome of petechial and gangrenous spots in the lower extremities associated with increasing renal insufficiency.[27] Urinalysis may show intermittent microscopic hematuria. A loud bruit over the abdominal aorta in a patient with unexplained and increasing azotemia may be a clue that showers of atheromatous emboli are lodging in small branches of the renal arteries. Occasionally, larger emboli may actually occlude a renal artery, causing acute flank pain and gross hematuria. An acute femoral artery occlusion can also occur.

Perhaps the most common sites of origin of symptomatic atheromatous emboli are the carotid arteries. A favorite location for large, bulky atheromas to develop is at the bifurcation of the common carotid into the external and internal carotid artery, causing a variable amount of stenosis. In most cases, a carotid bruit can be heard just below the angle of the jaw.[28] The transient ischemic attacks associated with carotid artery disease are thought to be more often the result of platelet-fibrin emboli than ischemia directly related to carotid stenosis. The signs and symptoms of carotid artery disease are discussed in detail in the chapter on cerebrovascular disease.

Therapy for atheromatous emboli is far from satisfactory. Recent attention has shifted from anticoagulant drugs to the antiplatelet agents. There is clinical evidence for the efficacy of aspirin in preventing transient ischemic attacks in men.[29] Various combinations of aspirin, dipyridamole, and sulfinpyrazone have been tried, but their overall effect is not yet established.

ACUTE ARTERIAL THROMBOSIS

The second major category of acute arterial obstruction involves in situ thrombosis. This event occurs almost always in a previously diseased arterial segment. As noted previously, hemodynamic evidence of arterial obstruction is not seen until the lumen is two-thirds occluded. Turbulent flow and stasis are present long before a weakening of the peripheral pulse can be appreciated. As atheromas develop along the wall of an artery, their irregular spicules act as a nidus for the aggregation of platelets, followed by the beginning of the intrinsic clotting process. Furthermore, as these atheromas erode the endothelial lining, collagen is exposed, which acts as a powerful stimulant of platelet aggregation. As blood flows in contorted fashion through an irregular lumen with jagged atheromas and exposed collagen, it is much like an archaeologist crawling through a cave filled with stalagmites and stalactites of varying size and shape. Indeed, it is surprising that acute thrombosis does not occur more often than it does under these circumstances. Thus, it is obvious that the risk factors for acute arterial thrombosis are very similar to those for chronic atherosclerosis. In many patients presenting with acute arterial obstruction superimposed on atherosclerosis, some evidence of a diabetic tendency can be found.

Most patients with acute arterial thrombosis of an extremity have had symptoms and/or signs of peripheral arterial disease before the acute event. For example, a patient with intermittent claudication may suddenly develop rest pain or numbness in the toes. In some cases, the vessel is so close to total obstruction before the acute events, and collateral circulation is so well established, that the patient notices only an increase in severity of his previous claudication. Careful examination after the event may show increasing pallor on elevation of the leg, slower return of color on dependency, and dependent rubor. However, an occasional patient may develop acute arterial thrombosis without prior signs or symptoms of arterial insufficiency, just as many patients have myocardial infarctions without prior angina. In this situation, it may be extremely difficult to distinguish thrombosis from embolism. A lack of an obvious source of embolism and the presence of diabetes mellitus favor a diagnosis of thrombosis, but one can never be certain without arteriographic evidence of advanced arteriosclerosis and/or exploration of the occluded artery.

Causes

Although most arterial thrombosis occurs as a complication of atherosclerosis, the possibility of other etiologies must always be considered, especially in young individuals and nondiabetics. Systemic lupus erythematosus (SLE) can involve arteries of all sizes from the aorta to digital vessels, and present with either acute or chronic arterial insufficiency.[30] Lupus vasculitis may lead to slow occlusion with the development of intermittent claudication or acute occlusion of a femoral or popliteal artery. Acute occlusion elsewhere may lead to cerebrovascular accidents, mesenteric infarction, and even myocardial infarction. This possibility should be kept in mind whenever acute arterial occlusion occurs in nondiabetic, nonhypertensive individuals with no obvious source of embolism, especially in women under the age of 40. An antinuclear antibody test and LE preparation are advisable for this type of patient. The presence of Raynaud's phenomenon or venous disease, especially migratory superficial phlebitis, is another hint that the patient may have SLE. Unfortunately, vasculitis in lupus does not appear to respond favorably to corticosteroid therapy.

Polyarteritis nodosa classically involves small- and medium-sized arteries, and may present with acute arterial occlusion in an extremity. Most patients are hypertensive and have involvement of other areas such as the mesenteric and renal arteries. Arteriography tends to show beaded arteries due to multiple areas of stenosis and poststenotic dilatation. A high proportion of current patients (perhaps 35% or more) have positive tests for hepatitis B surface antigen.[31] Presumably, what was once a hypersensitivity reaction to sulfonamides and other drugs is now often the result of an immunologic reaction to infection with the hepatitis B virus. Corticosteroid therapy and control of hypertension are the cornerstones of therapy, and the chances of remission are excellent. In resistant cases, immunosuppressive drugs such as azathioprine may be helpful.

Arterial thrombosis is often iatrogenic. Repeated arterial punctures for the determination of blood gases and insertion of arterial lines for monitoring of blood pressure can result in intimal tears and thrombosis. Cardiac catheterization is associated with the risk of traumatic thrombosis or medial dissection of major arteries, sometimes necessitating immediate surgical repair. Injury to an artery may not be immediately apparent. A small intimal tear may not compromise blood flow at first, but a thrombus may form within 24 to 48 hours and occlude the vessel. Furthermore, small clots formed during the procedure may require a day or two to coalesce.

The brachial pulse is frequently lost when it is used for catheterization and angiographic procedures, but the loss may go unnoticed because of excellent collateral circulation. Patients may later complain of decreased effort tolerance in that arm. Some angiographers and invasive cardiologists have adopted a procedure of passing a Fogarty catheter routinely before closing the arteriotomy site. This has resulted in an improved rate of preservation of the brachial pulse.

DISSECTION OF THE AORTA

Although it usually presents with other clinical clues, a dissecting hematoma may simulate acute, large vessel, arterial thromboembolism. Dissection almost always begins in the thoracic aorta and is secondary to cystic medial necrosis. Only a relative handful of cases of primary dissection of a peripheral artery has been reported. The dissecting hematoma may extend from the aortic wall into any branch, occluding the artery by compression. Thus, almost any ischemic syndrome can be produced, but the arterial occlusion is always proximal. Distal pulses are not lost unless the femoral or subclavian pulse is also missing.

A major pulse such as the femoral is often lost but returns several hours later as the false channel develops a second communication with the true lumen, allowing decompression of the blood-filled media (so-called re-entry phenomenon). The loss of several proximal pulses and their spontaneous return are important clues to the diagnosis of aortic dissection.

There are times when a dissection may present with one proximal arterial occlusion and no other signs or symptoms to suggest the diagnosis. In this situation, an embolectomy may be performed, and an occluded vessel with no thrombus or atheroma is found. A "dry" embolectomy strongly suggests the diagnosis of a dissecting hematoma and is an indication for aortography.

The treatment of a dissection is dictated by its location and extent, the severity of cardiac compromise, and the location and extent of any arterial occlusions. The general indications for surgery and medical therapy are discussed elsewhere. If limb-threatening ischemia is present, a local decompression and oversewing of the medial layer of an iliac or subclavian artery may be necessary.

ARTERIOSPASM

At times, severe arteriospasm may produce large-vessel occlusion in an extremity. This occurs regularly as part of the syndrome of phlegmasia cerulea dolens, which is severe iliofemoral thrombophlebitis with arteriospasm.[32] The name is descriptive of the extremity, which is painful and cyanotic. The etiology of the arteriospasm is not clear. Ordinarily, alpha sympathetic discharge would not be expected to cause large-artery spasm since most of the alpha receptors are located at the arteriolar level. In phlegmasia, spasm may be a result of direct injury from the inflammatory reaction and massive edema.

The venous thrombus in this syndrome is usually as high as the common iliac vein, and is massive, extending distally through the femoral vein. Edema of the leg and thigh is very severe and extends to the inguinal area. In most cases, the dorsalis pedis and posterior tibial pulses are obliterated, and even the popliteal and femoral arteries may be occluded by spasm. The foot and lower leg are cold and mottled.

The clinical course is quite variable. Spasm may disappear within 24 hours or less with no sequelae, or may persist longer and produce extensive gangrene of the foot. In most cases, tissue loss is minor and superficial, but phlegmasia can occasionally lead to amputation.

The distinction between phlegmasia cerulea dolens and arterial thromboembolism is usually easy to make because intrinsic arterial occlusion does not cause edema. Nevertheless, mistakes have occurred, and patients have undergone unsuccessful arterial embolectomies for this disorder. This is still another reason for a "dry" embolectomy.

Treatment of phlegmasia cerulea dolens consists of a combination of heparin and interruption of the inferior vena cava. If the arteriospasm persists in severe form for more than 24 hours or intense cyanosis suggests the possibility of incipient and extensive tissue breakdown, an attempt at vasodilatation by caudal block or use of alpha blocking agents may be indicated. Every patient who develops phlegmasia cerulea dolens should be evaluated for the presence of an abdominal malignancy.

Trauma

A second cause of large-vessel arteriospasm is trauma. Blunt or penetrating trauma of an extremity may cause spasm, either through inflammatory swelling around the vessel or by direct injury to the vessel, as in the case of a fracture or joint dislocation. Because of its tenuous position stretched across the back of the knee, the popliteal artery is particularly vulnerable to injury. Fractures of the lower femur and dislocation or even transient subluxation of the knee joint may lead to intimal tears, transection of the vessel, or merely severe arteriospasm. An intimal tear is a very serious complication and, in one series, 20% of the patients with serious knee dislocations had to have amputations because of ischemia.[33] It is extremely important to palpate the distal pulses carefully in any patient who has suffered significant trauma in the vicinity of the knee.

The absence of dorsalis pedis and posterior tibial pulses is always of concern. If there are no signs of cutaneous ischemia, one can observe carefully for signs of circulatory impairment. Pulses usually return within 24 hours if arteriospasm is the only problem. If progressive signs of ischemia develop, arteriography becomes urgent to locate the exact level of occlusion, and surgical exploration is necessary. If arteriography shows a smooth tapering of the vessel and the popliteal artery looks healthy but narrow at surgery, it may be wise to wrap the artery in papaverine and withdraw. If the artery is injured, repair and removal of the thrombus are necessary. Results of immediate surgery are often disappointing, and it is best to treat conservatively unless there is significant ischemia. It is much easier to perform arterial surgery at a later date when the popliteal space is no longer filled with edema and hematoma.

Ergots

A third cause of large-vessel arteriospasm is the use of ergot derivatives. Methysergide, an agent widely used to prevent migraine headaches, has caused coronary, mesenteric, and femoral arteriospasm.[34] In each case, the occlusion quickly disappeared when the drug was stopped. However, even transient spasm of vital arteries can lead to serious consequences, especially in patients with underlying atherosclerosis. With the discovery of the efficacy of propranolol in preventing migraine, use of methysergide should rarely be necessary.

TREATMENT OF ACUTE ARTERIAL OCCLUSION IN AN EXTREMITY

The development of the Fogarty balloon catheter has made arterial embolectomy a relatively simple procedure.[35] This thin, soft, rubber catheter can be inserted into an artery through a simple arteriotomy and passed in antegrade or retrograde direction for a considerable distance. From the femoral artery, it can be passed into the terminal aorta or tibial arteries. When it has passed the thrombosed area, a soft balloon is inflated near its tip and the catheter is pulled back to the arteriotomy site. Like a large brush, the catheter sweeps the thrombus out of the artery. With gentle maneuvering of the catheter, one is unlikely to tear the intima or cause medial dissection.

With the availability of this technique, it seems reasonable to take a rather aggressive approach to acute arterial occlusion. This technique is usually recommended in any patient with acute arterial embolism to a major artery in a lower extremity. Results are excellent, with low morbidity. The procedure can be performed under local anesthesia even during the first few days of a myocardial infarction.

The alternative is to watch the circulatory status of the foot and leg very carefully, intervening only if serious ischemia develops. Unfortunately, this often entails a rather subjective judgment. A foot may appear quite viable at the beginning, but then become very pale or mottled 12 to 24 hours later. Ischemic neuropathy may develop insidiously, and infarction of the calf muscle may go unnoticed for some time. Furthermore, even if the foot remains viable, the patient may have disabling claudication in the future.

The upper extremity has a greater capacity for collateral circulation, but we still tend to encourage embolectomy in most patients. Follow-up studies of patients who have lost brachial pulses during cardiac catheterization have shown a high incidence of claudication and arm fatigue. In a seriously ill or chronically debilitated patient, a conservative approach for an upper extremity occlusion may be reasonable when the hand shows no signs of serious ischemia such as cyanosis or marked pallor.

SMALL-VESSEL SYNDROME

Small-vessel (small-artery and arteriole) disease may be the end result of a variety of disease processes with distinct diagnostic and therapeutic implications. It is important to consider these entities when cutaneous ischemia is out of proportion to obvious large-vessel disease. The hallmark of the small-vessel syndrome is discrete, usually distal, cyanosis or gangrene in the presence of palpable pulses. The digits are most often involved, and this kind of ischemia is often called the "blue toes" syndrome. The process is often repetitive, and patients may report multiple episodes of painful blue toes. Even when pulses are absent, it is reasonable to assume that localized, distal ischemia is a sign of small-vessel occlusion.

With less severe episodes, the patient may notice nothing, but a digit may be cool and exhibit pallor on elevation. If this silent occlusive process continues long enough, an entire hand or foot may exhibit signs of chronic ischemia, such as pallor on elevation and dependent rubor, even though distal pulses are strong.

When the small-vessel syndrome involves a single extremity, thromboembolism from a peripheral aneurysm becomes a strong diagnostic possibility. Careful palpation of the subclavian artery in the supraclavicular fossa for an upper extremity lesion, and of the femoral and popliteal arteries for lower extremity ischemia, is extremely important. In the case of the popliteal artery, it may be difficult to be certain whether a somewhat prominent pulsation really represents an aneurysm or merely a tortuous vessel. Furthermore, a partially clotted aneurysm may not pulsate widely. When there is any clinical doubt, an ultrasound examination of the popliteal artery is indicated.

When the small-vessel syndrome cannot be ascribed to an aneurysm, one must look upon it as a possible harbinger of systemic disease, and a systemic evaluation is indicated. Diagnostic possibilities include the following:

1. Essential thrombocytosis
2. Polycythemia
3. Cryoglobulinemia
4. Cryofibrinogenemia
5. Disseminated intravascular coagulopathy
6. Collagen-vascular disease
7. Diabetes mellitus
8. Atheromatous emboli
9. Bacterial endocarditis

Thrombocytosis

Essential thrombocytosis is a disease that is often overlooked. It is a myeloproliferative disease in which there is hyperplasia, primarily of the megakaryocytic series. Platelet counts range from 700,000 to several million/mm^3 with a marked increase in megakaryocytes in the bone marrow and occasional appearance of giant platelets on peripheral smear. The disease has an incidence approximately one-fourth that of polycythemia vera. Clinically, there is sometimes overlap with other myeloproliferative disorders. The hematocrit and hemoglobin concentration may be slightly elevated, and leukocytosis up to 25,000/mm^3 may be present. However, neither the bone marrow aspirate nor the peripheral smear shows an increase in immature granulocytes. In long-term studies, patients with thrombocytosis have generally not developed any other myeloproliferative disorders.[36]

Clues to the diagnosis of this disorder include splenomegaly, hyperuricemia, and spurious hyperkalemia, but none of these need to be present. High serum potassium levels occur because potassium is liberated in large quantities from platelet degradation during clot formation. Plasma potassium levels are normal.

Essential thrombocytosis poses problems of hemorrhage and thrombosis, and the relative severity of each has varied among reported series. Bleeding appears to be correlated in the laboratory with decreased platelet aggregation, particularly epinephrine-induced aggregation. Some patients have had cerebral hemorrhage as the first clinical manifestation. In contrast to essential thrombocytosis, patients with high platelet counts secondary to infection or inflammatory disease have normal platelet aggregation, and rarely bleed.

The first thrombotic manifestation of essential thrombocytosis is usually digital infarction, but cerebral ischemia or superficial phlebitis may also occur very early.[37] Lesions on the extremities may be multiple and prominent, or quite surreptitious. Since ischemia worsens with vasoconstriction, the patient with multiple lesions may be erroneously thought to have Raynaud's phenomenon. Often, a small area of cyanosis or pallor at the extreme distal end of a single digit is the only evidence of the disease. Rarely, the platelet disorder leads to occlusion of a posterior tibial or dorsalis pedis artery.

Early diagnosis of essential thrombocytosis is extremely important because of its potentially dire consequences and its amenability to therapy. Any patient with a small-vessel syndrome in the extremities or cerebrovascular disease in the absence of hypertension, diabetes mellitus, and hyperlipidemia should have a platelet count. Busulfan in small doses is the usual treatment, and platelet counts generally return to normal within a few weeks. In most cases, long remissions occur after cessation of therapy, and many patients require no further treatment. However, platelet counts should be obtained several times a year and treatment reinstituted if the platelet count rises about 600,000/mm.[3] Platelet aggregation determinations return to normal as the total count decreases. If a patient presents with cerebral symptoms, platelet-pheresis on an emergency basis is indicated. Some investigators have advocated the use of antiplatelet drugs for digital ischemia, but this is potentially dangerous because futher impairment of platelet aggregation may lead to serious hemorrhage. We do not advocate their use.

Other Causes

Polycythemia, by increasing blood viscosity, can lead to small-vessel occlusions and also has a propensity to cause mesenteric and cerebral venous thrombosis. Cryoproteins may cause thrombotic manifestations very similar to those of essential thrombocytosis. Cryofibrinogenemia may sometimes have a fulminant course, causing sudden and extensive gangrene of several digits. These entities are discussed in more detail in other chapters.

The most common cause of acute small-vessel syndrome, especially in older individuals, is a shower of atheromatous emboli. Patients with chronic ischemia and palpable peripheral pulses are often diabetic, with evidence of atherosclerosis elsewhere. Nevertheless, even in the presence of diabetes and known atherosclerosis, other causes of small-vessel syndrome must be excluded in every case.

REFERENCES

1. Coulshed N, Epstein EJ, McKendrick CS, et al. Systemic embolism in mitral valve disease. *Br Heart J* 32:26, 1970.

2. Duchak JM Jr, Chang S, Feigenbaum H. The posterior mitral valve

echo and the echocardiographic diagnosis of mitral stenosis. *Am J Cardiol* 29:628, 1972.

3. Cope GD, Kisslo JA, Johnson ML, et al. A reassessment of the echocardiogram in mitral stenosis. *Circulation* 52:664, 1975.

4. Steele PP, Weily HS, Davies H, et al. Platelet survival in patients with rheumatic heart disease. *N Eng J Med* 290:537, 1974.

5. Steele PP, Rainwater JO, Genton E. Favorable effects of sulfinpyrazone on thromboembolism in patients with rheumatic heart disease. *Clin Res* (Abstract) 27:205, 1979.

6. Markiewicz W, Stoner J, Landon E, et al. Mitral valve prolapse in one hundred presumably healthy young females. *Circulation* 53:464, 1976.

7. Brown OR, Kloster F, DeMots H. Incidence of mitral valve prolapse in the asymptomatic normal. *Circulation* 5-2(suppl 2):11-77, 1975.

8. Barnett HJ, Jones MW, Boughner DR, et al. Cerebral ischemic events associated with prolapsing mitral valve. *Arch Neurol* 33:777, 1976.

9. Feigenbaum H. *Echocardiography.* Philadelphia, Lea and Febiger, 1976, p 119.

10. Weinstein L, Rubin RH. Infective endocarditis. *Prog Cardiovasc Dis* 16:239, 1973.

11. Gregoratos G, Karliner JS. Infective endocarditis: Diagnosis and management. *Med Clin North Am* 63:173, 1979.

12. Gladstone JL, Friedman SA, Cerruti MM, et al. Treatment of Candida endocarditis and arteritis. *J Thorac Cardiovasc Surg* 71:835, 1976.

13. Dillon JC, Feigenbaum H, Konecke LL, et al. Echocardiographic manifestations of valvular vegetations. *Am Heart J* 86:698, 1973.

14. Hirschfeld DS, Schiller N. Localization of aortic valve vegetations by echocardiography. *Circulation* 53:280, 1976.

15. Barron KD, Siqueira E, Hirano A. Cerebral embolism caused by nonbacterial thrombotic endocarditis. *Neurology* 10:391, 1960.

16. Kloster FE. Diagnosis and management of complications of prosthetic heart valves. *Am J Cardiol* 35:872, 1975.

17. Fairfax AJ, Lambert CD, Leatham A. Systemic embolism in chronic sinoatrial disorder. *Am J Cardiol* 35:872, 1975.

18. Schlichter J, Hellerstein HK, Katz LN. Aneurysm of the heart: A correlative study of one hundred and two proved cases. *Medicine* 33:43, 1954.

19. Kreamer R, Kerber RE, Abboud FM. Ventricular aneurysm: Use of echocardiography. *J Clin Ultrasound* 1:60, 1973.

20. Feigenbaum H. *Echocardiography.* Philadelphia, Lea and Febiger 1976, p 360.

21. Borer JS, Bacharach SL, Green MV, et al. Real-time radionuclide cineangiography in the noninvasive evaluation of global and regional left ventricular function at rest and during exercise in patients with coronary artery disease. *N Engl J Med* 296:839, 1977.

22. Meister SG, Grossman W, Dexter L, et al. Paradoxical embolism: Diagnosis during life. *Am J Med* 50:292, 1972.

23. Seward JB, Tajik AJ, Spangler JG, et al. Echocardiographic contrast studies: Initial experience. *Mayo Clin Proc* 50:163, 1975.

24. Pieroni D, Varghese PJ, Rowe RD. Echocardiography to detect shunt and valvular incompetence in infants and children. *Circulation* 48 (Suppl IV):81, 1973.

25. Gifford RW Jr, Hines EA Jr, Janes JM. An analysis and follow-up study of 100 popliteal aneurysms. *Surgery* 33:284, 1953.

26. Friedman SA, Hufnagel CA, Conrad PW, et al. Abdominal aortic aneurysms: Clinical status and results of surgery in 100 consecutive cases. *JAMA* 200:1147, 1967.

27. Richards AM, Eliot RS, Kanjun VI, et al. Cholesterol embolism: A multiple-system disease masquerading as polyarteritis nodosa. *Am J Cardiol* 15:696, 1965.

28. Grindal AB, Toole JF. Surgical treatment of carotid and vertebral artery disease. *Ann Intern Med* 81:647, 1974.

29. The Canadian Cooperative Group: A randomized trial of aspirin and sulfinpyrazone in threatened stroke. *N Eng J Med* 299:53, 1978.

30. Alarcon-Segovia D, Osmundson PJ. Peripheral vascular syndromes associated with systemic lupus erythematosus. *Ann Intern Med* 62:907, 1965.

31. Gocke DJ, Hsu K, Morgan C, et al. Association between polyarteritis and Austria antigen. *Lancet* 2:1149, 1970.

32. Brockman SK, Vasko JS: Phlegmasia cerulea dolens. *Surg Gynecol Obstet* 121:1347, 1965.

33. Shields L, Mital M, Cave EF. Complete dislocation of the knee: Experience at the Massachusetts General Hospital. *J Trauma* 9:192, 1969.

34. Daniell HW. Vasospastic reaction to methysergide maleate simulating Leriche syndrome: Ineffective treatment with adrenergic blockade. *Ann Intern Med* 60:881, 1964.

35. Green RM, DeWeese JA, Rob CG. Arterial embolectomy before and after the Fogarty catheter. *Surgery* 77:24, 1975.

36. Hussain S, Schwartz JM, Friedman SA, et al. Arterial thrombosis in essential thrombocythemia. *Am Heart J* 96:31, 1978.

37. Silverstein MN. Primary or hemorrhagic thrombocythemia. *Arch Intern Med* 122:18, 1968.

3 Abnormalities of Vasomotor Tone

Sandor A. Friedman

The cutaneous circulation is subject to enormous variations in blood flow through vasoconstriction and vasodilatation of precapillary arterioles. Blood flow to the digits may reach 100 ml/100 gm of tissue per minute during maximal vasodilatation, and fall to unrecordable levels during intense vasoconstriction.[1] This elastic quality is essential in maintaining a constant internal temperature. All of the major heat-losing mechanisms—convection, radiation, and sweat evaporation—require vasodilatation. On the other hand, a normal individual can survive for prolonged periods in subfreezing environments because of intense vasoconstriction, even at the expense of skin nutrition. Frostbite will often occur before hypothermia, unless vasoconstrictive ability has been paralyzed by a vasodilating agent.

At low temperatures above freezing (0° to 10°C), the peripheral circulation behaves differently. Intense vasoconstriction occurs first, but is followed shortly by oscillating short cycles of vasoconstriction and vasodilatation.[2] This mechanism protects the skin against necrosis while still maintaining body temperature. At constant temperatures of 15° to 25°C, continuous vasoconstriction occurs.

Vasoconstriction is mediated primarily through sympathetic nerve stimulation of alpha adrenergic receptors in cutaneous arterioles, and to a lesser extent other agents, including a direct effect of cold on vascular smooth muscle. Vasodilatation is mainly passive, occurring in the absence of vasoconstrictive influences. In addition, there is a small role for beta adrenergic receptors which, on stimulation, will cause vasodilatation. Although usually not a major factor, beta receptor influences may be significant in conditions of marginal blood flow. In the forearm, cholinergic sympathetic fibers and local formation of bradykinin may also contribute to vasodilatation. Heat and cold (0° to 10°C) can also cause vasodilatation directly, even in the sympathectomized extremity. The mechanisms are not clear but may include effects on catecholamine sensitivity and release of vasoactive substances.

The major stimuli to vasoconstriction are cold, emotional tension, and fall in blood pressure. Alpha adrenergic stimulation secondary to cold operates predominantly through spinal cord reflexes. The latter two stimuli operate through much more complicated mechanisms.

Blood pressure is maintained by a complex set of reflexes affecting muscle, cutaneous, and splanchnic arterioles. When a normal individual arises from the lying or sitting position, the carotid sinus immediately senses a lower distending pressure and decreases its stimulation of the vagus nerve and its inhibition of the vasomotor center in the brain stem.[3] As a result, the sympathetic nervous system is activated, resulting in peripheral vasoconstriction and a transient increase in heart rate, which prevent a sustained fall in blood pressure (Figure 3-1).

The other mechanism for maintaining blood pressure during changes in posture involves the renin-angiotensin system. Assumption of the erect position transiently decreases distending pressure in the juxtaglomerular apparatus of the kidneys, leading to secretion of increased amounts of renin. Renin activates angiotensin, a powerful vasoconstrictor.

Most of the conditions to be discussed in this chapter result from abnormalities in the autonomic nervous system or unusual sensitivity of the peripheral arterioles.

ORTHOSTATIC HYPOTENSION

There is little, if any, fall in blood pressure as a normal individual rises from the supine to standing position. In many people, systolic

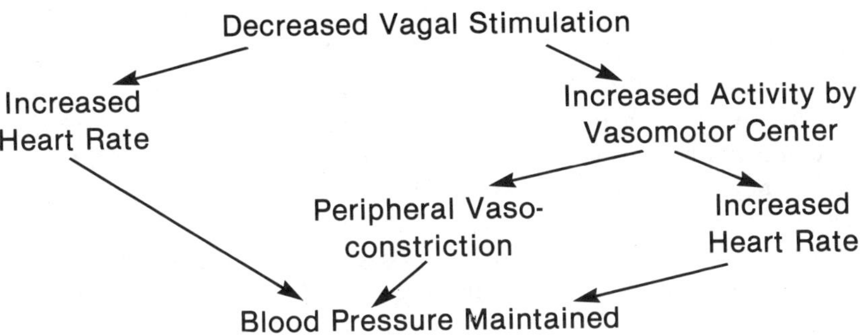

Figure 3-1 Carotid sinus mechanism for blood pressure control.

blood pressure actually rises about 10 mm Hg on standing. A fall of more than 20 mm Hg in systolic pressure is certainly abnormal. This orthostatic decrease in blood pressure is among the most common causes of dizziness and light-headedness.

To find minor orthostatic changes, it is necessary to study a patient carefully on a tilt table that can be instantly changed from the horizontal to vertical position. However, symptomatic, clinically significant, orthostatic hypotension can be detected in the following way:

1. Keep the patient supine for at least ten minutes,
2. Check the blood pressure several times to make sure that it is stable,
3. Ask the patient to stand up quickly, and
4. Take the blood pressure continuously for five minutes.

Symptoms of orthostatic hypotension include light-headedness, true vertigo and even syncope. The diagnosis is often overlooked because the majority of patients cannot relate their symptoms clearly to changes in posture. Some patients may be erroneously thought to have hypoglycemia because they complain of severe dizziness when they first arise in the morning. Furthermore, orthostatic hypotension may be a contributing factor to a variety of cerebral and brain-stem symptoms, such as vertigo and diplopia, and even precipitate transient ischemic attacks in patients with cerebral artery disease.

Causes

When the diagnosis of orthostatic hypotension has been made, the etiology of the unstable blood pressure must be found. Orthostatic hypotension can be divided basically into three categories: blood volume depletion, autonomic dysfunction, and idiopathic. With contraction of blood volume, a normal sympathetic nervous system attempts to restore blood pressure to normal through an increase in cardiac output and arteriolar constriction. Heart rate rises as blood pressure falls. The major causes of orthostatic hypotension in this category include: adrenal insufficiency, overuse of diuretic agents, salt-losing nephritis, gastrointestinal fluid losses, and hemorrhage. In the case of adrenal insufficiency, postural hypotension may be the earliest clue to the diagnosis, appearing before abnormalities in serum electrolytes and occasionally even in hypoadrenalism secondary to pituitary insufficiency.

With autonomic dysfunction, heart rate does not increase as blood pressure decreases. The three major causes of autonomic-induced orthostatic hypotension are: use of antihypertensive drugs, diabetic peripheral neuropathy, and central nervous system disease. In many patients with diabetes mellitus, who are also under treatment for hypertension, one often sees severe orthostatic hypotension due to the additive effects of neuropathy and medication.

It is important to check standing and supine blood pressures regularly in all patients being treated for hypertension. Even if the patient has no complaints, a postural fall of more than 40 mm Hg is cause for concern and modification of the antihypertensive medication. Drugs such as guanethidine, which inhibits the peripheral sympathetic nervous system at the postganglionic level, and reserpine, which depletes synapses of catecholamines, tend to lower the standing pressure significantly more than supine pressure. They must be used sparingly in older people and should be the first drugs eliminated if significant orthostatic hypotension develops. Drugs, such as alpha methyl dopa and clonidine that cause vasodilatation through a central nervous system action, also cause orthostatic hypotension quite frequently. Propranolol may occasionally cause this problem by decreasing cardiac output and preventing a reflex increase in heart rate when the patient stands. However, propranolol does not interfere with alpha receptors and actually blocks beta receptors in arterioles so that this complication is uncommon. A direct vasodilating drug, ie, hydralazine, may cause postural hypotension by competing with the effect of alpha receptors on arteriolar walls. However, hydralazine does not prevent reflex increases in cardiac output and heart rate. The responses of patients to all of these agents are quite variable, and it is not easy to predict with assurance which agent or combination of agents will be tolerated best. With trial and error based on an understanding of each drug's mechanism of action, the physician can usually arrive at a drug regimen that produces normotension without significant orthostatic changes.

Diabetic neuropathy is the leading noniatrogenic cause of orthostatic hypotension. The mechanism is not clear. It was originally assumed to result from failure of efferent sympathetic nerve fibers. However, several studies have shown that most patients with diabetic neuropathy—even those with postural hypotension—show an adequate vasoconstrictive response to cold exposure.[4] On the other hand, the cardiovascular response to the Valsalva maneuver is blunted.[5] Reflex increase in heart rate during the hypotensive phase, and decrease in heart rate when the pressure rises at the end of the maneuver, are either absent or slight. Respiratory variations in heart rate are also attenuated.[6] Taken as a whole, these facts tend to point away from efferent sympathetic fibers and toward the afferent side of the carotid sinus reflex in the pathogenesis of orthostatic hypotension. The vagus nerve may be involved in diabetic neuropathy since both blood pressure control and respiratory variations in heart rate involve vagal reflexes.

Decreased function of the renin-angiotensin system may also play a role in diabetic neuropathy. Beta-adrenergic stimulation of the kidneys is a major factor in controlling renin secretion. Several studies in diabetic patients have shown a tendency toward a hyporeninemic-hypoaldosterone state and inappropriately small rises in plasma renin levels with assumption of the upright position.[7] In fact, some patients with diabetes mellitus have a tendency to hyperkalemia because of low aldosterone levels resulting from a suppressed renin-angiotensin axis.[8]

When diabetic patients develop postural hypotension, they gradually exhibit signs of peripheral neuropathy in their lower extremities. Ankle jerks are absent, and there is almost always significant loss of vibratory sensation in the toes, and usually the ankles. In most cases, neuropathy is quite marked by the time orthostatic hypotension appears. In patients receiving insulin, it may be difficult to distinguish the symptoms of hypoglycemia from those of orthostatic hypotension. Both possibilities must be carefully evaluated.

Another important cause of autonomic dysfunction is cerebrovascular disease. Basilar artery insufficiency may lead to ischemia of the vasomotor center and severe fluctuations in blood pressure. This, of course, has an adverse effect on cerebral blood flow and leads to a vicious cycle of more cerebral ischemia and larger falls in blood pressure. Every patient with cerebrovascular disease must be carefully evaluated for postural hypotension because it is one of the important reversible factors.

The Shy-Drager syndrome, an idiopathic degenerative process starting in middle age, causes diffuse dysautonomia, a Parkinson-like syndrome, and cerebellar ataxia secondary to destruction of olivopontine-cerebellar pathways. Severe postural hypotension, impotence, and bladder dysfunction are early signs. The disease is inexorable and incurable.

Other autonomic causes of orthostatic hypotension include parkinsonism, Guillain-Barré syndrome, pheochromocytoma, and aging itself. Pheochromocytomas, by producing large amounts of circulating catecholamines, suppress the autonomic nervous system. If output suddenly diminishes, severe hypotension may occur. A pheochromocytoma should be suspected in untreated hypertensive patients with standing pressures lower than supine pressures. Aging affects efferent sympathetic nerves. It is known that nerve conduction velocity decreases with age, and some people over the age of 65 do not respond to a cold stimulus with adequate vasoconstriction.[9] There may also be other factors contributing to orthostatic hypotension in the elderly.

After consideration of known causes, there are still a small number of patients who have unexplained orthostatic hypotension. This group is heterogeneous and may include patients with a variety of poorly understood mechanisms. Some of these patients have abnormally low renin levels in the upright position, suggesting a primary failure of the renin-angiotensin axis. The others have high renin levels, indicating an attempt at compensation for defects outside of this system. Recently symptomatic orthostatic hypotension, responsive to beta sympathetic blocking agents, has been described in association with mitral valve prolapse.[9a]

In general, orthostatic hypotension due to idiopathic autonomic dysfunction can be divided into preganglionic and postganglionic abnormalities. With preganglionic lesions, catecholamine stores are intact at the terminal synapse, and basal plasma norepinephrine levels are normal. Response to norepinephrine infusion is also normal. In postganglionic conditions, there is an exaggerated response to norepinephrine. Basal levels of norepinephrine are decreased.

Treatment

The treatment of orthostatic hypotension is often quite simple. In many cases, symptoms occur only when the patient first arises, and teaching him to change position slowly may suffice. If orthostatic symptoms persist while he is standing or walking, elastic support for the lower extremities is the first therapeutic modality. Generally well-fitted, firm elastic stockings or leotards, by decreasing peripheral venous pooling, will decrease positional changes in blood pressure.

If the patient is receiving antihypertensive agents, judicious changes in medication may eliminate the problem. A rising blood urea nitrogen level may suggest overly zealous use of diuretic agents. Occasionally, one encounters patients with severe diabetic neuropathy or cerebrovascular disease in whom the goals of normotension and avoidance of postural hypotension are mutually exclusive. In this situation, it may be necessary to settle for less than complete control of hypertension.

For patients whose symptoms persist despite these simple measures, drug therapy may be necessary. However, this should be a last resort, reserved for those patients who really cannot function because of marked central nervous system symptoms, and have a demonstrated fall of more than 40 mm Hg in systolic pressure when they stand up slowly. A salt-retaining steroid may be helpful by increasing blood volume. If cardiac function is good, this volume expansion will be well-tolerated and will increase cardiac output in all positions. In patients with even mild heart disease, this therapy may precipitate congestive heart failure. Adrenergic, vasoconstricting agents, ie, ephedrine and levodopa, may be helpful but may also precipitate ventricular arrhythmias. Indomethacin is sometimes effective, probably through prostaglandin inhibition. Beta-blocking agents may be effective by blocking sympathetic vasodilatory fibers and increasing the ratio of alpha adrenergic to beta adrenergic activity.

In summary, orthostatic hypotension is a frequently overlooked cause of dizziness and a contributing factor to the symptoms of cerebrovascular disease. When recognized, its cause is easily ascertained and its effects easily overcome, or at least alleviated.

RAYNAUD'S PHENOMENON

The reversible arteriospasm, originally described by Raynaud in 1874, is an entity that has fascinated vascular physiologists for many decades.[10] Unfortunately, the terms Raynaud's phenomenon and Raynaud's disease are often used too loosely, leading to confusion and misdiagnosis. It is important to adhere to a specific and arbitrary definition of Raynaud's phenomenon in order to avoid unnecessary and expensive laboratory work.

Raynaud originally described a syndrome in which an individual's digits turned extremely pale (white) followed by intense cyanosis on exposure to cold (Figure 3-2). The individual's subsequent exposure to room temperature caused the digits to become intensely erythematous and hot, and then finally to return to normal. These symptoms usually involve hands predominantly, but also feet and sometimes the ears and tip of the nose. Basically, this is a syndrome of increased vasomotor tone, and there are many patients who manifest this problem without showing all three color changes. Many people who respond to cold with intense vasoconstriction may have only a phase of pallor or cyanosis and may not have subsequent erythema. Pallor represents a phase of virtually no blood flow to the skin, while cyanosis corresponds to unoxygenated blood stagnating in cutaneous capillaries. The later erythema results from reactive hyperemia, a phase of increased blood flow due to ischemia-induced vasodilatation. Patients with the highest vasomotor tone may develop pallor on exposure to cold and not have significant hyperemia on rewarming.

Symptoms associated with Raynaud's phenomenon are variable. Some patients will complain of nothing more than a mild feeling of coldness in their hands, while others may complain of pain and/or numbness. There is often excruciating pain during reactive hyperemia. Correlation between severity of symptoms and magnitude of color changes is poor. In fact, many people without Raynaud's phenomenon experience more severe symptoms on exposure to cold than some pa-

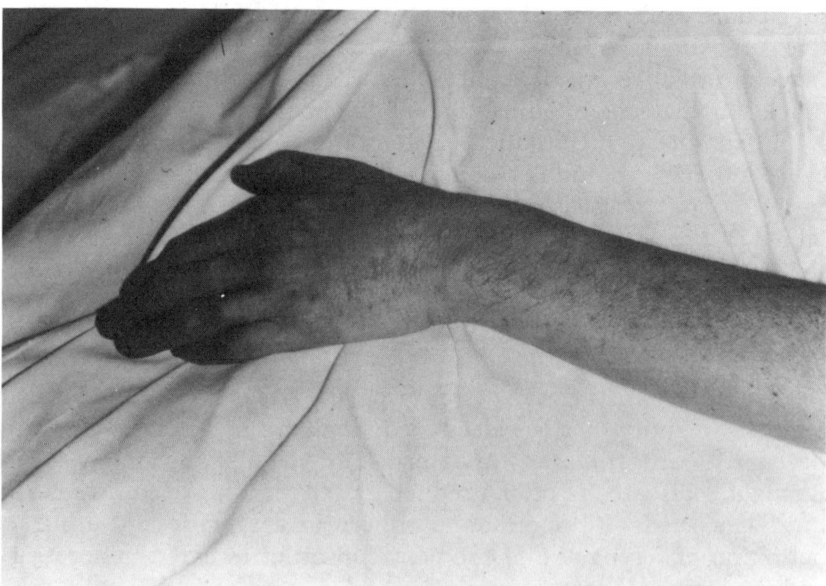

Figure 3-2 Intense phase of cyanosis in a patient with severe Raynaud's phenomenon.

tients with Raynaud's phenomenon. Yet the former should not be confused with patients having Raynaud's phenomenon. It is only the color changes that make the diagnosis.

Patients with Raynaud's phenomenon usually have high vasomotor tone much of the time. Their hands tend to be cool and sweaty even at room temperature, and they may have episodes of color change during emotional tension. With long-standing Raynaud's phenomenon, sclerodactyly may develop. The skin of the digits becomes adherent to underlying tissue through fibrosis. Wrinkles are lost, and the skin cannot be lifted off the bone. Sclerodactyly is often minimally present, and one must carefully examine the dorsal skin over the distal phalanges in order to notice it. This finding in association with cool hands confirms the diagnosis of Raynaud's phenomenon. In the presence of warm hands, sclerodactyly may be evidence of diabetic peripheral neuropathy.

Often, the physician attempts to confirm the diagnosis of Raynaud's phenomenon by immersing the patient's hands in ice water. This is usually not necessary. If the patient gives a clear history and has cool hands, one is generally safe in making the diagnosis. If the history is vague or unreliable, ice water immersion may confirm the diagnosis. However, this may not be adequate in all cases. It may be necessary to apply the conditions under which the patient ordinarily notices color changes.

From a physiological point of view, Raynaud's phenomenon is quite puzzling. Plethysmographic studies reveal virtually no measurable blood flow in the digits of any severely vasoconstricted individual, and yet most people do not develop intense pallor or cyanosis. It is not clear then what makes people with Raynaud's phenomenon different. The answer may lie in the difficulties and relative inaccuracies of digital blood flow measurements. There may be immeasurable, small differences in blood flow between normal individuals and those with Raynaud's phenomenon on exposure to cold. The cyanotic phase may occur partially because of venular constriction.

The most common form of Raynaud's phenomenon is of unknown etiology and is called Raynaud's disease. This disorder begins early in life, often by teenage, and almost always by age 40 (in 80% of cases).[11] It is five times as common in women as in men.

The pathogenesis of Raynaud's disease is still a puzzle. Debate continues over whether the increased tendency to vasospasm is a primary disorder of the autonomic nervous system or a matter of hypersensitive digital arterioles. The presence of migraine in 14% and hypertension in 9% of cases of Raynaud's disease[12] can fit with either theory. Early investigations incriminated the sympathetic nervous system because sympathectomy initially appeared to produce complete relief from this disease.[13] However, symptoms generally reappear within two years, suggesting increased sensitivity to circulating catecholamines. Physiologic studies have revealed no differences between patients with Raynaud's disease and normal subjects in brachial arterial and venous plasma concentrations of norepinephrine and epinephrine.[14] Heightened digital vessel sensitivity to cold cannot explain the occurrence of attacks in response to emotional stimuli. It is possible that the disease involves several physiologic disorders including increased release, decreased diffusion, and consequent re-uptake of norepinephrine at sympathetic nerve endings, as well as enhanced alpha-receptor and digital arteriole sensitivity.

Raynaud's Disease *vs* Raynaud's Phenomenon

Raynaud's disease is more annoying than dangerous. Patients rarely develop ischemic ulcers or atrophy of the fingers, although sclerodactyly eventually occurs. This disorder is not associated with any systemic diseases and has an excellent prognosis. Symptoms usually respond well to rather simple measures.

Since Raynaud's phenomenon can be caused by a number of diverse disorders, the diagnosis of Raynaud's disease remains one of exclusion. All the secondary forms of Raynaud's phenomenon must be ruled out to make a secure diagnosis of this primary disorder. Even after extensive evaluation demonstrates no other abnormalities, it may be several years before one can be sure of the diagnosis. Raynaud's phenomenon may be the first clinical sign of diseases that will not otherwise become manifest for five years or more. However, if the patient is under the age of 20 when Raynaud's phenomenon begins and has an initial negative work-up for systemic disease, it is very unlikely that he or she has anything more than Raynaud's disease.

There are several features which would cause the suspicion that an underlying disorder is present. The first is age. The older the patient at the onset of Raynaud's phenomenon, the more likely there is an underlying disease. Raynaud's phenomenon beginning after the age of 40 is usually a secondary disorder. Severity and persistence of arteriospasm are also clues. Patients who develop color changes at temperatures above 15°C are more likely to have Raynaud's phenomenon than Raynaud's disease. Development of ischemic ulcerations or digital gangrene rarely occurs in Raynaud's disease, and finally, spasm or occlusion of medium-sized arteries never occurs in Raynaud's disease. Absence of a radial pulse indicates the presence of another disorder, and an absent ulnar pulse strongly suggests that possibility.

Causes of Raynaud's Phenomenon

The differential diagnosis of Raynaud's phenomenon is extensive and can be divided into several categories: hyperactivity of the sympathetic nervous system, hypersensitivity of digital arterioles, and sludging of elements within the circulation.

The first category, hyperactivity of the sympathetic nervous system, includes: thoracic outlet syndrome, hypothyroidism, and immobilization of an extremity.

Thoracic outlet syndrome The thoracic outlet syndrome is associated with a narrow outlet between the thorax and upper extremity. It is related to a variety of anatomical problems and causes clinical syndromes involving the subclavian artery, subclavian vein, and brachial plexus. It leads to Raynaud's phenomenon by compressing and irritating sympathetic nerve fibers from cervical ganglia, which travel with the brachial plexus. It is the first diagnosis to consider when a patient has Raynaud's phenomenon of one arm only. Rarely is it bilateral. The diagnosis and treatment of thoracic outlet syndrome will be considered in more detail in another chapter.

Hypothyroidism Hypothyroidism has recently been recognized as a cause of Raynaud's phenomenon.[15] In fact, it may sometimes be the earliest sign of thyroid deficiency. Since many cases of hypothyroidism are related to Hashimoto's thyroiditis, there was initially some speculation that both Raynaud's phenomenon and hypothyroidism might be manifestations of an autoimmune disease. Thyroid replacement therapy, however, appears to eliminate the vasospastic episodes. Recently, Raynaud's phenomenon has also been described in hypothyroidism secondary to pituitary insufficiency.[16]

The mechanism of Raynaud's phenomenon in hypothyroidism is not entirely clear. Decreased activity or decreased basal metabolic rate may lead to vasoconstriction and decreased blood flow. This is not likely, however, to explain Raynaud's phenomenon in patients with very mild hypothyroidism in whom metabolic rate is not appreciably lowered. A more plausible explanation involves adrenergic receptors. It is well known that many of the manifestations of hyperthyroidism are mediated through increased sensitivity of beta receptors to adrenergic stimulation. This explains tachycardia, vasodilatation, and sweating. Conversely, hypothyroid individuals may have hyposensitive beta receptors, leading to bradycardia and high vasomotor tone. Animal studies have shown increased vasoconstriction secondary to norepinephrine administration in hypothyroidism.[17]

Immobilization Immobility of a limb for prolonged periods due to nerve or muscle disease or fracture may lead to severe arteriospasm. Subsequent exposure to cold will often result in pallor and cyanosis. If distal pulses are absent, it may be difficult to assess the relative roles of arterial disease and arteriospasm in producing ischemia. A trial of vasodilating agents, in conjunction with protection of the limb from cold, is advisable in that situation.

Arteriolar hypersensitivity The second category, hypersensitivity of digital arterioles, includes:

- Digital trauma
- Collagen diseases
- Scleroderma
- CRST syndrome
- Post-cold injury
- Thromboangitis obliterans
- Primary pulmonary hypertension

Digital trauma An occupational history is important in evaluating patients with Raynaud's phenomenon. Digital vessels are superficial and subject to both acute and chronic trauma. Since these arterioles have extremely reactive walls, it is not surprising that they may react to injury with spasticity. People in occupations requiring repeated impact of their fingers upon solid objects may develop Raynaud's phenomenon. This includes principally operators of vibrating tools such as pneumatic drills and occasionally typists. Since this occupational injury is quite unusual, however, an etiologic diagnosis based solely on occupation must be one of last resort after a full work-up for other causes.

Acute trauma of a finger or toe may lead to localized Raynaud's phenomenon. Even an insect bite in proximity to a digital vessel can lead to a localized syndrome of cold-induced vasospasm. This problem may disappear after a few days or weeks but may also last for many years. In general, the prognosis is one of gradual improvement.

Collagen Diseases The collagen diseases represent a major cause of Raynaud's phenomenon. Both systemic lupus erythematosus (SLE) and rheumatoid arthritis may be associated with this syndrome quite early in their course. In fact, there is little relationship between the presence of arteriospasm and severity of the collagen disease.

In the case of lupus, several years may pass with Raynaud's phenomenon the only finding. With time, the patient may develop systemic signs or symptoms, or perhaps only disease localized to the extremities. Some patients may develop large, medium, or small artery disease. Femoral and popliteal pulses may be lost with resultant intermittent claudication. Venous thrombosis may also occur. There may be a syndrome of migratory superficial phlebitis, or deep vein thrombosis with resultant deep vein insufficiency, and signs of venous stasis.

These patients may also have small-vessel occlusions and develop digital ulcers and gangrene.

In rheumatoid arthritis, there is no definite relationship between severity and duration of joint involvement and onset of Raynaud's phenomenon. Patients with very mild joint disease may have severe vasospasm. In rheumatoid vasculitis, patients may also have digital gangrene, as well as ischemic ulcers on other areas of the extremities.

Scleroderma Scleroderma (progressive systemic sclerosis) is the classical setting for Raynaud's phenomenon. As in Raynaud's disease, SLE and rheumatoid arthritis, young women are afflicted more often than men. The average age of onset of scleroderma was 42.9 in one series.[18] In this disease of unknown etiology, progressive fibrosis and atrophy occur in subcutaneous tissues, leading to a binding down of the skin. In the early edematous phase, the subcutaneous areas are swollen, and the skin is immovable and thick. As more atrophy ensues, the subcutaneous areas become thinner, calcinosis may occur, and the skin is strung taught over bone and tendon. This process may lead to contractures of fingers and toes, difficulty in opening the mouth, and generalized stiffness with limited mobility. It is important to remember that sclerodactyly alone is not specific for scleroderma. If similar changes occur proximal to the hands or feet, or on the trunk, then the diagnosis of scleroderma is obvious. Often a great deal of muscle atrophy results, especially in the proximal areas, and the patient may be extremely weak. In fact, the process can simulate polymyositis clinically and even histologically.

The very first sign of scleroderma is usually Raynaud's phenomenon. It may predate other manifestations by several years, even several decades. Even if the patient has not noticed color changes, the hands are usually cold and sweaty. Cyanosis is very easily precipitated in a cold environment. The absence of high vasomotor tone in the hands virtually rules out the diagnosis of scleroderma. As fibrosis develops in subcutaneous areas, small vessels are compressed and occluded. Furthermore, a low-grade vasculitis leads to more occlusive disease. As a result, the patient with scleroderma generally has a combination of arteriospasm and fixed arterial occlusive disease affecting the digits. These changes result in thinning of the fingers, marked sclerodactyly, pale, ischemic ulcers, and gangrenous changes. Autoamputation of the distal ends of digits is not uncommon. Ischemic ulcers may occur in other areas of the extremities also, sometimes in areas of subcutaneous calcinosis.

Internal organ involvement in scleroderma is variable. Clinical problems include dysphagia due to impaired esophageal motility, malabsorption syndrome due to impaired small bowel motility, renal failure, and cardiac and pulmonary abnormalities. The most common symptoms arise from the gastrointestinal tract, particularly the esophagus. Dysphagia, especially of liquids, may often be an early symptom of scleroderma. In fact, esophageal manometry may show significant abnormalities in patients without esophageal symptoms. Most of these patients will never develop dysphagia.

Symptomatology from lung involvement is not common and generally occurs as a late manifestation of scleroderma. The diffusion capacity may be low early in scleroderma, but clinically significant lung disease is unusual. In its full-blown manifestation, however, lung involvement can produce severe restrictive disease of the interstitial type. Cardiac involvement is usually located in the conducting system. Heart block and bundle branch blocks are the most common findings.

Renal disease is the most ominous development in scleroderma. Once it begins, it tends to progress rapidly to uremia over a period of a few months. Hypertension is the key to this renal failure and represents a major danger signal. Once hypertension develops in a patient with scleroderma, renal failure usually ensues rapidly. Even with vigorous antihypertensive treatment, the outlook becomes bleak.

There is no good correlation between severity of cutaneous disease and likelihood of internal organ involvement. Patients may have minimal cutaneous disease, or perhaps only Raynaud's phenomenon, and still develop severe visceral involvement. Conversely, there are many patients with severe stiffness and skin ulcers who never have internal problems. Survival in scleroderma depends greatly on the presence or absence of internal organ disease. In one series, patients with cardiac, pulmonary or renal involvement had a seven-year cumulative mortality of 50%.[19] Being white and female are good prognostic factors. In the same series, 80% of white females under age 45 survived seven years.[19]

The pathogenesis of scleroderma is not known, but certain facts have been established. Histologically, one finds a low-grade vasculitis in some areas with mild cellular infiltration of small blood vessel walls. In many areas such as the kidney, the vascular histology is very similar to the arteriosclerosis that is seen with long-standing hypertension.

From a functional point of view, there is evidence which implicates arteriospasm and exaggerated arteriolar reactivity in the pathogenesis of scleroderma. The early onset of Raynaud's phenomenon is one example. Studies of renal blood flow have been performed in patients with scleroderma before, during, and after induced attacks of digital arteriospasm. Renal blood flow decreases during these episodes, and returns to normal with vasodilatation of the hands and feet.[20,21] There is also epidemiologic evidence that a disproportionate number of patients with scleroderma die in the winter months as compared to summer months. Perhaps chronic ischemia leads to permanent vessel changes and fibrosis of surrounding tissue. Abnormalities in tryptophan metabolism, with high levels of serotonin and kynurenine, may also play a role.[22]

Unfortunately, there is no effective therapy for scleroderma. Corticosteroids have not been helpful. Vasodilators may give some relief from Raynaud's phenomenon and aid in the healing of ischemic ulcers. If a patient with scleroderma develops frequent skin ulceration and gangrene or internal organ involvement, moving to a warm climate may be advisable.

CRST syndrome The CRST syndrome consists of Raynaud's phenomenon, subcutaneous calcinosis, sclerodactyly, and telangiectasia. Since all of these features may be seen in scleroderma, many authorities believe CRST is merely a variant or forme fruste of the latter. In fact, many of these patients have esophageal motility abnormalities and occasionally dysphagia. Telangiectasia and calcinosis are usually quite prominent on the digits and elsewhere.

Post-cold injury Patients who suffer cold-related injuries to an extremity may develop Raynaud's phenomenon. This is another common cause of unilateral arteriospastic disease. Sometimes only one or two digits will be involved. The initial insult actually may be frostbite, or just a prolonged and appropriate episode of arteriospasm in response to severe cold or a damp, moderately cold environment. In some way, digital arterioles apparently become sensitized to cold, and Raynaud's phenomenon may persist for many years.

Circulating factors The third category of Raynaud's phenomenon is related to circulating factors. These include: cryoglobulinemia, cryofibrinogenemia, cold hemagglutinins, and thrombocytosis.

Cryoglobulins are serum proteins that precipitate at low temperatures.[23,24] Cryofibrinogen is a plasma component that precipitates at low temperatures, and is usually a complex of fibrinogen and fibrin monomer. Both can be demonstrated in vitro by refrigerating the patient's serum and plasma. Cryoproteins precipitate at the bottom of the test tube, and then return to solution when the test tube is heated. Precipitation in both the plasma and serum tubes indicates the presence of cryoglobulin, while precipitation only in the plasma tube proves that cryofibrinogen is present. The temperature characteristics of these substances may vary from patient to patient. Some cryoglobulins may begin to precipitate at room temperature while others will not precipitate until the temperature is near freezing. Quantitative measurements of these proteins are possible but laborious. A simple and useful estimate of their quantity is the cryocrit (the volume percentage of precipitate in the specimen). The upper limit of normal for cryofibrinogen is a cryocrit of about 2.5% The presence of even small amounts of cryoglobulin is abnormal.

The most common cause of cryofibrinogenemia is an active clotting process. Whenever a fibrin clot develops, secondary fibrinolysis liberates fibrin-split products, including fibrin monomer. The latter combines with fibrinogen to produce cryofibrinogen. Thus, small quantities are often present during the early stages of acute myocardial infarction, pulmonary embolism and strokes, and in patients forming thrombi over an extended period of time, ie, left atrial thrombi in mitral stenosis. In fact, the small amounts of cryofibrinogen seen in normal people probably represent fibrinolysis of subclinical thrombi. Pregnancy is also associated with a small amount of cryofibrinogen. In none of these conditions does the level of cryofibrinogen generally reach a level of clinical significance.

The second major cause of cryofibrinogenemia is disseminated intravascular coagulation (DIC). This process, of course, liberates a great deal of fibrin monomer. The diagnosis of DIC is based on demonstrating the presence of fibrin monomer in the absence of a primary thrombotic process, ie, a myocardial infarction. Since these fibrin-split products act as an antithrombin, the thrombin time is usually prolonged, and bleeding may occur. The disseminated thrombosis in this disorder may consume enough of the coagulation factors to produce thrombocytopenia, hypoprothrombinemia, and a prolonged partial thromboplastin time. This, in turn, can lead to more hemorrhage. DIC tends to occur acutely in septicemia and shock, and chronically in patients with malignancies. Sometimes, the only chemical manifestation of DIC is the presence of cryofibrinogen in high titer. Raynaud's phenomenon may result from the cryofibrinogenemia, and digital thrombosis may occur because of a combination of cryofibrinogen and the DIC itself.

Cryofibrinogenemia is rarely seen as an isolated condition of unknown cause. These patients may have Raynaud's phenomenon, and are subject to widespread thromboembolic disease. Whether the condition is also an incomplete expression of DIC is not known.

Cryoglobulinemia is seen in malignancies, particularly multiple myeloma, and in collagen diseases, particularly SLE. It can also be seen as a primary disorder. The abnormal protein in the latter condition is usually a mixed cryoglobulin (complex of I_gG and I_gM). This complex causes an antigen-antibody reaction within small blood vessel walls, leading to a vasculitis that may include glomerulitis, peripheral arterial disease, cerebrovascular accidents, and widespread visceral involvement. Recently, hepatitis B surface antigen has been found in the serum and/or cryoprecipitate of a number of these patients.[25] Thus, mixed cryoglobulinemia may be an autoimmune complication of hepatitis B infection. Management of cryoglobulinemia depends on appropriate treatment of the underlying cause. Therapy for idiopathic cryoglobulinemia has, for the most part, been unsuccessful. Case reports of remissions produced by corticosteroids, dicumarol, and melphalan have appeared but have not been duplicated. Digital arterial occlusions with gangrene occur frequently. Raynaud's phenomenon may be the first manifestation of cryoglobulinemia.

Cold hemagglutinins are I_gM cold antibodies against red blood cells, usually against the I antigens.[26] Cold hemagglutinins are found occasionally in collagen diseases and lymphomas, and are present in low titer in mycoplasma pneumonia. There is also an idiopathic cold hemagglutinin disease associated with hemolytic anemia, purpura, and splenomegaly. Raynaud's phenomenon is a prominent feature of the latter, but is rarely seen with mycoplasma infections.

A high platelet count secondary to myeloproliferative disease (over 800,000) can cause a clinical picture very similar to Raynaud's phenomenon. The cyanotic stage tends to last somewhat longer after exposure to cold, and the patient may have a blotchy cyanosis of his hands or feet in a warm environment. More often this entity makes its first clinical appearance with unexpected digital gangrene. Thrombocytosis will be discussed more fully in another chapter.

Management of Raynaud's phenomenon For any patient with bilateral Raynaud's phenomenon, the following laboratory work is advised in addition to a thorough history and physical examination:

- Plasma thyroxine level
- Antinuclear antibody test and LE preparation
- Testing for cryoglobulin, cryofibrinogen and cold hemagglutinins
- Test for rheumatoid factor
- Platelet count
- Cineesophagram and, if available, esophageal motility studies
- Diffusion capacity

The treatment of Raynaud's phenomenon involves simple measures as well as drug therapy. Keeping warm is the most important principle. This means, not only protecting the hands and feet from cold, but also the body as a whole. The warmer the body, the less reflex vasoconstriction will take place. Often, patients with Raynaud's phenomenon have a great deal of difficulty in early spring or late fall because they do not dress warmly enough. In winter, they are more aware of the need for warm clothing. These patients should never smoke.

The second measure is judicious use of vasodilator drugs. Some patients experience severe arteriospasm only in very cold weather and need only a mild vasodilator at the coldest times of the year. Provided they live in a warm climate all year, they may need no drug therapy. Others need vasodilators all year because they experience problems even with mild cold exposure as, for example, when washing dishes or bathing.

In using vasodilating agents, one generally begins with relatively weak agents and escalates the pharmacotherapy gradually until a satisfactory result is obtained. The goals are to prevent ischemic breakdown of skin, minimize symptoms, and allow the patient to perform normal activities of daily living. Many patients have no symptoms during their attacks of arteriospasm, and function relatively well even though their hands often feel cold. Drug therapy for them may be quite minimal. On the other hand, a patient with scleroderma and painful ischemic ulcers may require vigorous attempts at vasodilatation.

Usually, a mild vasodilating drug is given that acts directly on arteriolar walls. The dosage is three to four times daily. If inadequate relief is obtained after a trial of several weeks, a strong alpha blocker, generally phenoxybenzamine hydrochloride, may be used instead. This agent must be used with caution because of its potential to produce orthostatic hypotension. Generally it is not used in patients with significant coronary artery or cerebrovascular disease. The dosage of this drug can be increased gradually from 10 mgs, three to four times daily, up to total daily doses of 80 to 120 mgs, watching carefully for therapeutic effects and signs of orthostatic hypotension.

Other helpful therapeutic agents, especially in hypertensive patients, include the postganglionic blocker guanethidine, methyldopa,[27] and rauwolfia compounds,[19] which deplete the body of catecholamines. In addition to orthostatic hypotension, one must watch for impotence due to guanethidine and significant mental depression from the rauwolfia drugs. In some difficult cases of Raynaud's disease, intraarterial injection of reserpine has been associated with remissions of symptoms in the injected arm for several months.[28] The mechanism of this effect is not understood.

Griseofulvin, an antifungal agent, has been effective in daily doses of 500 to 1,000 mgs. In one series, there was subjective and objective improvement in six of seven patients.[29] Digital temperatures in these patients were found to remain higher during exposure to ice water after griseofulvin administration. This drug may act directly on digital arterioles.

A recent study has suggested a possible therapeutic role for biofeedback techniques.[30] Nineteen of 20 patients were trained to abort attacks of Raynaud's phenomenon at environmental temperatures below 4°C.

Finally, beta-blocking agents clearly increase the frequency and severity of vasospastic attacks, and should be avoided in patients with Raynaud's phenomenon.[31]

Surgery is an alternative to drug therapy. Cervical sympathectomy and/or removal of the first and second throacic ganglia have been used extensively for Raynaud's disease. Initially, the results may be excellent, often with complete disappearance of arteriospasm. With time, however, symptoms return and by the end of two years, many patients are no better off than they were before surgery. The reason for this transient response is not entirely clear, but it may be related to development of postdenervation hypersensitivity of the digital arterioles to circulating catecholamines. There may also be some regrowth of sympathetic fibers into the upper extremities from the lower sympathetic ganglia. When cervical sympathectomy is attempted for Raynaud's phenomenon secondary to scleroderma or other collagen diseases, even the initial results are often disappointing. Cervical sympathectomy is not recommended except in the most intractable cases of Raynaud's disease, and only after warning the patient that the symptoms will probably return later.

POST-TRAUMA SYNDROME

The post-trauma syndrome is a very curious disorder. Injury to an extremity occasionally leads to a constellation of findings including pain, weakness, muscle atrophy, and arteriospasm.[32] Because of the apparently prominent role of the sympathetic nervous system, this syndrome has been named post-traumatic reflex sympathetic dystrophy. The patient may complain of diffuse achiness and paresthesias throughout the extremity, not specifically in the area of trauma. Examination often reveals a swollen, cold extremity with pallor and patchy cyanosis of the foot. The foot is usually sweaty, and distal sensation may be somewhat impaired. Peripheral pulses are generally present although vasoconstriction may eliminate the dorsalis pedis pulse. The patient is reluctant to use the extremity. If a leg is involved, he limps, and with time, significant muscle atrophy is inevitable. A vicious cycle of pain, disuse, and atrophy leads to more arteriospasm and disability. The arteriospasm worsens in a cold environment.

The pathogenesis of this syndrome is puzzling. There is a poor correlation between severity of trauma and onset of this syndrome. In fact, sometimes rather mild or even inapparent trauma sets it off. Whenever a limb is not used, its blood flow decreases through sympathetic nerve-induced vasoconstriction. It is the immobilization following trauma, therefore, that begins the vicious cycle of sympathetic discharge and progressive atrophy.

This syndrome must be considered in the differential diagnosis of an ischemic limb. Presence of pulses, increased sweating, and diffuse ischemia without a sharp line of demarcation, point to increased sympathetic discharge. If the inactivity persists for many weeks, muscle stiffness may develop, and then the syndrome can be mistaken for a herniated disc. In contrast to disc disease, sensory loss is not in a nerve root distribution, and the pain does not radiate from the back in post-trauma syndrome.

The aim of treatment is to break the vicious cycle leading to progressive disability. Adequate analgesia and physiotherapy represent the cornerstones of therapy. The patient must be encouraged to use the limb in order to reverse muscle atrophy. Vasodilating agents increase blood flow and help to alleviate discomfort. In many cases, weak vasodilators are effective, but it may be necessary to employ stronger agents. Judicious use of local nerve blocks is an alternative to vasodilators. Sometimes, one or two stellate ganglion blocks for an upper extremity, or caudal anesthesia for a lower extremity, may reverse the process of excess sympathetic discharge. The block sometimes dramatically and mysteriously breaks the cycle, eliminating the chronic pain and allowing the patient to exercise the limb.

OTHER VASOCONSTRICTIVE SYNDROMES

Acrocyanosis and livedo reticularis are two less common syndromes that involve vasoconstriction. In acrocyanosis, the hands, and sometimes the feet, are diffusely cyanotic and cold almost all the time with little change in response to environmental temperature. The syndrome appears mostly in women, develops in the first three decades of life and is totally benign. Ulceration and sclerodactyly do not occur, but the patient may notice mild pain and swelling during cold weather. Although it may be frightening to the uninformed observer, patients with acrocyanosis rarely have serious symptoms and usually require relatively little therapy.

Livedo reticularis is a disorder of vasoconstriction occurring generally on the shins and feet. It appears as a local area of mottling or reticular blue discoloration. Although most cases are idiopathic, livedo reticularis may occur as a manifestation of periarteritis nodosa, SLE, cryoglobulinemia, and cholesterol emboli from the abdominal aorta.[33] In its secondary form, the reticular discoloration usually persists no matter what changes occur in environmental temperature. The idiopathic form has two variants: 1) cutis marmorata, in which the mottling disappears in a warm environment, and 2) livedo reticularis idiopathica, in which the mottling is more intense and does not disappear in a warm environment. There is a high incidence of hypertension in the idiopathic form.[34]

Livedo reticularis is usually a benign disorder, but occasionally ulceration and gangrene occur. Some patients note aching, coldness, and soreness that may be disabling. In such cases, lumbar sympathectomy may afford a great deal of symptomatic relief, although it does not eliminate the reticular pattern.

Vinblastine-Bleomycin Toxicity

There have been several reports of a Raynaud-like syndrome in patients receiving combinations of vinblastine and bleomycin for testicular carcinoma.[35,36] In one series, 22 of 60 patients (37%) experienced digital pallor on exposure to cold.[36] Five patients suffered fingertip ulcers, and ten patients had persistent hand cyanosis. The syndrome was more common in cigarette-smokers than non-smokers. Gangrene has not been described, and symptoms generally abate with cessation of therapy. Since vinblastine is neurotoxic, this syndrome may be the result of a drug-induced autonomic neuropathy.

RAYNAUD'S PHENOMENON AND ANGINA

A recent study has revealed a highly significant statistical relationship among Raynaud's phenomenon, migraine, and variant angina pectoris,[37] a syndrome apparently related to coronary artery spasm.[38] Of a group of 62 patients with variant angina, 16 (26%) had migraine and 15 (24%) had Raynaud's phenomenon. These patients were compared to matched groups of noncoronary patients and patients with more classical coronary disease in whom the prevalence of Raynaud's phenomenon was only 3% and 5% respectively.

It is well known that beta-blocking agents, used in the treatment of angina, can precipitate Raynaud's phenomenon. However, these agents cannot account for the findings because almost all the patients with classical coronary disease were receiving beta-blockers, and the onset of migraine and Raynaud's phenomenon preceded by many years the development of variant angina in nearly every case. These results suggest the possibility that migraine,[39] Raynaud's phenomenon,[40] and variant angina share an underlying defect that leads to inappropriate vasospasm.

ERYTHROMELALGIA

Symptomatic intense vasodilatation of the hands and feet is a rare condition called erythromelalgia. Patients complain of a burning sensation in their hands or feet and may be quite uncomfortable. Examination repeatedly reveals very warm and erythematous hands and/or feet. The increased cutaneous blood flow tends to persist even in a cold environment. The idiopathic form of this disorder is not well understood, but is related to decreased vasomotor tone. Treatment is symptomatic and aspirin is usually effective. Erythromelalgia also occurs occasionally in polycythemia vera, where it is probably a function of increased blood volume.

A transient erythromelalgia may develop after a successful arterial bypass graft. With restoration of distal perfusing pressure to an ischemic area comes a dramatic reactive hyperemia. This hyperemia may last for several days, or even a few weeks, while the patient complains of a burning sensation.

REFERENCES

1. Felder D, Russ E, Montgomery H, et al. Relationship in the toe of skin surface temperature to mean blood flow measured with a plethysmograph. *Clin Sci* 13:251, 1954.

2. Lewis J. Observations upon the reactions of the vessels of the human skin to cold. *Heart* 15:177, 1930.

3. Wallin BG, Sundlof G, Delius W. The effect of carotid sinus nerve stimulation on muscle and skin nerve sympathetic activity in man. *Pfluegers Arch* 358:101, 1975.

4. Friedman SA, Freiberg P, Colton J. Vasomotor tone in diabetic neuropathy. *Ann Intern Med* 77:353, 1972.

5. Sharpey-Schafer EP, Taylor PJ. Absent circulatory reflexes in diabetic neuritis. *Lancet* 1:559, 1960.

6. Watkins PJ, MacKay JD. Cardiac denervation in diabetic neuropathy. *Ann Intern Med* 92 (Part 2):304, 1980.

7. Christlieb AR. Renin-angiotensin-aldosterone system in diabetes mellitus. *Diabetes* 5:820, 1976.

8. Schambelan M, Stockigt JR, Biglieri EG. Isolated hypoaldosteronism in adults. A renin-deficiency syndrome. *N Eng J Med* 287:573, 1972.

9. Gorgy AN, Ben David S, Friedman SA. Vasomotor tone in the aged. *Arch Neurol* 29:439, 1973.

9a. Santos AD, Puthenpurakal K, Mathew AH, et al: Orthostatic hypotension: A commonly unrecognized cause of symptoms in mitral valve prolapse. *Am J Med* 71:746–750, 1981.

10. Raynaud M. New researches on the nature and treatment of local asphyxia of the extremities. In Barlow T (trans): *Selected Monographs,* London, The New Sydenham Society, 1888.

11. Blain A, Coller FA, Carver GB. Raynaud's disease: A study of criteria for prognosis. *Surgery* 29:387, 1951.

12. Gifford RW Jr, Hines EA Jr. Raynaud's disease among women and girls. *Circulation* 16:1012, 1957.

13. Adson AW, Brown GE. The treatment of Raynaud's disease by resection of the upper thoracic and lumbar sympathetic ganglia and trunks. *Surg Gynecol Obstet* 48:577, 1929.

14. Kantos HA, Wasserman AJ. Effect of reserpine on Raynaud's phenomenon. *Circulation* 39:259, 1969.

15. Shagan BP, Friedman SA. Raynaud's phenomenon in hypothyroidism. *Angiology* 27:19, 1976.

16. Shagan BP, Friedman SA. Raynaud's phenomenon and thyroid deficiency. *Arch Intern Med* 140:832, 1980.

17. Koehn MA, Schindler WJ, Stanton HG. Thyroid state and vascular reactivity in rats. *Pro Soc Exp Biol Med* 126:861, 1967.

18. Farmer RG, Gifford RW Jr, Hines EA Jr. Prognostic significance of Raynaud's phenomenon and other clinical characteristics of systemic scleroderma: A study of 271 cases. *Circulation* 21:1088, 1960.

19. Medgger JA Jr, Masi AT, Rodnan GP, et al. Survival with systemic sclerosis (scleroderma): A life-table analysis of clinical and demographic factors in 309 patients. *Ann Intern Med* 75:369, 1971.

20. Cannon PJ, Hassar M, Case DB, et al. The relationship of hypertension and renal failure in scleroderma (progressive systemic sclerosis) to structural and functional abnormalities of the renal cortical circulation. *Medicine* (Baltimore) 53:1, 1974.

21. Kovalchik MT, Guggenheim SJ, Silverman MH, et al. The kidney in progressive systemic sclerosis: A progressive study. *Ann Intern Med* 89:881, 1978.

22. Sternberg EM, Van Woert MH, Young SN, et al. Development of a scleroderma-like illness during therapy with L-5-hydroxytryptophan and carbidopa. *N Eng J Med* 303:782, 1980.

23. Lerner AB, Watson CJ. Studies on cryoglobulins I: Unusual purpura associated with the presence of a high concentration of cryoglobulin. *Am J Med Sci* 214:410, 1947.

24. Lerner AB, Barnum CP, Watson CJ. Studies on cryoglobulins II: The spontaneous precipitation of protein from serum at 5°C in various disease states. *Am J Med Sci* 214:416, 1947.

25. Levo Y, Gorevic PD, Kassab HJ, et al. The association between hepatitis B virus and essential mixed cryoglobulinemia. *N Eng J Med* 296:1501, 1977.

26. Mitchell ABS, Pegrum GD, Gill AM. Cold agglutinin disease with Raynaud's phenomenon. *Prog R Soc Med* 67:113, 1974.

27. Vardi DP, Lawrence AM. Suppression of Raynaud's phenomenon by methyldopa. *Arch Intern Med* 124:13, 1969.

28. McFayden IJ, Housley E, MacPherson AIS. Intraarterial reserpine administration in Raynaud's syndrome. *Arch Intern Med* 132:526, 1973.

29. Charles CR, Carmick ES. Skin temperature changes in Raynaud's disease after griseofulvin. *Arch Dermatol* 101:331, 1970.

30. Jacobson AM, Hackett TP, Surman OS, et al. Raynaud's phenomenon: Treatment with hypnotic and operant technique. *JAMA* 225:739, 1973.

31. Frohlich ED, Tarazi RC, Dustan HP. Peripheral arterial insufficiency; A complication of beta-adrenegic blocking therapy. *JAMA* 208:2471, 1969.

32. Pak TJ, Martin GM, Magness JL, et al. Reflex sympathetic dystrophy: Review of 140 cases. *Minn Med* 53:507, 1970.

33. Kazmier FJ, Sheps SG, Bernatz PE, et al. Livedo reticularis and digital infarcts: A syndrome due to cholesterol emboli arising from atheromatous abdominal aortic aneurysms: *Vasc Dis* 3:12, 1966.

34. Barker NW, Hines EA Jr, Craig W McK. Livedo reticularis: A peripheral arteriolar disease. *Am Heart J* 21:592, 1941.

35. Teutsch C, Lipton A, Harvey AH. Raynaud's phenomenon as a side effect of chemotherapy with vinblastine and bleomycin for testicular carcinoma. *Cancer Treat Rep* 61:725, 1977.

36. Vegelzang NJ, Bosl GJ, Johnson K, et al. Raynaud's phenomenon: A common toxicity of vinblastine and bleomycin therapy. *Clin Res* 28:785A, 1980 (Abstract).

37. Miller D, Waters DD, Warnica W, et al. Is variant angina the coronary manifestation of a generalized vasospastic disorder? *N Eng J Med* 304:763, 1981.

38. Meller J, Pichard A, Dack S. Coronary arterial spasm in Prinzmetal's angina: A proved hypothesis. *Am J Cardiol* 37:938, 1976.

39. Edwards J. Cerebral blood flow in migraine. *Headache* 17:148, 1977.

40. Robertson D, Oates JA. Variant angina and Raynaud's phenomenon. *Lancet* 1:452, 1978.

4 Arterial Aneurysms

Sandor A. Friedman

A true aneurysm is a localized dilatation of an artery secondary to weakening and stretching of its wall. Usually, the process of aneurysm formation is actually an exaggeration of the aging process in which smooth muscle and elastic tissue in the medial layer of the vessel are gradually replaced by collagen (arteriosclerosis). Stenoses and sharp bends in the arterial anatomy accelerate this dilatation by creating turbulence and increasing pressure against the wall.

Arterial aneurysms are quite common. Fomon et al,[1] in a review of 7642 consecutive autopsy records, found evidence of 249 aneurysms of the aorta or its major branches (3.3%). In subjects over age 25, the incidence was 4.5%, not including peripheral aneurysms. The abdominal aorta was the most frequent site (77 cases), followed by the ascending aorta (55 cases).

Once established, an aneurysm is subject to a vicious cycle of increasing dilatation. As blood flows through the ectatic segmenr, forward velocity decreases and turbulence increases. This results in thrombus formation and increased wall pressure which, in turn, causes the aneurysm to dilate further. This process may continue until rupture of the aneurysm or the development of serious thromboembolic episodes. Clinical manifestations depend very much on the location and shape of the aneurysm. Saccular aneurysms are subject to greater lateral pressure and, therefore, expand and rupture more quickly than fusiform lesions. Proximal aneurysms are more likely to rupture and less likely to produce embolic episodes than distal aneurysms.

This chapter will review current concepts in the diagnosis and management of the most common true aneurysms. Congenital cerebral aneurysms, which are etiologically and clinically quite distinct from other aneurysms, will not be discussed in this review.

ANEURYSMS OF THE THORACIC AORTA

With the decreasing prevalence of tertiary syphilis, arteriosclerosis has become the major cause of aneurysms in the thoracic aorta. A review from the Mayo Clinic identified arteriosclerosis as the cause of 78 of 107 thoracic aneurysms (73%), and lues in 19%.[2] Luetic aneurysms are almost always located in the ascending aorta. Other causes included closed chest trauma (5%), dilatation distal to aortic valvular stenosis, and Marfan's syndrome. Rare congenital aneurysms are generally located near the ligamentum arteriosum.

Most patients with thoracic aneurysms are asymptomatic, and the diagnosis is often made incidentally from a routine chest roentgenogram. In the Mayo Clinic series, 17% of the patients had pain at the time of diagnosis, but it was quite nonspecific in character, involving either the upper back or chest. When clinical signs and symptoms occur, they vary significantly with the location of the aneurysm.

Lesions of the ascending aorta rarely cause symptoms, but may lead to a number of clinical signs. Careful palpation of the chest with the patient leaning forward and holding his breath in expiration may reveal a pulsation along the upper right sternal border. Percussion may even identify an area of dullness corresponding to the pulsation. Since aneurysms in this area often lead to stretching and dilatation of the aortic valve ring, an early diastolic murmur of aortic regurgitation is often present. In contrast to aortic valvular disease, the aortic closure sound is loud, and the murmur is generally heard best at the aortic area and along the right sternal border. In some cases, a loud aortic second sound may be the only clinical clue to the presence of the aneurysm. When aortic insufficiency occurs, a systolic ejection murmur may be present, and is often louder than the diastolic murmur.

Aneurysms of the transverse aorta may produce signs and symptoms because of their proximity to mediastinal structures. Patients can develop hoarseness due to recurrent laryngeal nerve compression; dyspnea with wheezing or stridor secondary to tracheobronchial compression; dysphagia, anemia, and weight loss because of esophageal involvement; and even superior vena cava syndrome. With the appearance of a mediastinal mass on chest x-ray (Figure 4-1) and any of those syndromes, it is not surprising that these patients are generally first thought to have bronchogenic or esophageal carcinoma. Careful palpation may reveal a pulsation along the upper chest just to the right or left of the sternum. Aneurysms of the descending aorta are the most treacherous because they are almost always silent until they rupture. Even when they occasionally become large enough to erode into a vertebra, pain is often mild or absent.

Not surprisingly, arteriosclerotic thoracic aneurysms are associated with diffuse arteriosclerosis. In the Mayo Clinic series,[2] 11 patients had abdominal aneurysms, and coronary, cerebrovascular, and peripheral arterial diseases were also very common. Chronic arterial hypertension is of major etiologic importance in most of these patients.

The most important diagnostic procedure is the chest roent-

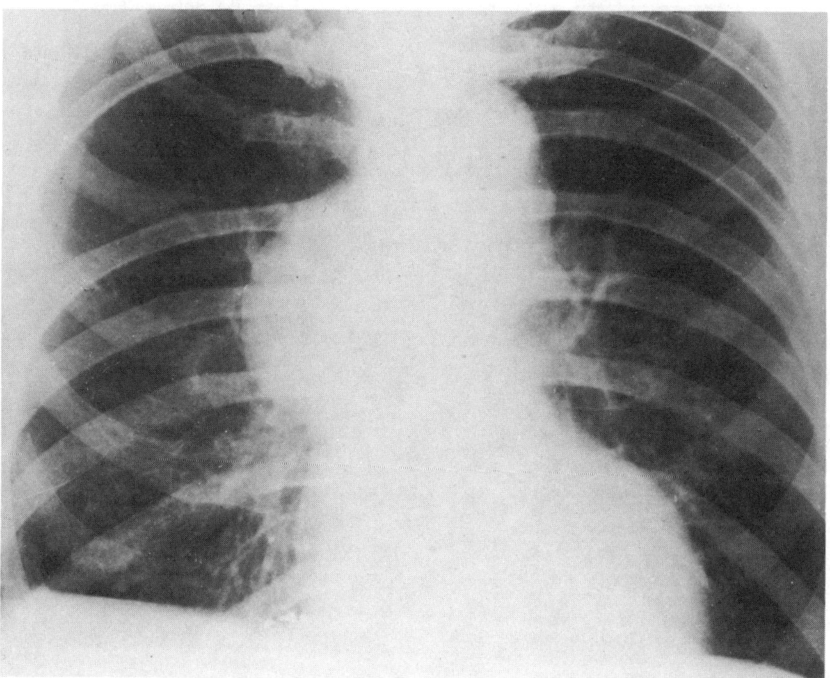

Figure 4-1 Aneurysm of the ascending and transverse portions of the thoracic aorta simulating mediastinal tumor.

genogram taken in several views. With lateral and oblique views, and tomograms, one can often distinguish between a true aneurysm, tortuosity or generalized aortic ectasia, and a mediastinal tumor (Figure 4-2). However, serious mistakes are possible so that further confirmation of the diagnosis is necessary. Fluoroscopy may reveal the expansile nature of the mediastinal shadow, but one must be wary of a transmitted aortic pulse through a nonvascular tumor. Therefore, unless the fluoroscopic findings are unequivocal, it is advisable to confirm the presence of an aneurysm with an angiographic procedure. If surgery is not contemplated, aortography with the intravenous injection of radiopaque material or a radionuclide such as technetium 99 will generally be sufficient for diagnosis. If surgical repair is under consideration, aortic catheterization is required in order to delineate clearly the size and extent of the aneurysm and properly visualize the brachiocephalic arteries. Whenever there is the possibility of an aneurysm, the angiogram should be done first, rather than procedures such as bronchoscopy and esophagoscopy, which might injure a dilated, contiguous aorta.

Decisions concerning therapy are difficult since medical treatment

A

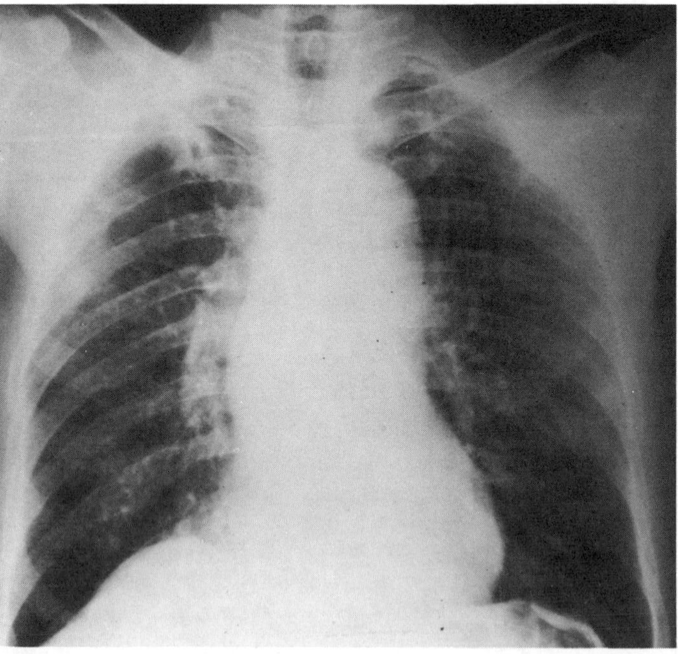

Figure 4-2 **A** Chest roentgenogram shows an enlarged aortic shadow. **B** Lateral view suggests the presence of an aneurysm of the ascending aorta; however, angiographic confirmation is necessary.

is limited. Lues can be treated with penicillin, and hypertension can be controlled, but the vicious cycle of aneurysmal expansion, once started, will continue. Before making a decision for or against surgical repair, one requires adequate knowledge of surgical risks, the natural history of the lesion, and the predicted longevity of the patient. The only modern prospective data concerning patients followed without surgery come from the Mayo Clinic series.[2] Forty-nine of 98 patients (50%) were still alive five years after initial diagnosis as compared to an expected rate of 90% for the normal population of the same age; 30% survived ten years. When the cause of death could be determined, it was found that 32% died of a ruptured aneurysm, and the remainder succumbed to other arteriosclerotic disease. The shape and location of the aneurysm did

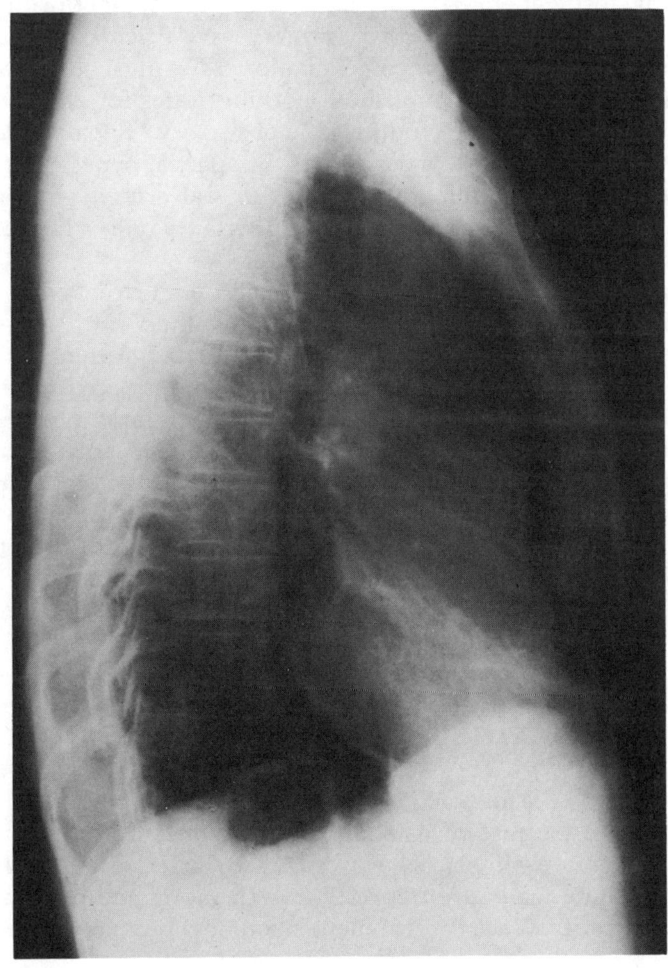

B

not affect the outcome, but mortality was approximately twice as high for patients with symptomatic lesions and those over 6 cm in diameter as for those with smaller lesions. In the autopsy series of Fomon and associates, only one of 84 aneurysms under 5 cm in diameter was ruptured, whereas the rupture rate was 15% for those lesions between 5 cm and 10 cm. Forty-three percent of those over 10 cm were ruptured.

Surgical handling of the aorta and techniques for extracorporeal perfusion have improved, but replacement of the thoracic aorta with a prosthetic graft is still associated with a high mortality rate even in the most experienced centers. In resection of the ascending or transverse aorta, adequate circulation must be maintained through both carotid arteries, at least one vertebral artery, and arteries supplying the lower portion of the body (especially the kidneys and spinal cord). Repair of ascending aortic aneurysms often requires replacement of the aortic valve. In the transverse aorta, surgery is particularly hazardous because the origins of the brachiocephalic vessels must be inserted into the prosthesis. Recently published mortality rates for elective resection vary from 14% to 20% for this kind of surgery.[3] Repair of descending aortic aneurysms is less dangerous, but partial bypass (left atrium to femoral artery, or femoral vein to femoral artery, with a pump oxygenator) is still necessary. A surgical mortality rate of 11% has been reported for repair of these aneurysms.[4]

On the basis of these data, it remains prudent to treat patients with small aneurysms conservatively and follow them with serial chest x-rays at 3- to 6-month intervals. On the other hand, patients with large lesions and/or clinical symptoms should be considered for surgical repair if their general medical condition is good. Early intervention is particularly appropriate for expanding aneurysms and large aneurysms in the descending aorta. It is important to remember, however, that patients with coronary artery and cerebrovascular disease may not tolerate major vascular surgery with its attendant blood loss, hypotension, and manipulation of the extracranial cerebral arteries. The decision for or against surgical repair must take all risk factors into account and be made on an individual basis.

ANEURYSMS OF THE ABDOMINAL AORTA

Aneurysms are most common in the terminal portion of the abdominal aorta because of its sharp bifurcation into the iliac arteries. These lesions are almost always caused by arteriosclerosis and frequently include the entire bifurcation of the aorta and proximal common iliac arteries. Since the turbulent blood flow produced by the sharp angulation extends over a relatively long segment, abdominal aortic aneurysms are more often fusiform than saccular.

The abdominal aortic aneurysm is not adequately emphasized in medical teaching and preventive medicine programs. It is clearly a clinical time bomb, and yet there is relatively little emphasis placed on its detection in contrast to many other cardiovascular disorders of less importance or reversibility. Palpation of the aortic pulsation may be the most neglected item in the art of physical examination. In one study of 100 consecutive patients referred for surgical repair of abdominal aneurysms, 19 lesions had been discovered fortuitously during a radiologic examination performed for other reasons.[5] In each case, the aneurysm was easily palpable. Ninety-eight percent of these aneurysms are entirely below the level of the renal arteries and thus readily amenable to surgical repair. Two retrospective studies have suggested that approximately one of every 250 people over the age of 50 succumbs from rupture of an abdominal aneurysm.[6]

Unfortunately, these aneurysms rarely cause symptoms until they are near or at the point of rupture. Approximately 10% of patients with unruptured aneurysms may sense vague chronic or intermittent pounding or abdominal palpitation, but abdominal or back pain almost always means rupture or impending rupture. When pain occurs, it is usually quite nonspecific and may vary considerably in location. Although it is usually in the upper abdomen or lower back and of a steady, sharp, or gnawing quality, it may also occur in the lower abdomen and even is occasionally colicky.

In the great majority of cases, the diagnosis can be made or strongly suspected through physical examination. Careful palpation of the abdominal aorta is one of the most important maneuvers in the routine health screening of healthy middle-aged people, especially those with a history of hypertension or other arteriosclerotic disease. The pulsation of the normal abdominal aorta is readily appreciated in the epigastric area in all but obese individuals. One must gain experience with this pulsation in order to appreciate when it is abnormal. An aneurysm is usually a pulsatile mass, which feels like a globular, hard tumor with an expansile quality. There is often lateral as well as anterior pulsation. With increasing tortuosity and uncoiling of the aorta, the aneurysm may shift to a position quite far from the epigastrium, particularly to the left upper quadrant and occasionally the right upper quadrant.

It is frequently difficult to distinguish clinically between generalized ectasia and tortuosity of the abdominal aorta and true aneurysm. One may find a wide pulsation without a mass. In thin individuals, a strong anterior pulsation in the epigastrium may be a normal finding. With aging and uncoiling, this pulsation may move laterally but still not represent an aneurysm. On the other hand, a wide pulsation in a heavier patient may represent an aneurysm. In fact, palpation of an abdominal pulse must raise the suspicion of an aneurysm in an obese individual. As a general rule, one should not be able to feel a normal aortic pulsation below the umbilicus except in very thin individuals.

About two thirds of abdominal aneurysms are associated with sufficient calcification of the medial layer to be detected on abdominal roentgenograms. The aneurysm may be seen as a curvilinear calcification on an anteroposterior view of the abdomen and on a lateral view as calcification just in front of the lumbar spine. A lateral x-ray taken with bone technique is quite useful because one can often see calcification of both anterior and posterior walls and thus obtain a reasonable estimate of the size, shape, and location of the aneurysm. Until recently, this film was the best noninvasive laboratory test for detecting and confirming the presence of an abdominal aortic aneurysm.

The advent of abdominal sonography has made the diagnosis of these aneurysms simple, safe, and extremely accurate. Ultrasound delineates the anatomy of the abdominal aorta in great detail (Figures 4-3, 4-4). With a series of transverse and longitudinal views, the sonographer can locate an aneurysm, distinguish it from generalized ectasia, and very carefully estimate its width, depth, and length. The sonogram also detects clot within the lumen of the aneurysm.

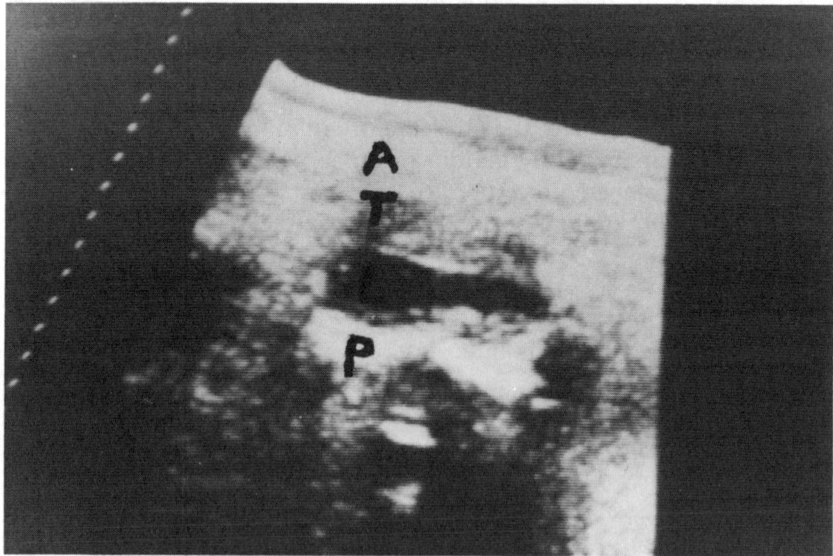

Figure 4-3 Sonogram shows thrombus in an abdominal aneurysm. An aortogram would underestimate the size of this aneurysm. (A = anterior wall, T = thrombus, L = lumen, P = posterior wall)

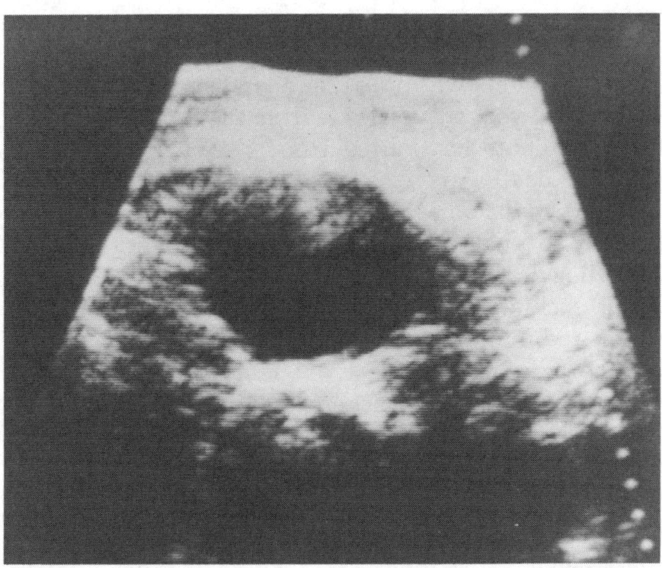

Figure 4-4 Sonogram shows thrombus protruding from the anterior wall of an abdominal aortic aneurysm.

Ultrasonography has relegated aortography to a minor role in the evaluation of patients with suspected abdominal aneuryms. In fact, aortography is far inferior to ultrasound as a diagnostic tool. Because of the frequent presence of a mural thrombosis, which may sometimes form a thick layer along the walls of the aneurysm, an aortogram may grossly underestimate the size of an aneurysm and even miss it completely (Figure 4-3). Often the aortographic diagnosis is made on the basis of an asymmetric narrowing of the aortic lumen secondary to thrombosis, rather than dilatation of its wall. The major role of aortography is in the visualization of the peripheral circulation beyond the aorta. If extensive peripheral arterial disease is present clinically, it may be important to see the distal run-off in order to choose properly the site of distal anastomosis of the graft used in surgical repair. Some surgeons prefer to have a preoperative aortogram in every case because they are concerned about the patency of the mesenteric circulation. Since the inferior mesenteric artery is generally sacrificed at surgery, major stenoses in the celiac axis and superior mesenteric arteries might result in postoperative intestinal ischemia. In most cases, however, this is a moot point because the inferior mesenteric artery is usually occluded before surgery. Serious gastrointestinal problems are rare after surgery for aneurysm.

Patients with abdominal aneurysms often have generalized cardiovascular disease. In one series, 47% had definite coronary artery disease; 43%, peripheral arterial obstruction; 8%, cerebrovascular disease; and 34%, hypertension.[5] Nevertheless, the findings in long-term studies of patients with this lesion lend support to an aggressive approach. The five-year survival rate from the time of initial diagnosis for untreated patients has varied from 17.2% to 36.4%.[7] Approximately half the deaths are caused by aneurysmal rupture. Several groups have shown that aneurysmectomy prolongs life. DeBakey et al[8] reported a 72% survival rate three years after surgery, and 58% after five years. Szilagyi and co-workers[1] compared treated and untreated patients after excluding those with advanced age, hypertension, and heart disease, and found a doubling of life expectancy in the operated group. The mortality rate for elective aneurysmectomy has gradually decreased. DeBakey and co-workers[8] had a 9% operative mortality rate in 1964. In 1966, a 4% rate was reported in a group of patients, 88% of whom had other cardiovascular disease.[5]

Close attention must be paid to blood pressure and urine output during and after surgery. Continuous electrocardiographic monitoring is advisable because arrhythmias and silent myocardial infarctions are common in patients with coronary heart disease. In particular, one must watch for signs of acute arterial occlusion in the lower extremities. Embolism from the aneurysmal sac or an atheromatous plaque can occur during aortic manipulation, and an embolectomy may be necessary on occasion.

Although it is generally agreed that most patients with significant aneurysms, even those with stable occlusive arterial disease, should undergo elective repair, there are some whom it is still wise to exclude. Surgery on lesions above the renal arteries is quite hazardous. Patients with severe angina, congestive heart failure, or frequent episodes of cerebral ischemia are poor candidates because of a higher surgical mortality rate and a relatively high probability of dying of coronary or cerebrovascular disease before aneurysmal rupture can occur. Some patients with unstable angina may be candidates for aneurysm repair after successful coronary artery surgery. Aneurysms under 5 cm in diameter rarely rupture before expanding further and are best left untouched if the patient has other significant cardiovascular disease. On the other hand, tender aneurysms of any size and those associated with unexplained abdominal or back pain should be repaired as soon as possible.

Ruptured Aneurysm

Rupture of an abdominal aortic aneurysm is most often fatal, but some patients may be salvaged with prompt and competent care. An early retroperitoneal leak may be temporarily tamponaded by clotted blood, but free rupture into the peritoneal cavity is rapidly fatal. The patient may develop back or abdominal pain with or without hypotension several hours before hemorrhage into the peritoneal cavity occurs. The sudden development of low-back or abdominal pain in a patient with a palpable aneurysm is an indication for immediate laparotomy. In an obese patient over the age of 60, the constellation of severe unexplained pain and shock should suggest the strong possibility of a ruptured aneurysm even if none is palpable. If there is no electrocardiographic evidence of an acute myocardial infarction, immediate surgical exploration may be warranted.

As long as the patient's systolic blood pressure remains above 60 to 70 mm Hg, it is probably inadvisable to replace blood volume rapidly until the aorta has been clamped above the site of perforation because a higher perfusion pressure may cause dislodgement of the tamponading thrombus. After aortic clamping, prompt restoration of effective blood volume is essential, using Swan-Ganz monitoring of the pulmonary artery and pulmonary wedge pressure as a guide. Mannitol may be given intravenously to induce diuresis and protect against renal failure. Arterial pH must be determined, and metabolic acidosis should be corrected with sodium bicarbonate. The postoperative course may be quite turbulent. Because of increased permeability in the inflamed mesenteric and peritoneal tissues, large amounts of fluid may be sequestered retroperitoneally during the first 24 to 36 hours. Abrupt declines in circulating blood volume produce shock and oliguria. Blood pressure, wedge pressure, and urine output should be monitored continuously as fluids are rapidly replaced. The appearance of acute renal failure may require dialysis (preferably hemodialysis) for several days. After the first 48 hours, the sequestered fluid begins to be reabsorbed, and the patient may develop congestive heart failure and sudden pulmonary edema if there is underlying heart disease. For this reason, prophylactic administration of digitalis soon after surgery is often advisable. Adequate oxygenation is important at all times. The patient may require intermittent use of a respirator during the first few days because the large abdominal incision, the orthopneic position, and the presence of acute respiratory distress syndrome may impair pulmonary function. If the patient survives the first five days with good cardiopulmonary and renal function, he is likely to recover, provided that wound dehiscence or retroperitoneal infection does not complicate the cardiovascular problems.

Other Complications

Several other complications of abdominal aortic aneurysms merit discussion although they are relatively infrequent. Because of the large amount of mural thrombus in the aneurysmal sac, peripheral embolization can occur and result in acute femoropopliteal arterial occlusion or small infarcts in the feet. It is possible that silent emboli contribute to the high prevalence of femoropopliteal occlusive disease in these patients. A bleeding diathesis secondary to consumption coagulopathy has also been reported in association with abdominal aortic and occasionally other aneurysms.[9] Any patient with laboratory evidence of disseminated intravascular coagulation, in the absence of sepsis or neoplasm, should be investigated for an occult aneurysm. Bacterial infection is a rare complication of arteriosclerotic aneurysms, most commonly aneurysms of the abdominal aorta. In one necropsy series, 6 of 178 arteriosclerotic aortic aneurysms were infected.[10] Salmonella has been the most frequent organism (35% of cases), followed by Staphylococcus (12%). Patients generally present with fever of unknown origin or prolonged, intractable sepsis. Rupture has occurred in 79%. Early surgical intervention, after institution of adequate antibiotic therapy, is necessary.

ANEURYSMS OF THE EXTREMITIES

Popliteal Aneurysms

Because of its unique anatomic location, the popliteal artery is the second most common site of arteriosclerotic aneurysm formation. Compression of the vessel by surrounding muscle as it leaves Hunter's canal in the lower thigh and more distally by the arcuate popliteal ligament, leads to slight poststenotic dilatation. This effect makes the vessel prone to aneurysmal dilatation as its media weakens and stiffens with age. Since the artery is stretched tautly across the popliteal fossa, it is also subject to lifelong trauma from extension and flexion of the knee joint. People in occupations that require a great deal of bending, such as house painters, may have an increased risk of developing popliteal aneurysms. Patients with popliteal aneurysms often have multiple lesions. In a study of 152 patients with popliteal aneurysms, 59% were found to have bilateral popliteal involvement, 35% had abdominal aortic aneurysms, and 29% had femoral artery aneurysms.[11]

The diagnosis of this lesion requires careful palpation of the popliteal pulse behind the knee. A patent aneurysm is usually recognized easily as an expansile tumor, but it is sometimes difficult to distinguish between generalized arterial dilatation and a local aneurysm, especially when all of the patient's pulses are prominent. A thrombosed aneurysm may be confused with a popliteal cyst. Sonography accurately distinguishes an aneurysm from other lesions and demonstrates the intraluminal thrombus.[12] Often, plain x-rays of the knee outline the calcified walls of the aneurysm.

Complications of popliteal aneurysm include thromboembolism, rupture, and compression. Rupture occurs in less than 10% of patent lesions and almost never when they are occluded. Compression of the popliteal vein may lead to edema, venous thrombosis, and pulmonary embolism. Occasional pressure on the posterior tibial nerve leads to pain and paresthesias along the calf and heel.

Thromboembolism is the most frequent complication. Gradual thrombosis of the lumen may cause intermittent claudication and progressive distal ischemia, while rapid occlusion may lead to rest pain and gangrene. Showers of emboli into the tibial and digital arteries are also quite common. The possible presence of popliteal aneurysm is the first diagnostic consideration in a patient with one or more focal areas of gangrene on a foot. In two series, evidence of thromboembolism was found in approximately two thirds of the patients at the time of initial diagnosis of popliteal aneurysm.[13,14]

A popliteal aneurysm is a treacherous lesion. Of 70 cases managed conservatively, Gifford and co-workers[15] reported thromboembolism in 11 patients, venous compression in 5 and rupture in 4 during a mean observation of 44 months. Eighteen limbs were eventually amputated, and 5 (11%) of the 45 patients with previously uncomplicated aneurysms had amputations. Wychulis et al[11] reported complications in 29% and amputation in 3% of patients with initially asymptomatic aneurysms.

Surgical excision with replacement by a graft is recommended for all but the most debilitated patients. Arteriography should be performed first to outline the distal arterial run-off. There were only two operative deaths in 107 cases from three surgical series. Crichlow and Roberts[13] reported patency of distal vessels in 77% and adequate blood flow in 81% of patients after a mean postoperative period of 4.8 years. Wychulis et al[11] reported excellent surgical results in patients with asymptomatic aneurysms, but an 11% amputation rate in 64 patients who underwent surgery after suffering serious thromboembolism. Patients with already occluded aneurysms should be treated like others with peripheral arterial disease.

Femoral Aneurysms

Femoral aneurysms behave similarly to popliteal aneurysms. Thromboembolism occurred in 23 of 89 patients in one series, and 7 of 44 treated conservatively required limb amputation.[16] Surgical repair is advisable for all patent lesions.

Subclavian Aneurysms

Chronic compression from a thoracic outlet syndrome is the most common cause of aneurysmal dilatation of the subclavian artery.[17] This aneurysm is generally small and rupture is rare, but it may be gradually occluded or shower emboli into the hand. One should think first of this lesion in any patient with upper extremity claudication or digital artery occlusion. Surgery must be directed at the aneurysm and the compressing structure in the thoracic outlet. Significant arteriosclerotic subclavian aneurysms are rare.

CAROTID ARTERY ANEURYSMS

Aneurysmal dilatation of the extracranial portion of the common and internal carotid arteries is quite unusual. One surgical group reported finding only three cases of carotid artery aneurysm during a 10-year period in which 300 aneurysms of the major arteries were identified.[18] Of major diagnostic importance is the differentiation of a true aneurysm from the rather common kinking or looping of the extracranial carotid arteries. The latter, of no clinical significance, was seen in 80% of 114 carotid angiograms performed on patients between 60 and 80 years of age. This kinking is particularly common in the region of the lower part of the sternocleidomastoid muscle on the right side of the neck. In contrast, carotid aneurysms almost always occur higher in the neck at the bifurcation of the common carotid artery. In difficult cases, the distinction can usually be made noninvasively with sonography.

When an aneurysm is present, physical examination usually reveals a fusiform pulsatile swelling in the upper neck. A bruit is frequently heard. Transient ischemic attacks secondary to thromboembolism are very common (perhaps 50% of cases). Surgical repair after angiographic confirmation of the diagnosis is usually recommended.

VISCERAL ANEURYSMS

The splenic artery is the site of the most common visceral aneurysm, followed by the renal arteries (about 1% of all aneurysms) (Table 4-1). Both of these lesions are usually found incidentally on abdominal x-rays as round calcifications. Splenic aneurysms usually result from idiopathic medial degeneration. They are the only aneurysms with a predilection for females and are most likely to occur as a complication of portal hypertension.[19] Rupture rate is high,

Table 4-1
Peripheral Aneurysms

Location	Usual Etiology	Age and Sex Distribution	Usual Mode of Presentation	Complications	Indications for Surgery
Popliteal and femoral	Arteriosclerosis	Mostly males over 60	Pulsatile mass Thromboembolism	Thromboembolism Venous compression Local expansion Rupture occasionally	Patent lesion Severe peripheral ischemia
Subclavian	Thoracic outlet syndrome	No prelidilection	Pulsatile mass Thromboembolism	Thromboembolism	Patent lesion Severe claudication
Splenic	Idiopathic medial degeneration	Mostly females, any age (mean in 50s)	Curvinlinear calcification in left upper quadrant Rarely palpable	Rupture in less than 10%	All lesions (excision with splenectomy)
Renal	Idiopathic	No sex predilection, mean age in 50s	Round calcification on x-ray Hypertension	Rupture (more likely in uncalcified lesions and during pregnancy) Hypertension (probably due to renal thromboembolism) Renal infarction	Uncalcified lesions and large calcified lesions Women in child-bearing age Renal infarction
Carotid	Arteriosclerosis	Usually over age 60	Pulsatile mass under the angle of the jaw	Strokes Transient ischemic attack	All lesions

especially during pregnancy, and surgical excision with splenectomy is always advisable. Overall, rupture can be expected in about 7% to 9% of patients followed conservatively. Pneumococcal vaccine should be administered postoperatively.

Renal aneurysms are more likely to rupture in pregnant women and when they are uncalcified.[20] They may also lead to renal infarction and renovascular hypertension. They are sometimes discovered during angiograms performed in the evaluation of hypertensive patients (Table 4-1).

Aneurysms of the superior mesenteric artery are quite rare and are almost always mycotic in origin. The usual source of infection is bacterial endocarditis. Rupture rate is exceedingly high, and immediate surgical repair is indicated even in the presence of active infection.

SUMMARY

Arterial aneurysms are extremely dangerous because they often have catastrophic consequences with few, if any, premonitory symptoms. Careful attention to arterial pulsations during routine physical examination is vital if these lesions are to be recognized early and repaired. In particular, the abdominal aortic aneurysm remains a significant public health challenge. With careful abdominal palpation and prudent use of sonography, it should be possible to decrease its toll.

REFERENCES

1. Fomon JJ, Kurzweg FT, Broadway RK. Aneurysms of the aorta: A Review. *Ann Surg* 165:557, 1967.

2. Joyce JW, Fairbairn JF II, Kincaid OW, et al. Aneurysms of the thoracic aorta. *Circulation* 29:176, 1964.

3. Crawford ES, Saleh SA, Scheussler JS. Treatment of aneurysm of transverse aortic arch. *J Thorac Cardiovasc Surg* 78:383, 1979.

4. Dillon ML, Young WG, Sealy WC. Aneurysms of the descending thoracic aorta. *Ann Thorac Surg* 3:430, 1967.

5. Friedman SA, Hufnagel CA, Conrad PW, et al. Abdominal aortic aneurysms: Clinical status and results of surgery in 100 consecutive cases. *JAMA* 200:1147, 1967.

6. Moore HD. Diagnosis of rupture of abdominal aortic aneurysms. *Lancet* 2:184, 1967.

7. Bernstein EF, Fisher JC, Varco RL. Is excision the optimum treatment for all abdominal aortic aneurysms? *Surgery* 61:83, 1967.

8. DeBakey ME, Crawford ES, Cooley DA, et al. Aneurysm of abdominal aorta: Analysis of results of graft replacement therapy 1 to 11 years after operation. *Ann Surg* 160:622, 1964.

9. Saltani B, Savrin R, Evans WE. Consumption coagulopathy associated with arterial aneurysms. *J Cardiovasc Surg* 273, 1979.

10. Sommerville RL, Allen EV, Edwards JE. Bland and infected arteriosclerotic abdominal aortic aneurysms. *Medicine* 38:207, 1959.

11. Wychulis AR, Spittell JA, Wallace RB. Popliteal aneurysms. *Surgery* 68:942, 1970.

12. Neiman JL, Yalo JST, Silver TM. Gray-scale ultrasound diagnosis of peripheral arterial aneurysms. *Radiology* 130:413, 1979.

13. Crichlow RW, Roberts B. Treatment of popliteal aneurysms by restoration of continuity: Review of 48 cases. *Ann Surg* 163:417, 1966.

14. Edmunds LH Jr, Darling RC, Linton RR. Surgical management of popliteal aneurysms. *Circulation* 32:517, 1965.

15. Gifford RW Jr, Hines EA Jr, Janes JM. An analysis and follow-up study of 100 popliteal aneurysms. *Surgery* 33:284, 1953.

16. Pappas G, Janes JM, Bernatz PE, et al. Femoral aneurysms: Review of surgical management. *JAMA* 190:489, 1964.

17. Dorazio RA, Ezzet F. Arterial complications of the thoracic outlet syndrome. *Am J Surg* 138:246, 1979.

18. Carrascal L, Marshiah A, Charlesworth D. Aneurysms of the extracranial carotid arteries. *Br J Surg* 65:590, 1978.

19. Stanley JC, Thompson NW, Fry WJ. Splanchnic artery aneurysms. *Arch Surg* 101:689, 1970.

20. Hageman JH, Smith RF, Szilagyi DE, et al. Aneurysms of the renal artery: Problems of prognosis and surgical management. *Surgery* 84:563, 1978.

5 Dissecting Hematoma

Sandor A. Friedman

Dissection of blood into the medial layer of an artery is a serious process which often ends in catastrophe. Long after it was originally recognized, dissection was considered a rare event for which no therapy was available. In the past 15 years, we have learned a great deal more about its prevalence, pathogenesis, prognosis, and treatment. The outlook for patients with dissecting hematoma has improved considerably and, even more importantly, we have learned how to prevent most cases.

Dissection is a diagnosis that is often missed because it is generally not even considered in the list of possibilities. Too often, it is discovered only at the necropsy table because symptoms and signs associated with it were ascribed to more common cardiovascular events. If one is to recognize a dissecting hematoma sufficiently early to save the patient, one must pay close attention to clinical details and retain a high index of suspicion whenever there are features atypical for other cardiovascular diseases. Once dissection is thought of, the diagnosis must be pursued vigorously. An aggressive diagnostic approach is justified because of the extremely dim prognosis for most untreated patients with dissections.

This chapter deals with the pathogenesis, diagnosis, and treatment of dissecting hematoma. An attempt is made to describe some of the pitfalls in diagnosis and explore dilemmas concerning therapy.

DEFINITION OF DISSECTING HEMATOMA

A dissecting hematoma is an intramural arterial hemorrhage that is propagated through the medial layer for a variable distance. It must be clearly distinguished from true and false aneurysm. The latter is an artery whose entire thickness has been perforated by a hematoma and is sealed temporarily. The greatest confusion occurs between dissection and true aneurysm. This error is more than semantic because it encourages misconceptions about the pathogenesis and treatment of both these conditions. The unfortunate term, dissecting aneurysm, has contributed significantly to this misunderstanding. A dissection is not a true aneurysm because it is not a general stretching and dilatation of the wall of the artery. At necropsy, it may have the gross appearance of an aneurysm only because of the distending effect of a large volume of blood in the medial layer. The clinical courses of these two conditions share little in common, and they must be considered separately.

Another misunderstanding is the false linkage of dissection with atherosclerosis. The two processes are entirely unrelated pathologically, and the presence of atheromas does not predispose an artery to dissection. The confusion has arisen because of the ubiquitous nature of atherosclerosis and the statistical fact that a dissecting hematoma is found with increased frequency in patients with coronary heart disease and other complications of atherosclerosis. This co-association occurs primarily because atherosclerosis and dissection share a very important risk factor—hypertension. In the former, hypertension is probably a secondary risk factor, playing a major role because of its synergism with other factors such as hyperlipidemia and diabetes mellitus. In the case of dissecting hematoma, on the other hand, hypertension has a primary role in pathogenesis.

PATHOGENESIS

The pathology of dissection is the same no matter what the cause. The medial layer of the artery becomes necrotic, and loss of smooth muscle and connective tissue leaves cystic spaces—hence the term cystic medial necrosis.[1] Once this occurs, the intimal lining of the vessel is left with no support and an intimal tear develops, allowing blood to flood into the cystic spaces of the media. It is the cystic nature of the pathology that allows the hematoma to remain within the arterial wall rather than to perforate immediately through the adventitia. The hematoma forms a false channel and can propagate in a number of different ways:

1. It can extend distally along the artery,
2. It can extend into some or all branches of the artery,
3. It can re-enter the artery through a second intimal tear,
4. It can stop propagating and clot after a short distance, or
5. It can perforate through the adventitia at any point.

Cystic medial necrosis is a lesion limited almost entirely to the thoracic aorta. There are only scattered case reports of peripheral dissections in renal,[2] carotid,[3] and mesenteric arteries. Even in some of the case reports of peripheral artery dissection, it is not entirely clear that the thoracic aorta was completely free of necrosis and hematoma.

The explanation for the location of dissection has to do with the important role of the proximal aortic wall in circulatory dynamics. The media of the thoracic aorta bears the major brunt of the propelling force of the left ventricle during each systole. Under normal conditions, delicate elastic tissue in this layer stretches during systole, absorbing and storing potential energy from the left ventricular thrust. During diastole, when left ventricular force is withdrawn, the aorta snaps back, creating a diastolic pressure. If the aorta lacked compliance, the force of the left ventricle would be spent totally in systole. The normal aorta acts much like a rubber band when force is applied to it, rather than a solid lead pipe. Not only does this resilient motion conserve energy, but it also protects the aortic wall from chronic trauma. By stretching with each systolic thrust, the aortic wall moves away from the force applied to it so that the actual pressure applied to the media is minimized. This action follows the engineering concept that a compliant, flexible object can often withstand a greater applied stress than rigid material even if the latter has greater tensile strength.

With aging, elastic tissue and supporting smooth muscle within the media of the aortic wall gradually atrophy and are replaced by collagen, which has less compliance. This change results in increasing stiffness and weakness of the aortic wall, which can no longer stretch efficiently. The media of the aorta is now subject to greater dynamic pressure during systole, accelerating the process of atrophy within that layer. This vicious cycle of gradual attrition may continue without clinical consequences for many years. In some patients, the process is reflected by changes in blood pressure. Less of the ventricular force is stored in systole so that systolic pressure rises, diastolic pressure may fall slightly, and pulse pressure increases significantly in many patients with advancing age.

In some patients, the media eventually fails to withstand the propelling force of the left ventricle, and cystic medial necrosis occurs. Obviously, the aortic wall is more likely to succumb to this complication if left ventricular force is great. The rate of rise of pressure against the aortic wall varies inversely with cardiac output, and thus congestive heart failure may actually protect against dissection of the thoracic aorta.

ETIOLOGIC FACTORS

Dissection of the aorta is found much more than it was in the past, and is certainly not a rare disorder. The liberal use of aortography has contributed to increased case finding by revealing evidence of dissection when it was not suspected, and providing a means of objectively verifying clinical impressions. There are very few epidemiologic studies of its incidence, but in one study of consecutive autopsies, dissecting hematoma of the aorta was found in one out of every 500 cases. Aortic dissection can occur at any age, but its peak incidence is in the sixth and seventh decades.

Hypertension

Hypertension is, by far, the most important risk factor.[4] The great majority of patients over age 45 (at least 75%) are hypertensive, and most have had long-standing hypertension prior to the event. They frequently have other stigmata of end-organ involvement such as hypertensive retinopathy and cardiomegaly. However, there is a spectrum of patients ranging from those with mild or no hypertension to those with marked hypertension and severe end-organ involvement. Patients with aortic dissection frequently have diabetes mellitus and atherosclerotic heart disease. These last two problems have no etiologic relationship to dissection per se, but merely reflect their high prevalence in patients with hypertension. It is possible that some of the normotensive patients with dissection were hypertensive at one time, but became normotensive as a result of a previous myocardial infarction.

The mechanism by which hypertension produces aortic dissection is still conjectural. There are at least two possible factors, and both may play a role in pathogenesis. First, the distending pressure against the aortic wall is increased. This, in turn, causes more stretching of the aortic wall and may eventually stress the resiliency of the elastic fibers to the breaking point just as a rubber band may snap when it is pulled too tautly. The increased pressure also accelerates the aging process of atrophy of muscle and elastic tissue. The end result is a stiffer aorta bombarded constantly by a higher pressure.

It is possible that hypertension interferes with nutrition of the aortic media. Vasa vasorum within the aortic wall may become tortuous, arteriosclerotic, and narrowed under the strain of an increased blood pressure. This would be analogous to hypertensive changes in arterioles throughout the body as seen in renal and skin biopsies and by direct visualization of the fundi.

Whatever the exact mechanism, prevention of dissection depends to a large extent on the detection and proper treatment of systemic hypertension. The treatment regimen must be carefully planned if it is to be successful. In fact, an injudicious drug regimen can actually be detrimental. The goal is to decrease the impact of blood against the aortic wall as measured not only by total pressure but also by the rate of rise of pressure during ventricular systole (dp/dt). The latter is determined by the ejection rate of the left ventricle. Thus, lowering cardiac output is beneficial, while raising it may predispose to dissection.

If one employs antihypertensive agents whose mechanism is direct vasodilatation of arterioles, cardiac output increases. Thus, drugs such as hydralazine may increase the chances of dissection, particularly if blood pressure is not well controlled. Beta blockers, on the other hand, are ideal agents for preventing dissection because they decrease the ejection rate of the left ventricle. Even if pressure is not perfectly controlled, the patient is afforded some protection. If a chest x-ray already shows a tortuous, uncoiled aorta, it may be particularly important to employ beta blockers and avoid direct vasodilating agents. We also believe that patients who are only partially compliant and who may be lost to follow-up are best treated in this way. There seems to be very little doubt that the overwhelming majority of cases of aortic dissection are presentable with strict and appropriate control of blood pressure.

CONNECTIVE TISSUE DISORDERS

The true connective diseases comprise a group of disorders in which many patients suffer dissections because the basic connective tissue of the aortic media is not sound. These patients experience dissections earlier in life than the hypertensive group. When there are defects in elastic tissue and smooth muscle, the aorta is not sufficiently distensible and lacks the tensile strength to withstand normal left ventricular forces.

Included in this category are Marfan's, Ellis-van Creveld, and

Ehlers-Danlos syndromes. By far the most common of these disorders is Marfan's syndrome. The classical patient with this syndrome is tall and thin with striking arachnodactyly and a high-arched palate. These features are not always present, but when they are, they may not be prominent. Many patients are of normal height and slender, with perhaps slightly long fingers, but they certainly do not appear to have an unusual body habitus.[5] Subluxation of one or both lenses is a frequent occurrence in Marfan's syndrome, and is often the first clinical clue. Spontaneous and incisional hernias, wound dehiscence after surgery and a tendency to joint dislocation and ligamental tears are also examples of poor connective tissue development in this disorder.

The thoracic aorta is subject to both true aneurysmal formation and dissection in Marfan's syndrome. When dissection occurs, it is usually more severe than in the hypertensive type. Multiple intimal tears and areas of medial necrosis may occur at the same time. Isolated stretching of the valve ring and degeneration of the valve leaflets may lead to severe aortic regurgitation and/or mitral insufficiency. Aortic insufficiency may also occur as a result of aortic ring dilatation in the course of dissection or aneurysm formation. Since dissection is a leading cause of death in Marfan's syndrome, it may be advisable to recommend lifetime therapy with beta blockers as a preventive measure.

With typical body habitus and/or lens subluxation, Marfan's syndrome is quite easy to recognize. When the body habitus is not classical, measurements of hydroxyproline excretion in the urine may be helpful. Since hydroxyproline is a major constituent of collagen, and collagen catabolism is increased, many of these patients have increased renal excretion of this amino acid.[6] The diagnosis of Marfan's syndrome should be strongly considered for any normotensive patient with aortic dissection, especially for those under the age of 40.

The Ehlers-Danlos syndrome can also produce true aneurysm and/or dissection of the thoracic aorta. Characteristics of this disorder are hyperextensibility of skin and joints, and frequent joint subluxations. These people are truly "double-jointed." Hydroxyproline levels may be elevated in this disorder also.

Homocystinemia

A third and rare cause of aortic dissection is homocystinemia, an inherited error of metabolism characterized by high blood levels of homocystine. Patients tend to have premature atherosclerosis and, in some cases, aortic dissection. They may be mentally retarded and share with patients with Marfan's syndrome the propensity for lens dislocation. However, unlike Marfan's syndrome, patients with homocystinemia tend to be short and squat.

Experiments in baboons have demonstrated increased platelet turnover and atherosclerotic-like lesions secondary to homocystine infusion. These changes can be prevented by simultaneous administration of dipyridamole.[7] Whether dipyridamole would protect against aortic dissection in patients with homocystinemia is not known.

Aortic Coarctation

Coarctation of the aorta is another cause of aortic dissection relatively early in life. In this congenital disorder, there is not only hypertension but also a slow transmission of systolic pressure beyond the thoracic aorta because of the obstruction to flow. This combination subjects the thoracic aorta not only to elevated pressure but also to a more continuous impact of left ventricular force.

Pregnancy

Aortic dissection is a rare complication of pregnancy.[8] The etiology is not known, but it is possible that sudden changes in intrathoracic pressure may play a role.

Idiopathic

Finally, it is important to recognize that aortic dissection occasionally occurs without a history of cardiovascular disease, hypertension, or connective tissue defects. One must never rule out the diagnosis of dissection because of the absence of obvious etiologic factors. For inexplicable reasons, the aortic media weakens and degenerates in some patients under the normal stresses of left ventricular function. Perhaps, they have occult connective tissue disorders that we are not yet able to diagnose, but this is purely speculative.

SYMPTOMS AND SIGNS

Because of the nature of the pathology, the symptoms of aortic dissection may be myriad. The findings depend partially on the location of the initial medial necrosis. The two "weak" areas of the aortic wall seem to be the portions just distal to the aortic valve and just distal to the left subclavian artery; thus, the intimal tear generally occurs in one of these two spots. Dissections beginning near the aortic valve are called proximal dissections, and those distal to the left subclavian artery, distal dissections.

In many series, proximal dissections have been reported more frequently than the distal type, but this is probably artifactual. Proximal lesions tend to produce more dramatic findings than distal ones, and are more easily diagnosed. Recent experience with aortography suggests that distal dissections may be quite subtle in their presentation and often missed. It seems quite probable that distal dissection is more common than proximal involvement.

The classic textbook description of excruciating chest and back pain radiating to the abdomen and extremities and accompanied by loss of several major pulses occurs in only a minority of aortic dissections. The dissecting hematoma is an unpredictable lesion affecting patients in many different ways. The clinical spectrum ranges from the symptomless patient to the patient in cardiogenic shock and coma. Pain occurs in the majority of patients, but a significant proportion (perhaps as high as 50%) may have no pain.[9]

Distal Dissection

Distal dissection usually presents with back pain. A knife-like midback pain without skeletal tenderness, particularly in a hypertensive individual, must alert the clinician to the possibility of this lesion. More often, however, the pain is not excruciating and may be of a pressing or nonspecific quality. It may be similar to the pain of myocardial ischemia, which sometimes localizes in the midback. Since many patients with distal dissection also have coronary artery disease, the pain of dissection is often mistakenly ascribed to coronary insufficiency or subendocardial infarction. Back pain may be the only symptom in a significant number of patients, even those with extensive distal dissection. If the pain disappears spontaneously within a few hours, the patient may not pay serious attention to it.

On occasion, pain may be in the lower back and, perhaps, gradually radiate up the back and even into the chest. Patients with low back pain often believe that they have muscle strain, especially if they have recently performed heavy lifting. It is the lifting, by suddenly increasing intrathoracic pressure, that may have been the precipitating event that led to the intimal tear. Unless one can demonstrate definite signs of musculoskeletal disease such as muscle tenderness, spasm, or neurological signs in the lower extremities, dissection must remain in the initial differential diagnostic list.

The other major symptoms of distal dissection are related to regional ischemia. As the hematoma extends distally, it may branch off into any major branch of the aorta. This may be symmetric or asymmetric. It may skip the celiac artery, but extend into the superior mesenteric or one of the renal arteries. It may also extend into one or both common iliac arteries. If the false channel obliterates the true lumen of the vessel, acute ischemia may develop. Thus, dissection must always be considered in the differential diagnosis of acute proximal artery occlusion.

It is obvious, then, that a variety of syndromes may herald the onset of aortic dissection. The patient may have abdominal pain, ileus and gastrointestinal bleeding secondary to mesenteric infarction, flank pain and hematuria secondary to renal infarction, signs of transverse myelitis due to spinal cord ischemia, or signs of acute aortoiliac obstruction. The first thought is often acute arterial embolism, and not infrequently the diagnosis of dissection is made only at exploratory abdominal surgery or after a Fogarty catheter fails to produce clot from an iliac artery. One should particularly think of dissection when more than one area of ischemia occurs within a period of a few days.

Another clue is spontaneous disappearance of ischemic symptoms or return of peripheral pulses. Although this can certainly occur with arterial embolism, it is more likely with dissection. This phenomenon may occur for several reasons:

1) A second, intimal tear may develop, allowing blood to reenter the vessel and provide distal perfusion. Thus, flow is from aortic lumen to false channel to lumen of the branch artery. In fact, this false channel may be even wider than the original lumen of the vessel. In many cases, this mechanism prevents ischemia from developing in the first place. For example, it is not rare to find, on aortography, an asymptomatic renal artery occlusion with the kidney perfused via a functioning false channel.
2) Distal disbursement of the hematoma may relieve luminal compression.
3) Retraction of clotted hematoma in the false channel may relieve compression. Because of the loss of supporting structure, progressive and rapid dilatation of the aortic wall may occur, producing a large saccular aneurysm. This complication is most likely to occur within the first six months and is associated with a very high rupture rate.
4) The most catastrophic complication of a distal dissection is arterial rupture. This can happen anywhere along the course of the false channel. Most often the rupture is near or at the site of the initial tear, producing a mediastinal hematoma or a left hemothorax. However, a retroperitoneal or intraperitoneal hemorrhage can also occur, simulating rupture of an abdominal aortic aneurysm.

Proximal Dissections

Proximal dissections are more likely to produce the widespread chest and back pain often described in classic descriptions. Substernal pain often simulates the pain of myocardial infarction. However, even here pain may be very mild and nonspecific or absent. Just as in distal dissection, the lesion may be recognized only by its cardiovascular consequences. In general, patients with proximal dissections are more likely to have serious complications, and the mortality rate is significantly higher than with distal lesions.

In addition to the complications already mentioned, proximal dissections cause a number of other problems. First, they may extend into the extracranial arteries and cause cerebral ischemia. All of the syndromes of carotid and subclavian artery disease may be found. Patients may present with acute cerebrovascular accidents or symptoms of basilar artery insufficiency. Both innominate and subclavian steal syndromes, indistinguishable from arteriosclerotic occlusive disease, may occur. In each one of these syndromes, of course, one or more proximal pulses are absent. If a patient develops hemiparesis, the contralateral carotid pulse should be missing or weak. In the case of a left hemiplegia, the innominate artery is involved, so that one would expect weak or absent right carotid and subclavian pulses and a diminished blood pressure in the right arm. With re-entry phenomena, cerebral symptoms may come and go, suggesting multiple transient ischemic attacks. Although there are often other clinical signs, a neurologic syndrome is often the first manifestation of proximal dissection.

A difference in blood pressure between the two arms is a frequent presenting sign of proximal dissection. In the absence of a prior history of peripheral arterial disease, dissection must be suspected whenever a patient with evidence of proximal arterial obstruction complains of chest pain. A subclavian or innominate artery obstruction may be easily missed unless the blood pressure is routinely taken in both arms.

Another important complication of proximal dissection is aortic valve involvement. Since the initial medial necrosis begins just distal to the valve, it may involve the valve ring, damage the supporting structure, and cause dilatation. The resulting aortic regurgitation may be very mild and asymptomatic and cause only a barely audible murmur, but it may also be devastating and produce acute left ventricular failure. Aortic regurgitation in this situation is usually clinically distinguishable from the regurgitation of primary valvular disease. In the first place, there is no evidence of aortic stenosis in cases of dissection. There may be a loud systolic ejection murmur because of increased flow across the valve in systole, but upstroke of major pulses is normal unless they have been cut off by the dissection. Second, valvular disease is usually associated with a muffled or absent aortic closure sound, while dissection tends to lead to an increase in this sound. However, in the late stages, the valvular apparatus may be so distorted that the leaflets do not move well, and then the aortic closure sound will begin to diminish. Third, valvular aortic incompetence is usually best heard along the left sternal border, while the aortic regurgitation of dissection is usually best heard along the right sternal border and at the aortic area.

If congestive heart failure develops, the signs are quite different from those of chronic aortic insufficiency. There is usually a very sharp drop in cardiac output. Wide pulse pressure is generally not seen, and the patient may actually develop cardiogenic shock. Intractable pulmonary edema and death may ensue very rapidly. This situation represents a true surgical emergency since medical treatment of the heart failure is usually of no avail.

Rupture of proximal dissections is quite common and almost always fatal. Hemorrhage is usually into the pericardial or left pleural cavity. Thus, one must immediately think of dissection as a diagnostic possibility whenever a patient develops cardiac tamponade. In a few cases, emergency surgery following relief of tamponade by pericardiocentesis has been life-saving. An unexplained left hemothorax should also prompt an urgent evaluation of the thoracic aorta.

Shock may dominate the clinical picture in either proximal or distal dissections, but is more common with proximal lesions even in the absence of pericardial tamponade. As mentioned above, acute aortic insufficiency can lower blood pressure. In addition, there may be hemorrhagic shock secondary to perforation anywhere along the arterial tree. Finally, a massive hematoma in the proximal aorta can compromise flow through the aorta. A clinical picture simulating shock can occur if blood flow is diminished to both femoral and subclavian arteries.

DIAGNOSIS OF DISSECTION

From the foregoing discussion, it is clear that dissection may mimic many other disorders, and one requires a high index of suspicion in many situations if one is not to miss this diagnosis. Perhaps the best way to approach the diagnosis of dissection is to list some of the clinical constellations that should suggest this diagnosis:

- The triad of chest pain, hypertension, and a murmur of aortic regurgitation.
- Chest pain and a missing femoral pulse, or a difference in blood pressure between extremities.

- Multiple areas of acute ischemia such as renal infarction and iliac artery occlusion.
- Unexplained back pain in a hypertensive individual.
- Cerebrovascular accident with a missing carotid pulse on the left side, or a missing carotid and subclavian pulse on the right side.
- Symptoms compatible with transient ischemic attacks.
- Acute onset of congestive heart failure and auscultatory evidence of aortic regurgitation.
- Acute arterial occlusion with spontaneous restoration of pulses.
- Chest pain and unilateral jugular vein distention (due to compression).
- Syndrome of acute ischemia in the abdomen without signs of low cardiac output or obvious source for arterial embolism.
- Acute onset of limb ischemia and loss of femoral or subclavian pulse without obvious source for arterial embolism.
- Syndrome of low cardiac output with low blood pressure, tachycardia, and peripheral vasoconstriction.
- Left hemothorax and hypotension.
- Sudden pericardial tamponade.
- Chest or back pain, hypertension, and a normal electrocardiogram.
- Chest pain and ptosis due to Horner's syndrome (caused by compression of the cervical sympathetic fibers).
- Chest pain, hypertension, and sudden hoarseness (caused by compression of the recurrent laryngeal nerve).
- Severe and sudden knife-like pain in the chest in the absence of a myocardial infarction or pneumothorax.

LABORATORY TESTS

Chest X-ray

Once dissection has been considered, it is essential to move judiciously toward making a definite diagnosis. The most important noninvasive test is a good posterior-anterior roentgenogram of the chest taken with the x-ray machine six feet from the patient. One looks for a prominent aortic shadow. If the aortic shadow is slender and free of uncoiling or tortuosity, it is highly unlikely that a dissection has occurred. However, even a slightly prominent aortic shadow in a properly taken x-ray is consistent with the diagnosis of dissection. In many cases of dissection, the aortic shadow is very prominent with marked tortuosity and a definite bulging of the ascending or descending segment or both, but the degree of aortic shadow abnormality is not well correlated with the severity of the dissection, especially when it is induced by hypertension. Most of the tortuosity seen on the roentgenogram represents merely arteriosclerotic stiffening, uncoiling, and ectasia secondary to aging and accelerated by long-standing hypertension. The actual false channel, except in the case of very large dissections, contributes only slightly to the total width of the aortic shadow.

Of course, the finding of an abnormal aortic shadow is very nonspecific, only supporting the diagnostic possibility of dissection in the appropriate clinical setting. Sometimes, a close look at the prominent shadow may suggest the appearance of a false channel. There may be a thin radiolucent line running through the aortic shadow near its lateral border. The area lateral to this line often corresponds to the false channel as seen by aortography. In other cases an area of calcification may be seen inside the aortic shadow. If the calcification is within the lateral or medial wall of the aorta, it indicates the presence of two lumens. However, this latter sign may be misleading because the calcification may be in the anterior or posterior wall, in which case it has no significance. A lateral view of the chest may confirm the position of the calcification and may also show a linear radiolucency suggestive of two lumens.

Electrocardiogram

Another useful test is the electrocardiogram, since the distinction between myocardial infarction and aortic dissection is often the major clinical problem. Theoretically, a proximal dissection may extend into one of the major coronary arteries and cause a myocardial infarction. As an isolated event, however, this is exceedingly rare. When dissection does affect a coronary artery, it is quite likely to affect other vessels as well, and also the aortic valve, making the diagnosis quite obvious. Thus, electrocardiographic evidence of an acute myocardial infarction in a patient whose only symptom is back or chest pain virtually rules out the presence of aortic dissection. On the other hand, nonspecific ST and T wave changes in the electrocardiogram are consistent with either diagnosis. In doubtful cases, serial electrocardiograms and serum enzyme studies are often useful. If acute infarction is ruled out and the pain is different from any that the patient has experienced in the past, aortic dissection becomes the most likely diagnosis.

Echocardiogram

Recent advances in M-mode echocardiography have made it a very useful tool in diagnosing proximal dissection.[10,11] In the echocardiogram of a normal aortic root, the anterior and posterior walls are seen as parallel dominant echoes, which move anteriorly in systole and posteriorly in diastole. The aortic valve echoes are seen within these two parallel echoes, separating in systole and coming together in diastole (Figure 5-1).

With dissection of the aortic wall, the layers of the aortic wall appear duplicated. Two dominant echoes separated by a space can be seen in the anterior and/or posterior wall rather than a single echo (Figure 5-2). These echoes remain parallel during all motions of the aorta. The space, representing the false lumen, may be silent or filled with soft, diffuse echoes if the hematoma has clotted.

There may also be other echocardiographic abnormalities, including fluttering of the anterior mitral leaflet secondary to aortic regurgitation. Widening of the aortic root suggests that the regurgita-

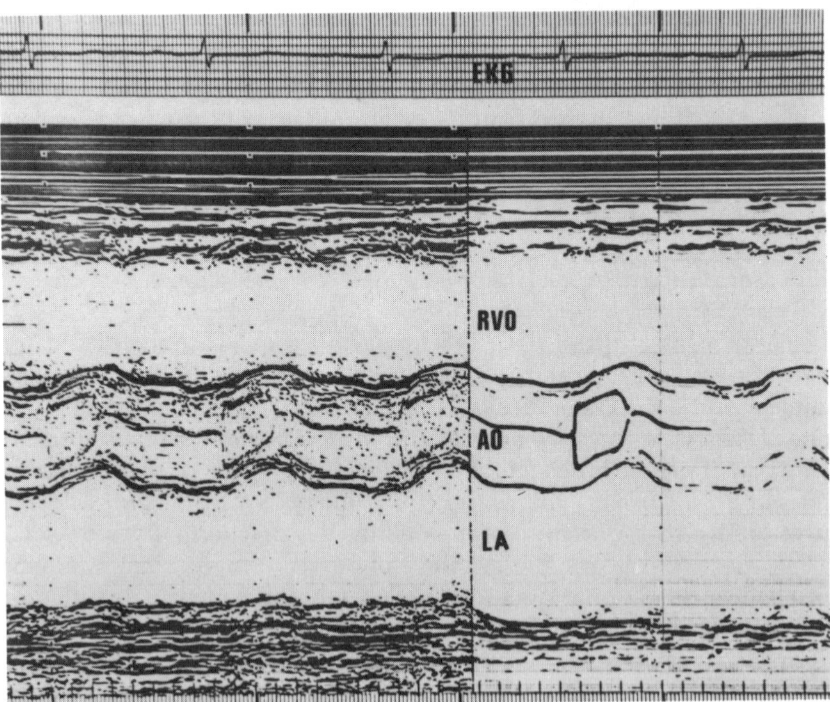

Figure 5-1 Echocardiogram of a normal aortic root. Note the aortic valve between two dominant parallel echoes.

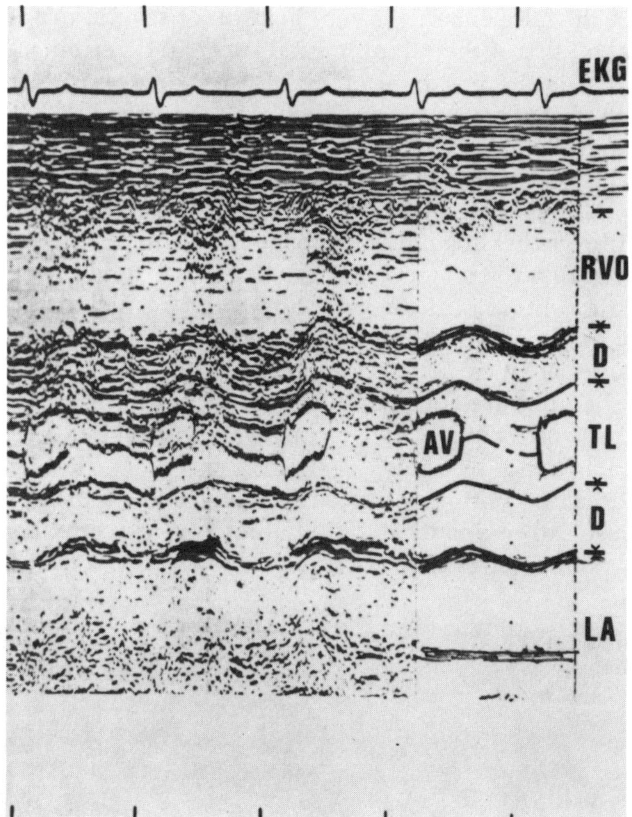

Figure 5-2 Echocardiogram of a patient with proximal aortic dissection. There is reduplication of the anterior and posterior walls of the aortic root.

tion is due to aortic ring dilatation, and early closure of the mitral valve indicates an acute process. If rupture has occurred, a hemopericardium may be seen. Although all these signs are helpful, proximal dissection can occur with a normal one-dimensional echocardiogram.

Aortography

The most definitive test for dissection is aortography. It is usually performed percutaneously by a retrograde route after the catheter has been inserted into a femoral artery and threaded into the ascending thoracic aorta. Diagnosis of dissection depends on demonstrating eccentric narrowing of the aorta, a false channel, or both. If only the former is seen, one cannot be sure where the dissection begins, only where the false channel is widest.

Finding the false channel is very helpful for several reasons. First, it localizes the site of the initial intimal tear and determines whether the dissection is the proximal or distal type (Figure 5-3). Second, it gives one an idea of acuteness and prognosis. Radiopaque dye running freely through the false channel suggests an actively dissecting lesion whose final prognosis is still quite uncertain. On the other hand, a false channel without dye indicates that the hematoma has clotted and suggests that fibrotic healing may have begun. This implies an improving prognosis because the dissection is less likely to extend further or lead to immediate rupture of the aorta. Third, with a small dissection, the aorta may not be narrowed. The diagnosis may depend on the demonstration of an extremely thin false channel which can be easily missed, if the films are not examined under a bright light. In fact, aortography may occasionally fail to uncover a dissection because the false channel cannot be seen.

In performing aortography for the diagnosis of dissection, one must exercise extreme caution. If the catheter is inadvertently inserted into the false channel and dye is then injected under pressure, the aorta

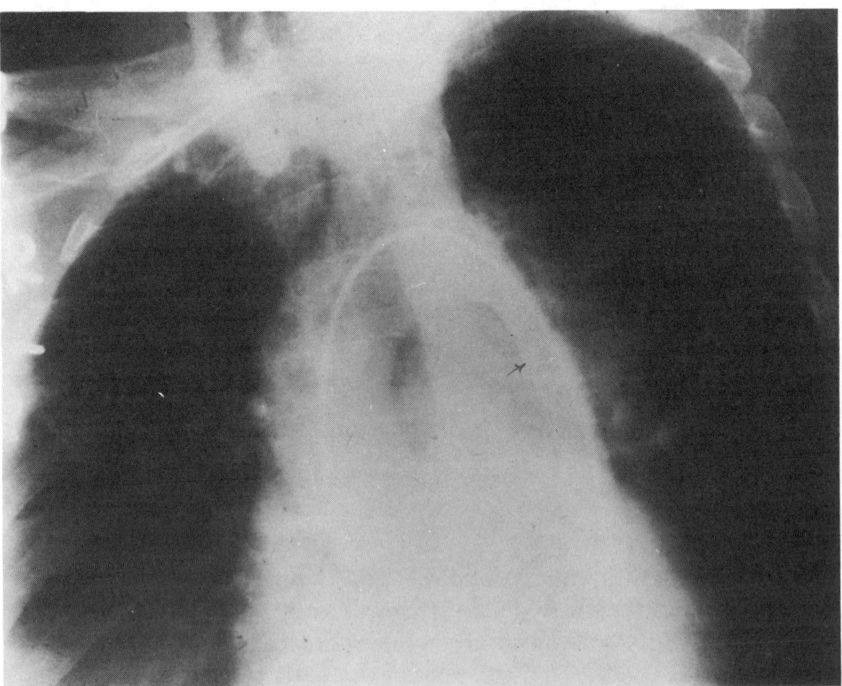

Figure 5-3 An aortogram demonstrates a wide false channel beginning distal to the left subclavian artery and compressing the aortic lumen. Some contrast material has extravasated into the false channel.

can quite easily be perforated. The catheter must be advanced slowly and withdrawn if resistance is encountered. The first injection should be by hand in order to establish that the catheter is not in the false lumen.

When should aortography be performed? In most of the situations described above, aortography should be performed immediately if the aortic shadow is abnormal on the chest roentgenogram. It is important to be sure of the diagnosis as soon as possible in order to institute vigorous therapy. Furthermore, if surgery is contemplated, it is necessary to determine whether the dissection is proximal or distal since the operative approach to these two lesions is quite different. If the patient presents only with chest or back pain and the main consideration is differentiation from acute myocardial infarction, one may institute medical therapy and allow 24 to 36 hours to rule out infarction.

TREATMENT OF DISSECTION

At one time, clinically diagnosed dissection was associated with a mortality rate of more than 50% within the first few weeks and 90% within one year. This gloomy outlook has been altered, partially by advances in medical and surgical therapy and partially because of better diagnostic methods. It is now known that cases uncovered several decades ago were really just the "tip of an iceberg," representing the more obvious and serious dissections. We now diagnose many milder cases, and we do not know what their natural prognosis would be since they are all treated. Since well-controlled studies of the treatment of dissections have not been performed, the exact efficacy of therapy is not known. It is apparent, however, that therapy has made a significant difference.

Immediate Therapy

The emergency treatment of dissection in the hypertensive patient calls for rapid lowering of the blood pressure to the normal range and simultaneously decreasing cardiac contractility.[12,13] The ideal method is to use a drug with rapid onset of action in an intravenous drip and to titrate the dose on a minute-by-minute basis. A ganglionic blocking agent is the best choice in this situation because it causes smooth and quickly reversible vasodilatation and, at the same time, blocks beta adrenergic cardiac reflexes so that the heart cannot increase its output.

Although nitroprusside has been advocated by some investigators, it is an inadvisable choice. As a direct vasodilator, which does not block the autonomic nervous system, it leads to an increase in cardiac contractility and dp/dt against the aortic wall. Blood pressure monitoring must be continuous. Urine output, neurologic status of the patient, and the electrocardiogram must also be watched closely. There is a small incidence of acute renal failure and cerebral and coronary ischemia with this therapy.

Since tachyphylaxis to ganglionic blocking agents often develops within 24 to 36 hours, it is important to begin oral antihypertensive medication at the outset and gradually increase the doses until the ganglionic blocker can be withdrawn. The oral drug of choice is a beta blocker such as propranolol, which is usually started in conjunction with a diuretic agent. If blood pressure is not completely controlled with reasonable doses of these agents, a third drug is added. We generally use methyldopa or clonidine.

In the case of distal dissections, many authorities believe that patients can be treated indefinitely with antihypertensive therapy as long as no complications occur. Blood pressure must be kept completely normal; the systolic pressure should not go over 140 mm Hg. We generally treat the patient similarly to one with an acute myocardial infarction, keeping him at bedrest for the first ten days and gradually increasing his activities during the first three months. Chest x-rays are obtained every month for the first four months and then three times a year.

Surgery

Surgical repair of a distal dissection becomes necessary if complications of dissection or hypotensive therapy develop. These include:

1) Acute renal failure,
2) Severe orthostatic hypotension,
3) Cerebral ischemia,
4) Development of a saccular true aneurysm in the area of original dissection, or
5) Extension of the dissection asymptomatically as shown by x-ray or clinically by cut-off of a regional circulation.

There are some authorities who believe that patients with distal dissections should have surgical repair after stabilization for a few months with antihypertensive therapy. In one surgical series, operative mortality was 22% and actuarial five-year survival was

57%.[14] A 52% survival rate at 3½ years has been reported with medical therapy alone.[12]

Patients with proximal dissections do not do as well with antihypertensive therapy, and the general consensus is that reparative surgery is indicated even in uncomplicated cases after a suitable period of medical therapy. If the patient presents with heart failure and severe aortic regurgitation, shock, or serious regional ischemia, immediate surgery is indicated. Surgical technique has improved in recent years, but is still difficult, often involving an aortic graft and replacement of the aortic valve, as well as obliteration of the false lumen. In one recent series, mortality rate was 34% for surgery performed within 14 days of the acute event and 14% when it was deferred beyond 14 days.[14]

Any aortic dissection in a normotensive individual is a much more serious matter than a comparable lesion in a hypertensive patient. Therapy with beta-blocking agents may still be helpful by decreasing cardiac contractility, but therapeutic options are much more limited. Early surgical intervention is usually indicated. The patients with connective tissue disorders often have multiple tears, and surgical mortality is very high.

REFERENCES

1. Erdheim J. Medionecrosis aortae idiopathica cystica. *Virchows Arch [Path Anat]* 276:187, 1930.
2. Bakir AA, Patel SK, Schwartz MM, et al. Isolated dissecting aneurysm of the renal artery. *Am Heart J* 96:92, 1978.
3. McNeill DH, Dreisbach J, Marsden RJ. Spontaneous dissection of the internal carotid artery. Its conservative management with heparin sodium. *Arch Neurol* 37:54, 1980.
4. Wheat MW Jr, Palmer RF, Bartley ID, et al. Treatment of dissecting aneurysms of the aorta without surgery. *J Thorac Cardiovasc Surg* 50:364, 1965.
5. Barrett JS, Helwig J Jr, Kay CF, et al. Cine-aortographic evaluation of aortic insufficiency. Unsuspected idiopathic aneurysmal dilatation of the aortic root as a possible indication of the Marfan syndrome. *Ann Intern Med* 61:1071, 1964.
6. Sjoerdsma A, Davidson JD, Udenfriend S, et al. Increased excretion of hydroxyproline in Marfan's syndrome. *Lancet* 2:994, 1958.
7. Harker LA, Slichter SJ, Scott R, et al. Homocystinemia vascular injury and arterial thrombosis. *N Eng J Med* 291:537, 1974.
8. Schnitker MA, Bayer CA. Dissecting aneurysm in young individuals, particularly in association with pregnancy with report of a case. *Ann Intern Med* 20:486, 1944.
9. Hirst AE, Johns VJ Jr, Kime SW Jr. Dissecting aneurysm of the aorta: Review of 505 cases. *Medicine* 37:217, 1958.
10. Moothart RW, Spangler RD, Blount SG Jr. Echocardiography in aortic root dissection and dilatation. *Am J Cardiol* 36:11, 1975.

11. Nanda NC, Gramiak R, Shah PM. Diagnosis of aortic root dissection by echocardiography. *Circulation* 48:506, 1973.

12. McFarland J, Willerson JT, Dinsmore RF, et al. The medical treatment of dissecting aortic aneurysms. *N Eng J Med* 286:115, 1972.

13. Palmer RF, Wheat MW Jr. Treatment of dissecting aneurysms of the aorta. *Ann Thorac Surg* 4:38, 1967.

14. Miller DC, Stinson EB, Oyer PE, et al. Operative treatment of aortic dissections. Experience with 125 patients over a sixteen-year period. *J Thorac Cardiovasc Surg* 78:365, 1979.

6 Venous Thrombosis

Marvin L. Sachs

The incidence of venous thrombosis and pulmonary embolism is a problem of impressive magnitude. Estimates are subject to the vagaries of varying diagnostic criteria and patient selection, but the heavy weight of the burden is not in dispute.[1] In the United States, the incidence of venous thrombosis is counted in millions of cases a year. Estimates of the overall prevalence of venous disease of all kinds range from 2% to 60% of the population in Western countries. Although extremes might be discounted, the prevalence of troublesome chronic venous disease of the lower extremities may be about 6% of people over 40,[2] many of whom have postphlebitic syndromes. Each year hundreds of thousands of people in the United States suffer pulmonary embolism, and the mortality is high.[3]

Patients confronted with the possibility that they may have a clot can be expected to be anxious. Some are thoroughly panicked, even if they are not physically sick. This reaction may derive from a previous illness involving a thrombotic process, but more often it comes from vague knowledge of the dangers of clots, or from stories heard about relatives, friends, or strangers who became ill or died because of clots. Heart attacks, strokes, and amputations may be blamed as readily on clots as phlebitis or embolism. Even contusions with hematomas, especially when they occur on the lower extremities, may be called clots and generate as much long-term fear and confusion as episodes of serious illness involving thrombi. When a patient is seen early in the course of any illness or injury in which a clot is suggested, however unlikely its presence may be, the physician faces a diagnostic and management problem of considerable difficulty. Recently, there have been advances in objective methods of assessing venous thrombosis that free the doctor from an excessive dependence on guesswork and allow a reasonably solid basis for advising aggressive therapy or presenting firm reassurance. For pulmonary embolism, diagnostic advances have been impressive also, but we are still dependent on difficult techniques of objective assessment.

VENOUS THROMBOSIS

Definitions Formally speaking, *phlebitis* means inflammation of a vein, *phlebothrombosis* means thrombosis of a vein, as does *venous thrombosis,* and *thrombophlebitis* means thrombosis and inflammation of a vein. The separate concepts of the pathology may have little clinical relevance, for inflammation of the wall of a vein can lead to thrombosis, and clot in a vein can lead to vein-wall inflammation. Because of this, and because a) deep venous thrombosis can occur with few if any symptoms or signs; and b) the classic symptoms and signs of inflammation are not diagnostically discriminating when thrombophlebitis is suspected; it becomes impractical and probably misleading to use the terms italicized above as separate diagnostic categories. In this chapter they will be used interchangeably. Distinctions also can be made between *clot* and *thrombus,* but they will not be observed here.

PATHOGENESIS AND PREDISPOSING FACTORS

In the middle of the nineteenth century, Virchow presented three major factors as the basis of intravascular thrombosis: vessel-wall injury or change, stasis of blood, and abnormal tendency for the blood to coagulate. This triad has held up well in modern concepts of pathogenesis.[1,4,5]

On the venous side of the circulatory system, vessel-wall injury often is the result of direct trauma, as in contusions or fractures. Vein walls may be damaged by infections in soft tissues traversed by the veins. Intravenous infusions of irritating substances can cause a chemical injury to the endothelium, and damage can occur from prolonged use of intravenous catheters. Noninfectious inflammation can occur, as in the migratory phlebitis of thromboangiitis obliterans.

Stasis of blood in veins as a concept of pathogenesis is extremely helpful, even though it is likely that slow blood flow alone is not a sufficient cause of intravascular coagulation. The association of stasis with inactivity or immobilization—as during an episode of illness, during or following surgery, while heavily drugged or unconscious, or when a cast is applied—ties in with other factors that might combine with sluggish venous blood flow to generate clotting.

Characteristics of the circulation and the blood itself contribute to stasis. The circulatory components concern pressure-flow relationships. Impediments to venous return to the heart, which affect the velocity of venous blood flow either generally or locally, can be as diverse as congestive heart failure, shock, old venous thrombosis with residual partial obstruction, or external compression of a vein (caused by a malignant tumor, a popliteal cyst, or a tight panty girdle). Sluggish venous return through the lower extremities can also be due to prolonged standing or sitting, venous valvular incompetence, and neuromuscular, skeletal or joint abnormalities that reduce the vigor of the muscle pump of the legs. Abnormalities of the blood that impair flow concern viscosity and include conditions such as polycythemia, sickling, sludging, dysproteinemia, and hyperlipemia.

The question of hypercoagulability of the blood is complex, controversial, and beyond the scope of this chapter. The literature contains good reviews of the current knowledge of thrombosis, coagulation, thrombolysis and fibrinolysis.[6,7] These concepts are dealt with in a later chapter.

Venous thrombosis differs from arterial thrombosis in several ways. The vessel wall is more likely to be free of disease or damage in veins than in arteries. Stasis alone is unlikely to cause a clot in veins; but in an artery in which an occlusion develops, thrombus usually forms in the segment distal to the occlusion, where there is no flow, at least to a point where collateral flow enters the vessel. Venous clots are likely to form where flow is sluggish, as in calf-muscle venous sinusoids or in valve-cusp pockets. Arterial thrombi are found in high-flow systems, but some form in eddies which exist beyond atherosclerotic lesions. Platelets tend to be more important in arterial thrombi, and venous thrombi usually have a larger fibrin component. Although their relative importance varies, initiating factors are the same: vessel wall damage, platelet adhesion, aggregation and activation, and activation of coagulation factors. Whether platelets or fibrin deposits accumulate first may depend on whether the endothelium is damaged or normal. The fate of early deposits depends on the stability of platelet aggregates and the activity of fibrinolytic mechanisms.

Table 6-1 lists a variety of factors known, or thought to be, predisposing to venous thrombosis. It is a heterogeneous collection, but most fit into the Virchow concept of pathogenesis. One of the most pervasive factors, which characterizes patients who are sick, old, injured, or have had an operation, is lack of physical activity.

A risk factor deserving special consideration is a history of previous thrombophlebitis or pulmonary embolism. A history documented with satisfactory proof implies, on the average, significant predisposition, but careful probing of the details of past episodes may allow reasonable separation of high-risk from low-risk histories. Three examples will illustrate this.

First, consider a patient who had several prior episodes of unequivocally established thrombophlebitis without specifically identified precipitating causes. This history would justify one to believe that this patient is predisposed to have still another episode of phlebitis. In the absence of other known risk factors, the past history of phlebitis forms the only basis of accepting the predisposition. The patient, however, may have an unknown coagulation abnormality, which is the real reason for the predisposition. This could mean that the episodes of phlebitis have no independent standing as a risk factor, but, by reflecting the hematologic abnormality, they have predictive power.

Now take another example: A healthy young patient, who acciden-

Table 6-1
Factors Known to Predispose to Venous Thrombosis

- Bedrest, inactivity, immobilization, paralysis, casts
- Injuries, fractures, surgery
- Older age
- Cardiac failure, myocardial infarction, stroke, shock
- Malignant disease
- Pregnancy, puerperium
- Estrogens, oral contraceptives
- Infection
- Obesity
- Varicose veins
- Tobacco
- Stress, physical and psychological
- Antithrombin-III deficiency
- Hyperaggregable platelets
- Polycythemia vera
- Cryofibrinogenemia
- Previous venous thrombosis or pulmonary embolism

tally fractures several vertebrae, is confined to a bed in a hospital where studies of the incidence of venous thrombosis are underway by the use of the tagged-fibrinogen technique. He develops a positive scan localized to the calf and is promptly treated with anticoagulants. Eventually, he makes a complete recovery with no residual venous damage, returning to an active life, as healthy as he was before the accident. The hospital record shows a diagnosis of thrombophlebitis, appropriately enough, which justifies the anticoagulation. Is this history, correct with respect to the diagnosis of phlebitis, to be used as evidence of the patient's predisposition to another episode? Would the risk of a subsequent episode of venous thrombosis be higher if the first episode, while he was immobilized with the fractures, had not been detected early but had progressed to extensive iliofemoral thrombophlebitis that left a severe postphlebitic syndrome? In that case, is it the vein damage and the venous insufficiency that might form a basis for predisposition to recurrence, rather than the venous thrombosis itself?

A third example rounds out the argument that a *history of phlebitis* must be more closely examined before assuming it indicates an above-average likelihood of developing deep venous thrombosis. A patient presents with pain and tenderness of a calf and has a history of six similar episodes, the first following a contusion and sprain, with a diagnosis each time of phlebitis and with hospitalization for anticoagulation therapy. A review of his records of the prior episodes shows that the diagnoses were not supported by any objective tests, and the symptoms and signs recorded were not specific for phlebitis. Is this *documented* history of phlebitis really significant with respect to a future episode of thrombophlebitis, or is it predictive only of recurrence of symptoms that might or might not be phlebitis? The crucial issue here is adequacy of diagnosis.

Another way of looking at a predisposition to venous thrombosis is to consider studies done to determine the incidence of venous thrombosis in various groups of patients. Risk factors have been determined from autopsy studies,[8] but most of the new data concerning this derive from prospective studies using the technique of scanning lower extremities (over several days) after patients have been given an injection of fibrinogen tagged with a radioactive marker. If clotting occurs, the tagged fibrinogen is converted to fibrin, which builds up in the vein, and the radioactivity at the site increases as the amount of fibrin increases. A handheld external scanner is placed at predetermined sites along the lower extremities and the readings of radioactivity measured and recorded at least once a day, along with a background count over the heart. Distinct increases in counts at one site from day to day, or with respect to adjacent sites, give evidence of clotting. This techinque is very sensitive and almost certainly picks up some small clots that are of no clinical significance, but it has provided valuable data for developing an understanding of the natural history of venous thrombosis. (It has also been an invaluable tool for evaluating prophylactic measures, as we shall see later).

Table 6-2 shows a summary of 20 studies done through 1974 of the incidence of lower extremity venous thrombosis, as determined by abnormal tagged-fibrinogen scans, in groups of patients considered at high risk.[9] One might expect the high incidence after hip fracture, but most surgical procedures reviewed had relatively high incidences. The high frequency in patients with myocardial infarction or stroke should not be surprising.

A reconstruction of information concerning risk factors, with unavoidable simplification and arbitrary groupings, leads to a revealing sense of risk of developing deep venous thrombosis, as shown in Table 6-3.[10] The calculated percentages shown cannot be accepted as being as precise as they appear, but the idea of a roughly predictable risk is important.

ANATOMY

Before dealing with problems of diagnosing venous thrombosis, a brief review of the anatomy of the veins of the lower extremities is pertinent (Figures 6-1 and 6-2).

Table 6-2
Reported Incidence of Abnormal Fibrinogen Leg Scans in *High-Risk* Patients*

Diagnosis	Incidence
Elective Surgery	
Major general abdominal surgery	14% - 33%
Thoracic surgery	26% - 65%
Gynecologic surgery	14% - 19%
Retropubic prostatectomy	24% - 51%
Transurethral resection prostate	7% - 10%
Emergency Surgery	
Hip fracture	48% - 74%
Childbirth	3%
Medical	
Myocardial infarction	23% - 38%
Stroke	60%

*Reprinted with permission from Gallus AS: ^{125}I-Fibrinogen leg scanning, in *Prophylactic Therapy of Deep Vein Thrombosis and Pulmonary Embolism:* Proceedings of National Heart and Lung Institute and American Heart Association Conference, April 1975, NIH No. 76-866, Department of Health, Education and Welfare, p 77-99.

Table 6-3
The Risk of Deep Venous Thrombosis in Eight Hypothetical Patients*

Age and other clinical factors present	Percent risk
1. Age 20 minor operation	0.8
2. Age 40 minor operation	2.9
3. Age 40 major operation	6.3
4. Age 60 minor operation	9.1
5. Age 60 major operation	18.3
6. Age 60 major operation + history of previous deep venous thrombosis	47
7. Age 80 major operation	43
8. Age 80 major operation + history of previous DVT, infection, varicose veins	96

*Reprinted with permission from Nicolaides AN, Gordon-Smith I: The prevention of deep venous thrombosis, in Hobbs JT (ed): *The Treatment of Venous Disorders.* Philadelphia, JB Lippincott Company, 1977, pp 211-235.

The *superficial veins,* the *greater* (or *long*) *saphenous* and the *lesser* (or *short*) *saphenous* and their tributaries, course through subcutaneous tissues. The greater saphenous vein enters the deep system at the femoral triangle and the lesser saphenous flows into the popliteal vein. These superficial veins may be readily visible, even prominent, in patients with minimal subcutaneous fat, who are examined with their legs in a dependent position. When dilated and tortuous, the veins become the typical varicosities of the lower extremities. Thrombosis of segments of superficial veins, except perhaps in the proximal portions, is not associated with serious pulmonary embolism.

The superficial veins drain into the deep system also through *perforating,* or *communicating* veins, which have *valves,* like all lower extremity veins. The orientation of valves is such that they prevent retrograde flow in the superficial and deep systems, and prevent flow from the deep system into the superficial system—if a full complement of valves is present and they function normally. The deep veins of the lower extremities are associated with the arteries that bear the same names. Unlike the superficial veins, they are not visible or palpable but for the most part, are surrounded by muscle. It is the compression of the deep system by muscle contractions that constitutes the venous muscle pump. The *anterior tibial, peroneal,* and *posterior tibial veins,* usually present in pairs, run generally along the routes of their respective arterial namesakes. The many interconnecting channels which form the *soleal veins* of the calf drain into the peroneal and posterior tibial veins. The soleal veins are commonly the site of localized thrombosis, which may explain why the peroneal and posterior

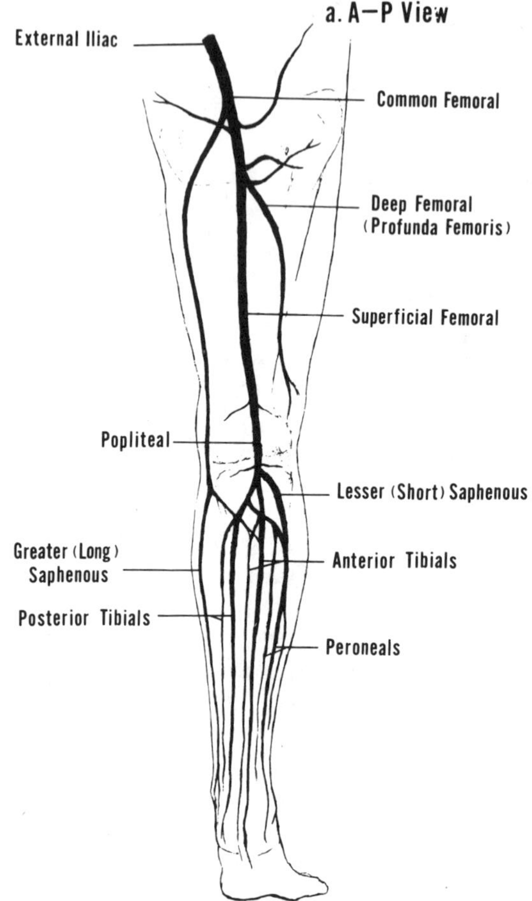

Figure 6-1 Major veins of the lower extremity, anterior view. Veins are in approximate anatomical positions. Valves and communicating veins are not shown.

tibial veins are more likely to be the site of clots than the anterior tibials. The gastrocnemial veins, also often the site of thrombosis, drain into the popliteal vein.

It is terminologically awkward that the common femoral artery divides into branches called deep femoral (profunda femoris) and superficial femoral, for both of these branches are deep vessels, and their names apply to the corresponding veins. Therefore, the *popliteal vein* becomes the *superficial femoral vein,* which is a deep vein. (The superficial femoral vein sometimes is called simply the femoral vein.)

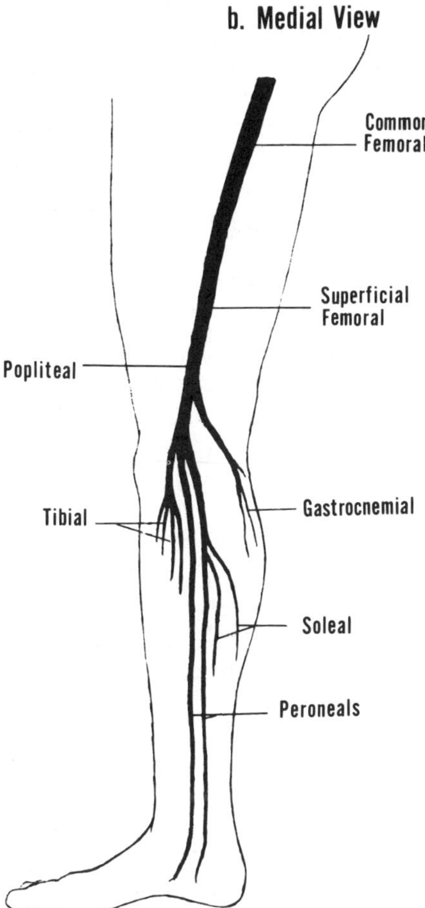

Figure 6-2 Major deep veins of the lower extremity, medial view. Valves and communicating veins are not shown.

It is joined by the *deep femoral vein* to form the *common femoral vein,* and this becomes the *external iliac vein.* The *internal iliac vein* merges with the external iliac, forming the *common iliac vein,* which joins with its contralateral counterpart to become the *inferior vena cava.* Interpretation of important diagnostic tests for venous thrombosis requires a clear notion of this anatomy, keeping in mind that anomalous variations occasionally are present.

With respect to the deep veins of the lower extremity, the term *proximal veins* has come into wide use in recent years. This refers to the popliteal vein together with the deep veins proximal to it, usually excluding the profunda femoris, the internal iliac, and the pelvic veins. The term *distal veins,* referring to the tibials, the peroneal, and soleal, and the gastrocnemial, is not so often used. These distal deep veins often are called *calf veins,* but some would limit calf veins to the soleal and gastrocnemial, calling the whole group of distal deep veins *leg veins.*

Perhaps the most troublesome difficulty with anatomical terms in the context of venous thromboembolism is the variable and inconsistent definition of *leg.* Such a fine, short word should be warmly welcomed by all, but it is unfortunately nearly useless today. Layman usually refer to the entire lower extremity when saying leg, sometimes excluding the foot. Physicians and surgeons often use this term the same way, but some will use it in a formal anatomical sense to mean that portion of the lower extremity between the knee and the ankle. When *calf* is appropriate, it has the same meaning for all. *Thigh* confuses no one. Occasionally, a patient will let the meaning of *foot* extend proximally an uncertain distance. In this chapter, *leg* will be used to refer to only the tissues between knee and ankle.

DIAGNOSIS

The implications of superficial thrombophlebitis are minor compared wth the potentially fatal complications of extensive deep venous thrombosis, and the diagnostic problems are much different.

Superficial Thrombophlebitis

If there have been no recent critical advances in the diagnosis of superficial thrombophlebitis, it is probably because none have been needed. Since these veins are often visible and, except in limbs that are extremely obese or edematous, almost always accessible to the examiner's fingers, the techniques of inspection and palpation usually suffice for establishing the diagnosis. A linear cord of more or less even diameter, usually tender and erythematous, along a course where a superficial vein is expected to be, is strongly suggestive. These findings may be so clear-cut as to make the diagnosis unequivocal. When no thrombus can be felt, and when the induration is not linear, other inflammatory conditions of the skin and subcutaneous tissue must be considered. Edema may be present along and near the thrombosed segment, but generalized edema of the limb implies another condition. Lymphangitis and cellulitis may occur along with superficial phlebitis, especially in cases with venous valvular insufficiency, stasis dermatitis, and ulceration. Only in unusual cases is venography needed to assess the presence of superficial venous thrombosis. A varicose vein is often a major predisposing factor to superficial phlebitis.

Deep Venous Thrombosis

Information derived from *physical examination* alone has long been known to lack sensitivity in diagnosing deep venous thrombosis. This is the obvious conclusion from autopsy studies that demonstrated clots in lower-extremity veins in high percentages of patients in whom this condition was not diagnosed or suspected antemortem.[11] In dying patients, much better sensitivity would be expected from the *history* simply by inferring from factors such as debility and prolonged immobility that most would have venous thrombosis. Among sick or postoperative patients in hospitals, an average of 30% to 50% might be expected to have at least small thrombi in deep veins, most of them undetectable by physical examination.

In viewing the other side of the inadequacy of clinical assessment, lack of specificity pertains as much to the history as to the physical examination. This is a more recently recognized fact, brought out by the use of adjunctive diagnostic methods, particularly appropriately conducted contrast venography,[12,13] Doppler ultrasound studies, [14,15] radioactive-tagged-fibrinogen scans,[16,17] and plethysmographic studies.[18,19] In most cases, even the most experienced clinical expert cannot expect to diagnose or exclude deep venous thrombosis with acceptable accuracy without assistance from one of these tests. It has been said that a coin toss is as valid as a history and physical examination in determining whether or not a patient has clot in a deep vein, but this is a naive distortion of the clinical realities. A physician who understands these matters will, in some situations, make correct decisions based only on history and examination. An extreme example is seen in the generally healthy, ambulatory patient who has a minor, acute illness not predisposing to phlebitis, and who has no symptoms or detectable abnormalities in the lower extremities. Such a patient confidently can be considered free of deep venous thrombosis without subjecting him to objective tests; or, put differently, objective venous studies cannot possibly be justified on all such patients, even though extremely rarely one of them will have a silent venous thrombosis.

This example points out the distinction between these classes of patients: the ambulatory, with no hint of thrombophlebitis; the ambulatory, with history or signs that raise a question of venous thrombosis; and nonambulatory patients. That a diagnosis of deep phlebitis in nonambulatory patients can be easily missed does not mean it will be missed in all patients.[20] But once the question of deep venous thrombosis is seriously raised, for any patient, it becomes appropriate if not mandatory to do an objective test.

Symptoms and Signs

Despite their lack of sensitivity and specificity, close attention must be paid to symptoms and signs, especially in ambulatory patients, for they often point to the diagnostic tests or therapies needed. Even if there were a totally safe, completely accurate, inexpensive, noninvasive test to rule phlebitis in or out, it still would be insufficient because other important conditions may be present, whether or not there were clots in the veins.

Pain and tenderness in the calf or at the femoral vein in the groin, when venous cords are palpable, are clues to the presence of phlebitis. Calf pain and tenderness alone, often present with muscle strains or tears, for example, are nonspecific features. Lower-extremity pain, suggestive of phlebitis, might be due to nerve compression from a herniated intervertebral disc, a ruptured Baker's cyst, or lymphangitis with cellulitis.

Swelling of a limb, especially when unilateral, suggests phlebitis but cannot establish the diagnosis. Muscle injuries, or cellulitis, are often associated with swelling. In bedridden patients, edema may be too slight to notice because the patient is horizontal. Careful measurements of the lower extremities may reveal changes of importance, right side as compared with left, or from day to day. To be relied on as serial data, a standard technique is necessary, such as measuring the circumference of each limb at the superior edge of the patella, the maximum circumference of the calf, and the minimum circumference of the ankle. Cardiac, renal, and hepatic disorders may cause peripheral edema, and a limb with veins damaged from long-past episodes of phlebitis is likely to be more edematous than a limb with normal veins. Lymphedema, whether congenital or due to obstructive processes in lymphatics or nodes, may be unequal in the two lower extremities, again reducing the utility of unequal swelling as a clue to fresh venous thrombosis.

Increased *warmth* of a limb, especially if it is swollen and painful, may hint at phlebitis but has little value as a discriminating sign. The same can be said of *erythema.* These are more suggestive of lymphangitis and cellulitis, as are *chills* and *high fever.* Patients who have had recurrent episodes of chills and fever, a red, swollen, and painful limb, who rapidly improved following the administration of an antibiotic, often speak of these illnesses as phlebitis, but they almost certainly are lymphangitis and cellulitis. (In such cases, examine carefully between the toes for athlete's foot, the common site of bacterial entry.)

Homans' sign[21] is commonly sought on examination when patients are suspected of having thrombophlebitis. It is defined as a resistance by the patient to passive dorsiflexion of the foot because of induced discomfort or muscle tension in the calf. Homans, himself, considered it useful but not specific for phlebitis, and careful observers since have agreed with him. It can be absent when deep venous thrombosis exists, and present when all the veins are free of clot. A variety of calf-muscle disorders can be associated with a positive Homans' sign.

With the patient lying flat, *dilatation of the superficial veins* of the lower extremity should be one of the more specific signs of deep venous thrombosis, particularly when unilateral. Unfortunately, reliable observation of venous dilatation is difficult.

Iliofemoral thrombophlebitis, particularly in its severe form, which is called phlegmasia alba dolens, can be correctly diagnosed more readily from signs and symptoms alone than can leg-vein thrombosis. The affected extremity may feel heavy and painful. Tenderness is likely to be elicited in the groin, probably in the thigh and calf. The limb is swollen, and the superficial veins are dilated. A slight-to-moderate elevation of body temperature is common, but the limb is not notably hot. Arterial pulsations usually are normal, but if swelling is great, some pulses may be hard to find. Lymphedema can mimic iliofemoral venous thrombosis after surgery on, or irradiation of, regional nodes, and the two conditions can coexist. Chills and high fever suggest acute lymphangitis and cellulitis. In some patients, however, there is always the possibility that chills and fever are due to a separate process such as acute urinary tract infection, pneumonia, or deep wound infection. Iliofemoral thrombophlebitis is a serious illness that demands immediate treatment.

Another type of phlebitis, fortunately uncommon, in which diagnosis by symptoms and signs is relatively accurate, is phlegmasia cerulea dolens. It is the most severe form of lower-extremity venous thrombosis. Clotting is so extensive that virtually all venous return is blocked, leading to massive edema, deep cyanosis, reduced or impalpable arterial pulses, gangrene, shock, and even death. This syndrome should never be confounded with acute arterial embolization or thrombosis, where pallor, cool skin, flat superficial veins, and absence of swelling are typical.

To summarize the value of clinical features in diagnosing deep venous thrombosis: a) One can select a few patients with such a likelihood of having clots in deep veins that a diagnosis can be suspected with accuracy by inference (as Table 6-3 indicates); b) in severe cases of extensive clotting (such as phlegmasia alba dolens or phlegmasia cerulea dolens), the symptoms and signs give good evidence of the diagnosis; c) even in these categories, confirmatory tests usually are in order, and in all other cases where phlebitis is suspected or must be excluded, objective tests are necessary, and d) lack of clues to the presence of venous thrombosis in the history or on physical examination in fully active, ambulatory patients excludes the diagnosis for all practical purposes.

Most of the conditions commonly misdiagnosed as phlebitis have been mentioned. Muscle tears or contusions, ruptured popliteal cysts, lymphedema, lymphangitis and cellulitis are among the most obvious. Arthritis of the knee, or referred pain from nerve irritation, especially in a chronically swollen limb, may suggest acute venous thrombosis. External venous compression, as by a malignant growth, a popliteal cyst or popliteal aneurysm, a cast or a severely constrictive garment, can cause swelling. Fear of clots, especially when the phobic patient becomes suspicious of visible normal or varicose veins, can lead to a hypersensitivity to sensing calf tenderness which may be misconstrued as a sign of phlebitis. All these conditions tend to occur in ambulatory patients, most of whom do not have the high-risk predisposing conditions common in sick, bedridden patients. Nevertheless, phlebitis does occur occasionally in patients who have other conditions that mimic phlebitis, and when suspicion indicates, objective tests should be performed.

The main objective studies are: contrast venography, radionuclide venography, Doppler ultrasound venous studies, plethysmographic studies, and radioactive-tagged-fibrinogen[22-24] scans.

Contrast Venography

At the present time, this must be considered the study most likely to determine definitively the presence or absence of deep venous thrombosis. Even if displaced in many cases by noninvasive methods (as has happened already at some medical centers), it remains important and valuable. It has the often-mentioned status of diagnostic gold standard, which, although a bit of an exaggeration, gives an impression of its value.

The method of performing contrast venography is crucial to the validity of the interpretation of the films. Although there may be other satisfactory techniques, the one described by Rabinov and Paulin[25] is widely accepted. It involves tilting the patient feet-down, with weight borne only on the foot that is not being injected. They recommend avoiding the use of a tourniquet so that muscle veins of the calf will fill, but others feel a tourniquet is helpful, at least in some cases. Errors of interpretation are much more likely to occur if the patient is horizontal, or if weight is borne on the limb being injected with the radiopaque contrast medium.

When discrete clots are outlined by the contrast, these filling defects make the diagnosis unequivocal (Figure 6-3). If the study is carefully and properly conducted, non-filling of veins, or segments of veins, may provide convincing evidence of clot, but the experienced radiologist will not always accept absence of filling as a positive study.

There are several problems with contrast venography. The first is the most obvious, that studies done by an inadequate technique may be misleading or uninterpretable, and the second is that considerable experience is needed for reliable interpretation of even the most adequate studies. The technique does not visualize the profunda femoris, the internal iliac, or the pelvic veins, and it does not always opacify the common femoral and external iliac veins well. Sometimes it is difficult to distinguish old from fresh occlusion.

Side reactions do occur but are uncommon. They include: inflammation of soft tissues if dye extravasates at the injection site; pain during injection and afterwards; hypersensitivity reactions to the dye; and postvenography phlebitis. The last of these is of uncertain incidence, estimates ranging from nil to 8% or 10%, but if relatively dilute dye is used and not allowed to remain long in the veins, and if care is taken to empty the veins completely of dye, this should be an infrequent occurrence.

Exactly what the rate of false positives and false negatives might be for contrast venography is unknown, but these rates, though low, cannot be zero. Comparison of venogram findings and results of radioactive-tagged-fibrinogen scans in humans show discrepancies, which also are found in animal studies that include direct examination of the veins.[26]

Radionuclide Venography[27-29]

The use of macroaggregated albumin or human albumin microspheres labeled with radioactive technetium (^{99m}Tc) as the medium to define lower extremity and lower abdominal venous channels is relatively new. The definition possible with this technique, in which a gamma scintillation camera makes the venograms, is poor compared with contrast venography, but the two techniques correlate well for proximal deep vein thrombosis. The radionuclide (or isotope) technique is especially suitable for patients who are sensitive to contrast dye and for those who also need perfusion lung scans. These can

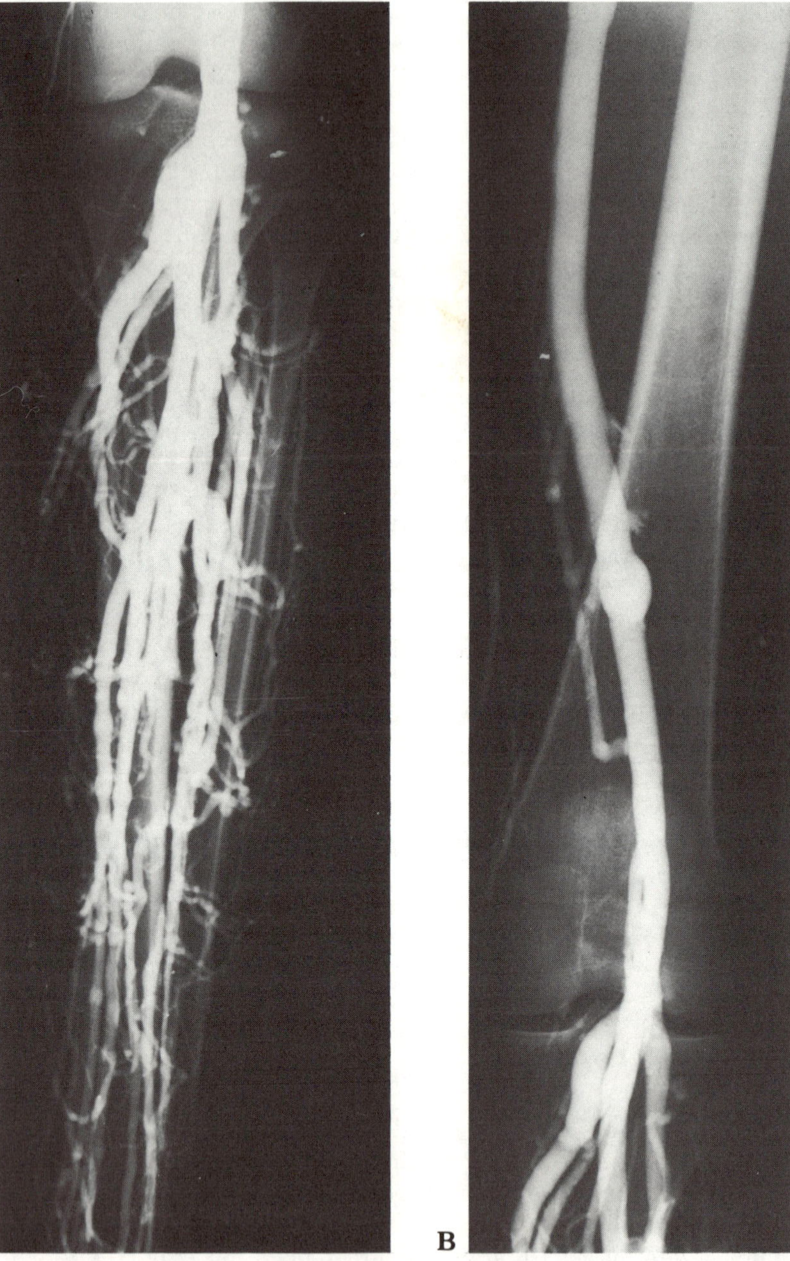

Figure 6-3 Contrast venograms. **A, B, C:** Normal venogram. Three views of the same limb, showing normal veins with no evidence of intraluminal clot. **D, E, F:** Abnormal venogram. Three views of the same limb in which deep venous thrombosis has occurred. Not all the deep veins fill. There are intraluminal fill-

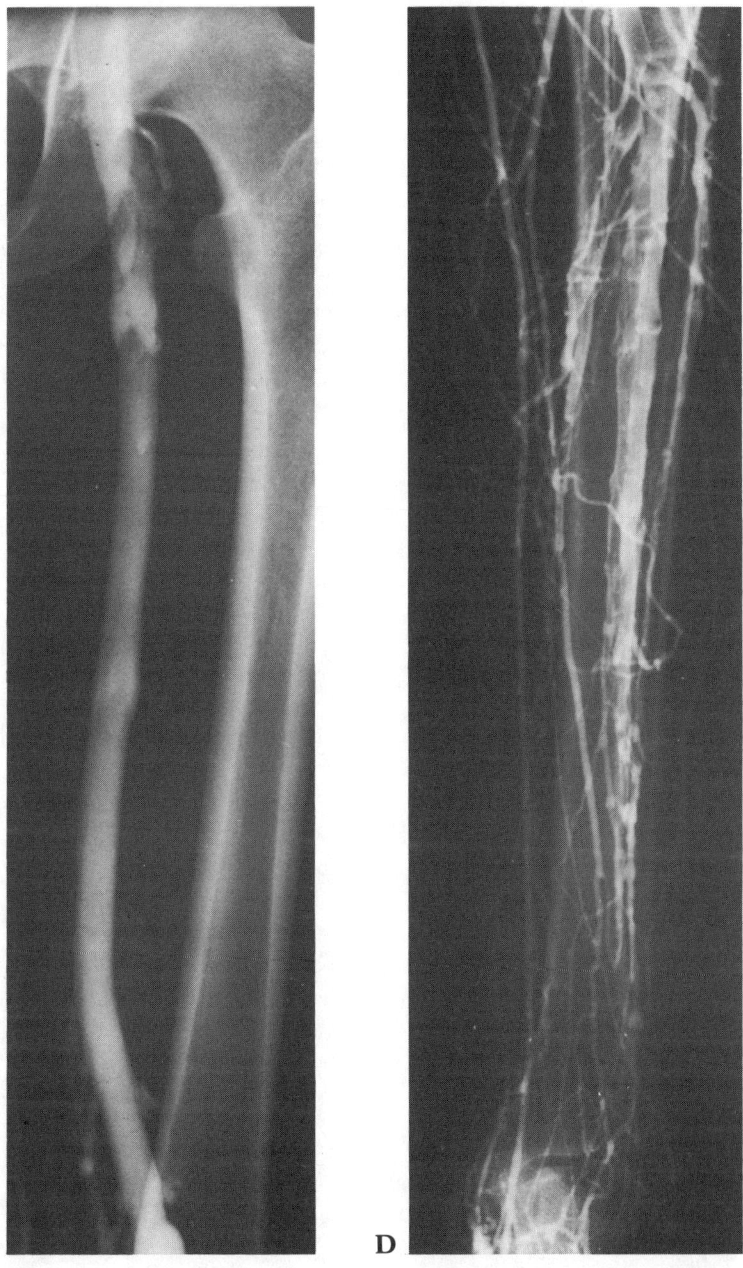

ing defects in the calf veins, the popliteal, and femoral veins. No contrast dye is seen in the superficial femoral vein above the distal thigh. (Radiographs courtesy of Dr E.J. Ring, Hospital of the University of Pennsylvania, Philadelphia).

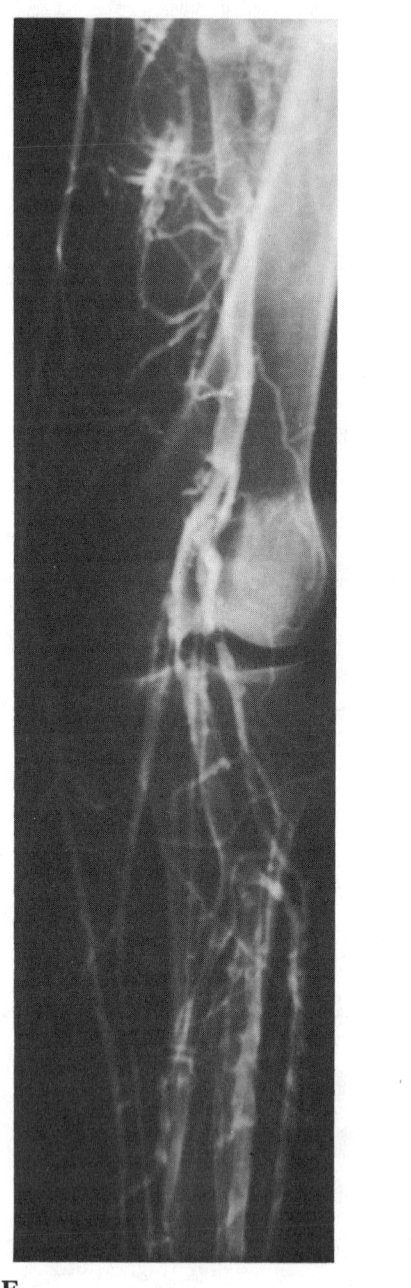

E

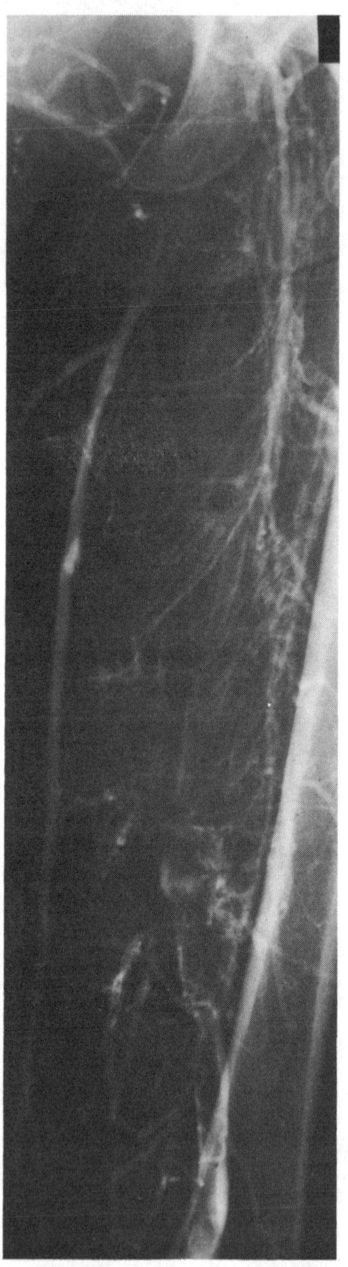

F

Figure 6-3—*Continued*

be performed as part of the same study, following the injection of the radioactive-tagged albumin particles in foot veins. The tagged albumin particles attach to some extent to thrombi, and this may give additional diagnostic information.

Doppler Ultrasound Venous Studies[30,31]

The principle of estimating velocity of a moving object by sensing frequency shifts of emitted or reflected, sonic or electromagnetic signals is well known. The classic, simple example is the change in pitch of a train whistle one hears while standing alongside the track as the train passes. In medicine, ultrasonic instruments are widely used. Continuous-wave ultrasound signals, usually in the range of five to ten million cycles per second (5MHz to 10MHz), can be aimed at blood flowing through arteries or veins, reflected back by the moving cells, and picked up by the instrument. The frequency shift is determined and translated into an audible signal or into an electrical signal that activates a graphic recorder. For venous studies, frequencies of 5 MHz to 6 MHz and audible presentation are the most convenient. Methods were developed and validated in the 1960s and 1970s by Sigel,[14,32] Strandness,[33] and others for using handheld Doppler ultrasound instruments to diagnose deep venous obstruction. By surveying posterior tibial, popliteal, superficial femoral, and common femoral veins for spontaneous venous signals and phasicity with respiration, and by seeking augmentation of signals by compression of the limb distally or by release of proximal compression, an experienced observer can determine with high reliability the presence or absence of thrombi in the proximal veins. It is more difficult to assess the calf veins, but Barnes[34] found that the absence of significant thrombi in the leg can be determined with high specificity (few false-negative examinations). However, the presence of calf-vein thrombi can be overdiagnosed (many false-positive examinations). There is some inconsistency among reported studies, probably due mainly to small but important methodological differences. Clots limited to soleal or gastrocnemial veins will be missed, however, as will clots in the profunda femoris, internal iliac and pelvic veins. The presence of large venous collaterals bypassing an occlusion may make the occlusion undetectable.

The great advantage of Doppler ultrasound testing for venous thrombosis is its convenience. The instrument is pocket-size and the studies can be done relatively quickly. Information can be obtained about venous valvular incompetence also. Doppler venous studies can be repeated frequently at little cost. The great disadvantage is that the technique is difficult to learn and demands considerable expertise.

Results obtained by this method should be discounted unless done by a thoroughly trained person.

Plethysmography

Studies of the peripheral circulation by various plethysmographic methods have generated valuable data for generations of investigators. The tests currently used to find deep venous thrombosis are modifications of classic techniques.[35] Most of them use temporary venous occlusion at the thigh, with monitoring of the volume of the calf. The calf-volume sensor can be an air-filled cuff, a mercury strain gauge, or electrodes that detect changes in electrical impedance—all of which pick up changes in the venous blood volume.[36-41]

Figure 6-4 illustrates the principles of venous-occlusion plethysmography. The patient is lying down, the exact position depending on the specific technique used. With the calf-volume sensor connected to a system for continuously recording an indicator of the volume, the thigh cuff is inflated to a pressure (approximately 40 to 55 mm Hg) sufficient to compress and block venous outflow but not impair arterial inflow, as shown in the middle panel of the figure. Blood accumulates in the veins distal to the thigh cuff, causing a rise in the tracing that reflects calf volume, and eventually reaching a plateau of maximum venous filling. The difference between the baseline and the maximum calf volume is called venous capacitance. The thigh cuff is then abruptly deflated, allowing the blood that has accumulated in the leg veins to flow out through the popliteal, femoral, and iliac veins into the inferior vena cava. If there is a thrombus obstructing this venous outflow tract, the leg veins will empty slowly, and this will be reflected in the leg-volume trace. Although the reduction in rate of venous outflow is the more important effect of thrombi in proximal veins, they may also cause a decrease in venous capacitance; the obstructing thrombus has already caused partial distention of distal veins, so there is less room for the accumulation of additional blood when the thigh cuff is inflated.

There are useful, commercially available air, mercury-strain-gauge and impedance plethysmographs. At the present time, the instrument most widely used and most thoroughly validated is the impedance plethysmograph. It has been developed by Wheeler and other investigators,[42-44] into a standardized technique for the diagnosis of lower-limb deep venous thrombosis. This method is highly accurate for finding or excluding thrombi obstructing the deep veins from the popliteal proximally, but it does not sensitively pick up leg-vein thrombi. When impedance plethysmographic tests are borderline or equivocal, usually it is because of inadequate venous filling after inflation of the thigh cuff. This

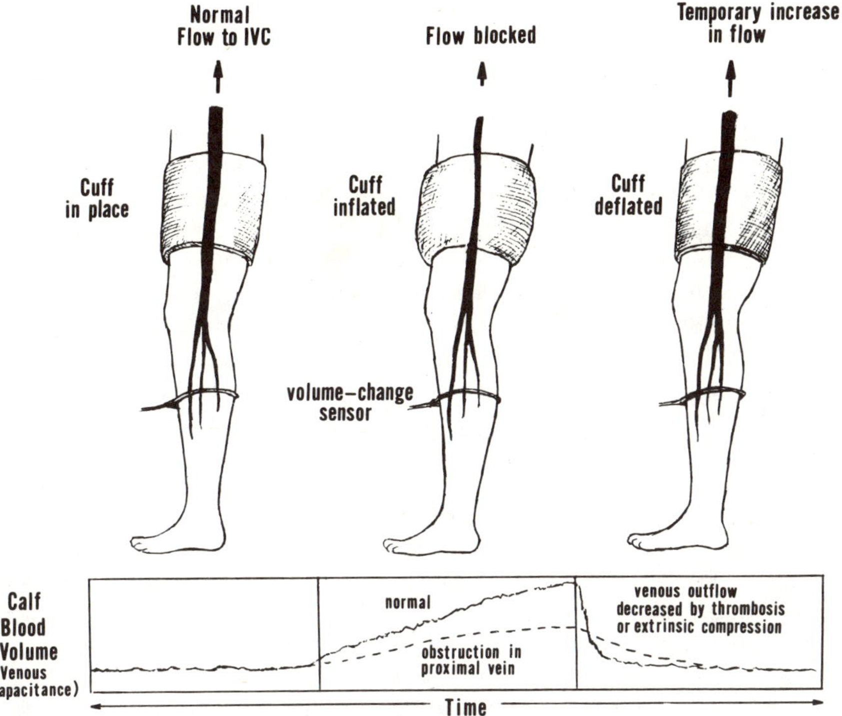

Figure 6-4 Impedence plethysmography in proximal vein occlusion. There is diminution of venous capacitance fluctuation with cuff inflation and deflation.

can be due to conditions such as restricted arterial inflow, obstructive arterial disease or arteriospasm, unrelieved calf-muscle spasm, residual old thrombosis in deep veins, or external compression of deep veins in the pelvis or in the popliteal space.

A special instrument for air plethysmography developed by Cranley and Grass,[45,46] called the phleborheograph, is more versatile than the conventional phlethysmographs mentioned above. Data so far available suggest it is extremely accurate when correlated with venographic studies,[47,48] and it is capable of more detailed analysis of the venous circulation. Studies done with it take somewhat longer and interpretation requires greater sophistication than with the other available instruments, but these disadvantages may prove minor.

In general, plethysmographic methods for diagnosing deep venous thrombosis are sound and reliable for proximal-vein clots, more or less unreliable for leg-vein clots. They are objective, and the interpretation of results usually is straightfoward. The instruments are portable in that they can be wheeled on a cart, but they lack the great convenience of the pocket-size Doppler ultrasound probe.

Radioactive-Tagged Fibrinogen Scans[9,49,50]

The isotope, ^{125}I, used to label fibrinogen, allows the use of a lightweight handheld ratemeter for counting the emissions. One injection suffices for counting for about a week. This study is especially reliable in detecting thrombi in the leg and the distal thigh. The closer one gets to the groin, the less reliable it is, and it cannot evaluate pelvic or abdominal veins. It can be misleading at sites of local trauma, infection, or recent surgery, and it does not separate clotting in superficial veins from clotting in deep veins. It should not be used in pregnant women or nursing mothers. Both false-positive and false-negative results can occur when scans are correlated with venograms. This test shows nothing about a clot that was formed before the tagged fibrinogen was injected; it reveals only new fibrin formation. Therefore, it has usually been used prospectively to screen for thrombus-formation in a patient considered at risk. These scans do have value, however, in diagnosing existing venous thrombosis in patients who are not fully anticoagulated, because usually there will be further deposition of fibrin on the existing thrombus. This diagnostic use of ^{125}I-fibrinogen scanning might be appropriate in patients suspected of deep calf-vein thrombosis who have normal plethysmographic and Doppler venous studies when venography is undesirable; for example, when the patient is hypersensitive to the contrast dye. These scans might also be indicated when new symptoms suggestive of phlebitis develop after a negative venogram has been obtained, and in trying to determine if a venographic abnormality represents old or new thrombus. Overall, ^{125}I-fibrinogen scans are most important in clinical investigation of the natural history of venous thrombosis in studies of prophylaxis of venous thrombosis, and in prospective screening of susceptible patients.

Other Diagnostic Tests

As yet, no definitive blood tests exist that will identify all thrombus-prone patients, but there are interesting analyses in the literature.[51-54]

Hypercoagulability may be revealed by low levels of antithrombin-III. This can be either an inherited disorder (with a high incidence of thrombotic episodes, sometimes fatal, even before age 45), or it can be an acquired one (as may occur with estrogen use). Increased platelet aggregability and increased platelet-coagulant activities may be important. Measurement of fibrin degradation products (fibrin-split products) provides useful information. Of all these, the antithrombin-III levels may be the most revealing single measurement, but the situation is so complex that generally available standard tests have yet to emerge.

From time to time *thermography* has been advocated as a diagnostic technique for the detection of deep vein thrombosis. A skin-temperature map of the lower extremities is made by a scanning camera that detects infrared radiation. Some investigators[55,56] report good correlations with venograms, but there exists a feeling that thermograms are difficult to interpret and that the results are often misleading. Thermographic studies have not been widely used, partly because the equipment is expensive. More extensive studies would be needed to establish the technique in this field.

Too little has been reported about newly developed *isotope techniques* for their value to be clear. Radioactive-technetium-labeled plasmin (^{99m}Tc-plasmin) has been given intravenously and scans made with a gamma camera. Good sensitivity for detecting established venous thrombosis was reported. The interesting advantage of this technique is having results in approximately 15 minutes.[57] Another technique requires injection of indium-isotope(^{111}In)-tagged platelets. Whole-body scans, done with a gamma camera, reveal platelet accumulations.[58] These types of studies deserve watching.

Combinations of Diagnostic Methods

Technological advances in diagnostic methodology impinge so heavily on medical practice that histories and physical examinations are sometimes downgraded. Their specific inadequacies, described above, do not negate their broad value when deep vein thrombosis is at issue. This is true even if a postitive or negative venogram report is in hand before the patient is seen by the physician who will be responsible for his care. The combination of symptoms and signs on the one hand, and an objective test on the other, can be sufficient even if the objective test is less definitive than a properly performed and interpreted venogram. A plethysmographic study or an expertly conducted Doppler ultrasound examination will often provide adequate corroboration or refutation of a clinical suspicion of phlebitis. Wheeler[59] reports successful screening by clinical and impedance-plethysmographic criteria, without venography, in the sense that follow-up revealed that pulmonary emboli were rare and those nonfatal. In cases of leg-vein thrombi, ^{125}I-fibrinogen scans are valid (with the exceptions noted before) but are inconvenient for outpatients. It could be argued that the Doppler examination or a plethysmographic method, or both, is the current practical screening method of choice for outpatients. If the results are equivocal, venography would be indicated. Where both ^{125}I-fibrinogen scanning and impedance plethysmography can be used, the combination can replace venography in some cases.[60] Impedance plethysmography adds substantially to the diagnostic value of tagged-fibrinogen scanning in hip surgery.[61] A variety of other combinations of tests has been reported to be useful in diagnosing venous thrombosis.[28,62,63]

Diagnostic Strategy

Algorithms are frequently proposed to specify diagnostic approaches. Some are extremely comprehensive and include interactions with management decisions[64]; others are much simpler and more practical as summary strategies.[65] Figure 6-5 shows a generalized approach to diagnosis which allows individual physicians to modify it continuously to suit their patients' requirements and the availability of special techniques in their communities.

An important question, which has no complete answer, arises after a diagnosis of thrombophlebitis is established: How far should one go to look for an occult predisposing disease? Where there is a clear precipitating factor, like an injury, and no past history or family history of recurring phlebitis, not much needs to be done. Minimum screening always includes a careful history and general physical examination, including digital examination of the rectum and in women, pelvic examination. It is reasonable to include a complete blood count, including platelet count, urinalysis, and examination of several stool specimens for occult blood. Patients with deep venous thrombosis would normally have a chest x-ray study as a baseline in case suspicion of pulmonary embolism develops. More controversial is the notion that even a first episode of unexpected phlebitis, including superficial phlebitis in a patient without varicose veins, signals a malignant, infectious, or collagen-vascular disease, requiring, among other tests, full urinary tract and gastrointestinal x-ray studies, and such blood studies as antinuclear antibodies and serum proteins. To many physicians, this will seem an extreme approach. It is sometimes felt that iliofemoral thrombosis is a stronger indication for a thorough search for underlying disease if it occurs on the right than if it occurs on the left. This is because of the presumed predisposition to stasis on the left due to impingement of the right common iliac artery on the left common iliac vein. Recurrent thrombotic episodes and familial tendency to throm-

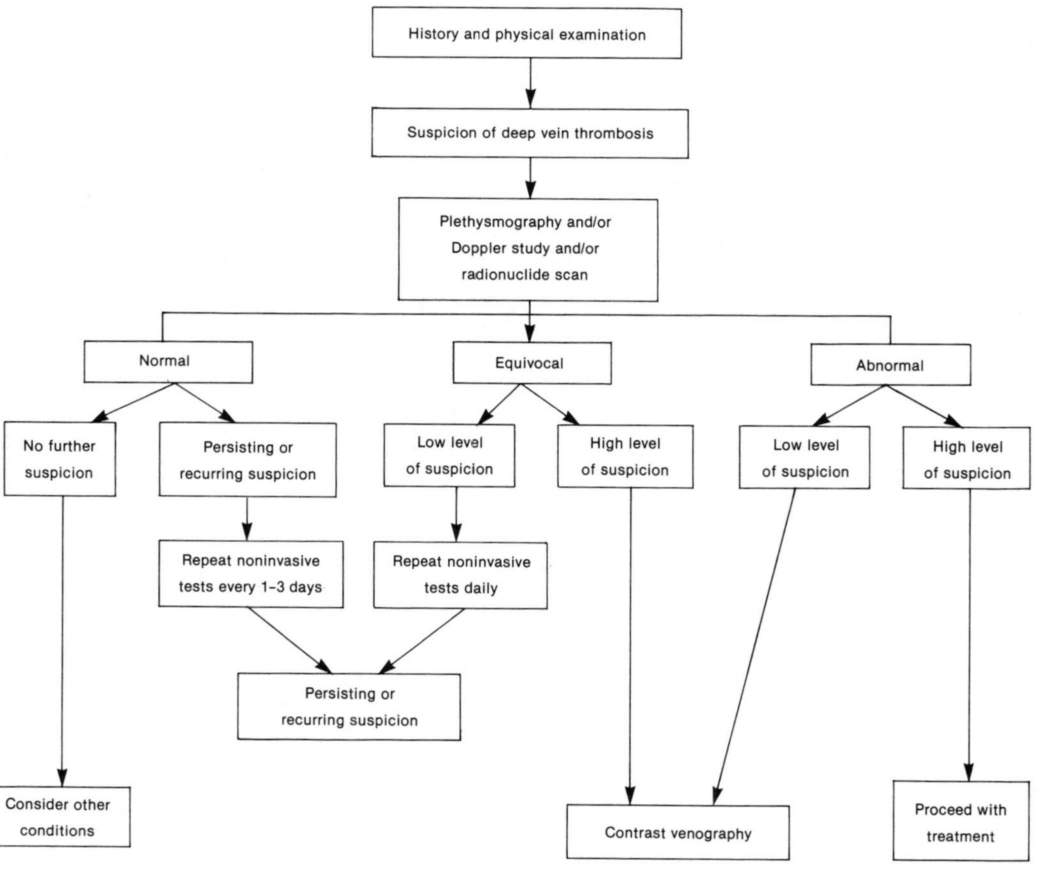

Figure 6-5 Algorithm for the management of patients with suspected deep vein thrombosis.

bosis require more detailed hematologic studies, including measures of platelet aggregability and of antithrombin-III levels. It is probable that severe psychological stress predisposes to thrombosis, and this should be kept in mind as a background factor, though a direct relationship is hard to establish.

TREATMENT

Superficial Thrombophlebitis

Except when thrombus is extending close to the popliteal or the femoral vein, or in otherwise intractable cases, full anticoagulation is not recommended for superficial phlebitis. Warm compresses and elevation usually help. Analgesics sometimes are needed. The use of nonsteroidal antiinflammatory drugs is often suggested, probably is not often needed, but can be helpful in some patients. If there is infection about the toes, or a stasis ulcer, there is a chance of coexistant lymphangitis, even in the absence of systemic symptoms or detectable lymphadenitis. In some such cases, this would justify the use of an antibiotic. Elastic support of the legs may give comfort to some patients but may not be tolerated by others if there is much tenderness.

When anticoagulation is contraindicated, ligation of the greater saphenous vein in the femoral triangle is appropriate, if the clot extends proximally beyond mid-thigh level. In the absence of such contraindication, full anticoagulation without ligation probably is the preferred treatment. Stripping of superficial veins which are the site of recurrent phlebitis should be undertaken reluctantly, and only after a thorough search for underlying predisposing disease. Whenever possible, superficial veins should be preserved for future use, if needed, in arterial bypass surgery.

Deep Venous Thrombosis

The keystone of therapeutic regimens for deep thrombophlebitis is anticoagulation, which is better understood as prophylaxis of complications than as treatment of the thrombosis. True treatment of phlebothrombosis is given only when agents that stimulate fibrinolysis are administered. There is increasing discussion and advocacy of more frequent use of fibrinolytic medications.[66] The traditions of practice may change fairly quickly to incorporate them, but at the present time the use of anticoagulant drugs is the accepted standard.[67]

Heparin[68] is the drug of choice for starting treatment, substantially because when an adequate amount has been given, its effect is immediate. Once the diagnosis of deep venous thrombosis is made, and contraindications to the use of anticoagulant therapy exluded, heparin should be given immediately to minimize extension of the clotting process. Beyond this, there is rampant controversy concerning heparin dose requirements and regulation, and appropriate duration of treatment. It is curious that a drug given to hundreds of millions of people over nearly half a century, extensively studied and generally considered indispensable, does not have more sharply defined and agreed-upon patterns of use.[69]

Heparin acts by accelerating the inhibiting action of antithrombin-III (also called antithrombin-heparin cofactor) on plasma proteases involved in coagulation. There is no test that indicates clearly what the minimum dose of heparin should be to induce adequate anticoagulation for an individual patient. Sophisticated assays exist that shed light on ways of regulating heparin therapy,[51] but in clinical settings the tests used are the plasma partial thromboplastin time (PTT), the plasma activated partial thromboplastin time (APTT), the whole-blood clotting time (Lee-White), and the whole-blood partial thromboplastin time.[70] Of these, the PTT and APTT are probably the most commonly used. The traditional measure of *adequate* heparin dosage is that amount which increases the PTT or APTT to about twice its control time, but this criterion is not solidly established. These measures can demonstrate that there is a definite circulating heparin effect, which is important, especially since large amounts of already formed thrombus may bind heparin and cause a need for larger than usual initial doses.

There is evidence that measurements of fibrin degradation products (FDP), which are derived mostly from fresh fibrin, or measurements of fibrin monomer, can be a guide to the adequacy of heparin anticoagulation.[71] Fibrin monomer should not be found after adequate doses of heparin have been given. Within two to five days of effective treatment, FDP should disappear from the blood. The use of tests for fibrin monomer and FDP, interpreted in this way, is not routinely established in most hospitals.

Since it is crucial to stop extension of thrombosis promptly, and since hemorrhagic complications of heparin are relatively uncommon during the first two days of therapy, large doses (40,000 to 60,000 units* in 24 hours, or more in cases of massive thrombosis) are sometimes recommended for the first two days, with reduction to 20,000 to 30,000 units daily thereafter.[72] After a secondarily administered oral anticoagulant is having an effect, the heparin dose

---

*In the United States, USP units are used. The International Unit is about 17% smaller than the USP unit.

might be further reduced. This approach implies that the PTT can be allowed to be far more than twice the control time in the first two days of heparin therapy, but after that it might be held to the traditional level. Unfortunately, there is no convincing evidence that bleeding complications can be avoided by the monitoring of heparin effect with conventional tests.

The preferred route of heparin administration is intravenous. Continuous uniform infusion is safer than intermittent bolus injection, and probably reduces the dose required per unit of time and the total dose. Subcutaneous administration can be successful, but absorption is often irregular. It is easier to use concentrated solutions of heparin (such as 20,000 units/ml) so that the volume of each subcutaneous injection is small, and the injections are usually given every six hours. Since it is desirable to treat patients with deep venous thrombosis in hospitals rather than at home, the continuous intravenous method of administration can reasonably be the first choice, but intermittent intravenous or subcutaneous injections are options. Heparin is not given intramuscularly because of the risk of hemorrhage at the injection site.

Practice varies with respect to the duration of heparin therapy. A few recommend starting with heparin and a loading dose of warfarin, stopping heparin as soon as the prothrombin time reaches *therapeutic* range, hoping that this will be on the third day of treatment, when the risk of bleeding from heparin increases. This is difficult to achieve, and may not give continuous effective anticoagulation. The more widely accepted approach is full anticoagulation with heparin for seven to ten days, perhaps extending this to two weeks or longer in cases of extensive thrombosis. Warfarin should be introduced five days before the anticipated withdrawal of heparin, because the prothrombin time may be prolonged a few days before all the clotting factors affected by warfarin are sufficiently depressed.

The chief complication of heparin anticoagulation is bleeding, for which there may be varying susceptibility among patients.[73] Although bleeding is more likely to occur when the PTT is greatly prolonged than when it is lower, this test is not a good predictor of bleeding in an individual at a particular time. One factor that can be associated with bleeding is heparin-induced thrombocytopenia. There is some merit in checking platelet counts along with PTT, prothrombin times, and routine blood counts before starting anticoagulation and in following the platelet counts after heparin is started. Deaths from bleeding during anticoagulation with heparin do occur; therefore, this drug must be used cautiously and carefully. When heparin effect must be neutralized, the antidote is protamine.

Hypersensitivity reactions to heparin occur but are rare. Occasionally, hair loss occurs. Long-term therapy with daily doses of about

Table 6-4
Oral Anticoagulant Drugs

Generic Name	Trade Name
Coumarin Derivatives	
Warfarin sodium	Coumadin
	Panwarfin
Dicumarol	
Ethyl biscoumacetate	Tromexan
Phenprocoumon	Liquamar
Acenocoumarol	Sintrom
Indandione Derivatives	
Phenindione	Hedulin
	Danilone
Anisindione	Miradon
Diphenadione	Dipaxin

20,000 units or more may be associated with the development of osteoporosis. Unlike the coumarin anticoagulants, heparin does not cross the placenta, and so it can be used in pregnancy.

The *coumarin compounds* are much more popular than the *indanedione drugs* for use as *oral anticoagulants* (Table 6-4), and *warfarin* has become the most widely used of the coumarin group. The coumarin derivatives work by interfering with synthesis of coagulation factors II (prothrombin), VII, IX and X, dependent on vitamin K.[74] They are not competitive inhibitors of vitamin K, but they interfere with its metabolism. It is as true of oral anticoagulants as it is of heparin that their place in medicine is incompletely worked out, despite a conviction that they are currently indispensible in some situations.

Control of warfarin dosage is by the prothrombin time. Since the rate of warfarin clearing varies from patient to patient, the dose required to prolong the prothrombin time also varies. Although an initial loading dose of 25 or 30 mg of warfarin will quickly prolong the prothrombin time, this is potentially hazardous for patients whose liver enzymes degrade the drug slowly. It is safer to give an initial dose of 15 mg, then 10 mg on each of the next two days, measuring daily prothrombin times. The first dose should not be given until a prothrombin time has been checked (in case the patient has unsuspected hypoprothrombinemia), and each day's dose should be withheld until the prothrombin time for that day is known. Control prothrombin times range between 10 and 13 seconds, and the desirable therapeutic range is one and one-half to two times control (between 18 and 24 seconds, for example, if the control is 12 seconds). By the third day of treatment (without large loading dose), the prothrombin time will have shown a distinct increase in most cases, and maintenance dosage of 5 to 7.5 mg daily is the likely requirement for these patients. If there has been no increase, or an increase of only one or two seconds, the patient needs larger doses and may require maintenance dosage of 10 or 15 mg daily. However, some of these patients will, after a time, require less warfarin. If the prothrombin time should reach therapeutic range in two or three days, the potential for bleeding exists because Factor VII has been depressed; but the other factors affected by coumarins have longer half-lives, and thrombus formation is not prevented until after approximately five days of treatment.

When warfarin is started during heparin therapy, the five-day overlap is desirable. There may be a change in prothrombin time when heparin is discontinued and so patients will need tests for another day or two. After patients leave the hospital, they need prothrombin times frequently, two or three times a week, until stable control is demonstrated. Then, the interval between tests usually can be extended to one, two, or even three weeks. Control will be erratic for a few patients, who will need to have more than one test a week. An unexpected large change in prothrombin time suggests a laboratory error, and the test should be repeated the next day.

Like heparin, coumarin drugs are dangerous and sometimes lethal; therefore, their use, which can be of great value, must be undertaken with meticulous planning. Outpatient anticoagulant therapy with a drug like warfarin cannot be done safely unless these factors are present: a) a physician who fully understands the drug and who is committed to continuous control of the dose, either personally or through a competent substitute; b) a patient who is responsible and who understands how to follow the physician's precise instructions, or a family member or other person who can give the prescribed doses and get the prothrombin tests done; c) a laboratory that does prothrombin times reliably and is accessible to the patient; and d) a system of communication between physician and patient which insures each knows what the prescribed dose is at all times. It is helpful to have prothrombin times done in the morning, with the results phoned to the physician who then calls the patient with instructions. Warfarin should be taken in the evening, about the same time each day. The patient should be instructed to call the physician if he has not already been notified of the results of the test, of any needed changes in warfarin dosage and of the interval before the next test should be done. The physician also should have a way of knowing if a patient failed to have a scheduled test, or if the test result and the instructions were not communicated. All this may seem fussy, but in the absence of such tight control the risks are high.

Other precautions must be taken when using oral anticoagulants for long-term therapy. The patient must report any bleeding immediately, and the physician must be alert to the development of new diseases that might cause bleeding. The diet must be relatively stable so that large variations of vitamin K intake do not occur; and heavy consumption of alcohol (especially binges), must be avoided. No new drugs should be introduced in the patient's regimen without advance clearance from the physician in charge of regulating the anticoagulant dose. This is the most practical way of dealing with the difficult problem of the interactions between coumarin anticoagulants and many other drugs.[75] Pregnant women and nursing mothers should not take coumarin drugs, and female patients should be advised to report the possibility of pregnancy to the physician regulating anticoagulation. Physical injuries can be risky for anticoagulated patients, and contact sports, or activities that might traumatize joints or soft tissues severely, should be avoided.

The optimum duration of anticoagulation after an episode of venous thrombosis is not clearly known. When warfarin is used for prophylaxis of recurrence, it probably should be given for at least one or two months in cases of calf-vein thrombosis, and for at least three to six months if the proximal veins were involved or if the extent of the thrombosis is uncertain. Patients who have recurrences shortly after stopping anticoagulation may have to be treated much longer. In some cases, years of anticoagulation may be appropriate, especially if there were several proved recurrences of deep venous thrombosis or if pulmonary embolism occurred. Long-term therapy occasionally will be frustrated by failure to control the prothrombin time, or by bleeding. Intercurrent illness or need for surgery may interrupt the regimen temporarily, and perhaps permanently.

There is controversy about a) the protection against recurrence offered by using heparin alone for treatment of the acute episode, followed by long-term heparin in low-dose regimen (5000 units subcutaneously every 12 hours), compared with b) the protection given by using heparin for the acute episode followed by long-term warfarin therapy.[76,77] The weight of evidence seems to lean toward the use of warfarin, for at least a few weeks, after which it is possible that a switch to low-dose heparin might be protective. Further studies are needed to resolve this.

The most serious complication of warfarin use is bleeding. When the anticoagulant effect of coumarin drugs must be reversed, the antidote is vitamin K_1. Hypersensitivity reactions are uncommon. Skin necrosis occurs rarely, possibly due to hypersensitivity since it is not dose-related. Development of bluish or purplish color of toes associated with warfarin also is uncommon and generally not of serious consequence.

An entirely different type of anticoagulant, used in Great Britain and in Europe but not available in the United States, is prepared from the venom of the Malayan pit viper, *Agkistrodon rhodostoma,* and is called *ancrod* (or arvin). It defibrinates blood, rendering it incoagulable,[78] and reduces the viscosity of blood, but bleeding complications are said to be extremely rare. It is given intravenously, intramuscularly, or subcutaneously, and it has been used successfully to treat venous thrombosis,[79] as well as to prevent it.[80] In the future it may prove to have a more important place in the management of thrombotic diseases than is now appreciated.

As mentioned before, the use of *fibrinolytic agents* to treat venous thrombosis is being more strongly advocated now. There is no doubt such drugs are often effective in clearing the vessels of clot. They may prove particularly helpful in cases of massive venous thrombosis or when venograms show a large tail of thrombus floating free. Since the most important studies using these agents concern pulmonary embolism, they will be discussed under that heading.

Surgical treatment of venous thrombosis largely concerns pulmonary emboli, and this too will be discussed later. Occasionally there may be justification for embolectomy in the lower extremity when thrombosis is massive, especially if done within three or four days of onset of the disease, but this operation has lost favor. There is no place for the stripping of superficial veins in the treatment of deep venous thrombosis. Interruption of the inferior vena cava is justified in cases of iliofemoral thrombophlebitis when anticoagulation is contraindicated.

General measures usually include bed rest to allow swelling to subside, to reduce the risk of dislodgement of a loosely attached thrombus, and to relieve discomfort. Heat applied to the affected limb may help relieve pain, but its full value is unclear. Care must be taken to insure that warm compresses are not hot enough to burn. They should be applied intermittently to avoid maceration of the skin and to allow examination of the extremity. Some of the other points mentioned concerning the care of patients with superficial phlebitis also apply to deep phlebitis, but not the use of antiinflammatory drugs. Elastic support while the patient is in bed and anticoagulated is unnecessary, and since the standard-size stockings provided routinely in hospitals do not fit most patients properly, they are best avoided. However, when the patient gets up, if there is a tendency for edema to collect in the affected limb, custom-fitted elastic stockings may be valuable.

The notion of *innocent* calf-vein thrombosis exposes a difficult issue in the management of deep vein thrombosis. On the one hand, we know calf-vein thromboses are detected by sensitive objective tests in patients who do not develop serious complications. On the other hand, we also know some cases of proximal vein thrombosis are extensions from the leg veins. Attitudes vary concerning the need for full anticoagulant treatment of distal, or leg, deep venous thrombosis. It is probable that many cases of soleal vein thrombosis resolve completely without treatment, but there is no way to ascertain in which cases extension will occur. It may even be safe to omit anticoagulation in some cases of tibial or peroneal thrombosis, but the current knowledge suggests it is wiser to treat these patients when the diagnosis is clear.

PROPHYLAXIS

Since certain groups of patients can be identified as susceptible to development of deep venous thrombosis, and since venous thrombi often form with no warning symptoms or signs and are *silent* in half the patients who die of pulmonary emboli, it is easy to understand the great enthusiasm for finding effective prophylactic regimens. The availability of reliable venographic and noninvasive techniques, especially the ^{125}I-fibrinogen scan used prospectively, has strongly stimulated investigative activity, despite substantial difficulties in designing and carrying out valid studies.[81] The main agents studied and found more or less useful are heparin (in low dosage), oral anticoagulants (in full dosage), *antiplatelet* drugs, dextrans, and certain physical methods or devices.

Low-Dose Heparin[10,82,83]

The effectiveness of low-dose (small dose, or mini-dose) heparin regimens for preventing venous thrombosis is now well documented in patients who have undergone elective abdominal or thoracic surgery. The dose used has been 5000 units subcutaneously every eight to 12 hours, and no appreciable difference was seen whether two or three injections a day were given. These low-dose regimens have not, however, been significantly helpful in patients who have undergone hip surgery. These patients tend to have low levels of antithrombin-III and so might need larger doses of heparin, which would increase the risk of bleeding. The thromboembolic complications of myocardial infarction are reduced by prophylactic use of low-dose heparin, but overall reduction in mortality has not been demonstrated. Of course, the sooner the prophylactic regimen is started the better, and evidence suggests heparin given before an operation as well as afterward, yields greater protection against thrombosis than if given only afterward. Bleeding complications are much less of a problem than with full-dose heparin, but bleeding can occur.[84] Aspirin taken concurrently may be a factor in inducing bleeding. It appears that patients vary in the amount of heparin they require for a happy combination of effective and safe antithrombotic effect, and measurement of antithrombin-III levels has been suggested as a guide to dosage.[85] The combination of *half-low-dose* heparin (2500 units per dose) with dihydroergotamine, a vasoconstrictor, has been shown to be more effective than heparin alone in preventing deep venous thrombosis in patients having total-hip-replacement surgery.

Despite impressive evidence of prophylactic efficacy in appropriately selected groups of patients, low-dose heparin has not been universally accepted, partly because of the risks and partly because the beneficial effects are not easily visible.[86]

Oral Anticoagulants for Prophylaxis

The possibility that relatively low doses of some oral drugs may have a place in prophylaxis has not been excluded, but the regimens now known to be effective are full-dose. Indandione drugs have been used,[87] but most experience has been with coumarin derivatives, particularly warfarin.[88] It is hardly surprising that there is reluctance to impose full anticoagulation on a patient with injuries or one who has just had a major operation, but where this has been done the efficacy of warfarin has been demonstrated, including cases of hip surgery. The risk of increased bleeding must be accepted when courmarin drugs are used this way. In hip surgery, one approach has been to delay administration of warfarin to the fifth postoperative day to reduce the risk of hemorrhage. This resulted in a slight reduction in venous thrombosis and a substantial reduction in pulmonary emboli, compared with a small control group; but there were significant hemorrhagic complications.[89] Extensive experience with coumarins in the management of patients with myocardial infarction has been inconclusive with respect to long-term benefit, although venous thrombosis was reduced in incidence. The major prophylactic use of oral anticoagulants, however, is in the medium-term or long-term prevention of recurrence of deep vein thrombosis and pulmonary embolism.

Antiplatelet Drugs

Excitement surrounds the possibility of successfully preventing venous thromboembolism by simple, relatively safe, oral medications such as aspirin, dipyridamole, sulfinpyrazone or hydroxychloroquine. The results of studies done so far, however, range from negative, to conflicting, to hopeful.[90–92] Dipyridamole appears to be ineffective, hydroxychloroquine and sulfinpyrazone somewhat effective.

Aspirin is the most interesting drug, partly because it is so familiar, partly because it has seemed to prevent transitory cerebral ischemic attacks (at least in men), and because it may have a beneficial effect on coronary artery disease. Aspirin renders inactive the enzyme, cyclooxygenase, needed to form thromboxane A_2, which is a powerful stimulator of platelet aggregation. The appropriate dose for antiplatelet effect in humans is uncertain. Dosage of 150 mg once or twice a week may be sufficient, but conventional dosage is one to four 325-mg tablets a day. Large doses also inhibit prostaglandin I_2 (prostacyclin), which is itself a potent inhibitor of platelet aggregation. This suggests the possibility that better results from aspirin in preventing thrombosis might have been found if the trials had used smaller doses. After total hip replacement, aspirin appears to be beneficial in preventing venous thromboembolism.[93]

Dextran,[94] a complex polysaccharide, is not always listed among the antiplatelet drugs even though it strongly affects platelet function, influencing adhesiveness and aggregation. In this regard, the fractions of higher molecular weight are more potent, but lower-molecular–weight fractions have been used in clinical trials, which have demonstrated efficacy in reducing incidence of venous thrombosis and pulmonary embolism after general and orthopedic surgery.[90,95,96] Dextran, given as an intravenous infusion, expands the blood volume, posing a problem for patients with overt or borderline cardiac failure. Allergic reactions occur. It does not seem suitable for widespread routine use but may be helpful in selected cases.

Physical methods[97] begin with simple measures. Elevations of the legs and early ambulation are classic parts of therapy, likely to help, but inadequate in themselves to prevent deep vein thrombosis reliably. Properly fitted elastic stockings may reduce the pool of blood in calf veins,[98] but they provide inadequate protection, and, more often than not, they fit poorly. Active exercise of the calf muscles against resistance will empty calf veins. However, this would have to be done frequently and around the clock, which though impractical, should be encouraged for its potential benefit. Passive leg exercises probably are of little value except to keep joints limber. In a few studies, electrical muscle stimulation has been shown to be effective, but rather painful, and thus best suited to anaesthetized patients.

Perhaps the most reliable method is intermittent external pneumatic compression,[99] for which there is a variety of devices on the market. Although one might expect these devices to be effective primarily by their hemodynamic effects,[99,100] evidence suggests they cause release of fibrinolytic factors from the compressed limb.[101,102] Naturally, interest has been strong in the use of these devices in patients for whom hemorrhage would be particularly dangerous, such as in those who have had strokes or have undergone neurosurgery, prostatic or ophthalmic surgery. In such situations, intermittent compression has been effective in reducing the incidence of thrombosis.[103-105]

COMPLICATIONS

The main complications of deep venous thrombosis are the postphlebitic syndrome, when vein walls and valves are damaged and venous insufficiency results, and pulmonary embolism. Another important complication, of unknown incidence, is a psychological disturbance now being referred to as thromboneurosis.

Postphlebitic Syndrome

If all cases of deep venous thrombosis were diagnosed and treated immediately after the thrombus first formed, there would be few cases of the postphlebitic syndrome. As it is, venous insufficiency is not expected if only some of the muscular calf veins are involved. Severe cases follow proximal vein thrombosis. The clots usually lyse or recanalize, so that permanent, total obstruction of the affected vein is uncommon, and valves can easily be destroyed. With the loss of functional valves, contraction of leg muscles, as during walking, cannot effectively reduce the venous pressure. Persistent venous hypertension at the ankle, especially when the valves in the perforating veins are incompetent, leads to edema, stasis staining of the skin, stasis dermatitis, and stasis ulceration.

Clinical features of the postphlebitic syndrome vary from nearly inapparent to severely disabling. A sense of heaviness or vague discomfort in the affected leg, perhaps also the thigh, relieved by elevation of the limb, is fairly common; but pain sufficient to require strong analgesics is unusual. Severe pain suggests a cause other than the postphlebitic syndrome, except perhaps in a few patients who seem to have unusually painful stasis ulcers. The severity of skin changes ranges from minimal brownish discoloration to marked inflammation, with intradermal edema, oozing of exudate, and ultimately ulceration. Pruritis may lead to scratching, which further damages the skin. Chronic severe eczematoid changes may occur. Skin that regenerates as an ulcer heals may be atrophic, and with recurrent ulceration and healing, scarring can become prominent. Surrounding cellulitis may be mild or severe, and chronic low-grade inflammation often results in considerable induration of skin and soft tissues.

Stasis ulcers usually occur about the ankles, rarely above mid-leg level, almost never on the feet, except just below the malleoli. Ischemic ulcers associated with obstructive arterial disease are typically distal to the sites of stasis ulcers and are especially likely to occur on the toes. Pressure sores occur whenever compression of soft tissues interferes continuously with blood flow for a long enough time. These ulcers are a special case of ischemic necrosis, unrelated to venous insufficiency except to the extent that venous stasis may interfere with healing. Ulcers due to *vasculitis,* inflammation and obstruction of microvessels, can occur anywhere on the lower extremities, often where stasis ulcers are found, but venous insufficiency is not a cause.

Varicose veins can develop as a result of venous thrombosis. Following superficial thrombophlebitis, the vein may dilate from the increased pressure associated with destroyed valves and from weakening of the structures of the vein wall by the inflammatory process. With sufficient venous dilatation, even undamaged valves become incompetent. After deep venous thrombosis, valves in the deep veins often are destroyed, which leads to venous hypertension. This can cause dilatation of the perforating veins at the ankles, rendering them incompetent and predisposing to local stasis dermatitis and ulceration. Whether or not thrombosed deep veins recanalize, collateral flow develops in superficial veins. This flow may be great enough to dilate the superficial veins beyond the point where the valves can remain competent. This sequence of events can result in superficial varicosities which are secondary to deep venous thrombosis. (Primary varicose veins, associated with congenital absence of a normal complement of venous valves, are much more prevalent than secondary varicose veins.) The sites of missing or incompetent valves can be determined by careful tourniquet testing (Trendelenberg test), and the Doppler ultrasound probe can be useful in demonstrating reflux through incompetent valves in the deep and the superficial systems. Thrombosis with inflammation is common in superficial varicose veins, often in short segments at the ankle or just below the knee. Pulmonary embolism would be exceedingly rare in such cases.

Treatment of the postphlebitic syndrome depends on its manifestations. Mild cases may require nothing more than occasionally elevating the legs to empty the veins. Edema, dermatitis, and ulceration all respond, sometimes slowly, to persistent elevation of the legs, which works by eliminating venous hypertension. The use of well-fitted elastic support or, especially with oozing ulcers, an Unna-type boot, may allow improvement and ambulation. There is little place for surgery in the treatment of the postphlebitic syndrome. Most of the varicose veins that need removal are primary varicosities, but sometimes, and only when the deep veins are open, secondary superficial varicose veins need stripping, excision, or injection. Many of the more serious aspects of the postphlebitic syndrome, particularily stasis ulcers, can be prevented by the regular use of well-fitted elastic stockings. Excellent discussions of the complexities of the postphlebitic syndrome and of its management can be found in the literature.[4,24]

Thromboneurosis

The thromboneurosis syndrome has not been fully characterized. It might be described as recurring anxiety, fear, depression, continuing disability, or a combination of these, deriving from knowing or presuming a clot is or has been present. The reaction is usually out of proportion to the seriousness of the illness and not always relieved by appropriate and reasonable reassurance. Probably in most cases the diagnosis of a thrombotic disorder has not been established, and so many patients with this syndrome never have had a clot. The syndrome intensifies with recurrence of symptoms or signs that the patient, or a physician interprets as due to a clot. Phlebitis is feared if the symptoms are in the extremities, and embolism if in the chest, but the patient may have little understanding of these conditions. Victims of this syndrome may be seen in emergency rooms and admitted for anticoagulation, unless objective tests are done to exclude a thrombotic disorder. Many such admissions may occur without a firm diagnosis of thrombosis ever being made. There may be a compensation or insurance claim pending, particularly if an injury was sustained, and this compounds the difficulties. Most of these cases could be prevented if the first episode were accurately diagnosed and correctly treated. However, a real episode of thrombophlebitis and perhaps also pulmonary embolism may have occurred, and a variety of subsequent symptoms may be interpreted as recurrence. When this happens, hospitalization and anticoagulation may follow even if there is no new thrombosis, unless objective tests are done to clarify the diagnosis.

THE INNOCENT VARICOSE VEIN

Another source of anxiety for many patients, which is extremely common, is the uncomplicated varicose vein, especially in women who have undergone several pregnancies, and in older individuals. Most often, these varicosities appear without the clinical signs of deep vein insufficiency, but patients may ascribe to them a number of nonspecific symptoms like numbness, tightness, and weakness, even though such symptoms are generally quite innocent. Except for the occasional patients with recurrent, incapacitating, superficial phlebitis or cutaneous hemorrhage (both of which usually can be prevented with good elastic support), venous stripping and ligation are usually not required. Stripping in this situation is merely a cosmetic procedure.

It is important to dispel the notion of surgical necessity when confronted with a patient with innocent varicosities. Often, reassurance is enough. If the patient wants surgery for cosmetic reasons, one must make sure the varicosities are not secondary to occult deep vein incompetence. The tourniquet test is an excellent clinical tool for this purpose. In this examination, the patient's leg is raised in order to empty the veins. The patient is then asked to stand quickly, and venous filling time is carefully measured. This standing maneuver is repeated after venous emptying with a tourniquet applied at various levels of the extremity. The tourniquet is tight enough to compress superficial veins, but deep, and communicating veins remain patent. If the deep veins are competent, the tourniquet prevents retrograde venous filling, and filling usually requires at least 45 seconds. The more quickly the veins fill, the more the deep vein incompetence.

Patients who should be dissuaded from varicose vein stripping include: 1) those with deep vein incompetence, 2) women intending to become pregnant, and 3) older individuals and those with significant medical problems. In the first two categories, recurrence of varicosities after surgery is quite likely.

Pulmonary thromboembolism, the most serious complication of deep venous thrombosis, is considered in the next chapter.

REFERENCES

1. Hume M, Sevitt S, Thomas DP. *Venous Thrombosis and Pulmonary Embolism.* Cambridge, MA, Commonwealth Fund/Harvard University Press, 1970.
2. Widmer LK, Mall TH, Martin H. Epidemiology and sociomedical importance of peripheral venous disease. In Hobbs JT (ed). *The Treatment of Venous Disorders.* Philadelphia, JB Lippincott Company, 1977, pp 3–12.
3. Wessler S. Venous thromboembolism: Scope of the problem. In *Prophylactic Therapy of Deep Vein Thrombosis and Pulmonary Embolism:* Proceedings of National Heart and Lung Institute and American Heart Association conference, April 1975, NIH No.76-866, Department of Health, Education, and Welfare, pp 1–10.
4. Juergens JL, Spittell JA, Fairbairn JF (eds). *Peripheral Vascular Diseases,* ed 5. Philadelphia, WB Saunders Company, 1980.

5. *Prophylactic Therapy of Deep Vein Thrombosis and Pulmonary Embolism,* Proceedings of a conference sponsored by National Heart and Lung Institute and American Heart Association, April 1975. NIH No.78-866, Department of Health, Education and Welfare.

6. Root WS, Berlin NJ (eds). *Physiological Pharmacology,* vol 5. New York, Academic Press, 1974, pp 3–174.

7. Kazmier FJ, Spittel JA. Coagulation, thrombosis, anticoagulants, and fibrinolysis. In Juergens JL, Spittell JA, Fairbairn JF (eds). *Peripheral Vascular Diseases,* ed 5. Philadelphia, WB Saunders Company, 1980, pp 107–137.

8. Havig Ö. Deep vein thrombosis and pulmonary embolism: An autopsy study with multiple regression analysis of possible risk factors. *Acta Chir Scand* (suppl 478), 1977.

9. Gallus AS. ^{125}I-Fibrinogen leg scanning. In *Prophylactic Therapy of Deep Vein Thrombosis and Pulmonary Embolism:* Proceedings of National Heart and Lung Institute and American Heart Association conference, April 1975, NIH No.76-866, Department of Health, Education and Welfare, pp 77-99.

10. Nicolaides AN, Gordon-Smith I. The prevention of deep venous thrombosis. In Hobbs JT (ed). *The Treatment of Venous Disorders.* Philadelphia, JB Lipincott Company, 1977, pp 211–235.

11. Hume M, Sevitt S, Thomas DP. *Venous Thrombosis and Pulmonary Embolism.* Cambridge MA, Commonwealth Land/Harvard University Press, 1970, pp 136–137.

12. Robertson B. Diagnosis of deep venous thrombosis. *Acta Chir Scand,* 387:(suppl) 27, 1968.

13. O'Donnell TF, Abbott WM, Athanasoulis CA, et al. Diagnosis of deep venous thrombosis in the outpatient by venography. *Surg Gynecol Obstet* 150:69, 1980.

14. Sigel B, Popky GL, Wagner DK, et al. Comparison of clinical and Doppler ultrasound evaluation of confirmed lower extremity venous disease. *Surgery* 64:332, 1968.

15. Barnes RW, Wu KK, Woak JC. Fallibility of the clinical diagnosis of venous thrombosis. *JAMA* 234:605, 1975.

16. Lambie JM, Mahaffy RE, Barber DC, et al. Diagnostic accuracy in venous thrombosis *Br Med J* 2:142, 1970.

17. Hicks BH. The value of clinical criteria for epidemiologic diagnosis of deep venous thrombosis. *Milbank Mem Fund Q 50* (pt 2):161, 1972.

18. Cranley JJ, Canos AJ, Sull WJ. The diagnosis of deep venous thrombosis: Fallibility of clinical symptoms and signs. *Arch Surg* 111:34, 1976.

19. Cooperman M, Martin EW, Satiani B, et al. Detection of deep venous thrombosis by impedance plethysmography. *Am J Surg* 137:252, 1979.

20. Hume M. Risk factors and the epidemiology of venous thrombosis. In *Prophylactic Therapy of Deep Vein Thrombosis and Pulmonary Embolism.* Proceedings of National Heart and Lung Institute and American Heart Association conference, April 1975, NIH No.76-866, Department of Health, Education, and Welfare, p 18–27.

21. Homans J. Venous thrombosis and pulmonary embolism. *N Eng J Med* 236:196, 1947.

22. Bernstein EF (ed). *Noninvasive Diagnostic Techniques in Vascular Disease.* St. Louis, The CV Mosby Company, 1978.

23. Bernstein EF (ed). *Noninvasive Diagnostic Techniques in Vascular Disease,* ed 2, St Louis, The CV Mosby Company.

24. Hobbs JT (ed). *The Treatment of Venous Disorders.* Philadelphia, JB Lippincott Company, 1977.

25. Rabinov K, Paulin S. Roentgen diagnosis of venous thrombosis in the leg. *Arch Surg* 104:134, 1972.

26. Kerrigan GNW, Buchanan MR, Cade JF, et al. Investigation of the mechanism of false positive ^{125}I-labelled fibrinogen scans. *Brit J Haematol* 26:469, 1974.

27. Barnes RW, McDonald GB, Hamilton GW, et al. Radionuclide venography for rapid dynamic evaluation of venous disease. *Surgery* 73:706, 1973.

28. Hendin RE, Yao JST, Quinn JL III, et al. Radionuclide venography (RNV) in lower extremity venous disease. *J Nucl Med* 15:171, 1974.

29. Dean RH. Radionuclide venography and simultaneous lung scanning: Evaluation of clinical application. In Bernstein EF (ed). *Noninvasive Diagnostic Techniques in Vascular Disease.* St. Louis, The CV Mosby Company, 1978, pp 374–381.

30. Strandness DE Jr. Doppler ultrasonic techniques in vascular disease. In Bernstein EF (ed). *Noninvasive Techniques in Vascular Disease.* St. Louis, The CV Mosby Company, 1978, pp 11–22.

31. Barnes RW. Doppler ultrasonic diagnosis of venous disease. In Bernstein EF (ed). *Noninvasive Techniques in Vascular Disease.* St Louis, The CV Mosby Company, 1978, pp 344–350.

32. Sigel B, Felix WR, Popky GL, et al. Diagnosis of lower limb venous thrombosis by Doppler ultrasound technique. *Arch Surg* 104:174, 1972.

33. Strandness DE Jr, Sumner DS. Ultrasonic velocity detector in the diagnosis of thrombophlebitis. *Arch Surg* 104:180, 1972.

34. Barnes RW, Russell HE, Wu KK, et al. Accuracy of Doppler ultrasound in clinically suspected venous thrombosis of the calf. *Surg Gynecol Obstet* 143:425, 1976.

35. Sumner DS. Volume plethysmography in vascular disease: An overview. In Bernstein EF (ed). *Noninvasive Techniques in Vascular Disease.* St. Louis, The CV Mosby Company, 1978, pp 68–92.

36. Sumner DS. Mercury strain-gauge plethysmography. In Bernstein EF (ed). *Noninvasive Techniques in Vascular Disease.* St. Louis, The CV Mosby Company, 1978, pp 126–147.

37. Young DG Jr, Cox RH, Stoner EK, et al. Evaluation of quantitative venous plethysmography for continuous blood flow measurement: III. Blood flow determination in vivo. *Am J Phys Med* 46:1450, 1967.

38. Nyboer J. *Electrical Impedance Plethysmography,* ed 2. Springfield, Illinois, Charles C Thomas, 1970.

39. Anderson FA Jr, Peura RA, Penney BC, et al. Simultaneous mechanical and electrical impedance plethysmography. In *Proceedings of the Second Annual New England Bioengineering Conference,* vol 2. Elmsford, NY, Pergamon Press, 1974,

40. Wheeler HB. Impedance plethysmography: Theoretical and experimental basis. In Bernstein EF (ed). *Noninvasive Techniques in Vascular Disease.* St Louis, The CV Mosby Company, 1978, pp 112–125.

41. O'Donnell JA, Hobson RW II. Comparison of electrical impedance and mechanical plethysmography. *J Surg Res* 25:459, 1978.

42. Wheeler HB, O'Donnell JA, Anderson FA, et al. Bedside screening for venous thrombosis using occlusive impedance plethysmography. *Angiology* 26:199, 1975.

43. Hull R, van Aken WG, Hirsh J, et al. Impedance plethysmography using the occlusive cuff technique in the diagnosis of venous thrombosis. *Circulation* 53:696, 1976.

44. Wheeler HB. Impedance phlebography: The diagnosis of venous thrombosis by occlusive impedance plethysmography. In Bernstein EF (ed). *Noninvasive Techniques in Vascular Disease.* St Louis, The CV Mosby Company, 1978, pp 359–373.

45. Cranley JJ, Canos AJ, Sull WJ, et al. Phleborheographic technique for diganosing deep venous thrombosis of the lower extremities. *Surg Gynecol Obstet* 141:331, 1975.

46. Cranley JJ. Air plethysmography in venous disease: The phleborheograph. In Bernstein EF (ed). *Noninvasive Techniques in Vascular Disease,* St Louis, The CV Mosby Company, 1978, pp 148–156.

47. Cranley JJ. Diagnosis of deep venous thrombosis of the lower extremity by phleborheography. In Bernstein EF (ed). *Noninvasive Techniques in Vascular Disease,* St Louis, The CV Mosby Company, 1978, pp 351–358.

48. Collins GJ Jr, Rich NM, Andersen CA, et al. Phleborheographic diagnosis of venous obstruction. *Ann Surg* 189:25, 1979.

49. Kakkar VV. The diagnosis of deep vein thrombosis using the ^{125}I-fibrinogen test. *Arch Surg* 104:152, 1972.

50. Hirsh J, Gallus AS. ^{125}I-Labelled fibrinogen scanning. *JAMA* 233:970, 1975.

51. Rosenberg RD. Hypercoagulability and methods for monitoring anticoagulant therapy. In *Prophylactic Therapy of Deep Vein Thrombosis and Pulmonary Embolism:* Proceedings of National Heart and Lung Institute and American Heart Association conference, April 1975. NIH No.76-866, Department of Health, Education and Welfare, pp 28–42.

52. Walsh PN. Role of platelets in the pathogenesis of venous thrombosis. In *Prophylactic Therapy of Deep Vein Thrombosis and Pulmonary Embolism:* Proceedings of National Heart and Lung Institute and American Heart Association conference, April 1975. NIH No.76-866, Department of Health, Education, and Welfare, pp 50–61.

53. Qureshi MB, Fratkin MJ, Roberts PS. Advances in the diagnosis of venous thrombosis. *Prog Clin Pathol* 7:317, 1978.

54. Wilson JE. Diagnostic methods for deep venous thrombosis. *Arch Intern Med* 140:893, 1980.

55. Cooke ED, Pilcher MF. Deep vein thrombosis: Preclinical diagnosis by thermography. *Br J Surg* 61:971, 1974.

56. Berqvist D, Efsing HO, Torgil H. Thermography: A noninvasive method for diagnosis of deep vein thrombosis. *Arch Surg* 112:600, 1977.

57. Ell PJ, Deacon JM, Jarritt PH, et al. A comparison between technetium-99m plasmin and iodine-125 fibrinogen in the detection of deep vein thrombosis. *J Nucl Med* 20:633, 1979.

58. Davis HH II, Siegel BA, Welch MJ. Scintigraphic detection of an arterial thrombus with In-111-labelled autologous platelets. *J Nucl Med* 21:548, 1980.

59. Wheeler HB. Personal Communication.

60. Hull R, Hirsh J, Sackett DL, et al. Combined use of leg scanning and impedance plethysmography in suspected venous thrombosis. *N Engl J Med* 296:1497, 1977.

61. Hull R, Hirsh J, Sackett DL, et al. The value of adding impedance plethysmography to ^{125}I-fibrinogen leg scanning for the detection of deep vein thrombosis in high-risk surgical patients: A comparative study between patients undergoing general surgery and hip surgery. *Thromb Res* 15:227, 1979.

62. Watz R, Ek I, Bygdeman S. Noninvasive diagnosis of deep vein throm-

bosis. A comparison between thermography, plethysmography and phlebography. *Acta Med Scand* 206:463, 1979.

63. Foti MEG, Gurewich V. Fibrin degradation products and impedance plethysmography: Measurements in the diagnosis of acute deep vein thrombosis. *Arch Int Med* 140:903, 1980.

64. Nicolaides AN, Lewis JD. The management of deep venous thrombosis. In Hobbs JT (ed). *The Treatment of Venous Disorders.* Philadelphia, JB Lippincott Company, 1977, pp 238–239.

65. Wheeler HB. A modern approach to diagnosing deep venous thrombosis. *J Cardiovasc Med* 5:217, 1980.

66. *Thrombolytic Therapy in Thrombosis.* National Institutes of Health Consensus Development Conference Summary, vol 3, no 1, 1980.

67. Sherry S. Therapy of deep vein thrombosis and pulmonary embolism: Medical approach. In *Prophylactic Therapy of Deep Vein Thrombosis and Pulmonary Embolism:* Proceedings of National Heart and Lung Institute and American Heart Association conference, April 1975. NIH No.76-866, Department of Health, Education and Welfare, pp 127–136.

68. Jaques LB. An old drug with a new paradigm. *Science* 206:528, 1979.

69. Spaet TH. Heparin therapy. *JAMA* 244:1243, 1980.

70. Estes JW. Heparin in clinical practice. *Arch Int Med* 137:1362, 1977.

71. Gurewich V. Laboratory diagnosis of thrombosis. *Arch Int Med* 137:1362, 1977.

72. Wessler S. Medical management of venous thrombosis. *Ann Rev Med* 27:313, 1976.

73. Walker AM, Jick H. Predictors of bleeding during heparin therapy. *JAMA* 244:1209, 1980.

74. Deykin D. Warfarin therapy. *N Engl J Med* 283:691–694, 801–803, 1970.

75. Koch-Weser J, Sellers EM. Drug interactions with coumarin anticoagulants. *N Engl J Med* 285:487–498, 547–558, 1971.

76. Hull R, Delmore T, Genton E, et al. Warfarin sodium versus low-dose heparin in the long-term treatment of venous thrombosis. *N Engl J Med* 301:855, 1979.

77. Bynum LJ, Wilson JE III. Low-dose heparin therapy in the long-term management of venous thromboembolism. *Am J Med* 67:533, 1979.

78. Ashford A, Ross JW, Southgate P. Pharmacology and toxicology of a defibrinating substance from Malayan pit viper venom. *Lancet* 1:486, 1968.

79. Sharp AA, Warren BA, Paxton AM, et al. Anticoagulant therapy with a purified fraction of Malayan pit viper venom. *Lancet* 1:493, 1968.

80. Lowe GD, Campbell AF, Meek DR, et al. Subcutaneous ancrod in prevention of deep-vein thrombosis after operation for fractured neck of femur. *Lancet* 2:698, 1978.

81. Hirsh J, Genton E. Low-dose heparin prophylaxis for venous thromboembolism. In *Prophylactic Therapy of Deep Vein Thrombosis and Pulmonary Embolism:* Proceedings of National Heart and Lung Institute and American Heart Association conference, April 1975. NIH No.76-866, Department of Health, Education and Welfare, pp 183–206.

82. Kakkar VV. The current status of low-dose heparin prophylaxis of thrombophlebitis and pulmonary embolism. *World J Surg* 2:3, 1978.

83. Thomas DP. Heparin in the prophylaxis and treatment of venous thromboembolism. *Semin Hematol* 15:1, 1978,

84. Gurewich V, Nunn T, Kuriakose TTX, et al. Hemostatic effects of

uniform, low-dose subcutaneous heparin in surgical patients. *Arch Int Med* 138:41, 1978.

85. Wessler S. Biochemical rationale for low-dose heparin in deep venous thrombosis. In *Prophylactic Therapy of Deep Vein Thrombosis and Pulmonary Embolism:* Proceedings of National Heart and Lung Institute and American conference, April 1975. NIH No.76-866, Department of Health, Education and Welfare, pp 173–182.

86. Wessler S, Gitel SN. Low-dose heparin: Is the risk worth the benefit? *Am Heart J* 98:94, 1979.

87. Sevitt S, Gallagher NG. Prevention of venous thrombosis and pulmonary embolism in injured subjects: A trial of anticoagulant prophylaxis with phenindione in middle-aged and elderly patients with fractured necks of femur. *Lancet* 2:981, 1959.

88. Hume M, Sevitt S, Thomas DP. *Venous Thrombosis and Pulmonary Embolism.* Cambridge, MA, Commonwealth Fund/Harvard University Press, 1970, p 334–343.

89. Coventry MB, Nolan DR, Beckenbaugh RD. "Delayed" prophylactic anticoagulation: A study of results and complications in 2,012 total hip arthroplasties. *J Bone Joint Surg* (Am) 55:1487, 1973.

90. Salzman EW. Prevention of venous thromboembolism with drugs that alter platelet function. In *Prophylactic Therapy of Deep Vein Thrombosis and Pulmonary Embolism:* Proceedings National Heart and Lung Institute and American Heart Association conference, April 1975. NIH No.76-866, Department of Health, Education and Welfare, pp 149–157.

91. Weiss HJ. Antiplatelet therapy. *N Engl J Med* 298:1344–1347, 1403–1406, 1978.

92. Hirsh J. Antiplatelet drugs in thromboembolism. *Postgrad Med* 66:119, 1979.

93. Harris WH, Salzman EW, Athanasoulis CA, et al. Aspirin prophylaxis of venous thrombolism after total hip replacement. *N Engl J Med* 297:1246, 1977.

94. Bygdeman S (ed). Thrombotic diseases with reference to the use of dextrans. *Acta Chir Scand* 387(suppl): 1968.

95. Evarts CM, Feil EJ. Prevention of thromboembolic disease after elective surgery of the hip. *J Bone Joint Surg* 53-A:1271, 1971.

96. Langsjoen PH, Murray RA. Treatment of postsurgical thromboembolic complications. *JAMA* 218:855, 1971.

97. Collins REC. Physical methods of prophylaxis against deep vein thrombosis. In *Prophylactic Therapy of Deep Vein Thrombosis and Pulmonary Embolism:* Proceedings of National Heart and Lung Institute and Amercian Heart Association conference, April 1975. NIH No.76-866, Department of Health, Education and Welfare, pp 158–172.

98. Husni EA, Ximenes JOC, Goyette EM. Elastic support of the lower limbs in hospital patients. *JAMA* 214:1456, 1970.

99. Sabri S, Roberts VC, Cotton LT. Effects of externally applied pressure on the haemodynamics of the lower limb. *Br Med J* 3:503, 1971.

100. Ah-See AK, Arfors K-E, Berqvist D, et al. The haemodynamic and antithrombotic effects of intermittent pneumatic calf compression on femoral vein blood flow. *Acta Chir Scand* 142:1976.

101. Allenby F, Boardman L, Pflug JJ, et al. Effects of external pneumatic intermittent compression on fibrinolysis in man. *Lancet* 2:1412, 1973.

102. Knight MTN, Dawson R. Effect of intermittent compression of the arms on deep venous thrombosis in the legs. *Lancet* 2:1265, 1976.

103. Turpie AGG, Gallus AS, Beattie WS, et al. Prevention of venous thrombosis in patients with intracranial disease by intermittent pneumatic compression of the calf. *Neurology* 27:435, 1977.

104. Skillman JJ, Collins REC, Coe NP, et al. Prevention of deep vein thrombosis in neurosurgical patients: A controlled, randomized trial of external pneumatic compression boots. *Surgery* 83:354, 1978.

105. Coe NP, Collins REC, Klein LA, et al. Prevention of deep vein thrombosis in urological patients: A controlled randomized trial of low-dose heparin and external pneumatic compression boots. *Surgery* 83:230, 1978.

7 Pulmonary Thromboembolism

Marvin L. Sachs

Accurate diagnosis and prompt, effective treatment of venous thrombosis is necessary to prevent complications, but it is fear of pulmonary embolism much more than fear of the postphlebitic syndrome that generates a sence of urgency and tension. In one estimate, 50,000 of 300,000 patients hospitalized for pulmonary embolism in the United States in a year died.[1] Dalen and Alpert[2] estimated that there are more than 600,000 cases of symptomatic pulmonary embolism per year in the United States, with approximately 200,000 deaths. About half of the deaths are due to massive pulmonary embolism and, of those, perhaps two-thirds die within an hour, precluding antemortem diagnosis and starting of therapy, except in rare situations. Of all patients with symptomatic pulmonary embolism who survive for more than an hour and who are not treated, about 30% die; of those who are fully treated with anticoagulants and other appropriate therapy, the mortality is greatly reduced, to less than 10%, and the long-term prognosis is good.

Wide variations in reported incidence of pulmonary embolism in autopsy series can be accounted for, in good part, by the characteristics of the pool of patients from which the series derives and by the meticulousness of the search for the emboli in the pulmonary arteries. Estimates gleaned from autopsy studies are also subject to the difficulty of deciding in which cases the found emboli were incidental and not primary causes of death. Nevertheless, there is evidence that during the last four decades the number of deaths from pulmonary embolism has been increasing, adjusted for population changes (at least in England and Wales, also probably true for other Western countries). This may be due to an increase in numbers of older people, but the main cause appears to be iatrogenic: advances in medical science and technology have made it possible to keep many seriously ill or injured patients alive much longer.

Geographical differences in incidence of thromboembolism are of great interest. In Europe and North America, this condition is seen more often than in many countries of Asia and Africa, where the incidence of venous thrombosis of the lower extremities is also lower. In South Africa the incidence of thromboembolism is said to be more than four times as great among whites as among Bantus. These differences suggest that environmental and dietary factors, and habitual levels of physical activity, especially among the sick and injured, may be important.[3]

PATHOLOGICAL FEATURES

Infarction of the lung was described in the early nineteenth century, and soon after, the association with clots in the pulmonary arteries was made. By mid-century, Virchow had defined pulmonary thromboembolism pathologically and experimentally, had shown the association with clots in the lower extremities and recognized its broad importance.

Large, or major, emboli may be 1.5 cm in diameter and 50 cm long, and when coiled up in the pulmonary arteries can block off blood flow nearly completely. Multiple emboli are common, perhaps the rule. The larger emboli, which are the ones most likely to be fatal, come from the femoral and iliac veins. Smaller emboli from calf veins, much less likely to be fatal, may be found in lungs that also contain major emboli. Minor, or very small emboli, may not cause detectable symptoms and do not cause death acutely. Frequent recurrences of small emboli, perhaps especially of microemboli, however, can lead to pulmonary hypertension and cor pulmonale. After lodging in the proximal arterial tree, large emboli may break up and distribute themselves distally. Emboli of all sizes, particularly if recently formed, are effectively lysed in the lungs, often completely, but scarring and plaques may result.

When considering the source of large pulmonary emboli, one must keep in mind that most come from *silent* deep venous thrombosis. The embolus may have arisen in the limb that is asymptomatic rather than in the one that is swollen and tender. Thrombi do form in the veins of the pelvis, arm, head, and neck, and in the right atrium, but these rarely cause life-threatening pulmonary emboli. Microemboli in the lungs are associated with severe burns, anaphylactic shock, hemorrhage, trauma, surgery in which pump-oxygenations are used, large transfusions, bacterial endotoxins, and irreversible shock.

Probably not more than 10% of pulmonary emboli lead to pulmonary infarction. Infarcts are hemorrhagic and usually occur in peripheral lung fields, more often in lower than upper lobes, somewhat more on the right side than the left. The hemorrhagic feature, which may be more prominent than necrosis, is associated with the hemoptysis sometimes seen. Since hemorrhage clears quickly in cases with little necrosis, chest x-ray findings may be transitory.

The impact of pulmonary embolism depends primarily on the size of the embolus, or total mass of emboli, particularly with respect to the proportion of blocked right ventricular output. When all output is blocked, death is immediate. Usually, the clinical features of pulmonary embolism are ascribed to the hemodynamic effects of obstructing thrombi; however, evidence suggests that humoral mechanisms can result in significant vasoconstriction and bronchoconstriction. There is a direct correlation between the extent of increased mean pulmonary arterial pressure and amount of pulmonary arterial obstruction, in patients whose hearts and lungs are normal before embolism occurs. In patients with chronic cardiopulmonary disease, this correlation is poor, for some of these patients will already have pulmonary hypertension and right ventricular hypertrophy.[4] In general, patients with preexisting cardiopulmonary disease tolerate pulmonary embolism less well than patients with normal hearts and lungs.

In recent years, a widely used classification of pulmonary embolism severity, based on angiographic assesssment of the degree of pulmonary arterial obstruction by clot, separated patients with proved pulmonary embolism into two groups: those with massive embolism, and those with submassive embolism. *Massive* refers to cases in which there are obstructions, or significant filling defects, involving two or more lobar arteries, or an equivalent amount of emboli in other arteries; *submassive* refers to obstructions, or filling defects, in at least one segmental pulmonary artery, with the sum of defects being less than that for massive embolism.[5]

CLINICAL FEATURES AND DIAGNOSIS

Asymptomatic pulmonary thromboembolism ranges from a completely benign condition in which small clots, perhaps even medium-size clots, are screened out of the circulation by the lungs and rapidly lysed, to a presentation of cor pulmonale with right ventricular failure in a patient who developed pulmonary hypertension as a result of previously unsuspected recurrent embolism. In neither case is there an issue of early diagnosis and prompt treatment of the thromboembolic process.

The hotly debated clinical issue concerns *symptomatic pulmonary embolism;* more precisely, patients who develop clinical features suggestive of the serious possibility of pulmonary embolism. When suspicion is great, the decision to invoke the necessary diagnostic strategy is easily made; but when suspicion is light, it can be an agonizing decision to put the patient through complicated and expensive testing. An alert physician will consider pulmonary embolism when there is only slight suspicion. In deep venous thrombosis, relatively simple and inexpensive noninvasive studies are available for screening, ie, tests like Doppler and plethysmographic studies that can be done in the office. Currently, the minimal screening test for embolism is the perfusion lung scan, or some would say ventilation and perfusion lung scans, and a chest x-ray study. Eventually, a simpler screening study, perhaps impedance plethysmography, may be found to be equally reliable, but this remains to be demonstrated.

Symptoms and Signs

Valuable knowledge was gained concerning the clinical features of pulmonary thromboembolism in the two-phase multicenter study known as the Urokinase Pulmonary Embolism Trial (UPET)[5,6] and the Urokinase-Streptokinase Pulmonary Embolism Trial (USPET).[7] A major conclusion found was that there is no specific combination of symptoms and signs for diagnosing pulmonary embolism, and the symptoms and signs most often encountered are nonspecific.

The findings of UPET and USPET concerning clinical features in 327 patients with angiographically proved pulmonary embolism are summarized and discussed by Bell et al[8] and shown in Table 7-1. From these findings, it might be argued that in the *absence* of chest pain, dyspnea, apprehension, and a respiratory rate greater than 16/min, pulmonary embolism is unlikely. Few physicians would be comfortable excluding the diagnosis on this basis if serious suspicion developed for other reasons; but if suspicion is minimal and these symptoms and signs are absent, one might justify avoiding a full-scale diagnostic work-up. The quality of the history, however, can be crucial. Patients may deny shortness of breath or difficulty in breathing, yet, when closely questioned, they may admit to a definite change in exercise tolerance with at least slight breathlessness when climbing stairs.

Table 7-1
Signs and Symptoms of 327 Patients with Pulmonary Embolism

	Total Series N = 327 %	Massive Emboli N = 197 %	*vs*	Submassive Emboli N = 130 %
Symptoms				
Chest pain	83	79		89*
Pleuritic	74	67		82**
Non-pleuritic	14	16		13
Dyspnea	84	85		82
Apprehension	59	65**		50
Cough	53	53		52
Hemoptysis	30	23		40**
Sweats	27	29		23
Syncope	13	20†		4
Signs				
Respirations >16/min	92	95		87
Rales	58	57		60
↑S_2P	53	58*		45
Pulse >100/min	44	48		38
Temperature >37.8°C	43	43		42
Phlebitis	32	36		26
Gallop	34	39**		25
Diaphoresis	36	42**		27
Edema	24	23		25
Murmur	28	28		27
Cyanosis	19	25†		9
Predisposing Condition				
Current venous disease	45	47		42
Immobilization	58	60		55
Congestive heart failure and chronic lung disease	38	36		40
Malignant neoplasms	6	8		5

*Statistically significant ($p < .05$)
**Statistically significant ($p < .01$)
†Statistically significant ($p < .001$)
(Based on chi-square test with continuity correction)
Reprinted with permission from Bell WR, Simon TL, DeMets DL: The clinical features of submassive and massive pulmonary emboli. *Am J Med* 62:355, 1977 (as corrected by personal communication with Dr DeMets).

Most patients who are ultimately shown to have pulmonary embolism present with several symptoms and signs which, although nonspecific, may singly or in combination suggest this diagnosis. Certain findings suggest massive embolism in patients who do not have significant cardiopulmonary disease: syncope, shock, enhanced pulmonic component of the second heart sound, cyanosis, and S_3 and S_4 gallop sounds. Pleural pain occurs more often in submassive embolism.

Factors which predispose to pulmonary thromboembolism are the same as those which predispose to deep venous thrombosis. The highest incidence is in sick, immobilized patients; infrequently the condition occurs in healthy young people, usually in association with an injury, operation or pregnancy. *Idiopathic* cases are reported in young people without identified predisposition,[9] but these are rare.

Laboratory Findings[10-12]

There is no simple screening laboratory test that reliably separates patients with acute pulmonary embolism from those with other illnesses. The white blood cell count is one of the more revealing tests, since it rarely is above 15,000 and, in about half of the patients with angiographically proven acute pulmonary embolism, it is less than 10,000. Platelet counts are almost always normal. Serum lactic dehydrogenase (LDH) is elevated in about 80% of such patients; however, the test is nonspecific, even when combined with normal serum glutamic-oxalacetic transaminase (SGOT). Measurement of serum bilirubin is not diagnostically helpful; when elevated, cardiac failure is likely.

Arterial Oxygen Tension

Since emboli in the pulmonary arterial tree cause blood to bypass ventilated alveoli and usually lead to tachypnea and bronchospasm, a decrease in the oxygen tension of systemic arterial blood (P_aO_2) would be expected. This certainly occurs in most patients with pulmonary embolism, but it also occurs in many other cardiopulmonary diseases. Many elderly patients who are not acutely ill normally have a P_aO_2 of 80 mm Hg or less (measured with patient breathing room air); whereas, normal P_aO_2 usually is considered 90 mm Hg or more. Obviously, a low P_aO_2 is not specific and cannot be used independently to establish a diagnosis of pulmonary embolism. But, is the P_aO_2 sensitive enough to exclude pulmonary embolism? It is relatively sensitive and in the past was suggested as a possible exclusionary test when greater than 80 mm Hg.[11] More extensive data from UPET,[5] however, have shown that P_aO_2 of 80 mm Hg or more was found in 11.5% of patients with proved pulmonary embolism. If the P_aO_2 is 90 mm Hg or more, the likelihood of pulmonary embolism is small but certainly not zero. A word of caution: the accurate measurement of P_aO_2 is demanding, and laboratory errors are easily made. The equipment must be in good order and the oxygen electrode calibrated before each determination.

Electrocardiogram[13]

Each patient suspected of having pulmonary embolism should have an electrocardiogram (ECG), not because it will make or exclude the diagnosis, which it cannot do, but because it may reveal cardiac problems that must be recognized, particularly myocardial infarction. In UPET, 87% of the patients with proved emboli had some kind of ECG abnormality, but none of these deviations from normal, singly or in combination, is diagnostically specific. Various arrhythmias were seen, but the great majority of patients had sinus rhythm. Left axis deviation was seen more often than right axis deviation. Clockwise rotation was seen in 28% of the patients, right bundle branch block (complete or incomplete) in 16%, and the S_1-Q_3-T_3 pattern of acute cor pulmonale in only 11%. In patients free of cardiopulmonary disease before an acute episode, ECG changes suggesting right ventricular strain signal the possibility of massive embolism.

Chest X-ray Studies

Standard posteroanterior and lateral chest roentgenograms can suggest pulmonary embolism but cannot establish it or exclude it. Chest films naturally are more likely to be abnormal in older patients with chronic lung or heart disease than in younger patients without these conditions who are suspected of having pulmonary embolism.

Fleischner[14] organized abnormalities seen in patients with pulmonary embolism. They include: elevation and decreased excursion of the diaphragm; basal atelectasis; pleural effusions; reduction in caliber of pulmonary vasculature on occluded side and increased filling on unoccluded side; dilatation of hilar arteries; dilatation of right atrium, superior vena cava, azygos vein, and right ventricle. Rarely would all these features be found in one patient. The most common UPET findings were pulmonary infiltration and high diaphragm, each occurring in 41% of the patients (not necessarily the same patients) with proved pulmonary embolism. Pleural effusion occurred in 28%, plump pulmonary arteries in 23%, atelectasis in 20%, focal oligemia in 15% and right ventricular enlargement in only 5%. Pulmonary infarction is likely to be associated with an infiltrate, classically a curved shadow along a pleural surface. Again, classical findings are uncommon, and infiltrates tend to be of a variety of configurations and densities, depending in part on the relative amount of hemorrhage.[15] Overall, the chest x-ray signs most suggestive of pulmonary embolism are infiltrates, elevated hemidiaphragm, pleural effusion, and atelectasis,[5,16] but even if all occur together they do not reliably make the diagnosis.

Radionuclide Lung Scans[17]

Perfusion lung scans for demonstrating aberrations in blood flow in parts of the pulmonary vasculature were introduced less than 20 years ago.[18] The first isotope used was ^{131}I, but now ^{99m}Tc is more commonly used, attached to macroaggregated albumin particles or to albumin microspheres. Scintigrams are made with a gamma camera. The tagged albumin particles are trapped in the pulmonary microvessels in proportion to the amount of blood flow through each part of the lung. Obstruction of a pulmonary arterial branch, as by an embolus, reduces blood flow to the lung tissue supplied by that branch. Thus, less of the radionuclide accumulates in this region of the lung, and this deficit shows up as a defect in the scintigram, or scan. Careful attention to technique is important. At least four views, anterior, posterior, and both laterals, should be taken; but there are important advantages to taking six views, adding both posterior obliques. Usually, perfusion lung scans are interpreted as being normal or as suggestive of a low, moderate or high probability of pulmonary embolism. Some authorities eliminate the category of moderate probability.

Perfusion lung scans are notoriously nonspecific, abnormalities being found in patients with almost every known kind of lung disease, including chronic obstructive pulmonary disease and pneumonia. Therefore, even a high probability scan is not diagnostic for pulmonary embolism. Since scans should always be compared with chest roentgenograms taken concurrently, the finding of perfusion defects where there are no abnormalities of the chest film enhances the specificity, at least for low-probability scans, but not sufficiently for reliable diagnosis of embolism.[19]

The high sensitivity of perfusion lung scans makes them of great practical value. A study of good quality will pick up even small pulmonary emboli, some that are missed even by pulmonary arteriography. Thus, a clearly normal perfusion scan is a reasonable basis for excluding the diagnosis of pulmonary embolism.[20] Keep in mind, however, that interpretation of perfusion scans is substantially subjective and associated with a rather high degree of inter-observer disagreement.[21] One would expect more consistent interpretations when scans are considered normal than when the degree of abnormality is at issue.

To enhance the specificity of lung scanning, ventilation scans are often done along with perfusion scans. The gas most often used is xenon (usually ^{133}Xe, but ^{127}Xe, which provides better imaging resolution, is available). Krypton (^{81m}Kr) has some advantages over xenon, but is expensive, and is not always readily available. An image of the lungs, taken after a single breath of the radioactive gas, shows regions of low activity, or poorly ventilated lung tissue. Valuable additional information is obtained by rebreathing the radioactive gas in a closed system until equilibrium of gas distribution occurs, then taking washout images. The gas rapidly disappears from portions of the lung that are normally ventilated, but it is trapped in regions with poor ventilation. Background emissions from trapped technetium are avoided, and better scintigrams are obtained, if ^{133}Xe is used when the ventilation scan precedes the perfusion scan. There are, however, advantages to doing the perfusion scan first, and one must be weighed against the other. For example, if the perfusion scan is normal, there is no need for a ventilation scan, and if it is abnormal, the location of defects can indicate the best projections for ventilation scanning.

Combination ventilation-perfusion scintigraphy, often referred to as V/Q lung scan, usually is analyzed in terms of *match* or *mismatch.* For this analysis, the ventilation and perfusion scans must be done one right after the other, and not separated by hours. Transitory abnormalities in the scans often occur (due to mucous plugs in bronchial branches, or to bronchospasm), which could lead to false impression of mismatch and diagnosis of pulmonary embolism.

In general, when the ventilation-scan defect and the perfusion-scan defect are in the same place (V/Q match), pulmonary embolism is very unlikely; and when the ventilation scan is normal and the perfusion scan abnormal (V/Q mismatch), especially with a normal chest x-ray study done at the time, pulmonary embolism is likely. Unfortunately, the situation is not always simple. The probability of correct diagnosis of pulmonary embolism by V/Q scanning depends on how many scan defects there are, how large they are, which of corresponding perfusion and ventilation defects is larger, and how each defect correlates with the standard chest x-ray study.[22,23]

The ventilation-perfusion scan combination is most helpful when the ventilation scan and chest x-ray study are normal and there are large perfusion defects. In this case, the probability that pulmonary embolism occurred is 90% or more. When the two scans match in patients with obstructive lung disease, there is a low probability of pulmonary embolism, perhaps less than 10%.

Pulmonary Angiography

Although visualization of the pulmonary vasculature has been done for nearly half a century, it is only in the past two decades that systematic studies have been used to define findings in cases of pulmonary embolism. Current technique involves the following: 1) a catheter is introduced into a peripheral vein and advanced through the right side of the heart into the main pulmonary arterial trunk, then, as necessary (often guided by the location of defects on the perfusion scan) into one or more of the pulmonary arterial branches; 2) contrast dye is injected selectively in each arterial site chosen for study; and 3) the opacification produced is rapidly filmed in different projections, as appropriate, often with magnification. An experienced angiographer and relatively sophisticated equipment are needed. Fatalities from the procedure are rare and morbidity is low, but it is not a totally benign study. The results are not always definitive, especially in patients with old or chronic heart or lung disease, but when clearly positive for emboli, pulmonary angiography provides the only absolute antemortem diagnosis now possible. Small emboli can be missed, but these are not likely in themselves to be clinically important, except to the extent that they might presage recurrence of embolization.[24]

Figure 7-1 shows an example of a diagnostically convincing pulmonary arteriogram. As is true of venograms, the most specific finding is an intraluminal filling defect. A variety of other findings occur, including abrupt cut-off of an arterial branch, localized oligemia, asymmetry of flow, reduction in caliber of vessels, plaques and webbing—some of which reflect old embolism or other disease. Expert interpretation is needed and even experts tend to agree with each other on reviewing the same angiograms.[21]

At the present time, pulmonary angiography is the only study accepted for resolving the diagnosis when pulmonary embolism is suspected and other studies fail to point strongly in a positive or negative direction. This poses a serious problem, since probably not more than 20% of the hospitals in the United States are fully staffed and equipped to do pulmonary angiograms reliably and whenever needed.

Search for Deep Venous Thrombosis

Since the great majority of pulmonary emboli come from the deep veins of the lower extremitites, and since lower-extremity deep venous thrombosis may be present even when the emboli formed elsewhere, it is rational to do noninvasive venous studies, such as plethysmography or Doppler ultrasound examinations. If pulmonary embolism is strongly

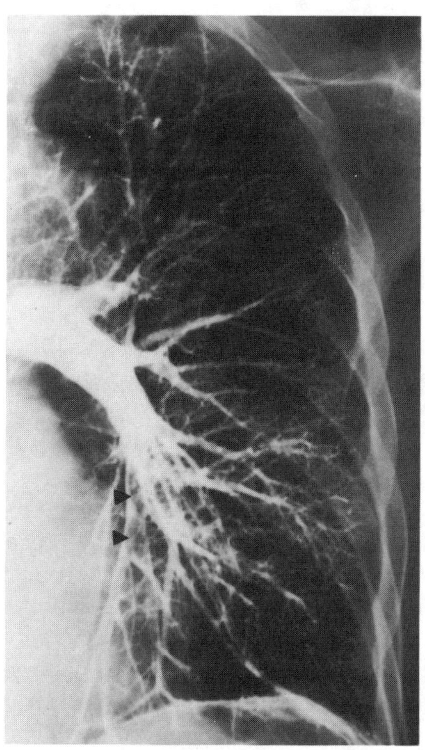

Figure 7-1 Pulmonary arteriogram. Markers point to intraluminal filling defects, which establish the diagnosis of pulmonary embolism. (Radiograph courtesy of Dr E.J. Ring, Hospital of the University of Pennsylvania, Philadelphia.)

suspected and these studies are positive, they help make the diagnosis, but when they are negative they do not overcome a strong suspicion of embolism. The exact role of these venous studies in the diagnosis of pulmonary embolism remains to be worked out, but they probably will be especially valuable, along with venography, in hospitals where pulmonary angiography is not available.

Diagnostic Strategies[22,25-27]

Current controversy among authorities concerning the wisest strategy for diagnosing pulmonary embolism suggests it would be imprudent and misleading to select a single scheme as best. A thorough clinical assessment in advance of ordering specific tests is absolutely necessary to identify the risk factors, and to decide if pulmonary embolism is suspected and, if so, the level of that suspicion.

Identified factors that predispose to deep venous thrombosis must be integrated with symptoms and signs, however nonspecific, that suggest pulmonary embolism, particularly unexpected breathlessness and even slight tachypnea. In a patient with such a clinical picture, suspicion is heightened by a normal white blood cell count, a normal chest x-ray study, and an electrocardiogram that does not suggest myocardial infarction but has one or more of the abnormalities known to occur with pulmonary embolism. Arterial oxygen tension of less than 90 mm Hg is consistent with the suspicion. An abnormal perfusion scan in such a case makes the diagnosis highly likely unless there is preexisting heart or lung disease, when a normal ventilation scan would confirm the suspicion. Alternatively, an abnormal impedance plethysmogram or venous Doppler study might persuade the clinician to treat for pulmonary embolism. This hypothetical case illustrates the kind of process that leads to a decision to treat without doing pulmonary angiography.

Probably the most widely accepted, simple strategy is promptly to get an electrocardiogram, standard chest x-ray study and perfusion lung scan in all cases where pulmonary embolism is suspected. A normal perfusion scan would be accepted as excluding pulmonary embolism. A high-probability perfusion scan would lead to a ventilation scan, and if normal, the patient would be treated for pulmonary embolism. Other lung scan findings lead to pulmonary angiography. This is an oversimplified statement of the clinical realities. This approach, when followed, it has been estimated, will require pulmonary angiography be done in only 36% of patients with pulmonary embolism and in only 11% of patients incorrectly suspected of pulmonary embolism. Not everyone follows a strategy that yields this incidence of pulmonary angiography. Even in sophisticated medical centers, where the technique is readily available and there is no shortage of expertise, the proportion of patients treated for pulmonary embolism who have pulmonary angiography ranges from about 15% to about 75%.[28]

It is sometimes easier to focus on the issue of overlooking or missing a diagnosis, especially of a dangerous condition, than on the issue of making the diagnosis when the condition does not exist. Concerning pulmonary embolism, the latter has aroused lively debate,[26,29] which has been centered around differing interpretations of the value of individual diagnostic studies for establishing the diagnosis, particularly in previously healthy people. Among the dangers to the patient of a false diagnosis are: the risk of bleeding induced by therapy with anticoagulants, or thrombolytic agents which can cause significant morbidity and even fatality; the burden of having such a serious diagnosis in one's medical history, and its consequences; difficulty in obtaining life insurance; and expensive hospital and post-hospital medical care. Perfect diagnostic discrimination is not to be expected, and good medical judgment may in some cases lead to treatment for probable pulmonary embolism; therefore, it is wiser in some cases to be clear with the patient, and in the written record, that the diagnosis was not proved.

TREATMENT

Heparin, in full anticoagulation dosage, is the keystone of treatment for pulmonary embolism. The main purpose of anticoagulation is prevention of additional thrombus formation and of recurrent embolization, which allows time for natural fibrinolytic processes to work. Heparin may also slightly enhance fibrinolysis, and it seems to influence restoration of cardiopulmonary function after massive embolism.

Administration of heparin should begin as soon as serious suspicion of pulmonary embolism develops and be continued while diagnostic tests are underway. An intravenous bolus of 5000 units should be given immediately and repeated every four hours. If pulmonary embolism is excluded, heparin is stopped; if it is confirmed, continuous intravenous infusion may be preferable.

When massive embolism is suspected, especially if the patient is in shock and in desperate condition, an initial immediate bolus of 10,000 to 15,000 units, should be given (and at least 60,000 units will be needed in the first 24 hours of treatment). Such patients need intensive supportive therapy. Oxygen, sometimes given with positive pressure, usually is required. Hypotension is managed by cautious use of vasopressors and careful regulation of fluid load. A central venous pressure line may be helpful. Use of a rapid-acting digitalis preparation may be justified, although it will not always help right ventricular failure. Sometimes aminophylline is useful. An indwelling catheter is necessary to monitor urine output. Constipation should be avoided.

Closed-chest cardiac massage may be effective in improving desperately ill patients with pulmonary embolism, probably by breaking up large clots in the proximal pulmonary arteries so that the fragments are distributed distally, allowing more blood to flow through, improving oxygenation and reducing the strain on the right ventricle. A conflict arises, however, when thrombolytic agents are used within about ten days of cardiac massage. They can be dangerous, at least when the massage was vigorous enough to cause rib fractures.

For these very sick patients, then, thrombolytic therapy is a serious option, and though much discredited, pulmonary embolectomy should not be totally abandoned.

Thrombolytic Therapy[5,30–33]

The administration of streptokinase or urokinase can hasten lysis of thrombi in deep veins or in the pulmonary arteries. Thus, these agents are extremely attractive for first-line therapy of thrombophlebitis and pulmonary embolism. That they have not yet been fully accepted, despite having such a highly desirable effect, attests to the level of concern about their safety, and no doubt to lack of familiarity with them among many physicians. Nevertheless, thrombolytic therapy must be recognized as an important advance although there is still much disagreement concerning its clinical indications.

There is much disagreement about the indications for thrombolytic therapy, ranging from declarations that there are not indications to advocacy of use in nearly all cases of deep venous thrombosis and pulmonary embolism that present no strong contraindications.

At this time, diagnosis of the following conditions justifies serious consideration for the therapeutic use of thrombolytic agents: iliofemoral thrombophlebitis, especially with extensive clotting; axillary-subclavian venous thrombosis, which can lead to long-term significant disability; and massive pulmonary embolism, especially if the patient is doing poorly after an hour or so of intensive conventional treatment.

Streptokinase is available in the United States under the trade names Streptase and Kabikinase. It is a non-enzymatic protein derived from cultures of streptococci. It forms a complex with plasminogen, and this activator complex converts plasma plasminogen to plasmin, which digests fibrin and leads to thrombolysis. *Urokinase,* available under the trade name Abbokinase, is an enzymatically active protein, commercially prepared from cultures of human fetal renal cells, which acts directly to split plasminogen to form plasmin. Pyrogenic reactions occur but they usually are not severe. Streptokinase is antigenic, urokinase is not. Retreatment with streptokinase within six months should be avoided, but treatment with urokinase can be repeated whenever needed. Urokinase is very expensive, a relative drawback, but the seriousness of the conditions for which it might be prescribed, in many cases, justifies the cost.

Standard regimens for the use of these agents have been established. For streptokinase, an initial loading dose of 250,000 IU in normal saline or 5% glucose is given intravenously over 30 minutes, followed by continuous intravenous infusion of 100,000 IU/hr for 24 to 72 hours (usually 24 hours for pulmonary embolism, sometimes longer for extensive deep vein thrombosis). Urokinase, used to treat pulmonary embolism, is given intravenously with a loading dose of 2000 IU per pound of body weight given over 10 minutes, followed by continuous intravenous infusion at a rate of 2000 IU per pound of body weight per hour for 12 hours. An active fibrinolytic state has been achieved if the thrombin time (in seconds) has been prolonged for two to five times the normal control value. Whole-blood euglobulin lysis time and prothrombin time are also used to monitor therapy. Before treatment, laboratory tests are used primarily to discover a preexisting hemostatic defect, during treatment to show that a lytic state has been reached, and after treatment to define a baseline for the use of heparin, which must follow to complete the therapy.

Thrombolysis can be effectively induced more completely and rapidly if the emboli, or thrombi in veins, are fresh. If treatment is not started until five days after embolism, or if the emboli were already about five or more days old, the results are not as good.

The UPET and USPET showed that thrombolytic therapy hastens lysis of emboli and effects a more rapid return toward normal of cardiopulmonary function than does heparin alone. The frequency of hemorrhagic complications, however, was high, mostly minor or easily controlled, but a few serious. If patients with preexisting risk of bleeding are excluded from those treated with thrombolytic agents, incidence of hemorrhagic complications will be reduced. Patients considered at risk are: those who are postpartum, have had major surgery or deep biopsies, or external cardiac massage within a week to ten days; those with intracranial disorders or an active bleeding site; those who recently had lumbar puncture, thoracentesis, paracentesis, or puncture of a blood vessel not controllable by external compression; those with severe hypertension, severe liver or kidney disease, bacterial endocarditis, or recent trauma with possible internal injuries; and those with uncorrected bleeding disorders. Excessive bleeding during treatment may require transfusion and discontinuation of the fibrinolytic activators. The antidotes are epsilon aminocaproic acid or kallikrein inactivator.

Because of the potential for bleeding complications, and because full proof is lacking that thrombolytic therapy reduces mortality, it is hardly surprising that this therapy has not been firmly established.[34] Cogent arguments can be made on both sides of the question of whether or not pulmonary embolism should be treated with fibrinolytic drugs.[35,36] More data will be needed to settle the point. Continuing comparison of the relative values of heparin and fibrinolytic therapies is needed so that specific indications for the newer drugs can be sharpened.

The use of activators of thrombolysis does not prevent the subsequent formation of thrombi, which may become emboli. Therefore, these agents should be followed by full anticoagulation with heparin. When the thrombolytic agent is discontinued, the partial thromboplastin time is followed until it falls to twice normal control. Then, continuous intravenous infusion of heparin is started, maintaining the PTT at this point of prolongation. Heparin usually is continued for about ten days, and during the last part of this period an oral agent like warfarin is added, planning an overlap with heparin of at least five days (as was described in the section on treatment of deep venous thrombosis). The duration of treatment with an oral anticoagulant following pulmonary embolism has not been established, but its continuation for six months or more seems reasonable, if control can be satisfactorily maintained. In some cases, where there is a known persisting predisposing factor, anticoagulation may have to be continued indefinitely.

Surgical Treatment

Attempts have been made to extract thrombi from pulmonary arteries by the use of suction or balloon catheters.[37] Although at times successful, this approach is not predictably reliable, and there are risks of cardiac damage and arrhythmia. The main surgical treatment is pulmonary embolectomy,[38] first reported in 1908 by Trendelenberg. A successful case was not recorded until 1924. Only relatively recently has some control of operative mortality been achieved, largely because of the availability of cardiopulmonary bypass. The indications for pulmonary embolectomy are controversial, but generally the procedure is seen as a desperate measure to save the life of a patient in shock due to massive pulmonary embolism. An agonizing problem: the clearer the indication for this procedure, the less likely the patient is to survive it. Some authorities doubt that pulmonary embolectomy has any place in the treatment of massive embolism, but others recognize a limited role, at least in those medical centers with superb and relevant professional and technical facilities that can be mobilized rapidly to handle such an emergency.

Interruption of the vena cava is not a treatment of pulmonary embolism but is a measure designed to prevent recurrence. It will be discussed below.

PROPHYLAXIS

Since 75% to 90% of thrombi that become pulmonary emboli arise in the deep veins of the lower extremities and the iliac veins, prevention of pulmonary embolism is largely the same as that of deep venous thrombosis.[39]

Kakkar et al[40] studied the use of a low-dose heparin regimen in preventing death from pulmonary embolism in postoperative patients. More than 4000 patients were included in the trial; approximately half were in the control group. The other half received 5000 units of heparin subcutaneously two hours before surgery and every eight hours thereafter for seven days. Cause of death was determined by autopsy. The study showed the group receiving heparin to have a statistically significant lower death rate from pulmonary embolism than did the control group. This is the largest such trial ever attempted, and it is not likely to be replicated soon. It should serve as a guide to all those who accept the conclusion. Thoughtful discussions on both sides of the question of the validity of this trial have been published.[41–44] Whether or not one accepts the *proof* that low-dose heparin reduces mortality from pulmonary embolism in patients undergoing major surgery, there is little doubt that its prophylactic use can prevent thrombophlebitis. Also, it is reasonable to assume this will reduce the frequency of pulmonary embolism.[45] As mentioned before, low-dose heparin has not been significantly helpful in cases of major bone surgery or urologic surgery, and it may be unacceptable for neurosurgery or eye surgery. There is some value to giving it preoperatively, perhaps during the whole time an inactive patient is being prepared for surgery.[46] Increased bleeding in wounds is a risk, which can be minimized by a dosage regimen of 5000 units subcutaneously every 12 hours.

All of the other methods of prophylaxis mentioned in the section on deep venous thrombosis apply in the prevention of pulmonary thromboembolism. Interruption of the inferior vena cava applies exclusively to prophylaxis of pulmonary embolism.

Interruption of Great Veins

The logic of blocking the venous channel through which an embolus must pass en route to the lungs is inescapable, but the advantages of so doing are difficult to weigh against the disadvantages. Homans advised tying off the common femoral vein[47] and later suggested ligating the inferior vena cava (IVC).[48] When disturbing complications of abrupt complete interruption of the IVC arose, a variety of procedures for partial interruption were developed. Subsequently, to avoid the need for general anaesthesia and major surgery, interest has grown in the use of devices placed in the IVC by a transvenous route.

Common femoral vein ligation, which can be done with local anaesthesia, is generally unpopular in the United States, but it has been used in patients too ill for major surgery.[49] This procedure must be done on both sides because of the likelihood that deep venous thrombosis will involve both lower extremities. Although at first glance it may seem a simple procedure, it requires substantial experience to sort out accurately the variable venous anatomy. The ligature must be placed proximal to the entry of the profunda femoris, distal to the circumflex and greater saphenous veins, and just distal to a large branch, in order not to leave a cul-de-sac with poor flow. Opinions differ concerning the incidence of resulting long-term, significant, lower-extremity venous insufficiency. An important limitation is the need to demonstrate that all thrombus is distal to the common femoral vein.

Inferior vena cava ligation produces impressive circulatory disturbances, including acute reduction in venous return and in cardiac output, and increase in distal venous pressure. On the average, the operative moratility was higher than with IVC plication, 14.3% compared with 9.9% respectively in one thorough review of the literature.[50] A wide range of mortality was reported, however, as well as variation in incidence of recurrent embolism, probably because of differences in patient selection. The indications for ligation of the IVC have been narrowing, and now are generally limited to these situations: septic emboli, not controlled by medical therapy; reduction in pulmonary arterial perfusion because of multiple small emboli; failure of IVC plication to prevent recurrence of embolism; paradoxical embolism to the systemic arterial circulation (as occurs, for example, through a patent foramen ovale).

Partial vena caval interruption began with suture-filter and suture-plication techniques. These methods, and the use of staples for plication, have been abandoned largely because the sutures and staples tend to pull out, and because thrombosis progresses through the sutures. Several clips have been devised to be placed around the IVC. The Adams-DeWeese serrated clip with one smooth edge, which creates several separated small channels, seems most favored. Blood continues to flow through the clipped segment, and all but very small emboli are stopped. Indications for its use will vary to some extent but will generally cover these situations: an episode of proved pulmonary embolism in a patient who cannot be treated with full anticoagulation; recurrent, proved pulmonary embolism after full anticoagulation for more than three or four days; massive pulmonary embolism despite well-established adequate anticoagulation; and when pulmonary embolectomy has been done. Clipping has been done in cases of iliofemoral venous thrombosis with one episode of pulmonary embolism even when it occurred before anticoagulation was established, but the morbidity and mortality of the procedure preclude its use routinely in such cases. A dilemma exists. Patients most prone to recurrent venous thrombosis and pulmonary embolism, such as those in heart failure, are most at risk when subjected to an operation to interrupt the IVC. Transluminally inserted vena caval filters help to resolve this dilemma.[37] Those first devised were unsuccessful. They were attached to the end of a catheter and intended for temporary use. The first transvenous approach to introduce a permanent filter was reported in 1967 by Mobin-Uddin and his colleagues.[51] The early version of the Mobin-Uddin umbrella filter sometimes migrated, but an enlarged version (28 mm in diameter) with barbed hooks has a very low incidence of migration and is associated with few incidences of recurrence of pulmonary embolism.[52] The small openings in the umbrella usually are closed off within a week. Another important device placed transvenously is the Kimray-Greenfield filter.[53] A cone-shaped cage, it has the advantage of being able to trap a large mass of thrombus without blocking flow completely. Although it may let a few more small clots pass than will the umbrella filter, follow-up studies show that some vena caval flow persists in 97% of the cases.

Transvenous insertion of vena caval filters is a major advance but the exact role it should play is uncertain. Originally justified to replace IVC ligation or plication in high-risk patients, it is thought of more frequently as being appropriate for patients who should easily tolerate the IVC clipping operation. Currently, the difficulty of ensuring proper placement of these filters is a major concern. For example, they have been put into renal and common iliac veins; and they cannot be removed, except by a major surgical procedure. Like IVC ligation or clipping, they are useless if the emboli are coming from the right side of the heart or via the superior vena cava. None of these approaches guarantees freedom from later pulmonary embolism through collaterals. There is a risk of consequent distal venous hypertension, common with IVC ligation, less common with clipping or with the umbrella filter, rare at least in principle with the Kimray-Greenfield filter.

Except where contraindicated, great-vein interruption is always followed by anticoagulation. As is true after pulmonary embolism, when the IVC has not been interrupted, it is difficult to know how long anticoagulants should be continued. It seems reasonable to judge this by the extent of the previous venous thrombosis, the severity of lower-extremity venous congestion, and the persistence or absence of other factors that predispose to venous thrombosis.

Another view of venous interruption, which suggests that 20% of patients with pulmonary embolism need surgical intervention, includes broader indications.[49] Patients to be considered for these procedures would have continuing predisposing causes for thrombosis, such as polycythemia, stroke, and malignancies, especially when combined with reluctance to use anticoagulants. Included, as well, would be all survivors of major embolism. Venous interruption would be advised for women who suffer pulmonary embolism early in pregnancy, as heparin therapy would not be feasible. In the continuing debate between liberal and strict indications for venous interruption there appears to be a trend away from surgical intervention.

SUMMARY

Venous thromboembolism offers a medical challenge because of its high incidence, potential serious consequences, and agonizing unpredictability. One extreme of the clinical spectrum, massive embolism and rapid death, has been on center stage. To see the whole spectrum in perspective, however, requires illuminating the other extreme, that of the remarkably efficient and adaptive normal mechanisms for hemostasis and thrombolysis. Probably everyone develops thrombi from time to time in small veins as a result of minor trauma or of illness with inactivity, and sometimes the thrombi will be large enough to break off and become emboli without any symptomatic notice. The lungs are a perfect filter and small emboli are rapidly lysed. It is only with larger venous thrombi, extending into proximal veins, that serious pulmonary embolism becomes of major concern.[54] Many patients develop soleal vein thrombi without ever showing evidence of extension. Other patients have more extensive deep venous thrombosis, from which they recover even without treatment, with or without postphlebitic venous insufficiency and certainly without symptomatic pulmonary embolism. We cannot, however, predict which patients will mobilize intrinsic fibrinolytic systems to overcome the thrombotic episode without medical help, nor can we usually predict which ones will develop serious complications without aggressive treatment. The difficulty of predicting, or of sorting patients, puts great pressure on the clinician and is intimately entangled with the problem of overdiagnosis of deep venous thrombosis and pulmonary embolism.[55]

The problem of underdiagnosis is concerned more with the lack of awareness of predisposing factors. Sufficient background and natural history of venous thromboembolism now is known to allow the alert physician confidently to adjust his level of suspicion for any patient, and to determine whether to institute prophylactic measures or diagnostic studies, or both.

Because nearly all emboli come from the lower extremities or iliac veins, the basic focus must be on the possibility of deep venous thrombosis in these vessels. In the absence of convincing findings in the history or physical examination—and these findings rarely are convincing when suspicion of thrombosis exists—objective studies are needed. Competently conducted noninvasive venous studies and contrast venography are essential to the good practice of modern medicine today. Their appropriate use should reduce both the risk of complications from true episodes of deep venous thrombosis and the risk of complications of anticoagulation in patients who really do not have deep venous thrombosis.

To introduce comparable clarity into the assessment of patients suspected of having pulmonary embolism is more difficult because selective pulmonary arteriography, the analogue of venography, is more complex, more expensive and less readily available. High quality perfusion lung scans, chest roentgenography, electrocardiography, noninvasive venous studies (or venography) should provide sufficient information to allow a reasonable decision concerning whether or not to treat a patient for pulmonary embolism in most cases, but unfortunately not in every one.

Whatever the quality and availability of all known diagnostic tests, in a few cases objective analysis will not yield a definite diagnosis or an unequivocally correct therapeutic action, leaving the physician dependent on his experience and judgment. As newer diagnostic methods are developed and safer therapies found, uncertainties will be fewer, but the need for clinical judgment is not likely to disappear.

The central role of heparin in the current treatment and prophylaxis of these conditions is striking, and most sharply exposed when its use is contraindicated. It often is thought of only as an anticoagulant, but if it were only that, low-dose regimens, to say nothing of ultra-low-dose regimens,[56] would have no power to prevent venous thrombosis. Much is known and much more needs to be learned about the various heparins and their many biological effects. Hopefully, this may lead to the safer use of heparin in treating and preventing venous thromboembolism. Despite the known problems, both full-dose and low-dose regimens, appropriately selected, are well established.

Streptokinase and urokinase have been shown to be effective in hastening the lysis of thrombi and thromboemboli, especially when they are fresh, and in helping improve cardiopulmonary function after massive pulmonary embolism. Their exact place in the management of venous thromboembolism is being debated but has not been settled.

For long-term anticoagulation, warfarin now is the most widely used drug in this country. Heparin might become a satisfactory substitute (with favorable effects the coumarins lack), but this has not been clearly shown. *Antiplatelet* drugs, such as aspirin, are tantalizing and almost certainly important, but so far they play no proven role in the management of venous thromboembolism.

Other measures to prevent deep vein thrombosis, particularly the intermittent compression boots, should be kept in mind for selected patients. Prophylaxis of pulmonary embolism requires alertness to the need for interruption of the inferior vena cava, and to the evolving indications and techniques for so doing.

Large medical centers are expected to have all the experts and instruments needed to carry out the studies and treatments discussed here, but it is impossible for *every* hospital to be so well staffed and well equipped. Nevertheless, a functional minimum should be provided even in smaller hospitals. One approach might involve a medical staff committee, concerned with the facilities and techniques needed to deal with this problem. As such a group works together, perhaps in communication with other medical centers, an exchange of knowledge and experience would be inevitable and beneficial.

It is obviously impossible to prevent, detect, or treat every case of deep venous thrombosis or pulmonary embolism that might or does occur. It is just as well; such a burden would be intolerable. Perhaps in the future, widely used public health measures will help to reduce the incidence. At the present time, medical involvement begins when suspicion of deep venous thrombosis or pulmonary embolism arises. This leads to appropriate prophylactic or therapeutic measures—or sometimes to no action: fatal pulmonary embolism is not a medical failure in a patient dying of an irreversible disease. But when recovery is possible, timely intervention to prevent or treat deep venous thrombosis or pulmonary embolism is usually successful, and the long-term prognosis is good.

REFERENCES

1. Wessler S. Venous thromboembolism: Scope of the problem. In *Prophylactic Therapy of Deep Vein Thrombosis and Pulmonary Embolism.* Proceedings of a conference sponsored by the National Heart and Lung Institute and the American Heart Association, April 1975. NIH No.76-866, Department of Health, Education and Welfare, pp 1–10.

2. Daien JE, Alpert JS. Natural history of pulmonary embolism. *Prog Cardiovasc Dis* 17:259, 1975.

3. Hume M, Sevitt S, Thomas DP. *Venous Thrombosis and Pulmonary Embolism.* Cambridge, MA, Commonwealth Fund/Harvard University Press, 1970 pp 9–24.

4. McIntyre DM, Sasahara AA. Hemodynamic and ventricular responses to pulmonary embolism. *Prog Cardiovasc Dis* 17:175, 1974.

5. The Urokinase Pulmonary Embolism Trial. American Heart Association, Monograph 39. *Circulation* 47(suppl 2):5, 1973.

6. Urokinase Pulmonary Embolism Trial. Phase 1 Results: A Cooperative Study. *JAMA* 214:12, 1970.

7. Urokinase-Streptokinase Embolism Trial. Phase 2 Results: A Cooperative Study. *JAMA* 229:12, 1974.

8. Bell WR, Simon TL, DeMets DL. The clinical features of submassive and massive pulmonary emboli. *Am J Med* 62:355, 1977.

9. Loehry CA. Pulmonary emboli in young adults. *Br Med J* 1:1327, 1966.

10. Sasahara AA, Cannilla JE, Morse RL, et al. Clinical and physiological studies in pulmonary thromboembolism. *Am J Cardiol* 20:10, 1967.

11. Szucs MM Jr, Brooks HL, Grossman W, et al. Diagnostic sensitivity of laboratory findings in acute pulmonary embolism. *Am Int Med* 74:161, 1971.

12. McGlynn TJ Jr, Hamilton RW, Moore R. Pulmonary embolism: 1979. *JACEP* 8:12, 1979.

13. Stein DD, Dalen JE, McIntyre KM, et al. The electrocardiogram in acute pulmonary embolism. *Prog Cardiovasc Dis* 17:247, 1975.

14. Fleischner FG. Observations on the radiologic changes in pulmonary embolism. In Sasahara AA, Stein M (eds). *Pulmonary Embolic Disease.* New York, Grune & Stratton, 1965, pp 206–213.

15. Dalen JE, Haffajee CI, Alpert JS et al. Pulmonary embolism, pulmonary hemorrhage and pulmonary infarction. *N Engl J Med* 296:1431, 1977.

16. Kelley MJ, Elliot LP. The radiologic evaluation of the patient with suspected pulmonary thromboembolic disease. *Med Clin North Am* 59:3, 1974.

17. Neumann RD, Sostman HD, Grottschalk A. Current status of ventilation-perfusion imaging. *Semin Nucl Med* 10:198, 1980.

18. Wagner HN Jr, Sabiston DC Jr, Ilio M, et al. Regional pulmonary blood flow in man by radioisotope scanning. *JAMA* 187:601, 1964.

19. Moses DC, Silver TM, Bookstein JJ. The complementary roles of chest radiography, lung scanning, and selective pulmonary angiography in the diagnosis of pulmonary embolism. *Circulation* 49:179, 1974.

20. Tow DE, Simon AL. Comparison of lung scanning and pulmonary angiography in the detection and follow-up of pulmonary embolism: The urokinase-pulmonary embolism trial experience. *Prog Cardiovasc Dis* 17:239, 1975.

21. Bell WR, Simon TL. A comparative analysis of pulmonary perfusion scans with pulmonary angiograms. *Am Heart J* 92:700, 1976.

22. McNeil BJ. A diagnostic strategy using ventilation-perfusion studies in patients suspect for pulmonary embolism. *J Nucl Med* 17:613, 1976.

23. Biello DR, Mattar AG, McKnight RC, et al. Ventilation-perfusion studies in suspected pulmonary embolism. *AJR* 133:1033, 1979.

24. Dalen JE, Brooks HL, Johnson LW, et al. Pulmonary angiography in acute pulmonary embolism: Indications, techniques and results in 367 patients. *Am Heart J* 81:175, 1971.

25. Sasahara AA, Genton E, Hirsh J, et al. Diagnosis of pulmonary embolism. In *Prophylactic Therapy of Deep Vein Thrombosis and Pulmonary Embolism.* Proceedings of a conference sponsored by National Heart and Lung Institute and American Heart Association, April 1975. NIH No. 76-866, Department of Health, Education and Welfare, pp 239–243.

26. Stein PD, Willis PW III, Dalen JE. Importance of clinical assessment in selecting patients for pulmonary arteriography. *Am J Cardiol* 43:669, 1979.

27. Adelstein SJ, McNeil BJ. A new diagnostic test for pulmonary embolism: How good and how costly? *N Engl J Med* 299:305, 1978.

28. Simon M. Personal communication.

29. Robin ED. Overdiagnosis and overtreatment of pulmonary embolism: The emperor may have no clothes. *Ann Int Med* 87:775, 1977.

30. Cudkowicz L, Sherry S. Current status of thrombolytic therapy. *Heart Lung* 7:97, 1978.

31. Marder VJ. The use of thrombolytic agents: Choice of patient, drug adminstration, laboratory monitoring. *Ann Int Med* 90:802, 1979.

32. Bell WR, Meek AG. Guidelines for the use of thrombolytic agents. *N Engl J Med* 301:1266, 1979.

33. Sasahara AA, Ho DD, Sharma GVRK. When and how to use fibrinolytic agents. *Drug Therapy* 9:111, 1979.

34. Genton E, Hirsh J. Observations in anticoagulant and thrombolytic therapy in pulmonary embolism. *Prog Cardiovasc Dis* 17:335, 1975.

35. Sasahara AA. The case for fibrinolytic therapy. *J Cardiovasc Med* 5:793, 1980.

36. Dalen JE. The case against fibrinolytic therapy. *J Cardiovasc Med* 5:799, 1980.

37. Greenfield LJ. Intraluminal techniques for vena interruption and pulmonary embolectomy. *World J Surg* 2:45, 1978.

38. Sautter RD, Myers WO, Ray JF III, et al. Pulmonary embolectomy: Review and current status. *Prog Cardiovasc Dis* 17:371, 1975.

39. Clagett GP, Salzman EW. Prevention of venous thromboembolism. *Prog Cardiovasc Dis* 17:345, 1975.

40. Kakker VV et al. Prevention of fatal postoperative pulmonary embolism by low doses of heparin. An internation multicentre trial. *Lancet* 2:45, 1975.

41. Kakkar VV. The current status of low-dose heparin prophylaxis of thrombophlebitis and pulmonary embolism. *World J Surg* 2:3, 1978.

42. Kakkar VV. Efficacy of low-dose heparin in preventing fatal pulmonary embolism: Results of an international multicenter trial. With discussions by Friedewald W, Sherry S, Freiman DG, Ebert R, Sevitt S, Bell WR, Sasahara AA, Halperin M. Fratantoni J, in *Prophylactic Therapy of Deep Vein Thrombosis and Pulmonary Embolism.* Proceedings of a conference sponsored by the National Heart and Lung Institute and the American Heart Association, April 1975. NIH No. 76-866, Department of Health, Education and Welfare, pp 207–235.

43. Nicolaides AN. Invited commentary. *World J Surg* 2:13, 1978.

44. Strandness DE Jr. Invited commentary. *World J Surg* 2:17, 1978.

45. Sherry S. Low-dose heparin for the prophylaxis of pulmonary embolism. *Am Rev Respir Dis* 114:661, 1976.

46. Heatley RV, Morgan A, Hughes LE, et al. Preoperative or postoperative deep-vein thrombosis? *Lancet* 1:437, 1976.

47. Homans J. Thrombosis of the deep veins of the leg, causing pulmonary embolism. *N Engl J Med* 211:993, 1934.

48. Homans J. Deep quiet venous thrombosis in the lower limb. *Surg Gynecol Obstst* 79:70, 1944.

49. Crane C. Venous interruption for pulmonary embolism: Present status. *Prog Cardiovasc Dis* 17:329, 1975.

50. Bernstein EF. The role of operative inferior caval interruption in the management of venous thromboembolism. *World J Surg* 2:61, 1978.

51. Mobin-Uddin K, Smith PE, Martinez LD, et al. A vena cava filter for the prevention of pulmonary embolism. *Surg Forum* 18:209, 1967.

52. Mobin-Uddin K. Invited commentary. *World J Surg* 2:55, 1978.

53. Greenfield LJ, McCurdy Jr, Brown PP, et al. A new intracaval filter permitting continued flow and resolution of emboli. *Surgery* 73:599, 1973.

54. Kakkar VV, Howe CT, Flanc C, et al. Natural history of postoperative deep vein thrombosis. *Lancet* 2:230, 1969.

55. Halberstam MJ. Pulmonary embolus: The unspeakable clot. *Modern Med* 48:12, 1980.

56. Negus D, Friedgood A, Cox SJ, et al. Ultra-low dose intravenous heparin in the prevention of postoperative deep-vein thrombosis. *Lancet* 1:891, 1980.

8 Thoracic Outlet Syndromes

Sandor A. Friedman

For the advantage of a specialized forelimb, man has paid a price. The relatively narrow area, bordered roughly by the supraclavicular area and shoulder, is subject to a great deal of tension and shearing during ordinary movements of the arm. Through this narrow tunnel travel the essential neurovascular structures that enable the arm, forearm, and hand to carry out their complicated and subtle functions. Given the marginal adequacy of the thoracic outlet, it is not surprising that symptoms secondary to neurovascular compression are quite common. A wide variety of clinical problems may occur in association with anatomical abnormalities in this area, but often the symptoms and signs are erroneously attributed to other causes. This chapter will review the diagnosis and treatment of the syndromes of thoracic outlet obstruction.

ANATOMY

The thoracic outlet corresponds roughly to the area from the supraclavicular fossa to the proximal axilla. It is bounded superiorly by the base of the neck, laterally by the clavicle and first thoracic rib, inferiorly by the clavicle and pectoral muscles, and medially by the costoclavicular joint. Abnormalities in the structure of the thoracic outlet can be divided into congenital and acquired structures. The former include the presence of a cervical rib,[1] anomalous origin of the first rib,[2] hypertrophy of a scalenus anticus muscle,[3] congenital fibrous bands from the seventh cervical vertebra to the first rib,[4] and abnormal insertion of a pectoralis minor muscle. Rare anomalies include variation in the position of the subclavian artery and vein, and fusion of the scalenus muscles.[5] Acquired abnormalities include soft tissue trauma with scarring, healed fractures of the clavicle, and deposit of adipose tissue in the supraclavicular areas. In many cases, symptoms arise from a combination of congenital and acquired abnormalities that may become more severe with age.

It is of interest that symptoms of thoracic outlet compression rarely occur in young children. Even with congenital abnormalities, the peak incidence occurs in young adults, particularly women. Developmental changes in the chest wall probably account for these observations. There is evidence that the anterior chest wall descends during the first two decades so that the clavicle is pushed in a downward direction and apparently moves farther in women.[6] The clavicle is often longer in women. Cervical ribs may not be fully developed until the third decade.[7]

DIAGNOSIS

The diagnosis of a thoracic outlet syndrome requires demonstration of compression as well as appropriate signs and symptoms that can be attributed to it. Compression is assessed by its effect on the subclavian-axillary arterial axis. Through a variety of provocative maneuvers, one must attempt to obliterate the radial pulse in order to make a diagnosis of a narrow thoracic outlet. The pulse will weaken in any individual who is subjected to these maneuvers. Thus, nothing less than total loss of the pulse is acceptable evidence for this diagnosis. When this obliteration has been demonstrated, the clinician must determine whether the patient's symptoms can be explained by thoracic outlet compression. It is important to remember that the majority of people with positive maneuvers for a narrow thoracic outlet never suffer from a thoracic outlet syndrome.

Loss of the radial pulse with any movement of the shoulder, arm, or neck is indicative of a narrow thoracic outlet. For this reason, it is important to take a careful history, and to be certain to examine the patient in the position that accentuates the symptoms. For example, if a baseball pitcher states that his arm suddenly feels very weak just as he is about to release the ball, one should attempt to palpate the radial pulse while he winds up and throws a ball. Loss of the radial pulse in this circumstance may be the only evidence of a thoracic outlet syndrome. The standard maneuvers may not always obliterate the pulse.

There are basically three standard maneuvers for demonstrating that the thoracic outlet is narrow. Each positive maneuver tends to localize the narrowing to a different postion of the thoracic outlet, but there is often a great deal of overlap among them. To perform the Adson maneuver, one extends the patient's neck as far as possible and turns it laterally toward the limb being tested. The radial artery is then palpated with the arm extended while the patient holds his breath (Figure 8-1). If the pulse is not obliterated, one should attempt the same maneuver with the neck turned away from the arm being tested. A positive Adson maneuver generally indicates considerable narrowing, and is well correlated with various arm symptoms. When it is the only positive maneuver, it suggests compression in the upper part of the thoracic outlet near the base of the neck. It is usually positive in patients with congenital causes of narrowing such as cervical ribs.

The costoclavicular maneuver consists of pressing the shoulder back as far as possible while the forearm is held up at a right angle to the upper arm (Figure 8-2). This test is quite nonspecific and is positive

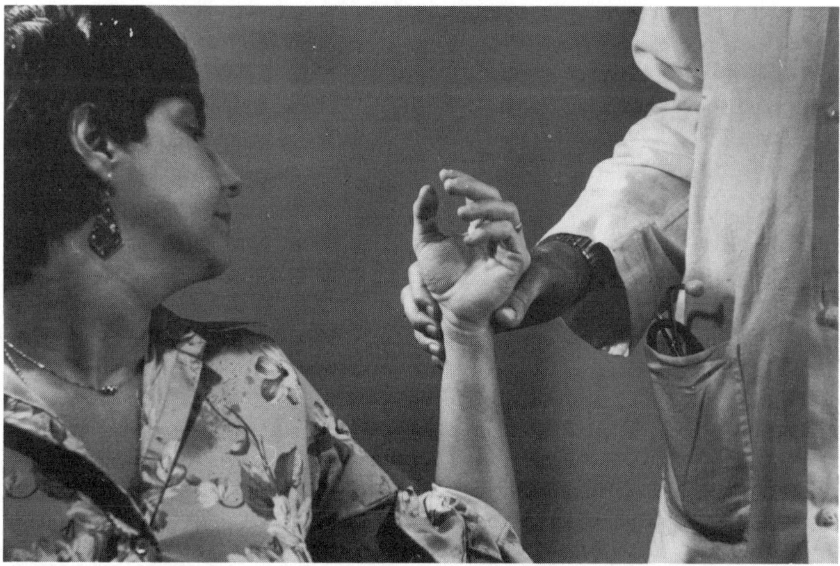

Figure 8-1 Adson maneuver. The neck is extended and turned toward the arm being examined.

in a rather large number of normal people, most of whom will never have any symptoms related to the thoracic outlet. When it is the only positive finding, it suggests narrowing in the area of the clavicle and costoclavicular joint. There is often compression between the clavicle and first rib.[8] Occasionally, simultaneous use of the Adson and costoclavicular maneuvers may obliterate the radial pulse when each maneuver performed individually is negative.

The third maneuver, hyperabduction of the arm, suggests narrowing in the lower portion of the thoracic outlet between the clavicle and pectoralis minor muscle (at the angle formed by the coracoid process and the insertion of the pectoralis minor).[9] It is the simplest and most reproducible maneuver (Figure 8-3).

These maneuvers are not easy to perform and are fraught with error. The patient must be cooperative and able to extend the neck and shoulders fully. Many older people with cervical osteoarthritis are not able to move the neck back far enough to elicit a positive Adson maneuver. False positive results may occur if a weak radial pulse is not detected by the examiner.

When the narrowing is located in the upper thoracic outlet, a positive Adson maneuver can often be corroborated by the loss of the subclavian pulse in the supraclavicular area. One can also auscultate the subclavian artery while the Adson or costoclavicular maneuver is

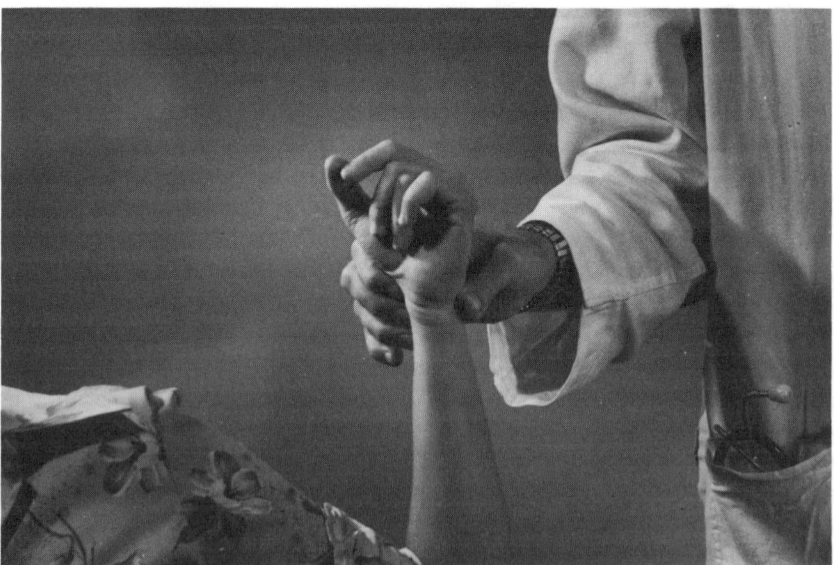

Figure 8-2 Costoclavicular maneuver. The shoulder is moved backward as far as possible while the radial pulse is examined.

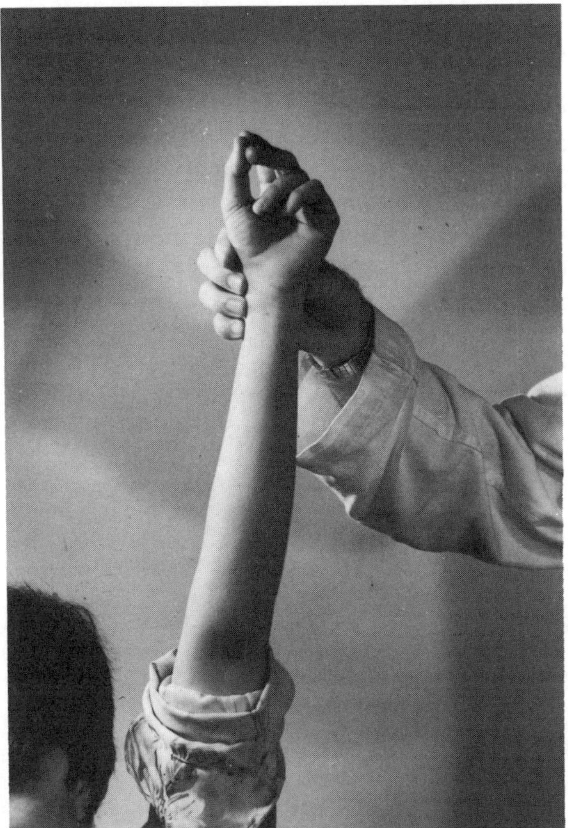

Figure 8-3 Hyperabduction maneuver. The arm is raised as the radial pulse is examined.

slowly and gradually performed. If there is significant narrowing, a bruit may appear shortly before full extension of the neck or shoulder, signifying partial compression of the vessel, and then disappear when full compression is achieved.

Onset of Symptoms

The development of clinical symptoms of thoracic outlet compression depends on many factors. The symptoms can occur in early adulthood or teenage when there is a congenital structural abnormality such as a cervical rib, or later in life as certain occupational movements strain a congenitally narrow tunnel. Poor posture and accumulation of adipose tissue lead to compression. Activity is a particularly important factor. If one puts very little strain on the upper extremities, symptoms may not occur despite a rather narrow thoracic outlet. In contrast, an athletic individual may develop difficulty with a wider outlet. Similarly, bad posture over the course of many years may lead to sufficient sagging of the pectoral and lower neck muscles to produce significant compression, while erect posture may prevent the onset of symptoms in an individual with a congenitally narrow outlet.

In short, there is a spectrum in the normal population from thoracic outlets that are severely narrowed by specific anatomical defects to those that are only slightly narrower than normal. A very significant percentage of people (10% to 20%) respond positively to a costoclavicular maneuver, indicating some degree of narrowing. The development of symptoms depends not only on the degree of narrowing but also on the lifestyle of the individual.

NEUROLOGICAL SYNDROMES

Thoracic outlet symptoms can occur from compression of the brachial plexus, subclavian artery, or subclavian vein. A variety of clinical syndromes can result, which may be confused with other conditions. Nerve root symptoms secondary to compression of the brachial plexus constitute the most common of the thoracic outlet syndromes. Narrowing anywhere along the course of the area can easily result in nerve impingement. The nerve root syndrome may appear for the first time at any age and can result from acquired as well as congenital defects. In some individuals, minor symptoms of nerve compression may appear from time to time during periods of intense physical activity and abate with rest. In its mildest form, nerve compression thus affects millions of people who may attribute their symptoms to a strained muscle. Many individuals, for example, who occasionally awake with paresthesia in a forearm and hand after sleeping on the arm, actually have a narrow thoracic outlet.

The ulnar trunk of the brachial plexus is most exposed to the nerve root compression; thus, symptoms and signs occur predominantly in the distribution of the ulnar nerve. Since cervical spondylosis also involves nerve roots that form the ulnar nerve, it is often difficult to distinguish a thoracic outlet syndrome from symptoms of cervical arthritis. Thoracic outlet syndrome is easily distinguished from a carpal tunnel syndrome because the latter affects only the medial nerve. An ulnar neuropathy can also be produced by chronic, insidious trauma to the ulnar nerve at the elbow, where it is very superficially placed. Occupations that require continuous pressure of the medial elbow against a hard surface may gradually damage the nerve. With this traumatic neuropathy, symptoms and signs are noted distal to the elbow, and a thick, cord-like, ulnar nerve can be palpated near the posteromedial corner of the elbow joint.

Patients with neurologic symptoms secondary to a thoracic outlet syndrome may first notice intermittent paresthesias in their first and second fingers, and feelings that the forearm and hand are asleep. As previously noted, these symptoms may initially awaken them from a sound sleep. Some patients complain that they cannot find a comfortable position for their arms when they lie down.

Shooting pain from the shoulder to the fingers, or even in the opposite direction, may be the major complaint. Although the patient may notice a predominantly medial distribution of the pain, it often involves the entire circumference of the arm. The pain may also occur anywhere between the shoulder and the hand, and mimic a local inflammatory process in the upper extremity or a shoulder-hand syndrome. Since this pain is worsened by stretching motions of the arm and extension of the shoulder, it may be mistaken for intermittent claudication. If the patient keeps his shoulder rigid and relatively motionless in order to avoid pain, he may actually develop a stiff shoulder that can be attributed to arthritis.

Raynaud's phenomenon is a characteristic finding in a small minority of patients with thoracic outlet syndrome.[10] It represents the result of irritation of cervical sympathetic fibers in the brachial plexus. Because vasoconstriction is related to overstimulation rather than hypersensitivity of digital arterioles, the episodes of coldness, cyanosis, and pallor often occur even in the absence of a cold environment. Stretching motions of the shoulder and neck may induce these episodes and, in severe cases, the hand may be cool and sweaty most of the time. One should always think first of thoracic outlet syndrome in any patient with unilateral Raynaud's phenomenon. This never occurs as an isolated finding. A diagnosis of thoracic outlet syndrome is not tenable without nerve-root pain and/or sensory loss.

In severe cases, motor function may be affected. Small muscles of the hand innervated by the ulnar nerve may be particularly affected. Atrophy of the medial interossei and hypothenar eminence may eventually occur, and the patient's grip may weaken.

Examination of the patient with brachial plexus compression often reveals decreased pin sensation along the medial side of the upper extremity and the dermatomes of the ulnar nerve. Although the compression is proximal, sensory loss may be confined to distal dermatomes, making distinction from ulnar peripheral neuropathy difficult. Sensory findings are identical to those that occur with nerve root compression secondary to cervical spine arthritis.

Major clues to the diagnosis of thoracic outlet syndrome include the following:

1. Pain radiating between shoulder and hand, but not including the neck,
2. A cold, sweaty hand or classic unilateral Raynaud's phenomenon,
3. Positive thoracic outlet maneuver,
4. Full mobility of the neck,
5. Ulnar sensory loss, and
6. Normal pulses in the extremity.

Unfortunately, many older patients with positive thoracic outlet maneuvers and signs and symptoms of ulnar nerve compression also have evidence of cervical spondylosis. Neck movements are often limited, and there may be significant radiologic evidence of degenerative arthritis. In fact, many of these patients are suffering from both problems, and it is often extremely difficult to assess the relative importance of each problem in the symptomatology.

Many patients have radicular pain without any objective neurologic findings. Measurement of ulnar nerve conduction time is particularly helpful in this situation in verifying the presence of compression, although it cannot distinguish between cervical spine and thoracic outlet problems.[11,12] However, a normal conduction velocity across the ulnar nerve tends to rule out the diagnosis of a neurogenic thoracic outlet syndrome. Delayed ulnar nerve conduction in association with normal median nerve conduction velocity clearly distinguishes a thoracic outlet syndrome from a carpal tunnel syndrome.

Because of its potential for producing a wide array of symptoms, brachial plexus compression should always be considered in the differential diagnosis of upper extremity symptoms. It is simple enough to perform the thoracic outlet maneuvers, and a positive result may uncover the cause of pain that may be masquerading as tendinitis or arthritis. More importantly, it may offer an alternative to cervical spine disease as a possible cause for radicular pain and paresthesias. This information may prevent the unwarranted performance of cervical myelography and even laminectomy.

ARTERIAL SYNDROME

Subclavian artery involvement is much less common than nerve compression, but is more likely to be diagnosed because it produces more dramatic and clear-cut symptoms. In general, thoracic outlet obstruction must be more severe for the development of arterial symptoms than for neurologic problems. There is a higher incidence of specific anatomical defects and of positivity of more than one thoracic outlet maneuver in the arterial syndromes.

Patients with subclavian artery compression may have ischemic pain on movement of the arm into a position that obliterates the radial pulse. Such motions may include putting the hand above the head, lifting packages, and throwing. Since arterial pulses and blood pressure are normal in the relaxed state, the examiner may initially have difficulty in explaining a symptom that appears to be due to intermittent claudication. In fact, in an occasional case the classic thoracic outlet maneuvers are negative. A careful elucidation of the circumstances leading to pain is the key to diagnosis. By palpating for peripheral pulses with the arm in a position associated with symptoms, one can make the diagnosis of thoracic outlet syndrome.

Often, the major symptom of subclavian artery compression is weakness or extreme fatigability of the arm. This also represents claudication, but it can be confused with a neurological problem. The weakness can be quite profound and prevent the patient from performing simple tasks such as combing the hair and lifting relatively light objects. The patient may complain of dropping objects suddenly because of extreme weakness. At times, the history can be quite suggestive of transient ischemic attacks. If brachial plexus compression is also present, transient paresthesias may add to the clinical impression of cerebrovascular disease. The proper diagnosis is made by finding normal muscle strength when the arm is relaxed and an absent radial pulse in the position associated with weakness.

Just as with the neurologic syndromes, occupation and lifestyle play an important role in determining the extent of symptoms. In some individuals with mild thoracic outlet narrowing, certain extreme motions of the arm may produce enough ischemia to inhibit successful completion of the task for which the motion was made. If the patient did not need to perform this function, he might never have any symptoms. For example, subclavian-axillary artery compression may cause ischemic pain when the arm is abducted to lift heavy objects. Thus, an otherwise aysmptomatic laborer may be disabled by compression not affecting an office worker.

There are several other ways in which thoracic outlet obstruction can affect the circulation of the upper extremity.[13] In fact, the possibility of thoracic outlet syndrome should be considered prominently in the differential diagnosis of arterial disease in an upper extremity. It is a more frequent cause of symptomatic arterial insufficiency than arteriosclerosis obliterans. In many cases, the patient notices position-related ischemic pain before developing other symptoms. Often, however, more serious features of circulatory impairment occur without this early warning.

Subclavian Artery Occlusion

Intermittent compression of the subclavian artery during the course of many years traumatizes the vessel and causes turbulent blood flow. Sometimes, the result is gradual thrombosis and occlusion of the lumen. A patient with this problem may be asymptomatic as this process of thrombosis takes place and may even remain free of symptoms when the vessel is totally occluded. The potential for collateral circulation with a slowly developing proximal occlusion is excellent in the upper extremity. If the individual does not vigorously exercise the arm, there may be no claudication, although a stress test would show a decreased capacity for heavy work in that extremity. On the other hand, an individual with more active arms may begin to have effort-limiting weakness, tiredness, or pain at an early stage of the thrombotic process. Sometimes, thrombosis occurs more quickly with resultant distal gangrene.[14] There have also been reports of cerebral embolism from proximal extension of a thrombus.[15]

Diagnosis of thoracic outlet syndrome in the face of subclavian-axillary artery occlusion is difficult. Examination of the arm reveals decreased or absent axillary, brachial, radial, and ulnar pulses as well as a lower blood pressure than that in the other extremities. The subclavian pulse is weak if the obstruction is in the upper thoracic outlet and normal if the problem is in the lower area inferior to the clavicle. A bruit may be present over the subclavian artery in the supraclavicular fossa. If the obstruction is only partial and easily palpable pulses are still present, the thoracic outlet maneuvers can be applied. However, total or almost total occlusion of the subclavian artery eliminates this major diagnostic aid.

The diagnosis in this case can often be inferred from the absence of any evidence of arteriosclerosis obliterans such as coronary heart disease or any risk factors associated with it. If the patient is relatively young (under the age of 45), thoracic outlet injury is the most likely explanation for subclavian artery occlusion, particularly if the diagnostic maneuvers are positive for the other arm. It is important also to rule out a collagen vascular disease before assuming the presence of thoracic outlet compression. If a chest roentgenogram demonstrates a cervical rib or aberrant first thoracic rib, the diagnosis is quite apparent.

If there is no abnormality on chest x-ray, the diagnosis can be assumed only by a process of elimination unless arteriography is performed. The latter, obtained with the arm in various positions, may demonstrate impingement on the subclavian artery as well as the exact location of the thrombus.

Subclavian Aneurysm

Chronic compression of the subclavian-axillary axis can also cause dilatation. Continuous trauma to the media of the vessel over a period of years can gradually damage its smooth muscle and lead to atrophy. As the atrophic muscle is replaced with collagen, the media loses its tensile strength, and aneurysmal dilatation occurs.[16,17] Thoracic outlet obstruction is clearly the leading cause of subclavian aneurysms. Arteriosclerotic dilatation of this artery is quite uncommon. Another mechanism involved in aneurysm formation is poststenotic dilatation. Just distal to the point of compression, there is turbulent blood flow in the subclavian artery, resulting in increased lateral pressure on the walls of the vessel and eventually aneurysmal dilatation.

When an aneurysm appears in this area, it is usually readily palpable in the supraclavicular fossa as a pulsatile mass and may reach a diameter of several centimeters. It is often accompanied by a bruit. There are times, however, when the aneurysm is located at the junction of the subclavian and axillary arteries and is, therefore, not readily accessible to palpation. This is more likely to occur with compression in the lower part of the thoracic outlet.

Subclavian artery aneurysms rarely rupture and may remain asymptomatic. They do, however, tend to fill with mural thrombus. One result is gradual narrowing and occlusion of the lumen. Sometimes, a subclavian aneurysm undergoes acute thrombosis and occlusion, causing limb-threatening ischemia. The patient develops severe pain in the arm and presents with a cold, cyanotic, or pale hand. Since the capacity for collateral circulation is excellent in the upper extremity, the arm may survive without therapy, but surgical intervention is often necessary. The patient is likely to be left with severe claudication if the arterial obstruction is not relieved.

Another problem with a subclavian aneurysm is distal embolization in a fashion similar to femoral and popliteal aneurysms. Showers of small emboli into the digital vessels are not uncommon. In fact, thoracic outlet obstruction is one of the most frequent causes of digital gangrene. Since arteriosclerosis rarely causes localized ischemia of the hand or fingers, one must examine carefully for a subclavian artery aneurysm in any patient with a small vessel syndrome in an upper extremity, particularly if there are repeated episodes of cyanosis or gangrene in the same hand. If an aneurysm is not palpable, it is important to search for a collagen-vascular disease, thrombocytosis, cryoglobulinemia, and cryofibrinogenemia. If these entities are not present, one should strongly consider performing arteriography to look for an occult aneurysm of the subclavian-axillary axis.

Since brachial plexus and arterial compression often coexist in the same patient, Raynaud's phenomenon and embolization may occur in the same extremity. One must, therefore, distinguish between paroxysmal episodes of vasospasm of the entire hand and attacks of localized ischemia with digital necrosis. The former do not require any therapeutic intervention unless they become severe and disabling while the latter is an indication for surgical intervention.

It is important to remember that thoracic outlet compression always occurs in the area of the distal subclavian artery and does not affect any of its major branches, which originate from the proximal, intrathoracic portion of the vessel. Thus, the vertebral circulation is never impaired by a thoracic outlet syndrome, and patient's symptoms are always confined to the upper extremity. If a patient complains of dizziness, diplopia, or other brain-stem symptoms and has circulatory insufficiency in an upper extremity, there is probably an intrathoracic subclavian artery obstruction proximal to the origin of the vertebral artery.

VENOUS COMPRESSION

The third and least common category of thoracic outlet compression involves the subclavian and axillary veins. When venous problems occur, they often arise suddenly and without any previous symptoms of brachial plexus or arterial compression. Thoracic outlet compression is a leading cause of subclavian vein thrombosis.[18] Many cases of so-called effort thrombosis are, in reality, examples of thoracic outlet obstruction. The typical history is of several hours of heavy physical work involving lifting, stretching, and hyperabduction of the arm, followed the next day by sudden swelling of the upper extremity. A high proportion of these patients have one or more positive thoracic outlet maneuvers. The stress of the labor compresses a vein that ordinarily is not disturbed by the narrow thoracic outlet. Venous narrowing leads to stagnation of blood and thrombosis.

Occasionally, pain accompanies this venous thrombosis, but most often there is only painless swelling of the forearm and upper arm. Examination reveals swelling with pitting edema and increased warmth. The veins of the dorsum of the hand are full and remain distended above heart level, indicating increased venous pressure. The absence of neck vein distention localizes the proximal extent of thrombosis to the subclavian rather than innominate vein. Any tenderness in the arm is usually secondary to muscle strain from the previous labor.

The differential diagnosis includes subclavian vein thrombosis secondary to the insertion of a transvenous pacemaker, migratory phlebitis associated with malignancy, collagen-vascular diseases and penetrating trauma to the subclavian vein. These other causes are usually quite apparent when they are present.

Contrary to old beliefs, pulmonary embolism with subclavian vein thrombosis is not rare. Patients must be anticoagulated and treated in the same manner as those with deep vein thrombi in the lower extremities. In fact, subclavian vein thrombosis is potentially more dangerous because there is no satisfactory surgical alternative for patients with contraindications to anticoagulation or repeated pulmonary emboli in the face of adequate anticoagulation.

The results of treatment with anticoagulation are fair, but recanalization of the vein is often incomplete. Many patients have mild-to-moderate chronic edema secondary to venous insufficiency.[18] Although this edema is generally not disabling, it may be annoying and cause a feeling of heaviness in the arm. A possible alternative therapy, which may avoid post-phlebitic symptoms, is thrombolysis with urokinase or streptokinase. This treatment is associated with a higher incidence of bleeding, and its overall efficacy for upper extremity venous thrombosis is not well established as yet.

Some patients with subclavian vein compression may notice intermittent swelling in the absence of venous thrombosis.[19,20] If their arm is not subject to straining movements, thrombosis may never occur. A common feature, for example, is occasional swelling of the arm in the early morning when the patient awakens. After he arises and moves the arm freely, the swelling gradually disappears within a few hours.

TREATMENT OF THORACIC OUTLET SYNDROMES

In managing a patient with thoracic outlet symptoms, the physician must take many factors into account. One must consider age of the patient, general health, the kind and severity of symptoms, lifestyle and occupation, and the cause of thoracic outlet narrowing.

Definitive therapy for thoracic outlet syndrome requires a surgical approach. If there is an easily identifiable structure causing the narrowing such as a cervical rib, one can be reasonably confident that its removal will result in significant relief of symptoms. For this reason, a roentgenogram of the chest in the apical lordotic position should be performed first in evaluating a patient with thoracic outlet syndrome for possible surgical exploration. This film will identify cervical ribs and an anomalous origin of the first thoracic rib. It must be emphasized that a short cervical rib extending only a few centimeters from its vertebral origin is not likely to cause significant compression by itself.

In the absence of a discrete radiologically identifiable cause for thoracic outlet narrowing, the surgeon cannot be certain of what he will encounter on exploring the area. In this situation, age of the patient at the initial onset of symptoms is an important consideration. In young individuals he is likely to find a specific cause for compression, but a middle-aged or older person who is just beginning to have paresthesias in his hands probably does not have a specific defect. His symptoms are often secondary to increased adipose tissue deposition and the chronic effects of a stooped posture.

Surgical exploration of a supraclavicular fossa without evidence of a specific defect may do more harm than good. Subcutaneous tissue is removed, but postoperative scarring may leave the whole area taut and actually narrow the thoracic outlet further. On the other hand, an operation aimed specifically at the removal of a cervical rib, and performed with a minimum of trauma, may offer the patient a great deal of relief. In removing a cervical rib, it is also advisable to release the head of the scalenus anticus muscle, since it may be contributing to the outlet obstruction. Even more important, however, is the removal of the entire first rib. This should be done in every operative case whether or not a cervical rib is present.

The kind of symptoms is also of crucial importance in deciding on therapy. Brachial plexus compression, the most common complication of a narrow thoracic outlet, is usually not a serious threat to the health of the extremity. Pain and paresthesias may be troublesome and even interfere with the patient's occupation, but there is rarely enough compression to lead to permanent neurological damage. Severe sensory loss and marked atrophy of hand muscles occur only occasionally. One must be conservative about surgery in these cases especially in older individuals. It is usually advisable for the patient to accept occasional shooting pains and paresthesias developing during sleep rather than submit to rather extensive and sometimes mutilating surgery. One must assess the magnitude of symptoms, the presence or absence of neurologic signs, and the degree of interference with occupation or lifestyle, in making a decision for or against surgery.

Arterial syndromes are another matter. They may frequently jeopardize the health of the extremity and often cause disabling symptoms. Intermittent claudication not only interferes with activities of daily living but carries the spectre of potential permanent damage to the artery. Thus, a more aggressive approach is warranted unless claudication occurs only with extreme movements that the patient can learn to avoid. One must not limit the patient too much for fear of losing shoulder mobility and even causing a shoulder-hand syndrome.

The development of a subclavian artery aneurysm is a definite indication for surgery. Repair of the aneurysm as well as removal of the offending structure in the thoracic outlet is necessary. There is usually a specific defect that can be found preoperatively or at surgery. Total occlusion of the subclavian artery should be treated like an arteriosclerotic occlusion. The need for surgery depends on the severity of symptoms.

An episode of venous thrombosis can be treated conservatively. Often only one episode occurs, and surgery is usually not necessary if there are no other symptoms of a thoracic outlet syndrome. If venous thrombosis recurs, or there is persistence of obstructive edema even after resolution of the thrombus, surgical resection of the obstructing lesion may be indicated. A venogram, in a position that obliterates the radial pulse, may be helpful in assessing such a patient for surgery. If the patient must perform manual labor and the offending structure is obvious and circumscribed, surgical intervention may be appropriate after one episode of venous thrombosis.

Because of the high incidence of residual edema, some authors have suggested that venous thrombectomy in conjunction with decompression surgery should be performed in the acute stage of venous thrombosis.[18,21] The efficacy of this approach has not been established.

There are helpful conservative measures that can be taken especially for obese, middle-aged and older individuals with mild-to-moderate neurological symptoms. Weight loss in an obese individual and learning to walk more erectly may have beneficial effects on symptoms. Daily lifting exercises can also be of considerable benefit.[22,23] The arms are lifted straight up and down with the shoulders erect. The patient is instructed to do this three to four times a day for about ten minutes at a time. After a week or two, he can perform the same exercise with one pound weights in each hand. He can gradually increase the weight to three to five pounds.

In summary, decisions concerning therapy for thoracic outlet syndromes are not simple. Surgical attempts to remove offending structures are most indicated in younger individuals with evidence of discrete obstruction and severe symptoms or potentially disabling complications.

REFERENCES

1. Adson AW, Coffey JR. Cervical rib: A method of anterior approach for relief of symptoms by division of the scalenus anticus. *Ann Surg* 85:839, 1927.

2. Etter LE. Osseous abnormalities of the thoracic cage seen in forty thousand consecutive chest photoroentgenograms. *Am J Roentgenol* 51:359, 1944.

3. Raaf J. Surgery for cervical rib and scalenus anticus syndrome. *JAMA* 157:219, 1955.

4. Law AA. Adventitious ligaments simulating cervical ribs. *Ann Surg* 72:497, 1920.

5. Nichols HM. Anatomic structures of the thoracic outlet. *Clin Orthop* 51:17, 1967.

6. Overton LM. The causes of pain in the upper extremities: A differential diagnosis study. *Clin Orthop* 51:27, 1967.

7. Brannon EW. Cervical rib syndrome: An analysis of nineteen cases and twenty-four operations. *J Bone Joint Surg* (Am) 45:977, 1963.

8. Falconer MA, Weddell G. Costoclavicular compression of the subclavian artery and vein: Relation to the scalenus anticus syndrome. *Lancet* 2:539, 1943.

9. Wright IS. The neurovascular syndrome produced by hyperabduction of the arms: The immediate changes produced in 150 normal controls, and the effects on some persons of prolonged hyperabduction of the arms, as in sleeping, and in certain occupations. *Am Heart J* 29:1, 1945.

10. Lewis T, Pickering GW. Observations upon maladies in which the blood supply to digits ceases intermittently or permanently, and upon bilateral gangrene of digits: Observations relevant to so-called "Raynaud's disease." *Clin Sci* 1:366, 1934.

11. Urschel HC Jr, Razzuk MA. Management of the thoracic-outlet syndrome. *N Engl J Med* 286:1140, 1972.

12. Sadler TR Jr, Rainer WG, Twombley G. Thoracic outlet compression: Application of positional arteriographic and nerve conduction studies. *Am J Surg* 130:704, 1975.

13. Dorazio RA, Ezzet F. Arterial complications of the thoracic outlet syndrome. *Am J Surg* 138:246, 1979.

14. Schein CJ, Haimovici H, Young H. Arterial thrombosis associated with cervical ribs: Surgical considerations; report of a case and review of the literature. *Surgery* 40:428, 1956.

15. DeVilliers JC. A brachiocephalic vascular syndrome associated with cervical rib. *Br Med J* 2:140, 1966.

16. Short DW. The subclavian artery in 16 patients with complete cervical ribs. *J Cardiovasc Surg* (Torino) 16:135, 1975.

17. Glass BA. The relationship of axillary venous thrombosis to the thoracic outlet compression syndrome. *Ann Thorac Surg* 19:613, 1975.

18. Swinton NW Jr, Edgett JW Jr, Hall RJ. Primary subclavian-axillary vein thrombosis. *Circulation* 38:737, 1968.

19. Charrette EJP, Iyengar KSR, Lynn RB, et al. Symptomatic nonthrombotic subclavian vein obstruction: Surgical relief in six patients. *Vasc Surg* 7:220, 1973.

20. Adams JT, DeWeese JA, Mahoney EB, et al. Intermittent subclavian vein obstruction without thrombosis. *Surgery* 63:147, 1968.

21. Drapanas T, Curran WL. Thrombectomy in the treatment of "effort" thrombosis of axillary and subclavian veins. *J Trauma* 6:107, 1966.

22. Peet RM, Henriksen JD, Anderson TP, et al. Thoracic-outlet syndrome: Evaluation of a therapeutic exercise program. *Proceedings of the Staff Meeting of the Mayo Clinic* 31:281, 1956.

23. Nelson PA. Treatment of patients with cervicodorsal outlet syndrome. *JAMA* 163:1570, 1957.

9 Pulmonary Arterial Disease

Sandor A. Friedman

The pulmonary arterial circulation differs in several important ways from systemic arteries. In the first place, it is a low pressure system and is extremely vulnerable to the effects of hypertension. In the systemic circulation, the effects of hypertension are variable and not necessarily well correlated with the exact blood pressure level. In fact, systemic hypertension is only a contributing factor in the development of atherosclerosis of medium and large arteries. It is of paramount importance in the pathogenesis of arteriolar subintimal fibrosis and endarteritis obliterans, but the severity of this lesion is extremely variable from patient to patient.

On the other hand, pulmonary arterial blood pressure is normally in the range of 20-25/10-15 mm Hg, and even relatively small increments above this level may affect the health of the arterial walls. Elevation of blood pressure is the principal, and perhaps, the only major factor in the development of atherosclerosis of the major pulmonary arteries and endarteritis obliterans of the smaller vessels. Furthermore, the onset of atherosclerosis is more predictable, better correlated with the severity and duration of pulmonary hypertension and relatively independent of the etiology of this hypertension.

A second important characteristic of the pulmonary circulation is its unique vascular reactivity. Vasoconstriction and vasodilatation of pulmonary arterioles occur as easily in the pulmonary as in the systemic circulation, but the stimuli are quite different. The pulmonary arterioles are the only ones in the body to constrict in response to hypoxia and then dilate in the presence of high oxygen tension.[1] This is in sharp contrast to systemic arterioles which dilate when hypoxic. Cerebral arterioles actually constrict when oxygen tension is very high.

Vasoconstriction of pulmonary arterioles in response to hypoxia is an extremely important protective mechanism in the body's oxygen delivery system. When a pulmonary segment or lobe is ventilated poorly secondary to any pathologic process, vasoconstriction of the local arterioles shunts blood flow away from that area and toward areas of normal alveolar ventilation. The effect is to minimize any disproportion between perfusion and ventilation, and thus prevent severe systemic hypoxia. Without this vasoconstriction, a severe lobar pneumonia, for example, might decrease red cell oxygenation by 20%, whereas the actual loss is much less.

When systemic hypoxia occurs, pulmonary vasoconstriction becomes harmful rather than protective. Generalized arteriolar constriction raises pulmonary arterial blood pressure and taxes the capacity of the right ventricle to maintain an adequate cardiac output. If hypoxia becomes chronic, pulmonary atherosclerosis occurs, increasing pulmonary peripheral resistance further and leading to right ventricular failure.

A third characteristic of the pulmonary circulation is its capacity for thrombolysis. In this regard, pulmonary arteries behave more like systemic veins than systemic arteries. Even after submassive pulmonary embolism, the last vestiges of thrombus are generally cleared from the circulation within 14 to 17 days, and sometimes as early as 7 to 10 days. This thrombolytic capacity may be related to high levels of plasminogen activators within the endothelium of the pulmonary microcirculation.[2] With the onset of significant atherosclerosis, this thrombolytic ability is gradually lost. Thrombosis in situ begins to occur because of increased peripheral resistance and circulatory stagnation, and the thrombi are not cleared. The result is higher pulmonary artery pressures and further deterioration of right ventricular function.

CAUSES OF PULMONARY HYPERTENSION

Before considering the specific etiologies of pulmonary hypertension, it is important to distinguish between two basic types—flow and resistance hypertension. Just as in systemic hypertension, blood pressure in the pulmonary arteries can be raised by an increase in cardiac output and/or an increase in peripheral resistance. Increase in blood flow through the pulmonary circulation usually leads to only a mild to moderate rise in pulmonary arterial pressure, and generally is associated with a better prognosis than pulmonary hypertension secondary to peripheral vasoconstriction. However, even this moderate increase in pressure, if prolonged over many years, will lead to pulmonary arteriolosclerosis and atherosclerosis. The severity of pulmonary hypertension produced by an increase in cardiac output depends largely on pulmonary vascular tone. The difference in natural course of interatrial and interventricular septal defects illustrates this principle very well. Although the former tend to cause more shunting of blood flow from the systemic to pulmonary circulation than the latter, they are rarely associated with severe pulmonary hypertension. Patients with ventricular septal defects appear to have a tendency toward pulmonary arteriolar constriction, which aggravates the effect of flow and greatly accelerates the development of severe pulmonary hypertension, atherosclerosis, and a right to left shunt.

Since there are many causes of pulmonary hypertension, it is useful to divide them into broad categories. Table 9-1 offers one useful classification:

Table 9-1
Causes of Pulmonary Hypertension

I) Increase in Pulmonary Blood Flow (early) and Increased Vascular Resistance (late)
  A. Interventricular septal defect
  B. Interatrial septal defect
  C. Patent ductus arteriosus

II) Increase in Pulmonary Vascular Resistance
  A. Left ventricular failure
  B. Mitral stenosis
  C. Intrinsic pulmonary disease
    1) Chronic obstructive pulmonary disease
    2) Restrictive lung disease
  D. Primary disorders of the pulmonary arteries
    1) Recurrent pulmonary embolism
    2) Primary pulmonary hypertension

SIGNS AND SYMPTOMS OF PULMONARY VASCULAR RESISTANCE

The symptoms of increased pulmonary vascular resistance are related to hypoxia secondary to impaired red cell oxygenation and decreased cardiac output. Dyspnea on exertion is characteristically present, but orthopnea is absent unless the basic cause of pulmonary hypertension is left ventricular failure or mitral valve disease. With dyspnea, the patient also notices easy fatigability and a tendency to lightheadedness, especially on exertion.

Chest pain that may mimic angina pectoris is not uncommon with moderate to severe pulmonary hypertension. The pain is usually in the retrosternal area and often described as a pressure sensation. Like the pain of coronary artery disease, this sensation is initiated and aggravated by exertion, but it also occurs at rest. Unlike angina, it may persist at times for as long as 30 minutes to an hour. The symptom is very similar to the chest pain associated with aortic stenosis.

Physical examination reveals signs of right ventricular strain with a loud pulmonary component of the second heart sound. At pulmonary

Table 9-2
Causes of Right Ventricular Hypertrophy and Their Recognizable Characteristics

Lesion	Murmur	Second Sound	Other
Interatrial septal defect	pulmonic ejection	wide, fixed splitting loud P2	occasionally mid-diastolic rumble of relative tricuspid stenosis
Mild pulmonic stenosis	pulmonic ejection	wide splitting with P2 muffled	ejection click
Moderate pulmonic stenosis	pulmonic ejection	wide splitting with decreased P2	atrial gallop
Severe pulmonic stenosis	long pulmonic systolic murmur	absent P2	atrial gallop
Tricuspid regurgitation	holosystolic murmur to right of apex	unchanged	murmur increases with inspiration
Interventricular septal defect	holosystolic murmur along left sternal border associated with thrill	wide splitting and loud P2	biventricular hypertrophy

artery pressures over 60 mm Hg, atrial gallops (S4) are common. When the pulmonary artery pressure reaches 100 mm Hg, the early diastolic decrescendo murmur of pulmonary regurgitation may be heard at the pulmonic area. Palpation of the chest may reveal a right ventricular heave along the lower left sternal border. In asthenic individuals or those with chronic obstructive pulmonary disease, this lift may be in the subxyphoid area. In patients without emphysema, it may be possible to percuss an area of dullness over the lower sternum. These signs indicate the presence of right ventricular hypertrophy, which is usually the result of increased pulmonary vascular resistance. The only other significant causes of right ventricular hypertrophy are interatrial septal defect, interventricular septal defect, pulmonic stenosis, and valvular tricuspid regurgitation. These lesions are easily recognizable by their characteristic auscultatory findings, summarized in Table 9-2.

If pulmonary hypertension persists and worsens, the eventual result is right ventricular failure. As the progression to heart failure occurs, the patient may develop relative tricuspid regurgitation. Its onset is heralded by pulsating neck veins and an appreciable systolic pulsation over the liver. The murmur may be very difficult to appreciate and is sometimes audible only during inspiration. Atrial fibrillation secondary to stretching of the right atrium may also occur.

LABORATORY EVIDENCE OF PULMONARY HYPERTENSION

Echocardiography is a sensitive tool for detecting early right ventricular hypertrophy and dilatation of the right ventricular cavity. A chest roentgenogram is somewhat less sensitive, but reveals prominence of the main pulmonary artery shadows in the early stages, followed later by narrowing of the peripheral pulmonary vascular markings. The electrocardiogram is a relatively insensitive tool for detecting acquired right ventricular hypertrophy because of the predominance of electrical forces from the left ventricle. Only in congenital heart disease, where the lesion is present when right ventricular forces still predominate, does the electrocardiogram detect early evidence of right ventricular hypertrophy. In acquired heart disease, right axis deviation is usually a sign of either very abrupt or very severe pulmonary hypertension.

EVALUATION OF A PATIENT WITH INCREASED PULMONARY VASCULAR RESISTANCE

When pulmonary hypertension is diagnosed, it is important to embark upon a stepwise, logical approach in order to arrive at the correct cause. The first step is to assess the possible role of left-sided failure in the pathogenesis of the pulmonary hypertension. Left ventricular failure usually begins with orthopnea and paroxysmal nocturnal dyspnea, but it may also present as fatigability and weakness due to low cardiac output. As the patient develops pulmonary atherosclerosis secondary to pulmonary venous hypertension, these symptoms may diminish and gradually be replaced by the characteristic dyspnea and fatigability of pulmonary hypertension. If the patient's left ventricular failure takes the form of a low cardiac output syndrome, one may erroneously assume that the pulmonary hypertension has nothing to do with left ventricular failure. Clinical examination may reveal clear lung fields at this stage, and left ventricular enlargement may not be appreciated.

Echocardiography is extremely useful in this situation by determining left ventricular size at a time when the chest roentgenogram is still ambiguous (Figure 9-1). If any confusion remains, Swan-Ganz catheterization can be performed. An elevated pulmonary artery pressure, associated with a normal pulmonary capillary wedge pressure, tends to exclude left heart disease as the cause of pulmonary hypertension. A word of caution is in order, however. If the patient has been recently treated with diuretics, wedge pressure may have decreased toward normal while pulmonary artery pressure remained normal.

Mitral Stenosis

Occult mitral stenosis can cause very severe pulmonary hypertension. Often only the murmur of relative tricuspid regurgitation can be heard. A loud first sound and the presence of atrial fibrillation are important clues. This lesion must always be excluded in the evaluation of any patient with pulmonary hypertension. Again, this can be easily accomplished in most cases with echocardiography.

Intracardiac Shunts

Unrepaired septal defects, particularly ventricular defects, can lead to pulmonary atherosclerosis and increased peripheral resistance. The ordinary auscultatory findings may no longer be present. Patients generally show signs of right to left shunting with intermittent or continuous cyanosis. A ventricular defect or patent ductus arteriosus is associated with left, as well as right ventricular enlargement. Radionuclide cardiac scan may reveal a right to left shunt in these patients.

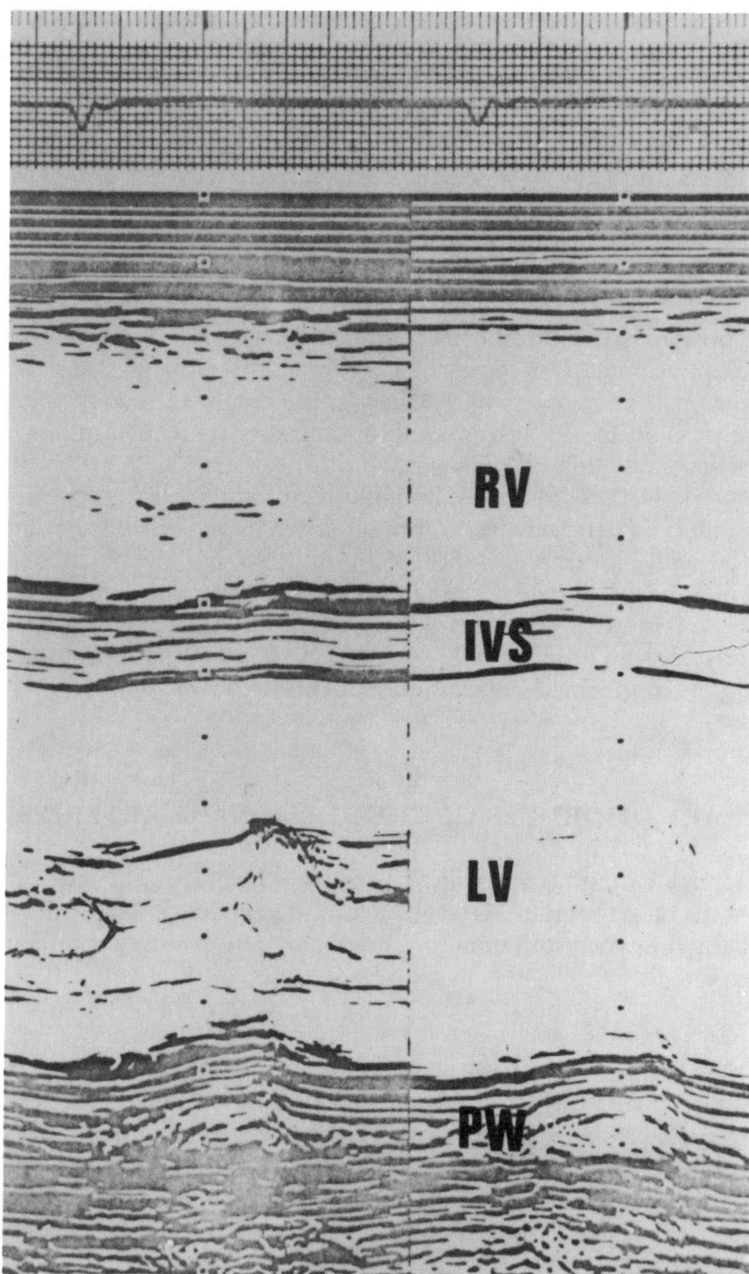

Figure 9-1 Echocardiogram of a patient with pulmonary hypertension secondary to arteriosclerotic heart disease. Note dilatation of both left and right ventricular chambers. Movement of the interventricular septum is attenuated because of infarction.

Interatrial septal defects can usually be recognized on echocardiography because of isolated right ventricular volume overload and abnormal motion of the ventricular septum.[3]

Chronic Lung Disease

Once left-sided disease has been excluded, the role of the lungs must be assessed. If the patient has chronic obstructive pulmonary disease, it is usually quite obvious from physical examination. Wheezing is present in the chronic bronchitic and decreased breath sounds in the emphysematous patients. In all cases of clinically significant chronic obstructive pulmonary disease, the diaphragms move poorly. By percussion of the lung bases in expiration and inspiration, one notices an excursion of 2 cm or less.

Restrictive lung disease is much more difficult to assess by clinical means alone. There may be prominent dry rales and obvious limitation of chest wall movement, but these findings are not always present.

Pulmonary function testing is mandatory in the evaluation of every patient with pulmonary hypertension. As a minimum, vital capacity, forced one-second vital capacity, and diffusion capacity should be performed to exclude the presence of significant lung disease.

PRIMARY DISORDERS OF THE PULMONARY ARTERIES

After all other lesions have been ruled out, one is left with a diagnosis of pulmonary artery disease. Then one must distinguish clinically between pulmonary embolism and primary pulmonary hypertension.

Multiple Pulmonary Emboli

The diagnosis of chronic pulmonary hypertension secondary to showers of small pulmonary emboli is one of the most difficult in clinical medicine and can never be made antemortem with certainty. When predisposing conditions such as prolonged immobility, obesity and hyperviscosity states are present, it is not difficult to suspect this diagnosis. However, some patients do not have obvious reasons for pulmonary embolism. A history of multiple, acute episodes of unexplained dyspnea is helpful in some cases, but the patient may not recall any symptoms before the onset of chronic dyspnea and fatigue. The diagnosis of multiple pulmonary emboli must be particularly considered in older individuals who tend to be more sedentary.

Pulmonary arteriography is not useful in making this diagnosis unless one is fortunate to see the patient at the time of an acute embolus. A negative angiogram cannot rule out the insidious showering of small emboli. Demonstration of venous thrombi in the lower extremities through venography, impedance plethysmography, or scanning with radio-iodinated fibrinogen is strong-supporting, but not confirmatory evidence. Lifetime anticoagulation or interruption of the inferior vena cava is indicated when this diagnosis is strongly suspected.

Primary Pulmonary Hypertension

There has been an increasing interest in recent years in the diagnosis and management of primary pulmonary hypertension, a disorder originally described in 1951.[4] At one time, this was thought to be an extremely rare disorder, probably caused by multiple pulmonary emboli. Indeed, necropsy findings in primary pulmonary hypertension and multiple pulmonary emboli are virtually identical. One sees widespread pulmonary atherosclerosis and small thrombi throughout the pulmonary arterial tree.

It appears now that primary pulmonary hypertension is uncommon but not as rare as previously thought. The disease is probably a disorder of pulmonary vasomotor tone, leading to prolonged arteriolarspasm. Atherosclerosis and thrombosis are secondary to prolonged hypertension. The disease has a marked predilection for women and always begins early in life, usually in the second, third or fourth decade. A history of progressive dyspnea is characteristic, and syncopal episodes are quite common. Syncope occurs mostly on exertion and is associated with cyanosis. Primary pulmonary hypertension is occasionally associated with Raynaud's phenomenon.

Physical examination reveals signs of cor pulmonale and clear lung fields. Chest roentgenogram shows straightening of the upper left heart border, prominence of both major pulmonary arteries, and attenuation of peripheral vascular markings. The left atrial indentation along the lower left heart border is normal (concave). By the time the diagnosis is made, right ventricular enlargement is usually evident on the film (Figure 9-2A, B). The electrocardiogram may show right axis deviation. Since a similar syndrome can occur in systemic lupus erythematosus and other collagen diseases, an antinuclear antibody test and LE preparation should be performed.

Unfortunately, the prognosis for patients with this disease is very poor. Most succumb from progressive pulmonary hypertension within two years. Recently, however, there have been hopeful reports about the use of vasodilators to treat this disorder. Pulmonary vascular resistance has decreased significantly in some patients after the intravenous administration of isoproterenol,[5] diazoxide,[6,7] hydralazine,[8] and phentolamine.[9] Chronic oral administration of these agents has been associated with lowering and stabilization of pulmonary vascular resistance for more than six months. It is not yet known whether this therapy will result in longer survival rates.

Because of these recent advances, it is imperative to measure pulmonary artery pressure and cardiac output in every patient with primary pulmonary hypertension in order to calculate peripheral

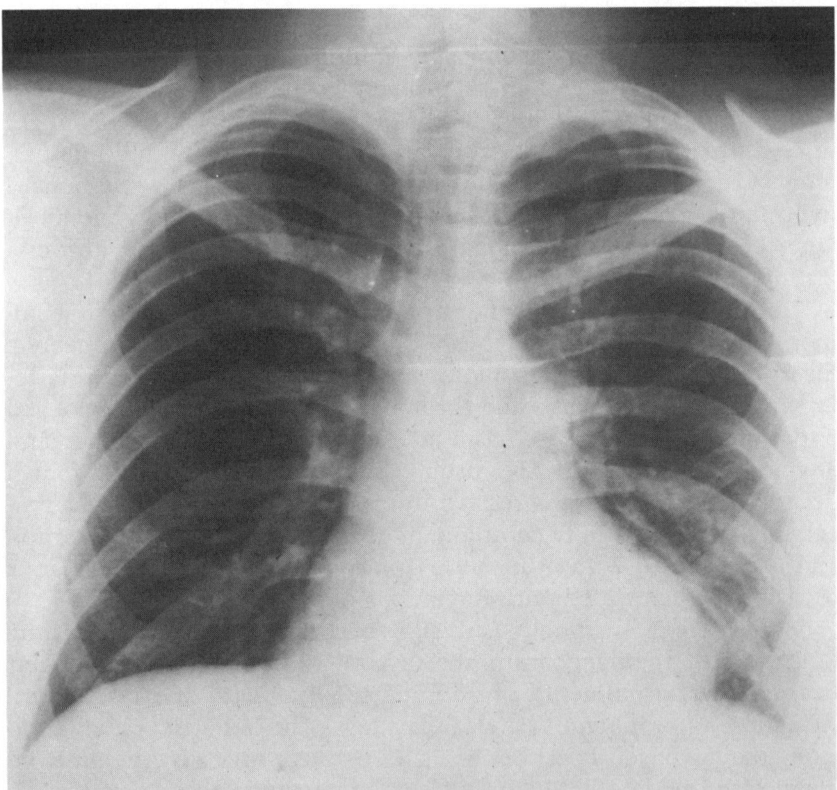

A

Figure 9-2A, B Chest roentgenogram of a patient with primary pulmonary hypertension. Note the convex appearance of the main pulmonary artery segment along the upper left heart border on the posterior-anterior view. The left atrial border is still concave. On the lateral view, note the encroachment of the right ventricle on the retrosternal space.

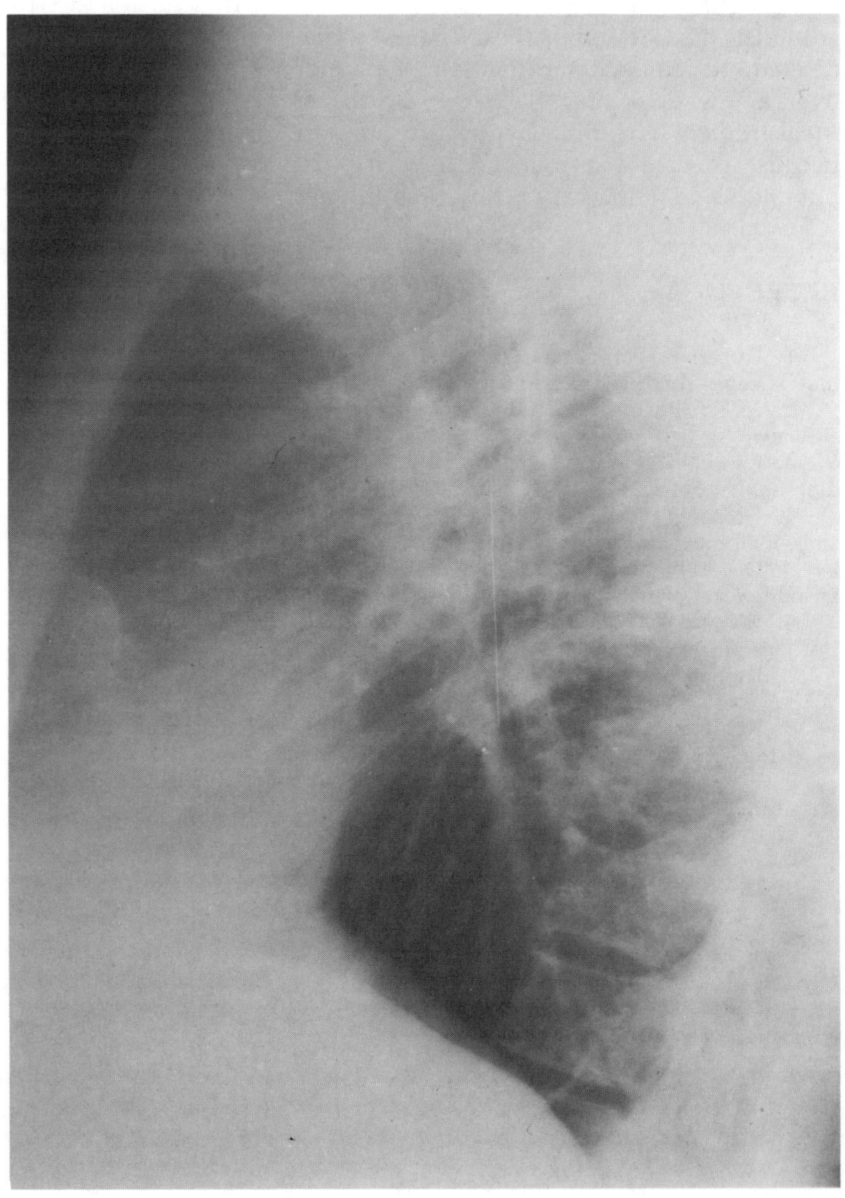

B

resistance. One must then assess the intravenous effect of several vasodilating drugs such as diazoxide, hydralazine and isoproterenol, on pulmonary vascular resistance. If resistance to flow decreases with administration of any of these agents, a trial with oral therapy is indicated. Repeated determination of pulmonary vascular resistance over a few days may be necessary to assess the proper dosage. Measurement of pulmonary artery pressure alone is not sufficient because a decrease in resistance may lead to an increase in cardiac output and leave pulmonary artery pressure unchanged.

REFERENCES

1. Dugard A, Naimark A. Effect of hypoxia on distribution of pulmonary blood flow. *J Appl Physiol* 23:663, 1967.
2. Ali SY. Purification and properties of tissue activator of plasminogen. *J Biochem* 104:1, 1967.
3. Radtke WE, Tawik AJ, Gau GT, et al. Atrial septal defect: Echocardiographic observations. Studies in 120 patients. *Ann Intern Med* 84:246, 1976.
4. Dresdale DT, Schultz M, Michtom RJ. Primary pulmonary hypertension. I. Clinical and hemodynamic study. *Am J Med* 686, 1951.
5. Daoud FS, Reeves JT, Kelly DB. Isoproterenol as a potential pulmonary vasodilator in primary pulmonary hypertension. *Am J Cardiol* 42:817, 1978.
6. Wang SW, Pohl JCF, Rowlands DJ, et al. Diazoxide in treatment of primary pulmonary hypertension. *Br Heart J* 40:572, 1978.
7. Klinke WP, Gilbert JAL. Diazoxide in primary pulmonary hypertension. *N Eng J Med* 302:91, 1980.
8. Rubin LJ, Peter RH. Oral hydralazine therapy for primary pulmonary hypertension. *N Eng J Med* 302:69, 1980.
9. Ruskin JN, Hutter AM Jr. Primary pulmonary hypertension treated with oral phentolamine. *Ann Intern Med* 90:772, 1979.

10 Vascular Disease of the Gastrointestinal Tract

Francis U. Steinheber

Although vascular diseases of the bowel have been clearly recognized since the turn of the century, it has been only in the last two decades that intensive interest has been focused on this subject, spurred on by advances in surgery and radiology.[1-3]

MESENTERIC CIRCULATION

A broad overview of the anatomy of the mesenteric circulation provides a useful background for understanding the clinical consequences of reduced blood flow to the gut.[4,5] The viscera receive their blood supply from three single vessels originating along the abdominal aorta: the celiac, superior mesenteric, and inferior mesenteric arteries. Although anastomoses between these vessels produce, in effect, a potential single functional vascular unit, the superior mesenteric artery (the central axis of this unit), is functionally an end artery supplying the entire mid-gut (Figure 10-1). The celiac and inferior mesenteric arteries receive abundant collaterals from visceral and non-visceral sources, and tolerate acute occlusion more readily. The celiac artery supplies the foregut as far as the duodenum, while the left colon and a variable portion of the distal transverse colon receive their blood supply from the inferior mesenteric artery. The remainder of the entire mid-gut derives its supply from the tributaries of the superior mesenteric artery.

A number of anastomoses link the axial superior mesenteric artery to the two vessels which flank it above and below. Through its inferior pancreaticoduodenal artery, the superior mesenteric artery joins the celiac artery at the level of the superior pancreaticoduodenal branch of its gastroduodenal division. The dorsal pancreatic arterial branch of the celiac artery's splenic division also forms a collateral pathway with branches of the superior mesenteric artery. The middle colic division of the superior mesenteric artery anastomoses with the left colic branch of the inferior mesenteric artery, establishing a major collateral

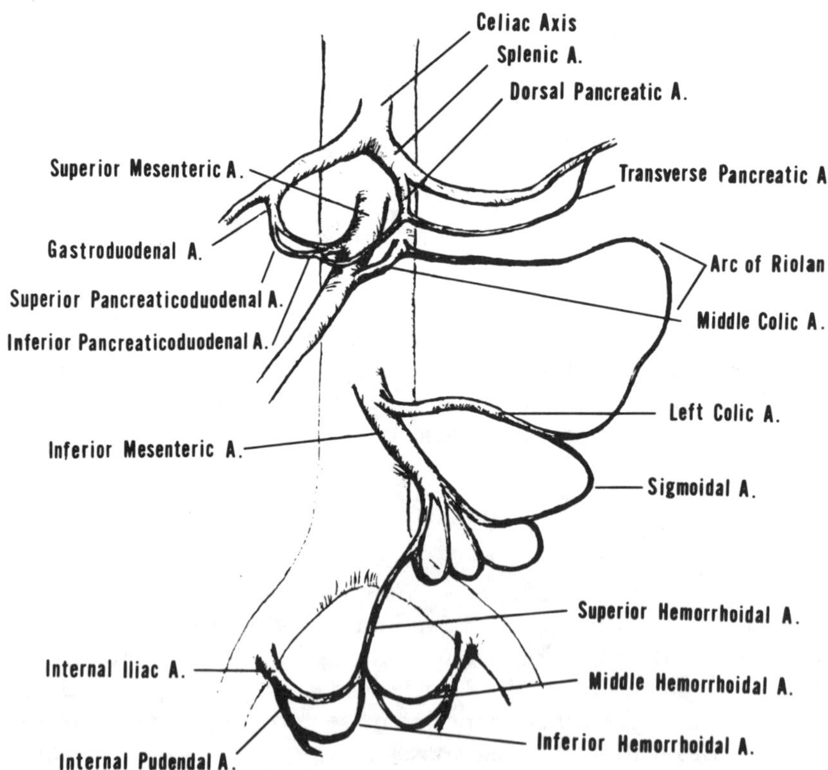

Figure 10-1 Mesenteric circulation illustrating major collateral pathways.

pathway between these two main arteries. This latter anastomotic link is referred to as the arc of Riolan, and constitutes a potentially crucial collateral pathway of flow to the superior mesenteric artery. As it enlarges, it is referred to as the "meandering artery" because of its sinuous course, and constitutes the largest, most effective collateral supply to the mid-gut. The inferior mesenteric artery terminates as the superior hemorrhoidal artery and communicates with the internal iliac system via the latter's middle hemorrhoidal branch and the inferior hemorrhoidal branch of the internal pudendal artery. Both the superior mesenteric and inferior mesenteric systems reach the colon via an arcade nearest the colon, which runs from cecum to sigmoid, known as the marginal artery of Drummond.

Dynamics of the Mesenteric Circulation

The splanchnic circulation receives about one quarter of the cardiac output, amounting to 1.5 to 1.75 L/min.[5-7] One half of this flow is distributed to the small bowel where the mucosa and submucosa receive three quarters of the total flow. In response to intestinal requirements during meals, blood flow increases 30% to 50%.[8,9] Yet, because only one fifth of the intestinal capillaries are open at any given time, mesenteric flow can be reduced by 75% without any discernable morphologic or functional changes.

Control of Splanchnic Flow

The amount of blood reaching the viscera is determined on a central basis by cardiac output, sympathetic nervous system and circulating catecholamines, and, at the microcirculatory level, by local regulatory factors.[7] The regulation of the arteriole at the microcirculatory level determines the total blood flow to the gut. The precapillary sphincter controls the amount of flow through capillaries and, therefore, directly affects the amount of diffusion from blood to tissue. The microcirculation responds to local vasodilator and vasoconstricting substances, metabolites, and neurotransmitters. Arterioles and precapillary sphincters are arranged in series and are independent in their responses to drugs. Precapillary sphincters exhibit a predominant beta adrenergic response, while arterioles are more responsive to alpha adrenergic stimuli. Nevertheless, both respond to a wide variety of local factors to maintain adequate flow to cells. Thus, when sustained sympathetic stimulation constricts arteriolar smooth muscle, lowering splanchnic blood flow, local mechanisms act to compensate by relaxing precapillary sphincters, thus opening new capillaries to provide nourishment to cells. This phenomenon of autoregulation, which permits a constant blood flow despite variations in pressure, is poorly understood and probably involves a complex interaction of local and circulating vasoactive influences including VIP, serotonin, and cholecystokinin among others.

The circulation of the villus is currently believed to be based on a countercurrent mechanism similar to that of the nephron. The essential component of such a system is parallel blood vessels with opposing flow. The central arteriole supplying the villus lies adjacent to veins returning blood in the opposite direction. Oxygen diffusion from the arteriole in response to concentration gradients results in a decreasing gradient of O_2 tension from base to villus tip, further aggravating ischemia during low flow states by depriving the villus of oxygen.

CLINICAL FORMS OF MESENTERIC VASCULAR DISEASE

When blood flow is gradually reduced in one or more mesenteric vessels, the interlocking of the three arterial systems permits the maintenance of adequate blood supply through development of competent collaterals. A high percentage of major stenoses and occlusions in asymptomatic patients has been found in both postmortem and angiographic studies.[10] The astounding capacity of the collateral network has been clearly demonstrated since Chiene's widely quoted postmortem description in 1869 of an asymptomatic patient with thrombosis of all three mesenteric arteries, and who died of other causes.[11] In recent times Lipchik and his associates described an asymptomatic 45-year-old patient with complete occlusion of the abdominal aorta documented on angiography.[12] In this case, retrograde flow from lumbar arteries filled the inferior mesenteric artery and, via collaterals, the branches of the superior mesenteric and celiac arteries. At autopsy the ostia of both these vessels were found to be occluded by thrombus. These and other similar examples,[13] while unusual, do illustrate the unique capacity of visceral circulation to maintain flow despite major vascular compromise.

Mesenteric vascular occlusion can lead to a variety of clinical responses including:

1. Development of collaterals adequate for normal function,
2. Development of collaterals sufficient to maintain viability but not function, and
3. Intestinal infarction.

CHRONIC INTESTINAL ISCHEMIA

In 1901 Schnitzler in Vienna described a premonitory phase of abdominal pain preceding fatal mesenteric infarction in a female patient, and likened it to claudication of the extremities.[14] Despite the fact that a number of observers in this country recognized the syndrome of abdominal angina early and emphasized its significance as a prodrome of intestinal infarction,[16] it was not until the report by Shaw and Maynard in 1958[17] of the first successful surgical relief of symptoms, that recognition of the syndrome had any impact on clinical practice. In the subsequent two decades, a number of reports have reemphasized this clinical syndrome and the beneficial results of surgical intervention.[18-20]

Clinical Features

Early observers noted the development of pain in response to nutritional demands of the viscera at mealtime, and likened this pattern to that seen after the exercise-related ischemia of the lower limb, and later of coronary artery disease.[14] The term ''intestinal angina'' or ''abdominal angina'' seemed to these observers to aptly characterize the postprandial appearance of symptoms, and has become generally accepted. As a rule, symptoms begin in middle or later life and patients often appear prematurely aged. A background of arteriosclerotic vascular disease is likely, which may include angina, cerebrovascular disease, and, especially, intermittent claudication.[20-22] The latter may occur in as many as half the patients.[22,23] Many patients have had previous inconclusive laparotomy.[22] Diabetes mellitus, hypertension, and a history of cigarette smoking are not uncommon in these patients.[22,23]

Pain characteristically begins 15 to 30 minutes following a meal, reaches a crescendo, and slowly abates after one to three hours. At its onset, pain may appear insidiously, at first only after a large meal, but it soon becomes an invariable response to food intake, increasing in severity and duration.[24] The pain is dull, aching, often crampy in nature, and central in location, with occasional radiation to either side or the back.[21] Bloating, flatulence, and anorexia frequently accompany the pain and, less often, nausea and vomiting. Postprandial somnolence and meteorism may be early symptoms in some patients. The patient soon learns to avoid distress by reducing the size of meals, often fearing even the smallest morsel despite hunger. On occasion the pain may awaken the patient at night.[25] The patient vainly seeks relief in a variety of almost gymnastic maneuvers which range from lying prone to squatting, assuming the fetal position, or sitting in a chair with legs drawn to the abdomen.[13,25] Attempts to vary eating habits may seem to bring temporary relief, but symptoms progress inexorably, often terminating in an acute episode of bowel ischemia or interrupted by another cardiovascular event.

The majority of patients experience weight loss, often of a substantial degree, averaging from 20 to 40 pounds.[15,20,21] In a small number of patients, alteration of bowel habits may dominate the clinical picture and lead the physician astray into a fruitless search for a gastrointestinal malignancy.[26] Disordered motility can manifest itself as either severe obstipation or diarrhea with as many as 6 to 20 stools daily.[20–22,27] When questioned, as many as one half of patients will notice that their stools float on water.[13] Table 10-1 indicates the percentage of patients with various symptoms in several large series.

Table 10-1
Incidence of Symptoms in Abdominal Angina

Symptoms	Connelly[15] 28 patients	Crawford[20] 40 patients	Reul[21] 25 patients	McCallum[22] 33 patients	Stoney[27] 35 patients	Total 161 patients (%)
Pain	28	39	23	29	34	153 (95)
Weight loss, range	24 (12–70 lb)	27 (9–75 lb)	9 (10–40 lb)	18 (10–60 lb)	30	108 (67)
Nausea/vomiting		8	3	8	3	22 (15)
Diarrhea	7	13	4	3	12	39 (24)
Constipation	12			3	8	23 (23)
Claudication	14			16		(49)
Coronary artery symptoms	11			12		(37)

Physical examination is more useful in excluding other causes of abdominal pain than in leading to a direct diagnosis. Hypertension and evidence of vascular disease elsewhere are common.[15] Crawford found signs of either aortoiliac obstruction or abdominal aortic aneurysm in one half of his patients.[20] An abdominal bruit can be heard in approximately two thirds of patients, but the significance of this finding is diminished by its frequent presence in asymptomatic patients.[22,28] There is some evidence that the phonocardiographic demonstration of a diagnostic component to the epigastric bruit increases the likelihood of significant vascular compromise.

Although only limited information is recorded in published series, laboratory signs of malabsorption are frequently found when sought.[1,29] Nonspecific decreases in serum proteins and carotene seem to be common. Steatorrhea, documented by a variety of methods, has been the most frequently observed abnormality, [29-33] but can be absent.[34]

Instances of isolated abnormal tests of absorption such as D-xylose, have been noted,[32] but many patients lack any evidence of malabsorption,[34] which is more likely to be present in those who have sustained acute ischemic injury than in the classic form of abdominal angina.[24] Tests of absorption, such as D-xylose, may return to normal after successful revascularization procedures, but at times only partial recovery occurs.[29,35] In the two instances where small bowel biopsy has been reported, abnormal histology, including significant villus changes, has been found. In both cases histology returned to normal following surgery.[13,30] The presence of occult blood in the stools has been noted in some reports.[18] A barium study of the upper gastrointestinal tract may show signs of stasis with dilation of loops and segmentation of the barium column, but is of no immediate diagnostic value.[31] Although the overwhelming majority of cases of abdominal angina are related to arteriosclerotic plaques at the origin of mesenteric vessels, rare causes include periarteritis nodosa, carcinoid, fibromuscular hyperplasia, Takayasu's disease, thromboangiitis obliterans, and one instance of polycythemia vera.[24]

Most data about the natural history of abdominal angina are scanty and inferential. Based upon Dunphy's report in 1936 that 60% of his patients with acute mesenteric infarction gave a prodromal history of ischemia,[16] an observation subsequently confirmed by a number of observers,[36-40] it seems reasonable to assume that the ultimate fate for most patients is catastrophic infarction. Symptoms can precede infarction by several months to years.[37] Rarely, arterial occulsion may result in an acute episode which spontaneously resolves without grave infarction, only to be followed by a period of accelerated symptoms. This seems to have been the case in several patients reported by Mavor.[33] Borrowing further from the cardiac analogy, this could be referred to as "crescendo abdominal angina."

There is no information available on the outlook for patients with minimally symptomatic disease. If experience with other ischemic diseases can be applied, then the spectrum of bowel ischemia must include patients whose symptoms are so minor that they never come to clinical attention. It is probable that mesenteric infarction may never occur in such patients. At present, there is no basis on which to speculate whether marginal collaterals can improve their efficiency to ameliorate ischemic symptoms.[41]

Mesenteric Steal

The confluence of the circulation of the lower extremities and the splanchnic circulation at their respective hemorrhoidal artery tributaries suggests that blood may be siphoned from the splanchnic bed to the arteries of the lower limb, or in a reverse direction. Several clinical reports raise the possibility that this can indeed occur. The patient described by Harris experienced intermittent claudication and progressive abdominal angina, and ultimately was able to eat only while lying supine.[42] Angiography demonstrated a large meandering artery and a large collateral between the superior hemorrhoidal artery and the internal iliac system. Another patient reported by Brooks noted increased claudication and ischemic digital pain after eating.[44]

While it is possible to find fault with these cases as examples of chronic mesenteric steals, the existence of the acute form of such a steal is on firmer grounds. The acute aortoiliac steal has been recognized since Connolly first described several patients developing acute intestinal gangrene following aortoiliac reconstruction, often developing after many months.[46] As circulation is restored to the extremities, a "steal" of blood from the mesenteric bed is assumed to occur via the well-developed collaterals. This has led to the suggestion that prophylactive revascularization should be included at the time of aortofemoral surgery if preoperative angiography demonstrates occlusive disease of the celiac and superior mesenteric arteries and the presence of a prominent meandering artery.[47]

Diagnosis

While the clinical picture may be sufficient to arouse suspicions of abdominal angina, the diagnosis requires angiographic confirmation. Before it is concluded that the pain is related to visceral ischemia, obstruction of at least two vessels should be demonstrated with the use of biplane angiography. The presence of prominent collateral vessels lends additional support. While most observers feel that visceral angina requires stenosis of a minimum of two vessels,[13,19,29] DeBakey noted that one third of his cases had involvement of a single mesenteric vessel.[22] Since in most of these cases this was the celiac artery, the diagnosis is open to some question. Moreover, occlusion of a single vessel is not uncommon at angiography.[20]

Despite a heightened clinical awareness, few clinicians will ever encounter a patient with abdominal angina. Therefore, although the entity is now well accepted and a diagnosis can be established by adhering to strict criteria, one should be reluctant to ascribe abdominal pain to this condition until a full investigation has been made. In a number of patients initially diagnosed as abdominal angina, other conditions have ultimately proved to be the source of pain.[19,41,43] Angiography merely records the anatomical defect but does not provide satisfactory information regarding effectiveness of splanchnic flow. Symptoms of ischemia appear only when collateral blood supply is unable to compensate for reduced blood flow through stenosed arteries. Demonstration of decreased caliber of vessels at best allows only crude guidelines. This is illustrated in the study by Dick.[45] Using precise quantitative measurements of the diameters of the main trunks of the three mesenteric arteries in a consecutive series of 100 patients undergoing angiography, and converting these figures to cross-sectional area, he found that this area was reduced to one third to two thirds of normal in all patients with abdominal angina. However, over 20% of asymptomatic individuals had similar degrees of narrowing. Moreover, as noted previously, many angiographic and postmortem studies indicate a high prevalence of significant stenoses in asymptomatic individuals.[10] For example, Crawford noted that one third of all patients studied by lateral aortography showed relatively high degrees of celiac axis obstruction, and one sixth of all patients studied for thoracoabdominal aneurysms had asymptomatic isolated obstruction of the superior mesenteric artery.[20]

Treatment

Vascular surgeons have increasingly espoused the virtues of remedial vascular surgery for abdominal angina with an enthusiasm rivaling that of cardiac surgeons for coronary bypass surgery. Certainly, the published results detailing successful relief of symptoms in over 90% of cases support their ardor.[13,18–21] However, since the criteria for defining the diagnosis of abdominal angina remain imprecise, the selection of patients for surgical reconstruction becomes a matter of judgment. The patient with typical symptoms and angiographic demonstration of occlusion of two major arteries and enlarged collaterals is certainly a reasonable candidate for surgery *if no other cause for the pain can be found.*[41,43] In the absence of such clear-cut evidence, especially in instances of single vessel disease, it would seem prudent to delay surgery in favor of cautious, close follow-up to allow time to observe the progression of the symptom complex.

Recently, Hansen[9] has made an attempt to put the diagnosis of abdominal angina on a more quantitative basis, using measurements of pre- and postprandial splanchnic blood flow. While resting blood flow was found to be equal in controls and patients with angina, postprandial flow rose in normals, but remained unchanged in the five patients with intestinal angina. While only preliminary, these results suggest that it is possible to develop a reliable test for quantitating the adequacy of the splanchnic circulation.

Although a variety of surgical procedures have been employed, bypass surgery utilizing a Dacron graft is the procedure of choice.[20-22,27] Some surgeons have successfully used endarterectomy with a venous patch graft.[13,20,27] In properly selected cases, a favorable outcome seems to be the rule.

While there have been a few initial attempts to apply percutaneous transluminal angioplasty to the treatment of chronic vascular insufficiency of the bowel, its future role as definitive therapy remains decidedly uncertain at this time.

Celiac Axis Compression Syndrome

This entity has been the cause for recurrent controversy since its first descriptions in the early 1960s.[48] With an almost biologic rhythm, a cycle of advocacy and rebuttal has appeared every few years since then as proponents rise to its defense, followed shortly by vigorous opposing arguments questioning its validity.[49-53] The basic conflict revolves about two points: the inconsistency of the clinical characteristics and the unresolved nature of the underlying cause.

The typical patient is a woman in her fourth decade or somewhat younger, with ill-defined complaints of upper abdominal pain, often of several years duration. Pain may be related to meals, but just as often consists of a constant, severe aching sensation inconsistently related to meals or position. Weight loss and alteration of bowel habits are inconstant features. In the majority of cases an abdominal bruit is often heard, but may be absent. Existence of the entity rests on the one objective finding of narrowing of the celiac trunk on abdominal angiography.

The theoretical objections against the existence of this syndrome are not easily dismissed.[51,53] The pain pattern is variable and uncharacteristic of intestinal ischemia.[20,51] Reduced caliber of the celiac trunk can be found on angiography in over one third of asymptomatic individuals, and is rarely responsible for alteration of splanchnic flow. A rich collateral blood supply easily accommodates obstruction of celiac flow. Both congenital absence of the celiac trunk and its complete resection at surgery are tolerated without ill effect.[55] Few reports provide detailed evidence of disturbed absorption.[51,56-58] Steatorrhea is absent in most cases,[57] while it is often found in cases of true abdominal angina.

Nevertheless, it is impossible to ignore the impressive number of patients who become symptom-free following surgery, averaging better than 80% in most series.[49,52,56] While certainly not wholly convincing, this suggests that there does exist a select group of patients who suffer from abdominal pain related to entrapment of the celiac trunk. It is doubtful, however, that the syndrome results from impaired splanchnic blood flow. Celiac compression is almost always related to entrapment of the vessel by the median arcuate ligament, and in most series decompression by transection of this ligament alone has been followed by relief of symptoms.[56] The initial proponents of the syndrome believed the pain was not ischemic in nature and ascribed it to fibrosis of the celiac ganglion[48] or to a hypothetical combination of vascular and neural phenomena.[49] A causal role of the ganglion is supported by the observation that improvement may follow simple resection of this ganglion. Only rarely has bypass grafting been necessary. Generally, most of the patients cited in the literature lack long-term follow-up, but more than one half have developed recurrence of symptoms with time.[59] Thus, the current status of this syndrome remains in doubt. Surgery is justified only after every effort has been made to exclude all other causes, and when angiography shows unequivocal evidence of celiac axis compression. Since some patients eventually become asymptomatic,[59] sufficient time should elapse before surgery is undertaken. Regardless of its status in the medical arena, it is clear that this syndrome has demonstrated enough staying power that it will continue to find its champions.

ACUTE INTESTINAL INFARCTION

Despite major advances in diagnosis and management, intestinal infarction continues to be a catastrophic event with mortality rates ranging from 70% to 90%. Although clinical features have changed little since early descriptions of this dread event, a discernible change in etiology has been noted over the past half century. The percentage of cases due to nonocclusive infarction has been gradually rising with a concomitant fall in the incidence of venous infarction. In Jackson's seminal monograph[60] on superior mesenteric artery occlusion in 1963, one third of the reported cases to that time were caused by mesenteric venous thrombosis, and only 12% were associated with nonocclusive mesenteric ischemia, whereas the latter now accounts for one third to one half of all cases in recent series.[39,61] The incidence of mesenteric emboli has remained steady at about one quarter of the reported cases.

Regardless of etiology, a common clinical picture evolves after acute interruption of mesenteric blood flow.[62] Patients are generally over the age of 50, frequently suffering from effects of cardiovascular disease, especially cardiac arrythmias and congestive heart failure.[40,62] Many are using digitalis and diuretics.[39] Pain is the outstanding feature in all forms of mesenteric infarction, although at times it may be less impressive than other clinical features. The pain is usually excruciating and intensely colicky in nature and variable in character and location, often appearing with explosive suddenness. The bowel initially responds to ischemia by intense smooth muscle reactivity leading to exaggerated bowel motility, while the villi of the mucosa are the first to suffer loss of viability with hypoxia. These changes are reflected at the onset in a high incidence of vomiting and explosive bowel evacuation. While occult blood is usually present, gross bleeding is evident in less than one quarter of cases.[39,61]

As loss of bowel viability and depth of infarction progress, vascular collapse ensues in response to a series of local and systemic reflexes, bacterial invasion and release of toxic metabolites, and cardiodepressant factors. On clinical examination the patient is generally in extreme distress with signs of cardiovascular instability. No one specific finding leads to a diagnosis, but the absence of significant abdominal findings in the face of severe abdominal distress should raise the possibility of this diagnosis. By the time the patient is seen, some abdominal tenderness is present, and ileus has already developed as evidenced by distension and decreased bowel sounds. In 20% of the cases a distinctive mottled cyanosis of the abdominal wall may be noted.[39]

Laboratory data are inconclusive but reflect the severity of the underlying process. The white blood count is elevated in 90% of cases, often greater than 20,000.[39,63,64] When the white count is normal, a marked increase in bands will be found. Hemoconcentration in response to exudation of protein-rich fluid into the ischemic bowel is reflected in a rising hematocrit, frequently above 50%.[39,65] A profound, often intractable, metabolic acidosis highlights the extensive tissue necrosis and hypoxia associated with bowel necrosis. Nonspecific elevations in transaminases, LDH, uric acid, and alkaline phosphatase are common. Serum amylase is elevated in 25% to 50% of patients, but levels above twice normal are found in only 5% of patients.[39,65,66] Patchy sloughing of ischemic mucosa probably accounts for the positive stool guaiac often found. Not unexpectedly, electrocardiographic abnormalities are frequently present.[65]

A bloody peritoneal fluid is found in three quarters of patients, underscoring the frequency with which transmural gangrene occurs by the time this diagnosis is considered.[61] Uncommonly, sigmoidoscopy may show a dark hemorrhagic mucosa with blue-black blebs, indicative of submucosal hemorrhage. Although the evolutionary changes in the gross structure of the bowel are evident in the appearances on x-ray, they are not specific.

A number of attempts have been made to detail the distinctive changes of bowel ischemia on the abdominal flat plate.[67,68] Although diagnostic findings are present in less than 10% of cases, specific changes can be found in 60% of cases. These consist of changes in bowel wall thickness, mucosal contour and configuration, all related to submucosal hemorrhage and edema. The airless abdomen, resulting from the initial period of bowel reactivity, will be found in less than 5% of cases. After paralytic ileus develops, dilated loops of bowel with a pseudoobstructive pattern are frequently found. On occasion, these dilated fluid-filled loops of bowel may simulate an abdominal mass or pseudotumor. Only at the advanced stages of gangrene will the diagnostic findings of mural gas, or gas in the portal vein, become radiologically apparent, and they are present in only 5% of cases[67,68] (Figure 10-2). Barium examination of the upper gastrointestinal tract defines more sharply the features delineated in the air studies. Thumbprinting, thickened, accordion-pleated valvulae, so-called "stacked coins" appearances, and signs of disordered motility may at times resemble other inflammatory conditions such as granulomatous diseases. The barium enema is appropriate only in cases of suspected ischemic colitis, when it is the most conclusive diagnostic study.

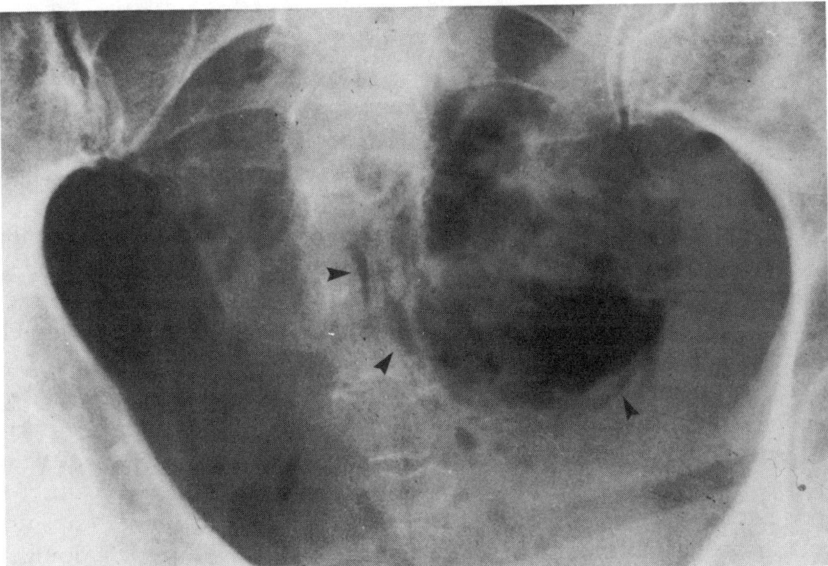

Figure 10-2 Flat plate of abdomen showing intramural gas.

As a rule, the greatest value of the flat plate of the abdomen is to exclude other causes of acute abdominal pain such as perforation or obstruction. The most pertinent information is to be found in visualization of the mesenteric arterial tree. Recently, emergency angiography has been advocated as the cornerstone of an aggressive diagnostic approach.[69,70] This permits the immediate detection of occlusions of the arterial trunks, as well as assessment of the entire arterial system for segmental obstruction or diffuse vasoconstriction seen in nonocclusive mesenteric infarction.

Based on this approach, Boley and his associates outlined a sequential program for the diagnosis and management of suspected mesenteric infarction and have achieved some noteworthy results. Briefly, their strategy is based upon the use of abdominal angiography as soon as resuscitative measures have stabilized the patient. If an occlusion of a main vessel or peripheral vasoconstriction is found, an immediate 25-mg bolus of tolazoline is administered directly into the superior mesenteric artery. In the presence of a significant occlusion, laparotomy is immediately undertaken to restore intestinal viability. Bowel is resected only if it is frankly necrotic after the return of blood flow. An infusion of papaverine is continued for the next 12 to 24 hours. If only peripheral vasoconstriction without occlusive disease is found on angiography in a patient who is not in shock or on vasoconstrictor support, a papaverine infusion at the rate of 30 to 60 mg/hr at a dilution of 1 mg/ml is immediately started into the superior mesenteric artery, using a constant infusion pump. This is continued for 24 hours at which point the angiogram is repeated, 30 minutes after discontinuing the papaverine. The decision whether to continue the infusion is then made, based on the clinical response of the patient and the angiographic findings. The infusion is discontinued only if the patient is stable and no further evidence of vasoconstriction is evident on angiography. In the authors' experience, infusions have been maintained for up to five days without adverse effects, although complications related to the catheterization did occur. The need for primary surgery and a second-look operation if surgery is undertaken, is evaluated on the basis of objective assessment of the patient's clinical course and the status of the bowel viability at the time of surgery. Any suspicion of peritoneal irritation or intestinal gangrene requires surgery. Anticoagulants are used only in the usual instances of mesenteric venous thrombosis. Guided by this approach, the authors have achieved an overall survival rate of 54%, a substantial improvement over the previously reported survivals below 30%. An abdominal condition other than mesenteric ischemia was ultimately found in 30% of patients, but in one half of these a correct diagnosis was made by angiography.

OCCLUSIVE MESENTERIC INFARCTION

The superior mesenteric artery supplies blood to the entire mid-gut. Despite potential collaterals, this vessel is a functional end artery, and acute interruption of blood flow will culminate in infarction of the mid-gut. Embolism and thrombosis account for about an equal number of the cases of acute occlusion in the large series by Ottinger,[66] although in some European studies thrombosis occurs up to four times more frequently.[40,64] Virtually all cases of acute occlusive infarction will involve the superior mesenteric artery, aside from the special circumstances in which the inferior mesenteric supply is interrupted at surgery.[71] The celiac axis is rarely a primary site of occlusion in such cases.[40] While involvement is limited to one artery in most instances, several vessels can be occluded simultaneously.

Although embolism and thrombosis are the usual pathological process, dissecting aneurysm and arteritis can be the precipitating event.[61] No matter what the nature of the occlusion, abdominal pain is the first symptom the patient experiences. It may be excruciating and seize the patient suddenly or, less commonly, evolve insidiously in a waxing and waning fashion with a vague colicky quality. It is surprising how long the pain may be present before the patient seeks hospitalization. Mavor[62] found that more than one third of his patients had severe pain for over 18 hours before admission to the hospital, and 13% for more than two weeks. Even more disturbing is his observation that more than one half of his cases had a greater than 12 hours wait before laparotomy, and a number waited several days.

The various causes of mesenteric ischemia cannot be differentiated on the basis of clinical features. These have been discussed previously. Vomiting seems to be a more common accompaniment of occlusive infarction but is of no diagnostic usefulness.[62,72] Angiography should be performed at the first suspicion of the diagnosis. The potential value of an aggressive therapeutic approach before peritoneal signs have set in is strikingly underscored by the survival of 9 of 10 such patients with ischemia of diverse etiologies in the previously discussed series by Boley and colleagues.[70]

Acute Arterial Embolism

Emboli to the superior mesenteric artery account for about 5% of all systemic emboli. The superior mesenteric artery originates from the abdominal aorta at an angle of about 45°, the least acute of the mesenteric vessels, an anatomical arrangement often cited as a reason for the fact that most mesenteric emboli lodge there. Peak incidence of mesenteric emboli occurs in the seventh decade, a decade earlier than thrombotic occlusions.[66] Most embolization occurs in the setting of cardiac disease. More than one half of the patients will have a history of myocardial infarction, while rheumatic heart disease serves as a background in less than one-quarter.[61] In some series, one third to one half of patients have had a previous episode of embolization.[61,69] Atrial fibrillation, often the first clue to the diagnosis, is present in one third of cases. In one out of three cases embolization occurs after hospitalization for another condition, which turns out to be for another embolus in 50% of these cases.[61] The source of the embolus in most instances is the left atrium, or a mural thrombus following an acute myocardial infarction. Other sites are not uncommon, however, as illustrated by one series where paradoxical embolization from deep leg veins occurred in 3 of 11 cases.[73] Other rare sources of emboli include bacterial vegetations from an infected valve, clots from valvular prostheses, abdominal aortic plaques often dislodged by catheters, and even tumor emboli from atrial myxoma or bronchogenic carcinoma.[74,75] While the onset of pain is apt to be more abrupt and recognized earlier because of the background medical illnesses, there is nothing in the clinical presentation to distinguish an embolic cause of ischemia from other causes. Ottinger and Austin noted tenesmus without diarrhea in three of their cases, a symptom they found to be associated only with embolization.[61]

Management

Embolic occlusions theoretically should offer the greatest opportunity for salvage of bowel viability. Unfortunately, results of therapy have not proved to be substantially different from that for other causes of bowel infarction. Nevertheless, since Stewart[76] first reported successful embolectomy in 1960, there has been an increasing number of survivals following surgery.[62,69] Early diagnosis by abdominal angiography and prompt surgical intervention offer the only hopes for improving survival in cases of proximal occlusion. The site of the embolus determines the extent of infarction and often is a pivotal factor in outcome. The majority of emboli lodge in the region of take-off of the middle colic artery or beyond (Figure 10-3). In about one half of the cases emboli lodge at this junction, while an equal number travel distal to it.[66] Occlusion at the origin of the main trunk is an uncommon occurrence.

Despite the potential opportunities for early diagnosis and treatment, mortality continues to remain high at 65% to 80%.[66] Undoubtedly much of this is attributable to the extensive and irreversible loss of

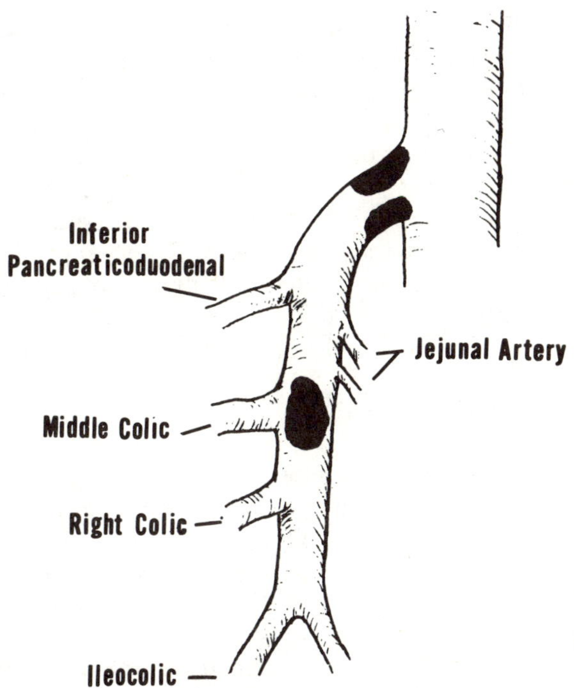

Figure 10-3 Superior mesenteric artery illustrating common sites of thrombosis and embolism.

bowel viability by the time of diagnosis, but the severe infirmity and serious cardiac disease of many of these patients are also major factors. However, some room for optimism can be found in the lower mortality rates of 18% to 56% in those series where early angiography was performed.[70,73] Outcome depends to a large extent on the level at which the embolus lodges. The use of heparin alone, for example, may be adequate treatment for peripheral emboli.[73] Despite the very high overall mortality in the large series by Ottinger,[66] all five patients who survived with simple resection alone had occlusions at the level of the ileocolic artery or beyond. The current recommended approach, therefore, is immediate surgery as soon as the diagnosis is confirmed. With distal emboli and limited areas of infarction, resection alone may suffice. In those occasional instances where no evidence of infarction is found and angiography shows distal emboli, it may be possible to avoid surgery. Proximal emboli must be removed. With restoration of flow, it is then possible to evaluate the viability of the bowel. In rare instances where complete viability is restored following embolectomy, no resection may be necessary. As is the general rule when dealing with cases of intestinal infarction, the decision to reoperate is usually made at the initial surgery, particularly when doubt exists about the viability of unresected bowel. Some recent reports suggest that the use of intraoperative Doppler ultrasound may be a more sensitive means of determining viability of ischemic bowel at the time of surgery. In Ottinger's series, the most frequent complication after embolectomy was rethrombosis at the arteriotomy site. Long-term follow-up is available in only a handful of cases. In at least half a dozen instances, however, reembolization has occurred.[75] Following embolectomy, malabsorption has been documented in a number of reported cases.[1,2] This gradually improved over a period of six months.

Arterial Thrombotic Occlusion

The peak incidence of arterial thrombotic occlusion occurs a decade later than embolic occlusion. Between one quarter to one half of mesenteric occlusive events are thrombotic in nature. Since arteriosclerotic changes are most marked at the origin of the superior mesenteric artery, thrombotic occlusions are most prone to occur at this location (Figure 10-3). Consequently, infarction tends to be massive.[62] Since the slow evolution of arteriosclerotic stenosis may permit the development of a collateral supply, often marginal in compensatory ability, a history of more protracted pain with delay in progression is more apt to be elicited in thrombotic occlusive disease. The frequency of a prior history of abdominal angina is unclear from published reports. Some observers have noted a prodromal phase in as many as 30% to 50% of all cases of acute thrombotic occlusion,[38-40] whereas others find this quite rare.[61] About one half of patients have a history of clinically significant heart disease.[61]

As with embolic occlusion, early diagnosis and surgical intervention offer the only means for improving survival. Because of the extent of bowel involvement and the technical difficulties in restoring intestinal flow, mortality rates remain over 90%.

Bypass grafting seems to be the preferable procedure because of the frequency of rethrombosis following thromboendarterectomy. While circulation to the bowel has been successfully restored in a number of patients, the long-term outlook remains poor.

Acute Venous Occlusion

While venous occlusion accounted for one out of every three cases of mesenteric infarction in earlier reports, at present less than 10% of mesenteric occlusions are venous in nature.[39,61] Patients tend to be younger than in arterial occlusive disease, generally between the ages of 30 and 60. A hypercoagulable state is often the setting for venous occlusion, such as cancer, sepsis, platelet defects, antithrombin III deficiency, trauma, or use of oral contraceptives.[77] Pain may appear abruptly, but in the usual case it develops insidiously over a period of 7 to 10 days as a poorly defined abdominal discomfort accompanied by anorexia and changes in bowel habits.[78] A number of patients with this slowly evolving form have had previous thrombophlebitis. A history of cirrhosis may be found in as many as 50% of patients, depending on the background from which the patients have been drawn.[62] Occasionally, venous and arterial thrombosis may coexist.[39] Other than the more protracted history and background of predisposing hypercoaguable states, no other clinical findings are useful for establishing the diagnosis. Although alteration of bowel habits is common, gastrointestinal bleeding occurs infrequently. Because the diagnosis is seldom suspected at the onset, serosanguineous peritoneal fluid is found in most cases at the time of diagnosis. The most solid diagnostic information is provided by abdominal angiography.[2] The characteristic features of venous infarction include spasm and prolongation of the arterial phase, delayed emptying of fine branches, and failure of opacification of the venous system. Prompt surgery with resection of infarcted bowel has been able to reduce the mortality to as low as 20%.[2] Anticoagulation is recommended as part of the management of venous infarction.

Segmental Small Bowel Infarction

Deprivation of blood flow to a localized segment of small bowel leads to a less dramatic clinical presentation than that of infarction secondary to a major vascular occlusion.[3] Since focal small bowel infarction occurs uncommonly except for bowel strangulation, and the symptoms are more subtle, the condition is more easily overlooked.

Clinical features reflect the nature of the ischemic process and the extent and severity of the necrosis. While abdominal pain is the overriding clinical feature, it can vary from a sudden onset of marked severity to a deceptive and less intense colicky pain. Strangulation obstructions account for the majority of cases, but a large number of insults may be responsible, including collagen vascular disorders, arteritis, emboli, and physical injury such as radiation, and ingestants such as potassium chloride tablets. If the necrosis extends transmurally, perforation and peritonitis may ensue. On the other hand, limited injury may be repaired without sequelae or may result in fibrosis with partial or complete obstruction.[79]

Symptoms of small bowel obstruction may appear long after the insult. In such cases x-ray shows a segmental stricture, often mimicking Crohn's disease. The most common ischemic strictures follow release of strangulated bowel from a hernia, where injury has been limited to the mucosa, stopping short of full mural necrosis.[79] Postoperative diarrhea, occasionally with blood, is the usual indication of such mucosal injury. Symptoms of obstruction usually follow surgery within 2 to 16 weeks. Whatever the cause of the ischemic stricture, local resection is adequate treatment in most cases.

NONOCCLUSIVE INFARCTION

Infarction of bowel without evidence of large vessel occlusion has emerged as the leading cause of intestinal infarction, approaching one half of all reported cases in this country, although less commonly elsewhere.[39,64,80] Two broad clinical patterns based on anatomical distribution have been recognizable. In the first, bowel infarctions lie within the region subserved by the superior mesenteric artery and involve predominantly the lower small bowel and right colon. In the second, perhaps larger group, vascular injury is limited to segmental areas of the colon and is now referred to as ischemic colitis. This will be discussed later.

The common factor underlying all cases of nonocclusvie infarction appears to be splanchnic vasoconstriction in response to diminished arterial perfusion on a central basis, although concommitant local factors may also play a role.[80] A substantial number of patients have severe organic heart disease and many have associated arrhythmias. The majority of patients are taking digitalis preparations.[39] Infarction often follows on the heels of another major illness such as shock or sepsis. In Renton's review of the literature,[72] pain was present in 55% of cases, a figure which suggests that the precarious medical condition of these patients and their cardiovascular instability attracts greater attention than any associated abdominal discomfort. Serosanguineous peritoneal fluid is present in the majority of patients by the time the diagnosis is made.

There are no distinctive features of nonocclusive infarction to distinguish it from occlusive infarction. The angiographic finding most suggestive of this diagnosis is a pruned appearance of the peripheral arterial tree, resulting from diffuse vasoconstriction. Mortality in this condition remains unacceptably high, approaching 90%, a fact which underscores the extent of bowel involvement, advanced state of necrosis by the time of diagnosis, and the underlying debility of most of these patients.[72,80] By the time peritoneal signs appear, the surgeon is left with the unhappy task of attempting resection of nonviable bowel in circumstances where the entire mid-gut is generally involved. Compounding the frustration is the virtual impossibility of distinguishing completely dead bowel from marginally viable regions. Such efforts are often ill-fated, prompting the suggestion that 8 to 12 hours should elapse before intervention to allow clearer demarcation of nonviable areas.[2] A second-look operation is almost always necessary if the patient survives. More experience is required before the use of intraoperative Doppler ultrasonography becomes an established method of determining viability of ischemic bowel.

The uniformly dismal results of resectional surgery have compelled surgeons to seek alternative methods of therapy. This has generated a number of approaches aimed at interrupting the cycle of factors perpetuating vasoconstriction. Some isolated successes have been reported with a number of techniques, including disruption of splanchnic autonomic nerves by splanchnic block,[81] and spinal epidural block.[82] The direct infusion of vasodilators as advocated by Boley and his associates[70] seems to hold the most promise as a realistic means for improving survival. While their overall survival with this method was 40%, an impressive figure itself, all five patients without peritonitis survived after vasodilator infusions. Results such as this encourage the belief that, with early diagnosis and prompt action, it is possible to achieve a substantial reduction in mortality.

ISCHEMIC COLITIS

In 1963 Boley and colleagues[83] reported five cases of transient diarrhea and rectal bleeding with distinctive but transient radiological findings, which they called "reversible vascular occlusion of the colon." In the decade preceding this description, scattered reports had appeared of idiopathic stricture of the colon, segmental colitis, and gangrene of the colon. During the same period vascular surgeons were beginning to recognize instances of ischemia of the colon which followed inferior artery ligation during aneurysmectomy. In 1966 Marston[84] first used the umbrella term of "ischemic colitis" to embrace all of these entities, proposing that they represented a spectrum of responses to a common underlying event, namely, deprivation of vascular supply to the colon. Numerous reports have appeared since then and the entity has flourished as a clinical syndrome.

Pathophysiology

The underlying susceptibility of the colon to vascular injury may in part derive from its intrinsically low blood flow and low priority for visceral supply after meals or systemic disturbances, actually declining in such circumstances. Blood supplies the colon via the marginal artery of Drummond, which originates from the ileocecal artery and straddles the entire length of the colon from ileum to sigmoid. This artery (Figure 10-4) is attenuated in the region of the splenic flexure where it lies at the greatest distance from the bowel than elsewhere. The region is also the watershed zone of the colon where the circulations of the superior and inferior mesenteric arteries coalesce as the "central anastomotic artery," a region of intrinsic vascular instability. The same spectrum of clinical, radiological, and histological responses to ligation of the inferior mesenteric artery can be observed in cases of spontaneous "ischemic colitis,"[71,84] supporting the theory of a common pathophysiological basis despite lack of conclusive proof of "ischemia." The term encompasses a broad range of disorders of blood flow from occlusion of the inferior artery or central alterations of blood flow, to disturbances at the microcirculatory level, presumed to underly the "spontaneous" variety where no clear precipitating event is present. These alterations can result from a variety of causes including trauma, abdominoperineal resection, arteritis, shock, increased blood viscosity, or raised intraluminal pressure secondary to obstructive lesions such as carcinoma, diverticular disease, hernia, or volvulus.[1,3] While emboli, thrombosis, and actual ligation of the inferior mesenteric artery can produce an identical picture, the surprisingly low incidence of such occurrences underscores the capacity of collateral circulation to compensate for acute occlusions at this site. At the Massachusetts General Hospital, only 20 instances of colon ischemia occurred in 1200 operations for aortoiliac reconstruction with interruption of the inferior mesenteric artery.[71]

Whether the episode is "spontaneous" or results from a definable insult, the clinical picture that emerges is solely dependent on the ultimate depth of tissue injury. Superficial injury leads to reversible submucosal edema with some denudation of mucosa, resulting in a transitory illness of several days' to several weeks' duration. Infarction penetrating into deeper layers without breeching the bowel wall is followed by a variable interval of more severe clinical symptoms, culminating in repair with stenosis (Figures 10-5A, 10-5B). Full-thickness gangrene leads to an overwhelming clinical illness with perforation and peritonitis. The outcome of an individual episode ultimately depends on a variety of factors influencing circulation to the affected region, but disruption of the inferior mesenteric circula-

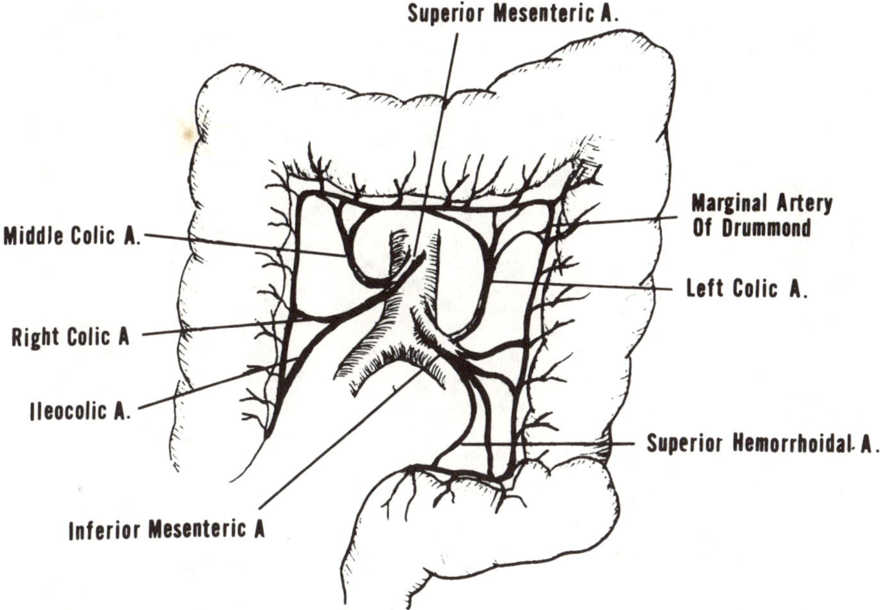

Figure 10-4 Blood supply of colon.

tion with inadequate collaterals tends to pursue a fulminant course to gangrene, as happened in two thirds of the cases in Ottinger's series.[71]

Clinical Features

Typically, the patient experiences a short episode of abdominal pain accompanied by diarrhea with blood. Within this setting, however, considerable variation exists. A history of pain may be absent in as many as 25% of patients,[85] and can range from severe, prolonged colic to discomfort so transient that it is revealed only after intense questioning. Only 60% of patients develop diarrhea,[85] and this is often mild in nature. In some instances constipation is a prominent complaint. One quarter of patients deny seeing blood in their stool. Bleeding massive enough to require surgery has been reported only once.[86]

Males and females are equally affected, and most patients are over the age of 70. In Boley et al's[3] series 90% of patients with no iatrogenic lesions were over and above this age. On the other hand, 20% of Marcuson's patients were under the age of 50.[87] Most series report a high frequency of predisposing conditions such as atherosclerotic disease, hypertension, or diabetes. An underlying obstructive lesion was pres-

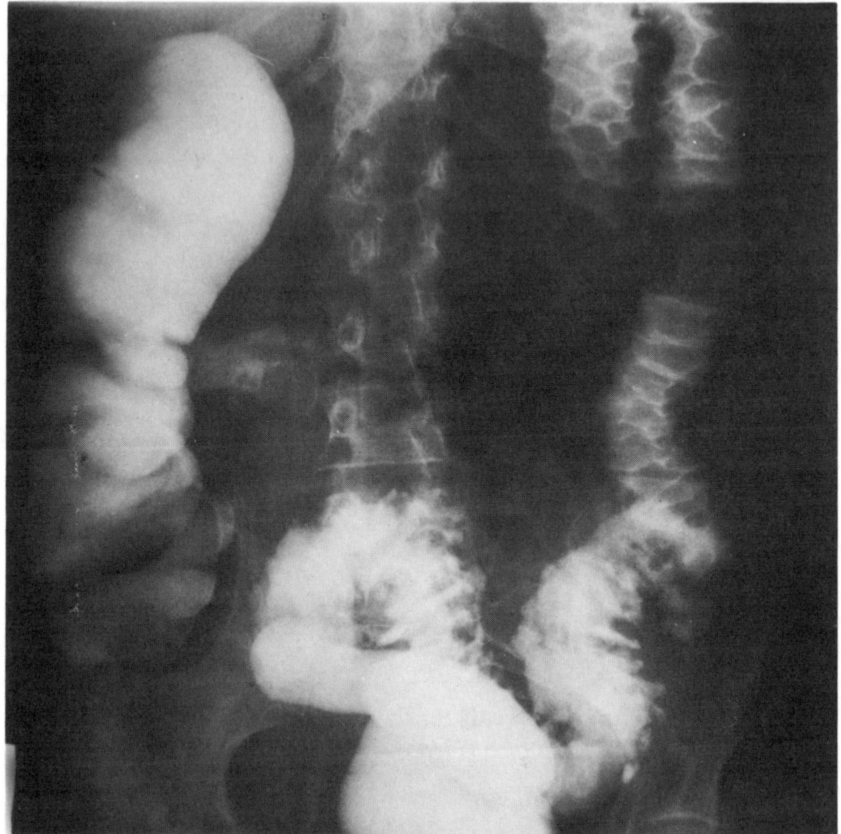

Figure 10-5A Barium enema in a 68-year-old woman with acute ischemic colitis involving splenic flexure. Note large "thumbprint" in descending colon.

ent in 20% of Boley's cases, of which one-half were carcinomas.[3] In patients below the age of 50, the episode is attributable to an underlying cause in as many as 75% of cases, twice the frequency found in patients above this age.[87] The use of oral contraceptives has been particularly incriminated in younger women.[88]

Physical examination reflects the degree of underlying tissue injury. Generally, little more than minimal fever and mild left lower quadrant tenderness is found, but severe toxicity and the presence of peritoneal signs point to the development of serious gangrene. Laboratory features usually are not helpful, merely reinforcing impressions gained by physical examination. Some degree of leukocytosis is common, as might be anticipated. In cases of rectal or low-sigmoid involvement, nonspecific findings of edema, granularity, and friability are seen on sigmoidoscopy, but only the presence of blue-

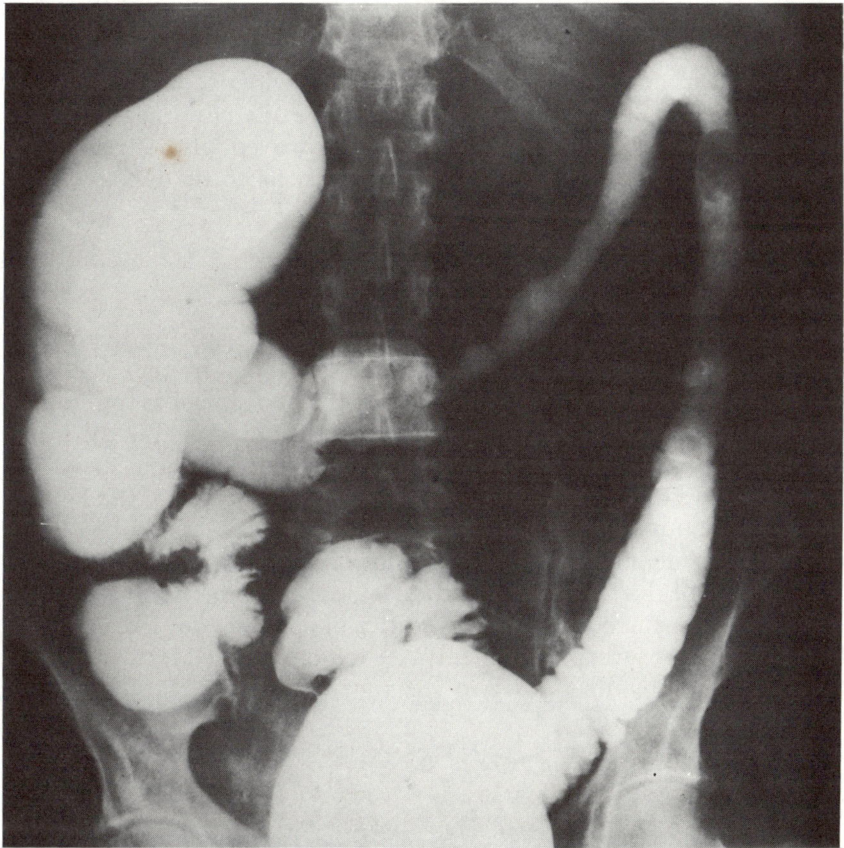

Figure 10-5B Same patient four weeks later. A stricture has developed in the same area.

black blebs of submucosal hemorrhage is diagnostic. While rectal involvement is usual in cases following surgical disruption of the inferior mesenteric artery, it is regarded as uncommon in most other instances. On the other hand, Williams[85] noted rectal involvement in 22% of his cases of spontaneous ischemic colitis. In contrast, Boley[3] found rectal involvement in only 6% of a mixed group of patients. A plain film of the abdomen may show nodular defects encroaching on the air-filled colon. The most precise information is to be found on the barium enema where these smooth nodular defects along the wall of the colon, referred to as "thumbprinting," are regarded as characteristic. Since these represent small areas of submucosal edema and hemorrhage which may rapidly resolve, a barium enema should be obtained within the first 48 hours.[89] Other radiologic findings such as edema, ulceration, and spasm often coexist but are nonspecific. Biopsy is useful only when findings are characteristic of ischemia, such as necrosis with hemorrhage, edema, and intravascular thrombi. Unfortunately, these are present in only 50% of the cases. While evidence of submucosal hemorrhage can be seen by colonoscopy, more often findings resemble inflammatory bowel disease, and this procedure entails definite risks, especially perforation. Angiography generally has little to offer.

Distribution of Involvement

In 80% to 90% of cases changes occur at the splenic flexure or beyond.[3,85,87] The descending colon is the most frequent site of involvement, although the splenic flexure may be almost as frequently involved. Figure 10-6 shows the frequency of involvement in the three largest series in the literature in the diagnostic locations used by Marcuson. Right colon involvement occurs in only 10% of the largest series where involvement is detailed, and only two cases of isolated cecal involvement could be found in the 288 cases from these series.[85] Ten percent of the total group had rectal involvement, although twice this number occurred in Williams' series of spontaneous ischemic colitis.[85] The latter series was the only one to note isolated rectal involvement, present by itself in two instances, and with discontinuous

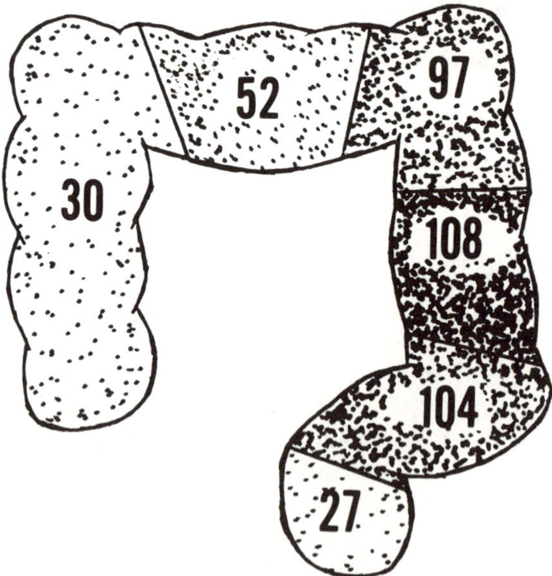

Figure 10-6 Frequency of involvement of various sites in ischemic colitis based on 288 patients pooled from three large series. Overlapping areas of involvement in a number of patients accounts for discrepancy in figures.

left colon involvement in another four. Others have noted rectal changes only in association with sigmoid involvement. In one series, 8 of 9 patients with spontaneous ischemic proctitis were men, a significant sex disparity when compared to ischemic colitis as a group.[90]

Course

A number of factors influence the outcome of an episode of ischemic colitis including the nature, rapidity, and duration of the insult, and the adequacy of collateral blood supply. Cases following ligation of the inferior mesenteric artery are more likely to run a fulminant course, two thirds of the patients developing gangrene. In contrast, in about one half the cases of spontaneous ischemic colitis, injury is limited, and resolution is the rule in most cases.[3] A protracted course develops in 25% of patients in whom inflammation persists for weeks to months, often culminating in stricture formation. Stricture developed in 25% of Williams's patients with spontaneous ischemic colitis. Approximately 25% of the patients will run a severe course. In 19% of Boley et al's series gangrene developed. Not unexpectedly, the mortality rate is high in these cases. Stricture formation does not automatically necessitate surgery, since documented obstruction is rare and many strictures heal over a period of months. While gangrene usually progresses rapidly in irreversible cases, in some instances a persistent inflammatory response may eventuate in gangrene.

Management

Since symptoms subside with 48 hours in most cases, only supportive therapy is required. Once the patient has been stabilized, a barium enema should be done at the earliest possible moment if ischemic colitis is strongly suspected. A worsening clinical condition and, especially, the evolution of peritoneal signs raises the question of bowel gangrene and calls for immediate surgical consideration. Patients with continuing symptoms beyond a period of several weeks present a difficult managment problem since medical therapy is of no avail in these circumstances. The need for surgery must be judged on the clinical status of the patient and the extent and severity of the ischemic lesions. In the event of progressive deterioration, surgery is the only resort.

Strictures developing during the course of ischemic colitis have until now been a frequent indication for surgical intervention. However, since many of these strictures have been shown to resolve over a period of six months, delay in this situation is justified if the patient remains stable.[87] Overt obstruction seldom occurs as a consequence of these strictures.[85] Previously, a strong suspicion of cancer has necessitated surgery in patients with ischemic strictures, particularly when a clear-cut history of an ischemic episode is lacking. The use of colonoscopy and biopsy to evaluate these areas has lessened the urgency for such intervention.

The physician is often faced with the dilemma of distinguishing ischemic colitis from a number of other inflammatory conditions including enteric infections, pseudomembrocolitis, and the idiopathic inflammatory bowel diseases. The abrupt onset of symptoms in an older patient with a history of predisposing vascular disease will usually alert one to the possibility of ischemic colitis. In addition, the lack of rectal involvement, negative stool cultures, distinctive changes on barium enema, and a transient course will generally suffice to establish the diagnosis. In a late stage, particularly if ulceration is present, differentiation from Crohn's colitis, and even occasionally ulcerative colitis, may be difficult. In these cases diagnosis becomes evident after spontaneous resolution in the absence of specific therapy. The milder nature of the pain, absence of severe toxicity, and stable clinical status of the patient generally prevent confusion with more extensive bowel ischemia. Necrotizing colitis[91] may be indistinguishable from the latter, but in either case surgery will be required. The outlook following recovery from an episode of ischemic colitis is excellent since only 5% of patients will experience a recurrence.[3]

REFERENCES

1. Boley SJ, Schwartz SS, Williams LF Jr. *Vascular Disorders of the Intestine.* New York, Appleton-Century-Crofts, 1971.
2. Williams LF Jr. Vascular insufficiency of the intestines. *Gastroenterology* 61:757, 1971.
3. Boley SJ, Brandt LJ, Veita FS. Ischemic disorders of the intestines. *Current Probl Surg* Vol 15, No 4, 1978.
4. Herlinger H. Angiography of the visceral arteries. *Clin Gastroenterol* 1:547, 1972.
5. Reynolds DG, Gurll NJ, Swan KG, et al. The clincial significance of gastrointestinal blood flow. *J Clin Gastroenterol* 1:353, 1979.
6. Bynum JA, Jacobson EF. Blood flow and gastrointestinal function. *Gastroenterology* 71:851, 1976.
7. Lanciault G, Jacobson ED. The gastrointestinal circulation. *Gastroenterology* 71:851, 1976.
8. Norryd C, Dencker H, Lunderquist A, et al. Splanchnic blood flow during digestion in man. *Acta Chir Scand* 141:1975.

9. Hansen HJB, Engell HC, Ring-Larsen H, et al. Splanchnic blood flow in patients with abdominal angina before and after arterial reconstruction. *Ann Surg* 186:215, 1977.

10. Bron KM, Redman HC. Splanchnic artery stenosis and occlusion. *Radiology* 92:323, 1969.

11. Chiene J. Complete obliteration of celiac and mesenteric arteries: Viscera receiving their blood supply through the extraperitoneal system of vessels. *J Anat [London]* (second series) 3(65):1868, 1969.

12. Lipchik EO, Rob CG, Schwartzberg BA. Obstruction of the abdominal aorta above the level of the renal arteries. *Radiology* 82:443, 1964.

13. Hansen HJB. Abdominal angina. *Acta Chir Scand* 142:319, 1976.

14. Schnitzler J. Zur symptomatologie des darmaterterienverschlusses. *Wein Med Wochenschr* 51:506, 1901.

15. Connelly TL, Garland PD, Smith RB, et al. Elective mesenteric revascularization. *Am Surg* 47:19, 1981.

16. Dunphy JE. Abdominal pain of vascular origin. *Am J Med Sci* 192:109, 1936.

17. Shaw RS, Maynard EP. Acute and chronic thrombosis of mesenteric arteries associated with malabsorption: Report of two cases successfully treated by thromboendarterectomy. *N Engl J Med* 258:874, 1958.

18. Morris G, DeBakey M, Bernhard V. Abdominal angina. *Surg Clin North Am* 46:919, 1966.

19. Rob C. Surgical diseases of the celiac and mesenteric arteries. *Arch Surg* 93:21, 1966.

20. Crawford, ES, Morris GC Jr, Myhre HO, et al. Celiac axis, superior mesenteric artery and inferior mesenteric artery occlusion: Surgical considerations. *Surgery* 82:856, 1977.

21. Reul GJ Jr, Wukasch DC, Sandiford FM, et al. Surgical treatment of abdominal angina. Review of 25 patients. *Surgery* 75:682, 1974.

22. McCollum CH, Graham JM, DeBakey ME. Chronic mesenteric arterial insufficiency: Results of revascularization in 33 cases. *South Med J* 69:1266, 1976.

23. Eidemiller LR, Nelson JC, Porter JM. Surgical treatment of chronic visceral ischemia. *Am J Surg* 138:264, 1979.

24. Dick AP, McC.Gregg D. Chronic occlusions of the visceral arteries. *Clin Gastroenterol* 1:689, 1972.

25. Bircher J, Bartholomew LG, Cain JC, et al. Syndrome of intestinal arterial insufficiency ("abdominal angina"). *Arch Intern Med* 117:632, 1966.

26. Gluecklich B, Deterling RA Jr, Matsumoto GH, et al. Chronic mesenteric ischemia masquerading as cancer. *Surg Gynecol Obstet* 148:49, 1979.

27. Stoney RJ, Ehrenfeld WK, Wylie EJ. Revascularization methods in chronic visceral ischemia caused by atherosclerosis. *Ann Surg* 186:468, 1977.

28. Watson WC, Williams PB, Duffy G. Epigastric bruits in patients with and without celiac axis compression: A phonoarteriographic study. *Ann Intern Med* 79:211, 1973.

29. Dardik H, Seidenberg B, Parker JG, et al. Intestinal angina malabsorption treated with elective revascularization. *JAMA* 194:1206, 1965.

30. Watt JK, Watson WC, Haase S. Chronic intestinal ischemia. *Br Med J* 3:199, 1967.

31. Meyers MA, Kaplowitz N, Bloom AA. Malabsorption secondary to mesenteric ischemia. *Am J Roentgenol* 119:352, 1973.

32. Papp JP, Sullivan BH Jr, Bloom AA. Malabsorption and mesenteric ischemia. *Cleve Clin Q* 32:227, 1965.

33. Mavor GE, Michie W. Chronic midgut ischemia. *Br Med J* 2:534, 1958.

34. Heard G, Jeffries JD, Peters DK. Chronic intestinal ischemia; successful aorta/superior mesenteric by-pass. *Lancet* 2:975, 1963.

35. Webb WR, Hardy JB. Relief of abdominal angina by vascular graft. *Ann Intern Med* 57:289, 1962.

36. McClenahan JA, Fisher B. Mesenteric thrombosis: *Surgery* 23:779, 1948.

37. Fry WJ, Kraft RO. Visceral angina. *Surg Gynecol Obstet* 117:417, 1963.

38. Purdue GD, Smith RB. Intestinal ischemia due to mesenteric arterial disease. *Am Surg* 36:152, 1970.

39. Pierce GE, Brockenbrough EC. The spectrum of mesenteric infarction. *Am J Surg* 119:233, 1970.

40. Hansen HJB, Christoffersen JK. Occlusive mesenteric infarction. *Acta Chir Scand* 472:103, 1976.

41. Marstan A. Intestinal arterial disease. *Proc Roy Soc Med* 64:1079, 1971.

42. Harris PL, Charlesworth D. Chronic intestinal ischemia due to aorto-iliac steal. *J Cardiovasc Surg* 15:122, 1974.

43. Reuter SR, Olin T. Surgery of the celiac and superior mesenteric vessels. *Radiology* 85:4, 1965.

44. Brooks DH, Bron KM. Postprandial rest pain and claudication of the lower extremity. A case report. *Surgery* 78:677, 1975.

45. Dick AP, Graff R, Gregg D, et al. An arteriographic study of mesenteric arterial disease. *Gut* 8:206, 1967.

46. Connolly JE, Stemmer EA. Intestinal gangrene as the result of mesenteric arterial steal. *Am J Surg* 126:197, 1973.

47. Connolly JE, Kwaan JHM. Prophylactic revascularization of the gut. *Ann Surg* 190:514, 1979.

48. Harjola PT. A rare obstruction of the coeliac artery. *Ann Chir Gynaecol* 52:547, 1963.

49. Dunbar JA, Molnar W, Beman FF, et al. Compression of the celiac trunk and abdominal angina. *Am J Roentgenol* 95:731, 1965.

50. Brandt LJ, Boley SJ. Celiac axis compression syndrome. A critical review. *Dig Dis Sci* 23:633, 1978.

51. Szilagyi DE, Rian RL, Elliot JP, et al. The celiac artery compression syndrome: Does it exist? *Surgery* 72:849, 1972.

52. Watson WC, Sadikali F. Celiac axis syndrome. Experience with 20 patients and a critical appraisal of the syndrome. *Ann Intern Med* 86:278, 1977.

53. Sleisinger MH. The Celiac artery syndrome—again? *Ann Intern Med* 86:356, 1977

54. Levin DC, Baltaxe HA. High incidence of celiac axis narrowing in asymptomatic individuals. *Am J Roentgenol* 116:426, 1972.

55. Appleby LH. The celiac axis in the expansion of the operation for gastric carcinoma. *Cancer* 6:704, 1953.

56. Stanley JC, Fry WJ. Median arcuate ligament syndrome. *Arch Surg* 103:252, 1971.

57. Watt JK. Coeliac axis stenosis. *Scot Med J* 17:298, 1972.

58. Garvin PJ, Sawyerr O, Cabal ET, et al. Malabsorption and abdominal pain secondary to celiac artery entrapment. *Arch Surg* 112:655, 1977.

59. Evans WE. Long term evaluation of the celiac band syndrome. *Surgery* 76:867, 1974.

60. Jackson BB. Occlusion of the superior mesenteric artery, in *American Lectures in Surgery.* Springfield, IL, Charles C Thomas, 1963.

61. Ottinger LW, Austin WG. A study of 136 patients with mesenteric infarction. *Surg Gynecol Obstet* 124:251, 1967.

62. Mavor GE. Acute occlusion of the superior mesenteric artery. *Clin Gastroenterol* 1:639, 1972.

63. Hildebrand HD, Zierler RE. Mesenteric vascular disease. *Am J Surg* 139:188, 1980.

64. Kairaluoma MI, Karkola P, Heikkinen E, et al. Mesenteric infarction. *Am J Surg* 133:188, 1977.

65. Slater H, Elliott DW. Primary mesenteric infarction. *Am J Surg* 123:309, 1972.

66. Ottinger LW. The surgical managment of acute occlusion of the superior mesenteric artery. *Ann Surg* 188:721, 1978.

67. Tomchik FS, Wittenberg J, Ottinger LW. The roentgenographic spectrum of bowel infarction. *Radiology* 96:249, 1970.

68. Scott JR, Miller WT, Urso M, et al. Acute mesenteric infarction. *Am J Roentgenol* 113:269, 1971.

69. Bergan JJ, Dean RH, Conn J Jr, et al. Revascularization in treatment of mesenteric infarction. *Ann Surg* 182:430, 1975,

70. Boley SJ, Sprayregen S, Siegelman SS, et al. Initial results from an aggressive approach to acute mesenteric ischemia. *Surgery* 82:848, 1977.

71. Ottinger LW, Darling RC, Nathan MJ, et al. Left colon ischemia. Complicating aorto-iliac reconstruction. *Arch Surg* 105:841, 1972.

72. Renton CJC. Non-occlusive intestinal infarction. *Clin Gastroenterol* 1:655, 1972.

73. Kaufman SK, Harrington DP, Siegelman SS. Superior mesenteric artery embolization: An angiographic emergency. *Radiology* 124:625, 1977.

74. Bergan JJ, Dry L, Conn J, et al. Intestinal ischemic syndromes. *Ann Surg* 169:120, 1969.

75. Williams LF. Vascular insufficiency of the bowels. *DM,* August 1970, pp 1–38.

76. Stewart DG, Sweetman WR, Westphal K, et al. Superior mesenteric artery embolectomy. *Ann Surg* 151:274, 1960.

77. Khodadi J, Rosencwajg J, Nacasch N, et al. Mesenteric vein thrombosis. *Arch Surg* 115:315, 1980.

78. Naitove A, Weismann R. Primary mesenteric venous thrombosis. *Ann Surg* 161:516, 1965.

79. Windsor CWO. Ischaemic strictures of the small bowel. *Clin Gastroenterol* Vol I, 1972.

80. Ottinger LW. Non-occlusive infarction. *Surg Clin North Am* 54:689, 1974.

81. Britt LG, Cheek RC. Non-occlusive mesenteric vascular disease: Clinical and experimental observations. *Ann Surg* 169:704, 1969.

82. Jackson BB, Lykins R. Serial epidural analgesia in mesenteric arterial failure. *Arch Surg* 90:177, 1965.

83. Boley SJ, Schwartz S, Lash J, et al. Reversible vascular occlusion of the colon. *Surg Gynecol Obstet* 116:53, 1963.

84. Marston A, Pheils M, Thomas MC, et al. Ischaemic colitis. *Gut* 7:1, 1966.

85. Williams LF, Wittenberg J. Ischemic colitis. *Ann Surg* 182:439, 1975.

86. Parks TG, Johnson GW, Kennedy TL, et al. Spontaneous ischaemic proctocolitis. *Scand J Gastroenterol* 7:241, 1972.

87. Marcuson RW. Ischaemic colitis. *Clin Gastroenterol* 1:745, 1972.

88. Cotton PB, Thomas ML. Ischemic colitis and the contraceptive pill. *Br Med J* 3:27, 1971.

89. Wittenberg J, Athanasoulis CA, Williams LJ, et al. Ischemic colitis. Radiology and pathophysiology. *Am J Roentgenol* 123:287 (1975).

90. Farman J, Betancourt E, Kilpatrick ZM. The radiology of ischemic proctitis. *Radiology* 91:302–307, 1968.

91. Heikkinen E, Larmi TK, Huttunen R. Necrotizing colitis. *Am J Surg* 128:362, 1974.

11 Disorders of the Renal Vasculature

Herman Rosen

The kidney has a disproportionately large blood supply for its size. Its blood flow is normally about 20% to 25% of the cardiac output, supplying a tissue mass that is less than 0.5% of the total body weight. The organization of this vast blood supply is of interest in any discussion of disorders of the renal vasculature.

VASCULAR STRUCTURE OF THE KIDNEY

Each kidney is supplied by a renal artery which arises from the abdominal aorta at about the level of the second or third lumbar vertebra, the left usually at a higher level than the right. The renal artery divides into an anterior and a smaller posterior division, which then enter the renal hilus. A separate segmental vessel supplies each of the five renal segments. The anterior branch of the renal artery gives rise to three segmental arteries—upper, middle, and lower—while the posterior branch supplies the posterior segment of the kidney and may also give rise to an apical segmental artery. In some cases, the apical segment is supplied by the anterior branch of the renal artery. Each segmental artery is essentially an end artery, there being no anastomosis between the segments.[1-3]

The segmental arteries divide within the renal sinus to form the interlobar arteries which run adjacent to the renal pyramids. At the corticomedullary junction, each interlobar artery divides into arcuate arteries which curve smoothly across the base of the renal pyramids. These arcuate arteries give rise to interlobular arteries which course straight toward the renal capsule. The interlobular arteries give rise to afferent arterioles, each supplying the capillary tuft of a glomerulus; each glomerulus is supplied by a sole afferent vessel. If this vessel is compromised, glomerular injury may ensue[4,5] (Figure 11-1).

The glomerular capillary network unifies to form the efferent arteriole which emerges from the glomerulus. In most cortical nephrons, the efferent arteriole then breaks up into a capillary plexus which surrounds a tubule, not necessarily from the same nephron from which it arose. Efferent arterioles from juxtamedullary nephrons are larger and give rise to parallel vessels which descend without branching into the pyramids of the medulla. These straight vessels are called arteriolae rectae spuriae, and give rise to capillary networks at

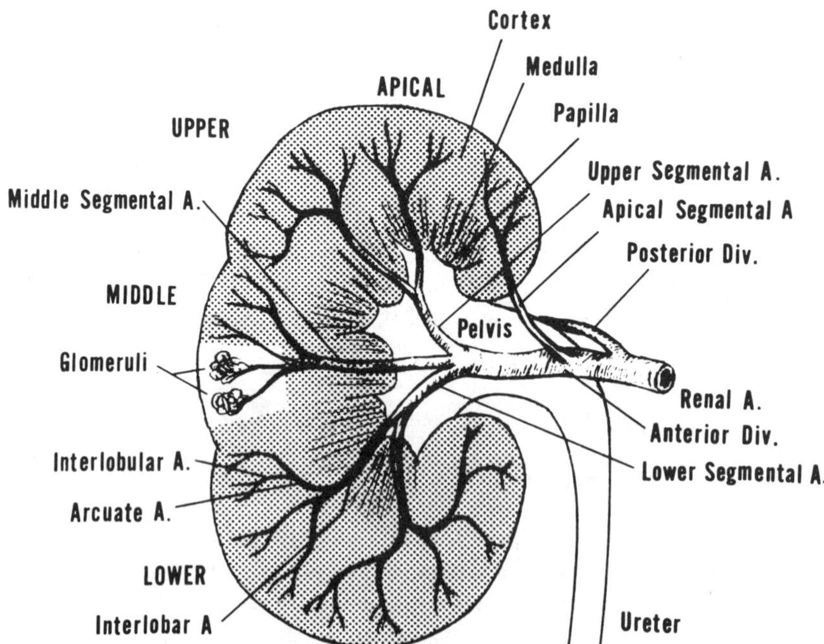

Figure 11-1 Arterial blood supply of the kidney.

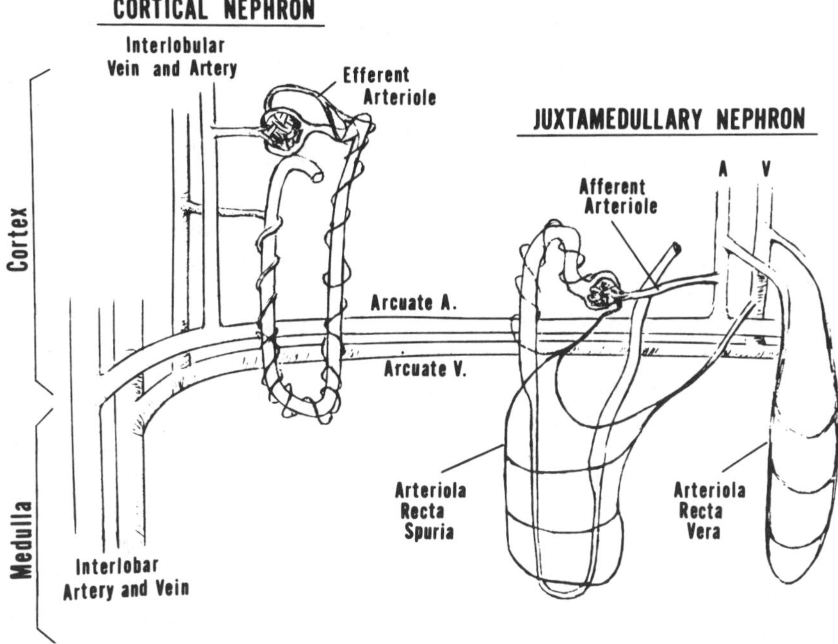

Figure 11-2 Pattern of blood vessels in the renal parenchyma showing types of vasa rectae and comparing postglomerular circulation in cortical and juxtamedullary nephrons.

various levels and supply the papillae with blood. Other straight vessels very infrequently arise directly from an intralobular artery close to the medulla without going to a glomerulus. These are called arteriolae rectae verae, and represent aglomerular shunt pathways which may have formed when glomeruli became sclerosed, leaving a direct communication between afferent and efferent arterioles. The vasa rectae lie close to their counterpart veins, forming a vascular countercurrent system. The tubular capillaries form interlobular veins which empty into arcuate veins.The arcuate veins receive blood from the venous vasa rectae and drain into interlobar veins, which in turn coalesce to form the main renal vein[6,7] (Figure 11-2).

RENAL VEIN THROMBOSIS

Thrombosis of the renal veins was described over 100 years ago and believed to be relatively rare. However, in the past few years, renal vein thrombosis has been increasingly recognized. More frequent diagnosis probably does not reflect a true increased incidence of this problem, but rather is a reflection of improved angiographic techniques and increased clinical suspicion.

When renal vein thrombosis occurs in infants, it is present in a catastrophic clinical setting. In these cases, thrombosis often occurs as a complication of severe dehydration due to diarrhea or vomiting. The sudden and complete blocking of the renal veins causes hematuria, severe flank pain, fever, leukocytosis, and proteinuria. Consumptive coagulopathy may be present. Renal failure with rising levels of serum creatinine and urea nitrogen as well as shock may supervene. Sonography shows enlarged kidneys, and urography shows no function. In these acute cases, the prognosis is exceedingly grave in spite of vigorous anticoagulation, rehydration, and supportive measures.[8,9]

In contrast to the acute form of renal vein thrombosis, the chronic form may have few localizing symptoms. There may be some hematuria, flank pain, or edema, but these manifestations or even renal insufficiency may be surprisingly absent. Presumably, collateral venous vessels can develop to accommodate the renal blood flow. Frequently, the first suspicion that renal vein thrombosis has occurred is when there is evidence of pulmonary embolism with no other obvious source for the clots. Clinical suspicion of this thrombosis is heightened when predisposing conditions are present. Such conditions include hypercoagulable states, severe dehydration, neoplasms in the region of the kidney, flank trauma, consumption coagulopathy, and polycythemic states. Renal vein thrombosis occurs in association with several glomerulopathies, especially membranous glomerulonephropathy and amyloidosis.[10-13]

The known association between the nephrotic syndrome and renal vein thrombosis merits special comment. For many years, it was felt that the nephrotic syndrome was a consequence of renal vein thrombosis since these conditions often coexist. The nephrotic syndrome was considered a secondary event because clinical conditions with elevated renal venous pressure such as constrictive pericarditis are often associated with proteinuria, at times heavy. In the past few years, however, physicians have been rethinking this relationship, and the bulk of evidence now indicates that renal vein thrombosis is a complication of, rather than the cause of, the nephrotic syndrome. It is now clear that there is a hypercoagulable state in the nephrotic syndrome. Plasma antithrombin III levels are depressed, presumably due to urinary loss of this normal circulating anticoagulant.[14] Also contributing to hypercoagulability may be a shrunken intravascular volume due to hypoalbuminemia and resultant hemoconcentration. In patients with unilateral renal vein thrombosis, ureteral catheterizations have shown proteinuria to be bilateral, eliminating local thrombosis as a cause of the proteinuria. Furthermore, patients with the nephrotic syndrome have been described in whom renal vein thrombosis was not initially present but subsequently developed.

The diagnosis of renal vein thrombosis is based upon clinical suspicion in the appropriate setting. When the thrombosis is sudden, the acute signs often point to the kidney and the diagnosis is readily considered. In the chronic form, renal vein thrombosis must be suspected and studies then done to confirm the suspicion. Abdominal films may show enlarged kidneys, but it should be noted that in long-standing thrombosis, the kidneys may atrophy. Sonography may similarly show renal size, or a clot may be appreciated in the vena cava. In approximately one third of cases of renal vein thrombosis, there is associated vena caval thrombosis. On excretory urography, there may be poor visualization of the collecting system and evidence of interstitial swelling with separation of the calyces. When present, notching of the proximal ureter due to venous collaterals is a useful sign. In some cases however, the urogram may be entirely normal.[15]

The definitive study for the diagnosis of renal vein thrombosis is selective renal venography. The risk of dislodging clots during the procedure may have been overestimated, since recent studies reveal few complications during venography. Because of the fear of producing pulmonary emboli with venography, many radiologists prefer arteriography with careful attention to the renal venous phase. However, arteriography is not as specific as selective renal venography. Inferior vena cavagrams are also not reliable for renal vein thrombosis, since interpretive artifacts may be produced by normal renal venous flow.

Treatment

In the management of patients with renal vein thrombosis, anticoagulation with heparin is initially indicated to prevent thromboemboli and prevent further extension of the clot within the kidney. Generally, after two weeks of heparin therapy, long-term anticoagulation with warfarin is begun, but the duration of administration is not clear. It seems reasonable to continue anticoagulation as long as risk factors for renal vein thrombosis persist. Nevertheless, anticoagulation in uremic patients requires special caution because of associated bleeding tendencies. Fibrinolytic therapy with urokinase has been tried in renal vein thrombosis, but sufficient experience with this therapy has not been obtained. Surgical thrombectomy is generally not done, since the smaller branches of the renal vein cannot be adequately declotted, and recanalization of the veins or drainage via rich collaterals may take place while the patient is receiving anticoagulant therapy.[16] Surgery may be warranted in specific situations such as acute thrombosis with severe symptoms, bilateral thrombosis, and thrombosis in a solitary kidney.

When renal disease is complicated by renal vein thrombosis, the prognosis worsens because of an increased risk of pulmonary embolism and a general tendency to a decline in renal function. Faced with radiographically documented renal vein thrombosis, the clinician must use keen judgment. In the presence of definite pulmonary emboli, anticoagulants appear indicated even though uremia is present. As for their effect on renal function, anticoagulants appear to offer little benefit in most cases. Occasionally, there is improvement during anticoagulation, with decreased proteinuria and increased renal function. Whether such improvement is the result of therapy or a spontaneous occurrence is difficult to say.[17]

RENAL ARTERIAL THROMBOEMBOLIC DISEASE

Obstruction of the renal arterial tree has an effect on the kidney that varies with the size of the vessel involved, the extent of the vessel occlusion, and the duration of the occlusion. When the renal artery or its main branches are severely involved, there is resultant infarction of the renal parenchyma. If vascular occlusion is not complete and some flow of blood can occur, or if vascular obstruction develops slowly, thereby allowing development of collateral circulation, there may be preservation of glomeruli and only relatively minor tubular damage[18] (Figure 11-3).

Occlusion of the larger renal vessels occurs mainly from embolism in patients with rheumatic heart disease and atrial fibrillation. It is not surprising that the kidneys are the most common sites of arterial emboli since they receive one fourth of the cardiac output. Other, less frequent sources for renal emboli include mural thrombi in myocardial infarction and vegetations in bacterial endocarditis. Athermatous emboli large enough to occlude the major renal vessels have been dislodged during surgery or arteriographic procedures. Thrombosis of the renal artery has been reported after extensive trauma. Certain medical conditions can be associated with thrombosis, such as systemic lupus erythematosus, polyarteritis, malignant hypertension, scleroderma, thrombotic thrombocytopenic purpura, and the hemolytic-uremic syndrome. In these illnesses, the thrombosis generally involves intrarenal arterial branches rather than the main renal artery.

Renal Infarction

Total arterial obstruction from any cause results in infarction in all or parts of the kidney with necrosis of both the cortex and medulla.

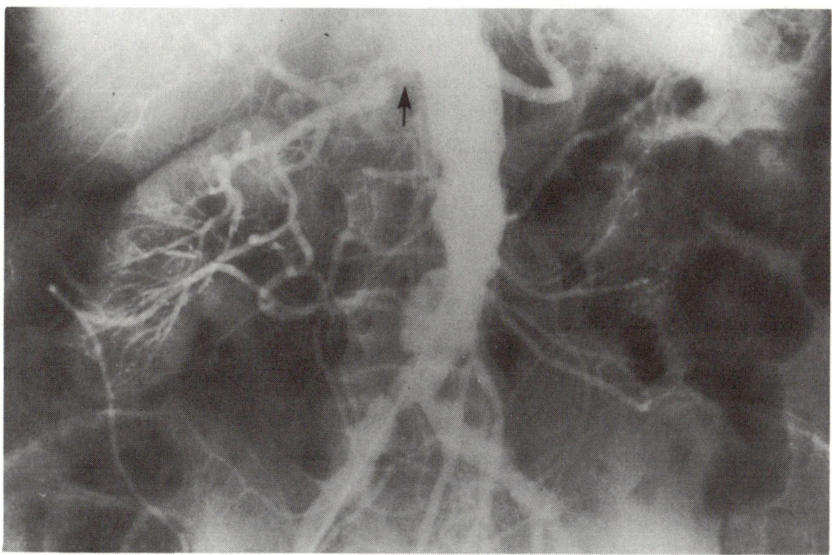

Figure 11-3 An aortogram showing severe renal arterial disease. The left renal artery is totally occluded, and collateral circulation fails to perfuse the infarcted left kidney. There is a high-grade proximal obstruction of the right renal artery (arrow) with extensive collateral circulation from branches of the superior and inferior mesenteric and internal iliac arteries.

Grossly, the infarcted area appears hemorrhagic in the earlier stages. Later, the renal mass shrinks as necrotic tissue is replaced by scar. When renal emboli are multiple and occur over a period of time, as in patients with mitral stenosis, various stages in the organization of the infarcts may be noted in the kidney. The cumulative effects of many infarcts may lead to a deformed kidney with many scars.

Renal infarction evokes severe flank and upper abdominal pain which may be steady or colicky in nature. There is nausea, vomiting, and low-grade fever. Hematuria may be surprisingly minimal, or massive bleeding and passage of clots may occur. Laboratory evidence of renal infarction includes elevation of the white cell count and of the plasma lactic dehydrogenase (LDH) level. The level of LDH peaks within several days after infarction and may remain elevated for several weeks. Unlike cases of pulmonary infarction with elevated plasma LDH levels, the urinary LDH in renal infarction is also very elevated.[19,20] The elevation of urine LDH is not specific for infarction and occurs in a variety of intrinsic renal diseases. There are also minor elevations of serum glutamic-oxaloacetic transaminase and alkaline phosphatase in renal infarction. It should be mentioned that renal infarcts are frequent findings at autopsy, although antemortem comments on this diagnosis are infrequent. Thus, many infarctions are silent or are otherwise undiagnosed.

It is of interest that transitory hypertension has been noted in some cases of documented renal infarction.[21] After two to three weeks, the blood pressure reverted to normal. This observation has also been noted in patients in whom therapeutic embolization of the kidney has been performed because of massive proteinuria or renal adenocarcinoma.[22,23] The etiology of this brief hypertensive period is not clear. It has been attributed to release of a pressor substance by the necrotic tissue and, indeed, renin levels are elevated during acute infarction of the kidney. It is also possible that the hypertension is related to the presence of ischemic but viable tissue around the border of the infarct.[24]

Diagnosis

When a patient presents with flank pain, nausea, vomiting, fever leukocytosis, and hematuria, many diagnoses come to mind. The clinician must first think of pyelonephritis, renal calculus, or subacute bacterial endocarditis, since these diagnoses are clinically more common than renal infarction. However, if the patient has atrial fibrillation, recent myocardial infarction, a history of previous emboli, or has had recent trauma, then renal infarction becomes more probable. Urinary LDH level may be elevated in all of these conditions, but infarction leads to the highest values. Blood cultures may be helpful in diagnosing endocarditis. Careful urinalysis and urine culture will show the presence of bacteria in patients with pyelonephritis, or crystals may be evident in the patient with a renal stone. The intravenous pyelogram should next be scheduled, since renal calculus or infarction can often be differentiated by this means. With major vessel occlusion, the kidney is not visualized and, with segmental artery occlusion, the calyx of the corresponding renal segment is not seen. Similarly, a renal scan in cases of infarction shows a defect in the area of necrotic tissue. In the case of a nonfunctioning kidney, retrograde pyelography may be needed to see if the collecting system is obstructed by a stone or mass, or if it is patent, as would occur in renal infarction. Final confirmation of renal infarction is achieved through demonstration of the occluded vessel on arteriography, and decreased or absent contrast material in the nephrographic phase.

Treatment

Treatment of major vessel occlusion by surgery remains controversial. There have been reports of prompt reversal of anuria and partial restoration of renal function following embolectomy.[25] However, patients with renal emboli generally have cardiac disease as well, and are a poor-risk group for major surgery. Mortality has been over 30% in the operated patients. Therefore, medical therapy with anticoagulants is probably the most prudent course, but needs to be further evaluated. There has been a report of removal of clot from the renal artery by a Fogarty catheter.[17] The efficacy of this procedure must also be assessed.

Atheroembolism

Occlusion of the smaller radicles of the renal artery occurs mainly by atheromatous emboli. This is likely to occur in individuals with severe erosive disease of the aortic intima, especially during aortic surgery or selective renal arteriography. Spontaneous atheroembolism also occurs.[26] Arcuate arteries and smaller vessels are likely to be involved. On pathological examination, the emboli have characteristic cholesterol crystals which appear as needle-shaped clefts on routine histologic sections. In established lesions, the embolus is engulfed by fibrous thickening of the vessel intima, occluding the lumen. When there are showers of atheromatous emboli, there is patchy necrosis of the renal substance, often wedge-shaped with the apex towards the medulla. There is reduction in renal mass in chronic cases.[27]

Massive atheroembolism causes oliguric acute renal failure which is generally irreversible. In patients with more subtle atheroembolism, there is progressive azotemia without oliguria, and eventual renal failure. Patients with erosive atherosclerosis of the aorta are usually over the age of 60. The diagnosis of atheroembolic disease is suggested when there is involvement of the kidney and other organs. Showers of emboli may lead to pancreatitis, retinal infarction, gastrointestinal bleeding, and gangrene of the toes. There are no characteristic laboratory findings in atheroembolism. The diagnosis is best established by biopsy or by fortuitous examination of tissue, such as amputated toes.

There is no treatment for atheroembolism and renal failure. Despite supportive measures, management of fluid and electrolyte disturbances, and dialysis, survival rates remain poor.

RENOVASCULAR LESIONS IN HYPERTENSION

Hypertension is a significant factor in the development of stroke, heart failure, and renal failure.[28] Effects of hypertension on the kidney are largely manifested in the renal vasculature. Most cases of hypertension have no clearly recognized cause and are classified as essential hypertension. A definable etiology is recognized in less than 10% of the hypertensive population, and their condition is known as secondary hypertension. Recognized causes of secondary hypertension include primary aldosteronism, pheochromocytoma, intrinsic renal disease, and renal artery stenosis.

Pathology

The intrarenal vascular lesions in chronic hypertension are those of hyperplastic arteriosclerosis in the larger vessels, and hyaline sclerosis in afferent arterioles and their respective interlobular arteries. The larger arteries down to arcuate-artery size show fibrous intimal thickening with fraying of the internal elastic membrane. The intimal proliferation may show concentric layers of connective tissue, and causes a reduction of lumen caliber. The vessel media is generally not altered in size, but some of the muscle may be replaced by collagen. This hyperplastic sclerosis is not like atherosclerosis, although the older literature may have confused this difference. Atheroclerosis has intimal lipid deposits which are not at all prominent in the renovascular lesions of chronic hypertension.[29]

The interlobular arteries show intimal thickening with considerable reduplication of the internal elastic lamina. The preglomerular arterioles show a hyaline or homogeneous, eosinophilic thickening of the entire wall, which occurs in a patchy distribution. On electron-microscopy, the vascular hyaline is seen to be a finely granular protein deposit, with some minute lipid inclusions, believed to be derived from plasma proteins which have been rendered insoluble by denaturation in the arteriolar wall. The lesion is predominatly in the afferent vessels, generally sparing the glomeruli and the efferent vessels. This arteriolar change is called arteriolosclerosis. It occurs in chronic hypertension, but is also seen in normotensive individuals beginning at about age 50. This lesion can be considered to be the result of an aging process which can be accelerated by hypertension. Except in diabetics where the lesion is exaggerated and more extensive in distribution, arteriolosclerosis before the age of 50 is a good indicator of hypertensive disease. The amount of hyaline sclerosis of preglomerular arterioles roughly parallels the duration of hypertension.[30] As the lesion advances, glomerular atrophy ensues. Eventually, tubular atrophy follows, and several atrophied nephrons cause a small, pitted scar on the kidney and a granular subcapsular surface (Figure 11-4). The renal cortex becomes thinner and the kidney contracted with the development of arteriolonephrosclerosis.

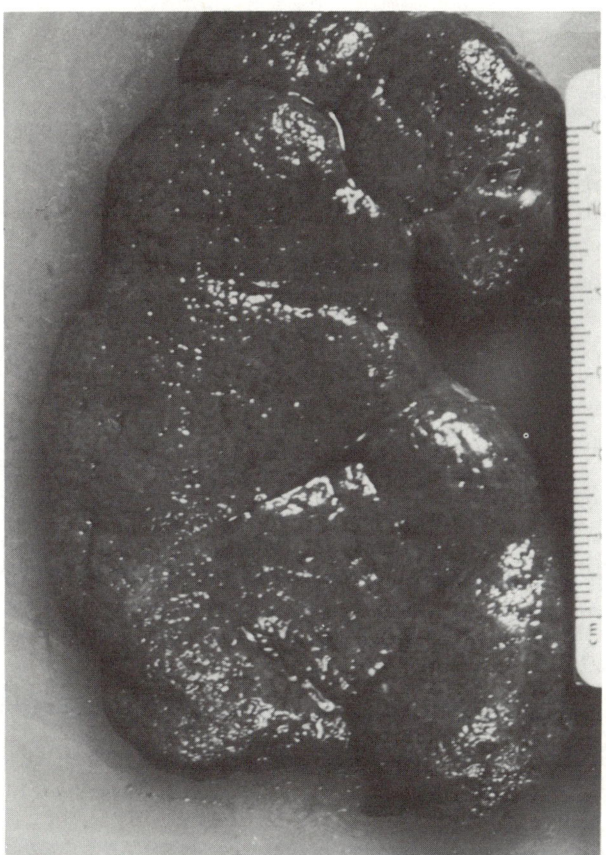

Figure 11-4 Kidney from patient with hypertension and arteriolonephrosclerosis, showing subcapsular granularity.

Clinical Manifestations

The natural history of essential hypertension has been studied by Perera in 350 patients.[31] Eighteen percent developed impaired renal function and 42% developed proteinuria. Uremia was a terminal event in 12%. As in most studies, cardiovascular complications were the most frequent: 50% developed congestive heart failure and 74% had cardiac hypertrophy. Several studies have now shown that antihypertensive treatment reduces the incidence of strokes, congestive heart failure, accelerated hypertension, and renal failure.[32] Nevertheless, hypertensive arteriolonephrosclerosis is still an important cause of end-stage renal failure. Approximately 5% of patients on chronic dialysis became azotemic as a result of hypertension.[33] Whether this continued incidence of renal failure in hypertension is due to inadequate treatment, delay in therapy, poor patients compliance, or other factors deserves important consideration.[34]

Malignant Hypertension

In about 1% of hypertensive patients, the disease develops an accelerated or malignant phase.[35] The blood pressure is high and target-organ damage from hypertension occurs rapidly. This phase can develop in the course of essential hypertension, especially when the blood pressure is poorly controlled, or it may be seen in secondary hypertension. It is most frequently associated with renovascular hypertension, acute glomerulonephritis, chronic renal failure, renal vasculitis, and preeclampsia.

Clinically, malignant hypertension is easily recognized. The diastolic blood pressure is over 130 mm Hg and sometimes as high as 180 mm Hg. Characteristically, there is papilledema along with retinal hemorrhages and exudates. Symptoms include headache, blurred vision, dizziness, nausea, vomiting, confusion, and somnolence. Neurologic deficit, seizure, and coma may occur. The accelerated hypertension may cause left ventricular failure with pulmonary edema, or acute myocardial infarction. Renal damage regularly occurs, and there is proteinuria and hematuria with rapid development of azotemia. Oliguria is often seen. The blood smear may show red cell fragments, suggesting microangiopathic hemolytic anemia.

On examination of the kidneys in accelerated hypertension, one finds necrosis of arteries, arterioles, and glomeruli superimposed on the intrarenal vascular lesions already discussed. The lesions are focal, and may be extensive or minimal in distribution. These lesions are called fibrinoid necrosis. Their etiology is complex. It is possible that sudden dilatation of small blood vessels due to elevated intravascular pressure causes disruption of the endothelium, permitting plasma and blood elements to penetrate the vessel wall. Examination of the walls of arterioles in this condition shows necrosis of myofibrillae in smooth muscle cells, presence of plasma and fibrin precipitation, and nuclear pyknosis and karyorrhexis.[36]

It is of interest that these changes of accelerated hypertension are not common in the elderly even though one frequently encounters very high blood pressure levels in that age group. It is possible that with aging there are fibrotic changes in the vascular musculature which strengthen the vessel wall and make it less susceptible to disruption by high intravascular pressure. Similarly, malignant hypertension is infrequent with chronic renal lesions other than arteriolonephrosclerosis. Many cases of scleroderma progress to malignant hypertension, and the renovascular lesions are indistinguishable. However, these changes can be seen in the interlobular arteries in scleroderma even without the development of hypertension.

The kidney in accelerated hypertension varies in size from case to case, depending on the length of the clinical course. There are many petechial hemorrhages on the surface. The glomeruli show fibrinoid necrosis in the capillary tufts in a patchy distribution. Most of the glomeruli, however, are generally unaffected or show minimal capillary thickening. This feature is useful in the differentiation of malignant hypertension occurring in essential hypertension from that noted in chronic glomerulonephritis. Although the glomerular changes in accelerated hypertension are not diffuse, there is a severe reduction in renal function frequently leading to uremia.

Untreated malignant hypertension has a grim prognosis. Various studies have shown a high mortality—as high as 80% in one year.[35,37] The major causes of death generally have been renal and cardiac failure. The results of treatment show great improvement in mortality and improvement or stabilization of renal function. In Perry's series[38] after treatment, the one-year mortality was 15%, and Woods[39] had 2 of 20 patients who survived for seven years. Thus, it appears certain that all patients with malignant hypertension deserve intense antihypertensive treatment.

RENAL VASCULAR LESIONS IN DIABETES MELLITUS

Diabetes mellitus is accompanied by considerable changes in the kidney, and vascular changes are especially prominent. Arteriosclerotic lesions are noted in the arteries and arterioles; these lesions are more extensive and severe in the diabetic than in the nondiabetic. The larger vessels demonstrate atheromatosis characterized by intimal fibrosis and lipid deposition. The vessel lumen is narrowed and blood flow impaired. Arteriolar involvement includes hyalinization of the intima and media. The glomerular capillaries show thickened basement membranes.[40] The arteriosclerosis of the major renal vessels in diabetes mellitus is often extensive and may contribute to renal insufficiency. Renal artery stenosis sufficient to cause secondary hypertension often occurs in diabetics. This increased severity of arteriosclerosis may be noted even in subclinical diabetes mellitus.

The arteriolar lesions are also more frequent, more extensive, and occur earlier in diabetics than in nondiabetics. Hyaline arteriolosclerosis is more severe in diabetics than in essential hypertension and often extends to involve the efferent arteriole. It is noteworthy that many diabetics exhibit arteriolar hyalinization but have normal blood pressure. Therefore, arteriolosclerosis is seen not only in hypertension or in the aging kidney. The presence of considerable hyaline arteriolosclerosis in a young patient, even without glomerular lesions, should strongly suggest the presence of diabetes mellitus.[41]

Glomerulopathy

The glomeruli in diabetes mellitus show several changes: a nodular lesion, a diffuse lesion, and an exudative lesion. The nodular lesion or intercapillary glomerulosclerosis consists of rounded, homogeneous deposits in the central and peripheral parts of the glomerular lobules. It is virtually specific for diabetes. The diffuse lesion consists of capillary wall thickening accompanied by an increase in the intercapillary mesangial substance. This lesion, while suggestive of diabetes mellitus, may also be seen in glomerulonephritis. The exudative lesion appears as a "fibrin cap" or smooth, eosinophilic, lipid-containing crescentic mass within a capillary at the periphery of a lobule. Similar lesions called "capsular drops" may be seen inside the glomerular capsule. Exudative lesions are not specific for diabetes and are seen in other conditions such as systemic lupus erythematosus, glomerulonephritis, and arteriosclerosis.

The thickening of the glomerular capillary basement membrane in diabetes appears to be part of a wider process which affects small vessels throughout the body.[42] This diabetic microangiopathy probably occurs following carbohydrate intolerance, but it is still controversial. It has particular significance in the retina and the kidney, where changes can be readily detected. The retinal expression of early microangiopathy is the microaneurysm, easily detectable on ophthalmoscopic examination. The renal expression is proteinuria. These changes generally portend the development of accelerated vascular damage.

Clinical Course

Patients without proteinuria tend not to develop renal failure. On the other hand, when the diabetic develops proteinuria of greater than 3 gm per day, renal failure generally ensues within six years.[43] The reason for the development of diabetic nephropathy in some but not all diabetics is not known. Approximately 6% of all deaths in diabetic patients are due to nephropathy; the proportion in diabetic patients below age 40 is even higher.[44,45] There is no clear treatment of the diabetic nephropathy. Insulin therapy does not alter the condition. Current management of diabetic nephropathy with renal insufficiency is essentially similar to that of other patients with renal disease. Pancreatic transplantation and the computerized artificial pancreas are a few avenues that are being explored in the hope of reducing the incidence of renal failure in diabetes.

RENAL ARTERY STENOSIS

The work of Goldblatt and co-workers has shown that renal artery constriction can lead to hypertension.[46] There has been considerable interest in this observation, resulting in improved diagnostic methods for renal artery stenosis. Enthusiasm has grown for repair of such lesions in the hypertensive patient. The incidence of hypertension caused by renal artery stenosis is not definitely known, but it is at least 2% of all hypertensives. Although renovascular hypertension is relatively uncommon, it is important because it is one of the most common curable forms of hypertension. In perhaps three fourths of carefully selected patients, repair of the renal artery stenosis can produce significant improvement or cure.

Pathophysiology of Renovascular Hypertension

Early experimental work on renal hypertension has shown that constriction of one renal artery by a metal clip with the other kidney intact causes hypertension. In this model (two-kidney clip model) the vascular changes of hypertension could be produced in the untouched kidney, but the clipped kidney was protected from the vascular changes. Upon removal of the ischemic kidney, there was a fall in blood pressure, but only if the contralateral nonischemic kidney did not have the vascular changes due to hypertension. In another model, it was also possible to produce sustained hypertension if one kidney was removed and a clip placed on the remaining kidney (one-kidney clip model).[47]

The mechanisms involved in the hypertension produced by these two models have become somewhat clearer with studies of the renin-angiotensin system.[48,49] Renin is produced in the kidney by a structure in the afferent arteriolar smooth muscle layer located adjacent to the glomerulus (juxtaglomerular apparatus). The release of renin is normally controlled by several factors such as renal perfusion pressure, tubular sodium concentration and beta-adrenergic stimulation, which act to cause renin release when blood volume is reduced. When in the circulation, renin is a proteolytic enzyme that acts upon an alpha globulin from the liver (angiotensinogen) to produce antiotensin I, a ten-amino-acid peptide that appears physiologically inert. Upon circulating through the lung, angiotensin I is changed by a converting enzyme to the octapeptide angiotensin II. The converting enzyme is present in large quantities in the lung, but there is experimental evidence that it is also present in the kidney.[50] Angiotensin II is the most potent vasoconstrictor in the body, and it also stimulates the adrenal cortex to produce aldosterone, a hormone that causes salt and water retention.

With regard to the role of the renin-angiotensin system in the experimental hypertension noted above, it has been shown that renin is rapidly released in large amounts from the ischemic kidney in both the one-clip and two-clip models. Hypertension can be prevented by prior administration of converting enzyme inhibitor (captopril) or angiotensin II antagonist (saralasin).[51] Therefore, it appears certain that angiotensin is important in the development of hypertension in both models. In the chronic situation, the role of long-term vasoconstriction is less clear, since values for renin, angiotensin, and aldosterone are often not elevated. Mechanisms for the maintenance of chronic renovascular hypertension are thus still speculative, but may involve a complex relationship between angiotensin and effective circulating blood volume.

Pathologic Changes

A variety of lesions can cause renal artery stenosis. The most common lesion in the older age group is arteriosclerosis. In the Far East, Takayasu's disease is a common cause of stenosis.[52] Arteriosclerotic obstruction is usually due to a plaque in the aorta, occluding the origin of the renal artery, and generally occurs in patients over 50 years of age with evidence of diffuse atherosclerosis. This lesion increases in incidence with advancing age and diabetes mellitus, and is more frequent in males. The lesion is usually eccentric, compromising the lumen. Thrombosis may be superimposed on this lesion, further compromising blood flow (Figure 11-5).

Another common cause of stenosis is fibromuscular dysplasia of the renal artery. This is a heterogeneous group of lesions that can be classified according to involvement of the intima, media, or adventitia. There is characteristic fibrous or fibromuscular hyperplasia of the renal vessels which can be bilateral and extend to involve the branches of the renal artery. The most common variety of dysplasia is medial fibroplasia with aneurysms, consisting of many stenotic fibromuscular

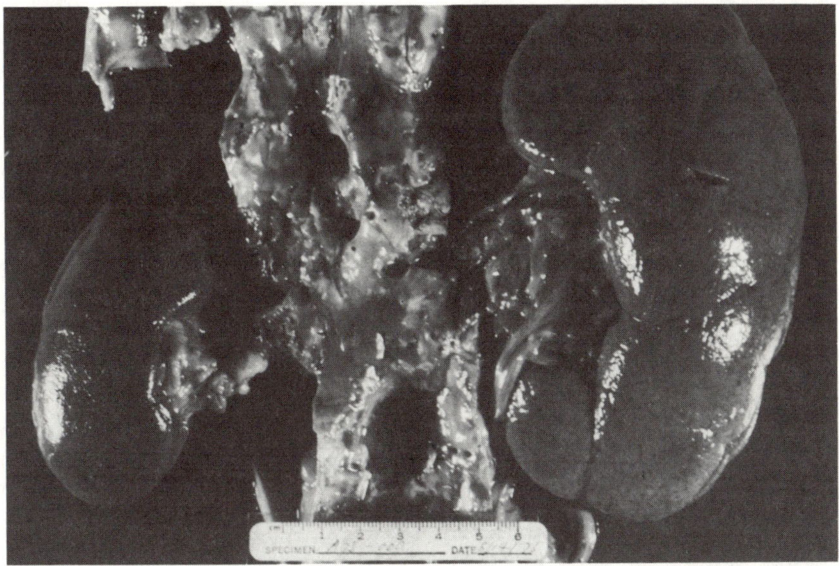

Figure 11-5 Kidneys from patient with renal artery stenosis showing narrowing of renal artery due to atherosclerotic plaque and unilateral reduction of kidney size.

ridges alternating with considerably thinned segments. On arteriography, the appearance of this deformity in the affected artery is that of a string of beads. Unlike atherosclerosis, this lesion is more common in females in their 20s and 30s, and usually affects the distal two thirds of the main renal artery or beyond. The distal involvement of the renal artery and the frequent bilateral nature of the lesion often make surgical revascularization impossible. Nevertheless, there are many renal dysplastic lesions that are amenable to surgery. The pathogenesis of the dysplasias is not known, but it is possible that intimal fibroplasia may be caused by organization of fibrin.

Clinical Features

Specific clinical features of renovascular hypertension are few. This type of hypertension should be suspected if the hypertension occurs before the age of 30 or after 45, since essential hypertension usually presents between those ages. The known absence of hypertension among family members may suggest that the condition is of the secondary type. Also, hypertension of acute onset, especially if symptomatic, should make the clinician think of secondary hypertension. A history of flank trauma or pain suggestive of renal infarction should make one suspect renovascular hypertension. The most helpful clinical feature of renovascular stenosis is an abdominal bruit, generally high-pitched and of long duration with accentuation during cardiac systole, located in the upper abdomen and transmitted laterally. The bruit may be especially suggestive of renal artery stenosis if unilateral. This finding should be distinguished from bruits arising from atheromata in the abdominal aorta, which are lower-pitched, systolic, and tend to radiate toward the iliac vessels.

Diagnostic Evaluation

There is no simple reliable screening test for renal artery stenosis. Plasma renin activity, generally after stimulation by diuretics, is often greatly elevated in renal artery stenosis, but this is not uniformly reliable.[53] A promising, more sensitive screening technique under investigation is to measure the degree of reactive hyperreninemia after angiotensin blockade by saralasin, or converting enzyme inhibition by captopril. The latter drug can be given orally. A significant rise in renin activity coupled with a fall in blood pressure of about 10% occurs in renovascular hypertension, malignant hypertension, and essential hypertension with elevated renin activity. Malignant hypertension is readily recognized on clinical grounds. The other two conditions can cause some clinical confusion. However, false negative responses to this protocol seem to be minimal.[54] It should be noted that this procedure uses investigational drugs which are not yet released for this clinical use.

An excellent screening procedure for renal artery stenosis is the use of excretory urography with rapid-sequence filming. In interpreting the urography, one looks for certain abnormalities. The most common abnormality seen in renal artery stenosis is unilateral reduction in renal size, a difference of 1.5 cm in size occurring in over 60% of adults with severe disease. One should examine early sequence films to see the appearance time of the radiographic contrast material. The ischemic kidney has delayed initial uptake of contrast as compared with the contralateral nonischemic kidney. In later films, the ischemic kidney has delayed excretion and greater concentration of the contrast material. One may also see ureteral notching due to collateral arteries crossing the ureter. Occasionally, one can see cortical irregularity suggestive of partial renal infarction. When care is taken in the performance and interpretation of urography, it is an excellent screening procedure for renal artery stenosis and provides positive signs of lateralization in about 80% of severe cases. The limitations of this technique are mainly in bilateral disease and mild stenosis.[55]

Radioisotope renal scanning, like urography, is also useful in diagnosing renal artery stenosis. This technique avoids hypersensitivity reactions to the radiographic contrast material, and also the development of dye-related acute renal failure seen in patients with diabetes mellitus or dysproteinemias. A shortcoming of this technique is the occasional false lateralization in bilateral intrinsic disease with asymmetric involvement of the kidneys.

To further evaluate the functional significance of renal artery stenosis, the separate function of each kidney can be measured by catheterization of each ureter. This technique involves an invasive procedure requiring anesthesia and carries with it a high morbidity. It, therefore, has been supplanted by other techniques.

If renovascular hypertension is strongly suspected because of clinical features or drug-resistant hypertension, and if the patient is a suitable candidate for artery repair, then more definitive, but invasive, studies are warranted. These studies may be indicated even if screening tests are negative. Indications for selecting patients for further studies are not definite and vary from center to center. Some of the points to be considered in this selection are discussed later under treatment. In the selected patients, the studies to be done are bilateral venous sampling for renin activity and renal arteriography. The concentration of renin in the vein from each kidney is compared with the other and with the peripheral blood. The probability of a surgical cure is good if: 1) the ischemic kidney has twice the renin level of the opposite kidney, and 2) the opposite kidney is not producing renin, ie, the level from the noninvolved kidney is no higher than in the periphery. To increase the diagnostic accuracy of differential renal vein studies, renin activity is ordinarily stimulated by administering diuretics or angiotensin blocking agents.[56] Renal arteriography is, of course, necessary to outline the anatomic impairment and aid in any surgical approach.

Treatment

Much controversy still exists over the treatment of renovascular disease. In the high-risk patient with cardiac disease or impaired renal function or in the patient with bilateral lesions, the indications for medical therapy may outweigh those for surgery. Drugs that inhibit renin generally are useful in therapy. Currently available drugs in this category include beta-blockers, clonidine, ganglionic blockers, methyldopa, prazosin, and reserpine. Although it increases plasma renin activity, captopril may also be efficacious.

If surgical repair is attempted in a suitable patient, nephrectomy should be avoided, if possible. Techniques include autotransplantation of the kidney to another vessel such as the hypogastric artery, saphenous vein bypass graft, or splenorenal shunt for the left kidney.[57] The outcome of surgery is difficult to evaluate since results vary from center to center. Starr et al[58] reported on long-term follow-up of 216 patients who had renovascular surgery for hypertension. Postoperatively, normal blood pressure was seen in 85%, but this percentage fell to 74% after 15 years. Other series have shown greater return to hypertension in later years, but claim also to have better preservation of renal function.[59] Hunt,[60] in a long-term study of 214 patients, noted progressive impairment of renal function in patients treated medically and treated surgically. His concept is that treatment for renal artery stenosis, either by medical or surgical means, does not cure but provides amelioration of a progressive disease process. In his prospective study of patients with angiographic evidence of renovascular disease treated either by drugs or surgery, 78% of the surgical group survived over 10 years, and 53% had diastolic blood pressure less than 90 mm Hg. Of the medically treated group, 40% survived 10 years and 34% were normotensive. Five percent of the drug-treated group went into chronic renal failure, while none of the surgical group did.[55]

These observations suggest that the treatment of choice for renovascular hypertension is surgical. However, medical management should certainly be tried if the patient is old or has other surgical risk factors present, such as coronary heart disease, cerebrovascular atherosclerosis, renal insufficiency, or aortic aneurysm. The ideal patient to work up for possible surgery is a young individual with recent onset of hypertension, clear evidence of unilateral renal artery disease, and good renal function. However, clinical medicine does not usually present easy choices. The clinician must weigh the factors in the individual patient because criteria for selecting medical or surgical management of renovascular hypertension have not been clearly delineated. An additional factor to consider is the availablity of a surgical team with extensive experience with renal artery revascularization.

There now have been reports of treatment of renal artery stenosis by percutaneous transluminal dilatation, using a balloon catheter to compress the lesion.[61] Although follow-up has been short so far, initial results have shown improvement in over 80% of patients. Angioplasty is not possible in patients with severely stenotic lesions through which the catheter cannot be passed, or severely calcified lesions that are too rigid to dilate.[62] Complications have included renal artery rupture and other problems of percutaneous angiography such as infection, bleeding, or partial renal infarction. The technique of balloon catheter angioplasty has the potential for being an alternative to surgery in suitable patients. Further studies of this technique need to be done to define the indications and long-term effects.

Most experiences with surgical correction have been with severe degrees of renal artery stenosis. Moderate or mild degrees of stenosis have generally been treated medically. The aim of therapy is to maintain normal blood pressure and preserve renal function. Studies of the natural progression of patients with mild or moderate degrees of renal artery stenosis would be of interest in assessing therapeutić results.

REFERENCES

1. Beeuwkes R III. The vascular organization of the kidney. *Ann Rev Physiol* 42:531, 1980.

2. Graves FT. *The Arterial Anatomy of the Kidney.* Baltimore, Williams and Wilkins, 1971.

3. Beeuwkes R III, Bonventre JV. Tubular orgainzation and vascular-tubular relations in the dog kidney. *Am J Physiol* 229:695, 1975.

4. Bulger RE. Kidney morphology. In Earley LE, Gottschalk CW (eds). *Strauss and Welt's Diseases of the Kidney,* ed 3. Boston, Little, Brown, 1979, pp 32–34.

5. Heptinstall RH. *Pathology of the Kidney,* ed 2. Boston, Little, Brown, 1974, pp 2–12.

6. Stein JH. The Renal circulation. In Brenner BM, Rector FC (eds). *The Kidney.* Philadelphia, WB Saunders Co, 1976, pp 215–219.

7. Leaf A, Cotran R. *Renal Pathophysiology.* New York, Oxford University Press, 1976, pp 1–8.

8. Beckmann CF, Abrams HL. Renal venography: Anatomy, technique, applications, analysis of 132 venograms, and a review of the literature. *Cardiovasc Intervert Radiol* 45, 1980.

9. Scrier RW, Gardenswartz MH. Renal vein thrombosis. *Postgrad Med* 67:83–87, 90–93, 1980.

10. Churg J. Coagulation and the kidney. *Monographs in Pathology.* Baltimore: Williams and Wilkins, 1979, pp 20, 140.

11. Trew PA, Biava CG, Jacobs RP, et al. Renal vein thrombosis in membranous glomerulonephropathy. *Medicine* 57:69, 1978.

12. Barclay GPT, Cameron HM, Loughridge LW. Amyloid disease of the kidney and renal vein thrombosis. *Quart J Med* 29, 1960.

13. Llach F, Arieff AL, Massry SG. Renal vein thrombosis and nephrotic syndrome. A prospective study of 36 adult patients. *Ann Intern Med* 83:8, 1975.

14. Jorgensen KA, Stoffersen E. Antithrombin III and the nephrotic syndrome. *Scand J Haematol* 1979, 22:442, 1979.

15. Clark RA, Wyatt GM, Colley DP. Renal vein thrombosis: An underdiagnosed complication of multiple renal abnormalities. *Radiology* 132:43, 1979.

16. Ross DL, Lubowitz H. Anticoagulation in renal vein thrombosis. *Arch Intern Med* 138:1349, 1978.

17. Kassirer JP. Thrombosis and embolism of the renal vessels. In Earley LE, Gottschalk CW (eds). *Strauss and Welt's Diseases of the Kidney,* ed 3. Boston, Little, Brown, 1979, pp 1385–1402.

18. Duncan DA, Dexter RN. Anuria secondary to bilateral renal-artery embolism. *N Engl J Med* 206:971, 1962.

19. Gault MH, Steiner G. Serum and urinary enzyme activity after renal infarction. *Can Med Assoc J* 93:1101, 1065.

20. London IL, Hoffster P, Perkoff GT, et al. Renal infarction. Elevation of serum and urinary lactic dehydrogenase (LDH). *Arch Intern Med* 121:87, 1968.

21. Ben-Asher S. Hypertension caused by renal infarction. *Ann Intern Med* 23:431, 1945.

22. Bracken RB, Johnson DE, Goldstein HM, et al. Percutaneous transfemoral renal artery occlusion in patients with renal carcinoma. *Urology* 6:6, 1975.

23. Almgard LE, Fernstrom I, Haverling M, et al. Treatment of renal adenocarcinoma by emboli occlusion of the renal circulation. *Br J Urol* 45:474, 1973.

24. Arakwa K, Torii S, Naito S, et al. Plasma renin activity as a more specific diagnostic aid for renal infarction. *Arch Intern Med* 125:830, 1970.

25. Kliger ME, Nisnewitz S. Renal artery embolectomy. *Am J Surg* 115:669, 1968.

26. Kaplan K, Millar JD, Cancilla PA. "Spontaneous" atheroemboli renal failure. *Arch Intern Med* 110:218, 1962.

27. Harrington JT, Sommers SC, Kassirer JP. Atheromatosis emboli with progressive renal failure: Renal arteriography as the probably inciting factor. *Ann Intern Med* 68:152, 1968.

28. Kannel WB. Some lessons in cardiovascular epidemiology from Framingham. *Am J Cardiol* 37:269, 1976.

29. Heptinstall RH. *Pathology of the Kidney,* ed 2. Boston, Little, Brown, 1974, pp 123–134.

30. Fishberg AM. Anatomic findings in essential hypertension. *Arch Intern Med* 35:650, 1925.

31. Perera GA. Hypertensive vascular disease; description and natural history. *J Chronic Dis* 1:33, 1955.

32. Veterans Administration Cooperative Study Group on Antihypertensive Agents: II. Results in patients with diastolic blood pressure averaging 90 through 114 mm Hg. *JAMA* 213:1143, 1970.

33. Bryan FA. *The National Dialysis Registry 6th Annual Progress Report,* 1974.

34. Alfrey AC. The renal response to vascular injury. In Brenner BM, Rector FC (eds). *The Kidney.* Philadelphia, WB Saunders Co, 1976, pp 1145–1192.

35. Kincaid-Smith P, McMichael J, Murphy EA. The clinical course and pathology of hypertension with papilledema (malignant hypertension) *Quart J Med* 27:117, 1958.

36. Hepinstall RH. Malignant hypertension. A study of fifty-one cases. *J Pathol Bacteriol* 65:423, 1953.

37. Keith NM, Wagener HP, Barker NM. Some different types of essential hypertension; their clinical course and prognosis. *Am J Med Sci* 197:332, 1939.

38. Perry HM Jr, Schroeder HA, Catanzaro FJ, et al. Studies on the control of hypertension. VIII. Mortality, morbidity and remissions during twelve years of intensive therapy. *Circulation* 33:958, 1966.

39. Woods JW, Blythe WB, Huffines WD. Malignant hypertension and renal insufficiency. *N Engl J Med* 291:10, 1974.

40. Churg J, Dachs S. Diabetic renal disease: Arteriosclerosis and

glomerulosclerosis. In Sommers SC (ed). *Kidney Pathology Decennial 1966–1975.* New York, Appleton-Century-Crofts, 1975, pp 503–528.

41. Heptinstall RA. *Pathology of the Kidney,* ed 2. Boston. Little, Brown, 1974, pp 929-962.

42. Siperstein MD, Unger RH, Madison LL. Studies of muscle capillary basement membranes in normal subjects, diabetic and prediabetic patients. *J Clin Invest* 49:1973, 1968.

43. Ducrey J, Febre J, Balani L, et al. Proteinuria in maturity-onset diabetes. *Schweiz Med Wochenschr* 105:138, 1972.

44. Watkins PJ, Blainey JD, Brewer DB, et al. The natural history of diabetic renal disease. *Quart J Med* 41:437, 1972.

45. Balodimos MC. Diabetic nephropathy. In Marble A, White P, Bradley RF, et al (eds). *Joslin's Diabetes Mellitus,* ed 11. Philadelphia, Lea & Febiger, 1971, p 526.

46. Goldblatt H, Lynch J, Hanzal RF, et al. Studies on experimental hypertension I. The production of persistent elevation of systolic blood pressure by means of renal ischemia. *J Exp Med* 59:347, 1934.

47. Wilson C, Byrom FM. The vicious circle in chronic Bright's disease: Experimental evidence from the hypertensive rat. *Quart J Med* 10:65, 1941.

48. Pickering GW, Prinzmetal M, Kelsall AR. The assay of renin in rabbits with experimental renal hypertension. *Clin Sci* 4:401, 1942.

49. Gross F, Schaechtelin G, Brunner H, et al. The role of the renin-angiotensin system in blood pressure regulation and kidney function. *Can Med Assoc J* 90:258, 1964.

50. Thurau K. Modification of angiotensin-mediated tubulo-glomerular feedback by extracellular volume. *Kidney Int* 8:202, 1975.

51. Laragh JH, Baer L, Brunner HR, et al. Renin, angiotensin and aldosterone in pathogenesis and managment of hypertensive vascular disease. *Am J Med* 52:633, 1972.

52. Heptinstall RH. Hypertension and vascular disease of the kidney. *Monogr Path* 20:281, 1979.

53. Simon N, Franklin SS, Bleifer KH, et al. Clinical characteristics of renovascular hypertension (cooperative study). *JAMA* 220:1209, 1972.

54. Case DB, Laragh JH. Reactive hypereninemia in renovascular hypertension after angiotensin blockade with saralasin or converting enzyme inhibitor. *Ann Intern Med* 91:153, 1979.

55. Hunt JC. Renovascular hypertension. In Earley LE, Gottschalk CW (eds). *Strauss and Welt's Diseases of the Kidney,* ed 3. Boston, Little, Brown, 1979, p 1357.

56. Strong CG, Hunt JC, Sheps SG, et al. Renal venous renin activity; enhancement of sensitivity of lateralization by sodium depletion. *Am J Cardiol* 27:602, 1971.

57. Bergentz SE, Ericsson BF, Husberg B. Technique and complications in the surgical treatment of renovascular hypertension. *Acta Chir Scand* 145:143, 1979.

58. Starr DS, Laurie GM, Morris GC Jr. Surgical treatment of renovascular hypertension. Long-term follow-up of 216 patients up to 20 years. *Arch Surg* 115:494, 1980.

59. Pinkerton JA Jr, Crouch TT, Sharma JN. Surgical treatment of renovascular hypertension. *Am J Surg* 138:759, 1979.

60. Hunt JC, Bernatz PE, Harrison EG Jr. Factors determining diagnosis

and choice of treatment of renovascular hypertension: Influence of location, severity, and type of stenosing lesions. *Circ Res* 21 (suppl 2):211, 1967.

61. Kuhlmann V, Vetter W, Furrer J, et al. Renovascular hypertension: Treatment by percutaneous transluminal dilatation. *Ann Intern Med* 92:1, 1980.

62. Russel RP, Whelton PK, Kaufman SL, et al. Transluminal angioplasty in renovascular disease (abstract). Annual Meeting of the American Society of Nephrology, Washington, DC, 1980, p 67A.

12 Ischemic Disease of the Brain

Sandor A. Friedman

Occlusive cerebrovascular disease has been the subject of a great deal of investigation and controversy during the past 15 years. With increases in median longevity, more people can be expected to suffer the ravages and disabilities associated with inadequate cerebral blood flow. Once considered a disease of elderly people, it is now frequently seen in symptomatic and asymptomatic forms in many patients in the fifth and sixth decades. This phenomenon may result from better diagnostic methods, but it is also possible that the stresses of industrialized society are leading to an increased incidence of hypertension and cerebral arteriosclerosis.

New methods enable physicians to diagnose cerebrovascular disease at earlier stages, but facts about prognosis and proper therapy lag behind. Data about the natural history of occlusive lesions are often contradictory and fragmentary, and proponents of various alternative therapies hold quite dogmatically to their opinions. Very few studies concerning therapy of cerebrovascular disease fulfill the criteria for well-designed, double blind research projects.

Yet, there is certainly a great deal known about the prevention of strokes, and a number of studies have begun to elucidate the significance of certain findings. This chapter will review what is known about occlusive cerebral arterial disease and indicate where controversy still exists regarding diagnostic evaluation and therapy.

INCIDENCE AND PREVALENCE OF CEREBROVASCULAR DISEASE

It is difficult to estimate the true incidence and prevalence of cerebrovascular disease because clinical diagnosis is often difficult. In the first place, we must differentiate between intracranial and extracranial occlusive disease in estimating the frequency of cerebral ischemia. Intracranial arterial disease is not associated with any specific physical signs and cannot be diagnosed in the asymptomatic state. This diagnosis can be made only after a stroke occurs or on the basis of symptoms compatible with a transient ischemic attack. The latter may be very subtle at the beginning. Rather than frank focal weakness or loss of vision, the patient may have episodes of forgetfulness, intermittent dizziness or incoordination, or occasional thickness of speech. He may not think much of these symptoms or seek help until they occur quite frequently or are associated with obvious motor weakness. Thus, in many respects, the diagnosis of intracerebral occlusive disease is really the tip of an iceberg.

On the other hand, intracerebral disease may easily be overdiagnosed. Metabolic or more centrally located circulatory problems may produce transient, focal neurologic symptoms and signs in the same way as cerebral arteriosclerosis. It is well recognized, for example, that hypoglycemia may produce a focal neurologic deficity, and many other metabolic encephalopathies may lead to disorientation and weakness that can be confused with transient ischemic attacks. Cardiac arrhythmias and even congestive heart failure can lead to a variety of neurologic deficits. In fact, any disorder associated with intermittent hypoxia can simulate transient ischemic attacks. It is not surprising that reliable figures concerning the frequency of early intracerebral arterial disease are not available.

Cerebrovascular disease is the most common category of neurologic disorder in adults and, in one series, was found in 25% of consecutive autopsies.[1] It has been estimated that 275,000 Americans die and another 300,000 are disabled each year as a result of strokes. At any given time, at least two million individuals are disabled from the effects of cerebrovascular disease; 30% of this group are under the age of 65. In the United States, approximately 70% of strokes result from atherosclerotic occlusive disease, 20% from cerebral hemorrhage and 10% from cerebral embolism. Embolism is relatively more frequent in younger patients and hemorrhage, in blacks. The peak incidence of cerebral thrombosis is between the ages of 60 and 80, whereas embolism peaks between ages 40 and 60. A United States Public Health Service survey for the 1950s reported annual death rates in the United States of 23.4 per 100,000 population from cerebral thrombosis and embolism, and 63.8 per 100,000 from cerebral hemorrhage.[2] These figures represented 21% of all deaths due to cardiovascular disease. Worldwide, the reported death rate from cerebral infarction varies from 4.7 per 100,000 in Norway to 65.6 per 100,000 in Scotland. Japan has reported a relatively low death rate from infarction (14.5 per 100,000), but an extremely high rate from hemorrhage (179.6 per 100,000). It is not clear whether the variations from nation to nation represent real differences in risk factors or varying reporting criteria. In all nations, males are more commonly afflicted with cerebrovascular disease than females, and this trend has increased during recent decades. Unfortunately, differences in demographic data from region to region have not yet enabled epidemiologists to expand our knowledge concerning risk factors.

Estimates of the incidence and prevalence of strokes have come from epidemiologic studies within specific communities. A survey performed in Middlesex County, Connecticut suggested an annual incidence of 2.3 cases per 1000 individuals for all forms of stroke, and one per thousand for cerebral thrombosis.[3] The incidence of strokes in men between ages 45 and 64 was 2.5 per 1000. Another study of cerebrovascular disease in the employees of two corporations yielded lower incidence figures for strokes in men of this age range (1.22 and 1.37 per 1000 respectively).[4] All of these incidence figures are lower than the death rate figures reported by the Public Health Service and demonstrate the difficulties in obtaining reliable and reproducible data.

A study of stroke prevalence was performed in a retirement community at Seal Beach, California.[5] In a group of 792 unselected elderly people, most of whom were in the seventh and eighth decades, the prevalence of previous stroke was 7.8%. It was 4.5% for subjects aged 60 to 69, and 12% for those between 70 and 79. Eleven percent of men and 4.8% of women had had strokes.

The incidence of extracranial cerebral arterial disease has been estimated on several occasions by listening for bruits in the neck. This method is also fraught with problems. Neck bruits sometimes represent transmission of aortic systolic murmurs or evidence of rapid circulation. In one study of a rural African population with a very low incidence of stroke, 17% of the subjects had carotid bruits.[6] Thus, a carotid bruit is diagnostic of arterial occlusive disease only in a population group with a relatively high incidence of atherosclerosis.

RISK FACTORS FOR CEREBROVASCULAR ATHEROSCLEROSIS

The risk factors for cerebral arteriosclerosis are basically the same as those for coronary and peripheral arterial disease. However, hypertension assumes a position of much greater importance with respect to the cerebral circulation. At least 80% of patients with occlusive cerebral arterial disease are hypertensive, and there is excellent evidence that the probability of stroke can be directly related to the severity of hypertension. Therapy of hypertension clearly decreases the risk of stroke but does not appear to affect appreciably the incidence of myocardial infarction of intermittent claudication. It seems, therefore, that elevation of blood pressure is an important factor in the pathogenesis of cerebral ischemia, but may be only a synergistic factor in other areas of the arterial circulation. The reasons for this apparent difference are not clear. It is known that markedly elevated blood pressure levels (diastolic over 120 mm Hg) may cause cerebral vasoconstriction. In addition to accelerating atherosclerosis, hypertension also leads to the development of subintimal fibrosis and endarteritis obliterans of small arteries and arterioles throughout the circulation. These small vessel occlusions may produce significant ischemia which is too distal to be relieved by collateral circulation. Narrowing of small arteries and arterioles can also accentuate the effects of atherosclerosis in larger vessels. It is probable that cerebral ischemia generally represents the combined effects of large vessel atherosclerosis and small vessel endarteritis.

Diabetes mellitus is probably the second most important risk factor. Thirty percent of patients with cerebral infarction are obviously diabetic, and many more can be shown, on careful testing, to have abnormal glucose tolerance. As in other areas, there is no correlation between the severity or control of glucose intolerance and the likelihood of developing cerebral arteriosclerosis.

Patients with cerebral ischemia often have a family history of strokes. This may be an independent risk factor, but it seems to modify the importance of some of the major causes of cerebral ischemia. For example, there is a tendency toward familial clustering of stroke-prone individuals within the hypertensive and diabetic population. In some families, there is a pattern of strokes even when most of the afflicted individuals have relatively mild hypertension. Other families seem to be free of strokes even though several members may have rather severe hypertension. The other major risk factors include hyperlipidemia, smoking, and polycythemia. Polycythemia is a more significant risk factor in the cerebral circulation than in other areas, possibly because of its association with hypertension.

NORMAL ANATOMY AND PHYSIOLOGY

The brain is supplied by a group of major arteries that anastomose at the base of the brain to form the Circle of Willis (Figure 12-1). Most of the blood flow to the anterior portion of the brain including the cerebral cortex, thalamus, and subcortical tracts is supplied by the two internal carotid arteries and their major branches. The two carotid arteries anastomose through the anterior communicating artery. The pons, medulla, cerebellum, and midbrain receive their blood supply from the basilar artery, formed by the merging of the two vertebral arteries. The basilar artery branches into two posterior cerebral arteries, each of which anastomoses with a posterior communicating artery arising from an internal carotid artery.

Unfortunately, only a minority of the normal population has a perfect Circle of Willis with no anatomic variations. Both anterior and posterior communicating arteries may be absent or very small, and other congenital variations may also be present. The degree of disability produced by occlusion of an internal carotid or posterior cerebral artery depends to a large degree on the patency of anastomotic vessels that can act as collateral circulation. Symptomatology in the steal syn-

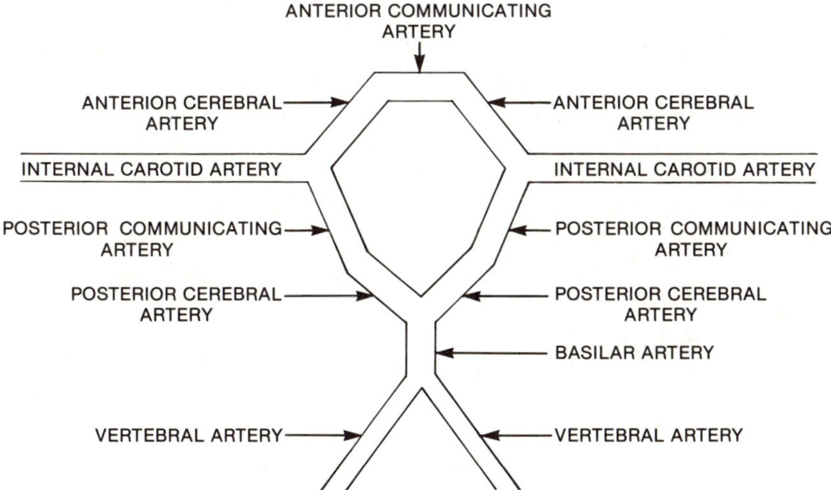

Figure 12-1 Diagram of Circle of Willis.

dromes (to be discussed later) also depends to some extent on the anatomic state of the Circle of Willis. Within the brain itself at the level of the middle cerebral and small arteries, there is also a variable potential for shunting blood flow through anastomotic channels that may normally be dormant. The outcome of a cerebral arterial occlusion depends to a large extent on the availability of these channels and the speed of the process. With sudden thrombosis, potential collateral circulation is not as valuable as in the case of a slowly occluding artery. Significant shunting of blood flow through collapsed dormant channels generally requires a certain critical opening pressure (usually about 40 mm Hg) for a period of time. The external carotid artery is an excellent source of collaterals when the internal carotid artery is occluded. Blood flows from orbital, nasal, facial, and occipital arteries into the distal internal carotid system. For example, blood can travel from the orbital to the ophthalmic to the middle cerebral artery.[7]

Autoregulation of Blood Flow

Under normal conditions, the total amount of cerebral blood flow is in the range of 50 ml to 60 ml per 100 g of brain tissue per minute, which amount to a total flow of 700 ml to 840 ml per minute. Measurements with electromagnetic flowmeters have shown that this flow is fairly evenly divided between each internal carotid artery and the vertebral-basilar axis. There is a definite tendency toward autoregulation in the cerebral circulation. Within certain limits, cerebral blood flow is maintained at a constant level, despite changes in perfusion pressure, by changes in vessel caliber. Cerebral arteries constrict when intraluminal pressure increases and dilate when intraluminal pressure decreases. This response is almost immediate in normal individuals and keeps blood flow almost constant at blood pressure levels up to 200/120 mm Hg. Above 200/120 mm Hg, cerebral vasoconstriction exceeds increases in perfusion pressure, and blood flow falls sharply. Chronic hypertension and cerebral arteriosclerosis stiffen arterial walls and impair this autoregulative process, narrowing the blood pressure range within which cerebral blood remains constant. It is for this reason that patients with cerebral ischemia are very sensitive to fluctuations in blood pressure and decreases in cardiac output.

Other factors in the regulation of cerebral blood flow include the partial pressures of oxygen and carbon dioxide. Elevation of PCO_2 causes cerebral vasodilatation, and reduction in PCO_2 leads to vasoconstriction and a rapid decrease in cerebral blood flow. It is for this reason that cerebral edema and papilledema occur in some patients with chronic respiratory failure. Syncope associated with the hyperventilation syndrome can also be partially explained on this basis. When the metabolic rate of cerebral tissue increases, more carbon dioxide is liberated, resulting in local vasodilatation.

Oxygen has an opposite but less pronounced effect. Increasing oxygen tension causes an immediate decrease in cerebral blood flow, whereas hypoxia leads to vasodilatation. Despite the vasoconstrictive influence of oxygen, however, inhalation of 100% oxygen improves its delivery to ischemic cerebral tissue. The effects of both carbon dioxide and oxygen decrease in the presence of long-standing hypertension and cerebral arteriosclerosis.

Arterial pH has an effect on cerebral blood flow that is independent of carbon dioxide tension. Acidosis leads to vasodilatation, and alkalosis causes vasoconstriction.

Autonomic innervation of the cerebral circulation is of uncertain importance. Sympathetic fibers from the stellate and cervical ganglia follow the course of the internal carotid and vertebral arteries. The internal carotid nerve originates in the superior cervical ganglion and terminates in the carotid and cavernous plexuses, which in turn supply fibers to the anterior and middle cerebral arteries. Experimental stimulation of the cervical sympathetic ganglia causes cerebral vasoconstriction and decreases carotid blood flow by 30%. Whether this stimulation is operative under normal physiologic conditions is not certain. Attempts to treat patients with cerebral ischemia by stellate ganglion blocks have not been successful. There is no evidence that parasympathetic fibers play a role in regulating cerebral blood flow.

SYMPTOMS AND SIGNS OF CEREBRAL ISCHEMIA

The deficits produced by occlusive disease of the cerebral circulation depend on the location, extent, and rapidity of the insult. Occlusion of a major vessel due to progressive atherosclerosis is often a slow process that allows time for collateral circulation to open. In this situation, a patient may remain asymptomatic if all other vessels are patent. This is particularly true of the internal carotid artery. Most strokes result from occlusion of smaller arteries. It is important to consider, however, what can occur with occlusion of each major vessel as a framework for correlating regional circulatory deficits and neurologic signs.

Internal Carotid Artery

The internal carotid artery provides blood flow to the homolateral eye through its ophthalmic branch, and to the frontal lobe and portions of the temporal and parietal lobes. Major effects of occlusion of this vessel include homolateral blindness, contralateral hemiplegia and hemianesthesia, homolateral Horner's syndrome, and aphasia, provided the artery supplies the dominant side of the brain. It can also cause contralateral homonymous hemianopsia.

Anterior Cerebral Artery

The anterior cerebral artery supplies the anterior limb of the internal capsule, the head of the caudate nucleus and the putamen through short perforating branches, the corpus callosum, and the medial and superior portions of the cerebral hemisphere. The area of the cortex controlling the legs, as well as the subcortical fibers from Broca's speech area, receive their blood flow from the anterior cerebral artery. Occlusion of this vessel, or more commonly one of its branches, can result in hemiplegia and hemianesthesia of the contralateral leg. If the dominant hemisphere is involved, the patient may become confused, aphasic, and somewhat stuporous.

Middle Cerebral Artery

The middle cerebral artery furnishes the blood supply of the lateral part of the cerebral hemisphere including the parietal cortex. In addition, through its lenticulooptic and lenticulostriate branches, it supplies the head of the caudate nucleus, anterior limb of the internal capsule, putamen, external capsule, and claustrum.

Occlusion of the middle cerebral artery can lead to a large infarction with contralateral hemiplegia, hemianesthesia, and homonymous hemianopsia. A lesion on the dominant side also produces aphasia. Weakness of the face and arm tends to be more severe than that of the leg. Lenticulostriate branches are totally occluded more often than the middle cerebral artery itself. The results of these branch occlusions are hemiplegia and a mixed communication problem, including varying severity of alexia, apraxia, agnosia, and anomia.

Posterior Cerebral Artery

The posterior cerebral artery supplies blood to the medial and inferior segments of the occipital and posterior temporal lobes and the optic thalamus. Occlusion of this vessel damages the occipital lobe and thalamus, resulting in contralateral homonymous hemianopsia and/or the thalamic syndrome. The latter may include transient hemiplegia, permanent loss of deep sensation and deterioration of superficial sensation, ataxia, tremor, chorioathetoid movements, and severe burning pain. Occlusions of branches of the posterior cerebral arteries produce portions of this clinical picture. The posterior cerebral artery branches into the thalamogeniculate, thalamo-perforating, and calcarine arteries. Obstruction of the thalamogeniculate branch produces only the thalamic syndrome, while occlusion of calcarine branches causes only homonymous hemianopsia. When the thalamo-perforating artery is involved, only the anterior part of the thalamus and certain subthalamic structures and pathways are affected. The major clinical sign is contralateral choreoathetosis. Sensation remains mostly intact because the ventrolateral nucleus of the thalamus (a major focal point for sensory pathways) is spared.

POSTERIOR CIRCULATION

The vertebral-basilar axis supplies the entire brain stem from the midbrain to the medulla, and arterial insufficiency in this portion of the cerebral circulation can lead to a variety of signs and symptoms involving cranial nerve function, sensation, motor function, and coordination. Since several areas of the brain stem participate in the control of fine motor skills and coordination, and there is much overlapping of basilar artery branches, it is usually difficult, if not impossible, to delineate precisely which vessels are occluded in patients with basilar artery insufficiency.

Total obstruction of the basilar artery itself is quite rare. If sudden occlusion does occur, the result is generally coma and severe neurologic damage. With partial obstruction, the patient may have transient ischemic attacks consisting of dysarthria, dysphagia, hemiplegia or quadriplegia, paresthesia, and disorders of eye movements and pupillary function. Third, fourth, or sixth nerve palsies may occur, and the pupils may be fixed and dilated as a result of third nerve palsy. If the third nerve nucleus is not involved, the pupils are likely to be miotic because of ischemic damage to the descending sympathetic pathways in the brain stem. Crossed paralyses, involvement of the ninth and tenth nerves with resulting dysphagia and loss of the gag reflex, and loss of sphincter control occur with basilar artery stenosis.

Most causes of brain stem ischemia result from occlusive disease of branches of the basilar artery. In order to apply some order to the myriad signs and symptoms that may occur, it is useful to divide basilar artery insufficiency into areas of anatomic damage. Each side of the brain stem can be divided conceptually into two neurovascular zones: paramedian and lateral. The paramedian area receives its blood supply directly from short, perforating branches of the basilar artery, and the lateral area is nourished by longer, surface arteries.

Damage to the paramedian area causes contralateral hemiplegia and ipsilateral paralysis of one or more cranial nerves. In the midbrain, the third nerve nucleus is often damaged, resulting in ptosis, lateral deviation of the eye, and a fixed, dilated pupil. Involvement of the medial lemniscus and red nucleus may cause contralateral hemianesthesia and choreiform movements. Paramedian damage in the pons causes sixth nerve and facial paralysis and rhythmic contractions of the palate, if the olivo-denato-rubral pathways are involved. In the medulla, the tongue is paralyzed because of damage to the twelfth nerve nucleus, and tactile sensation may be lost on the paralyzed side.

Occlusion of the surface arteries causes ischemia of the cerebellum as well as the lateral portions of the brain stem. The lateral area of the midbrain receives its blood supply from the superior cerebellar artery. When flow through this vessel is compromised, the patient develops contralateral hemiplegia and sensory loss, ipsilateral cerebellar dysfunction, and a choreiform disorder.

The lateral area of the pons is nourished by the anterior inferior cerebellar artery. Its occlusion leads to ipsilateral deafness due to damage of the eighth nerve nucleus, facial paralysis, Horner's syndrome, contralateral loss of pain and temperature sensation, and ipsilateral loss of touch sensation on the face due to fifth nerve nucleus damage, as well as nystagmus and ipsilateral cerebellar ataxia. The posterior inferior cerebellar artery (a branch of the vertebral artery) supplies the lateral medulla. Occlusion of this vessel or its branches involves the ninth and tenth nerve nuclei and many cerebellar tracts, and may lead to a great number of neurologic findings including the following:

1. Ipsilateral cerebellar dysfunction,
2. Contralateral hemianesthesia of the entire body,
3. Ipsilateral facial hemianesthesia,
4. Nystagmus,
5. Ipsilateral palatal muscle weakness,
6. Dysphagia,
7. Dysarthria, and
8. Horner's syndrome.

In the great majority of clinical situations, one cannot identify discrete anatomic areas of involvement of the vertebral-basilar circulation. Patients may have a mixture of findings including cranial nerve involvement and bilateral pyramidal tract dysfunction. In general, discrete cranial nerve dysfunction, especially of the ninth and tenth nerves, cerebellar ataxia, nystagmus, bilateral limb weakness, and the absence of aphasia should suggest the diagnosis of brain stem infarction.

SMALL VESSEL DISEASE

Microinfarctions between 0.5 mm and 15 mm in size are the most common lesions found in necropsy studies of the brain. They appear as irregular holes, often called lacunae, throughout the internal capsule, cerebellar white matter, brain stem, and basal ganglia. Many of these lesions are due to thickening and subintimal fibrosis of small arteries and arterioles, and occur most frequently in hypertensive individuals. Clinical signs and symptoms secondary to lacunar infarcts generally do not occur before the seventh and eighth decades in normotensive individuals, but appear 10 to 20 years earlier in hypertensive patients.

Patients with lacunar disease may have a variety of neurological findings secondary to dysfunction throughout the brain. A progressively broad-based ataxic gait is characteristic of this syndrome, but sudden episodes of hemiplegia also occur. Also common are dysarthria, incoordination of the hands, and basal ganglia abnormalities that simulate Parkinson's disease.

Small vessel ischemia can also lead to gradual frontal lobe atrophy, manifested by a dementing process, hyperactive jaw jerk, and the presence of sucking, grasping, and palmar-mental reflexes. This diagnosis should always be one of last resort for any patient with a chronic organic brain syndrome. Metabolic causes must be ruled out, and computerized axial tomography (CAT) should be performed to search for mass lesions and hydrocephalus. With small vessel disease, the CAT scan shows cerebral atrophy and may identify areas of infarction.

TRANSIENT ISCHEMIC ATTACKS

Acute cerebral ischemia can assume two forms: a transient ischemic attack or cerebral infarction. In general, a transient attack is defined as the appearance of focal neurologic signs secondary to cerebral ischemia, and their disappearance within less than 24 hours. Most such episodes resolve within a few hours and often a few minutes. Cerebral infarction is arbitrarily defined as an ischemic episode that persists longer than 24 hours. While the neurological findings are still changing, the infarction is called a stroke in evolution; stable abnormalities represent a completed stroke.

It must be emphasized that these definitions are quite arbitrary.

It is difficult to determine with any reliability when encephalomalacia has actually occurred. Some patients gradually recover full neurologic function within several days after the acute insult. Has encephalomalacia occurred, or can an area of brain tissue remain viable with marginal collateral circulation and then recover physiologic function as arteriolar blood flow improves? This question is unanswerable and is similar to the difficulties encountered in distinguishing prolonged angina or coronary insufficiency from a myocardial infarction. Analogous to coronary artery disease, it is not unreasonable to suspect that there is an intermediate stage between ischemic injury and actual necrosis of brain tissue. Unlike the situation with coronary disease, there are no simple laboratory methods to aid in making this distinction. The wide availability of CAT scanning, however, has facilitated the diagnosis because it enables the clinician to visualize all but very small areas of infarction and to distinguish them from hemorrhage. Difficulty still arises in distinguishing between very small infarcts and prolonged transient ischemia. The distinction is of more than academic importance because it has therapeutic implications.

Cerebral arterial disease is not the only cause of transient, focal neurological findings. Other disorders can independently produce identical findings or act synergistically with occlusive arterial disease. It is extremely important to investigate carefully for any extracerebral factors that may contribute to transient ischemic attacks because most are treatable or preventable.

Cardiac Arrhythmias

One of the most common and insidious causes of cerebral ischemia is a transient cardiac arrhythmia. Since patients with cerebrovascular disease often have concomitant arteriosclerotic heart disease, they may be subject to paroxysmal brady- and tachyarrhythmias. There is a very significant coincidence of sick sinus syndrome and atrioventricular node dysfunction and cerebrovascular disease. A short run of sinus bradycardia or occasional sinus arrest might not affect a normal individual, but such a transient decrease in cardiac output may be enough of an insult to produce focal neurologic dysfunction in an area of the brain supplied by a stenotic artery. In one study, significant arrhythmias were found in 28% of patients suffering from transient ischemic attacks.[8] Most of these arrhythmias would have gone undetected without a careful investigation.

Continuous cardiac monitoring for at least 24 hours is mandatory for every patient who has had a transient ischemic attack. Even then, infrequent arrhythmias may not appear, and repeated monitoring may be indicated when the index of clinical suspicion is very high. Patients who have ischemic attacks without any major risk factors for cerebral arteriosclerosis, and those with electrocardiographic evidence of a diseased cardiac conduction system (bifascicular, trifascicular, and bundle branch blocks) fall into this category. This diagnostic procedure should certainly be performed before embarking on cerebral angiography or treating the patient with anticoagulating or antiplatelet drugs. A permanent pacemaker, when indicated, may eliminate any further difficulty. If the patient continues to have transient ischemic attacks with a properly functioning cardiac pacemaker, further investigation and treatment is indicated.

With tachyarrhythmias, the problem may be more complicated. Antiarrhythmic drugs are of variable efficacy from patient to patient, and runs of ventricular tachycardia may or may not be totally eliminated when these agents are employed. If the patient continues to have ischemic episodes, blood levels of these drugs must be checked to be certain that the dose is adequate. The cardiac rhythm must be monitored again to determine whether the arrhythmia is still occurring. The presence of scattered, multiple, premature ventricular contractions without documentation of ventricular tachycardia is not an adequate explanation for transient ischemic attacks and should not forestall further investigation.

Orthostatic Hypotension

Another important contributing factor to attacks of cerebral ischemia is orthostatic hypotension. Since autoregulatory ability is lost in patients with cerebral ischemia, a fall of 30 or 40 mm Hg in systolic pressure may be sufficient to produce inadequate perfusion for an area supplied by a stenotic vessel. Since brain stem ischemia is one of the causes of orthostatic hypotension, the latter is a particularly frequent aggravating factor in ischemic episodes secondary to insufficiency of the basilar artery and its branches. From the history alone, it is usually difficult to determine the presence of orthostatic hypotension in these patients. Blood pressures in the supine and standing positions must be carefully and frequently checked in every patient with symptomatic cerebrovascular disease, particularly in those receiving antihypertensive medications. The application of elastic stockings or leotards may be extremely helpful in preventing cerebral ischemia if significant orthostatic hypotension is found.

Hypoglycemia

A third important factor is hypoglycemia, which can produce focal neurological signs even in the absence of cerebrovascular disease. Since many patients with cerebrovascular disease are overtly diabetic, they may be receiving insulin or oral hypoglycemic agents. As a patient ages, appetite often decreases, and requirements for these agents may decrease. If blood sugar levels are not followed closely, hypoglycemic episodes may occur. If the patient is taking a beta blocking agent for hypertension, peripheral symptoms such as palpitation may be masked, thus making the diagnosis of surreptitious hypoglycemia even more difficult.

Hypoxia

Problems in the oxygen delivery system may also play a role in producing transient ischemic attacks. Exacerbations of chronic obstructive lung disease, recurrent pulmonary emboli, congestive heart failure, and anemia may produce cerebral hypoxia which occasionally dominates the clinical picture. Phosphate depletion due to poor nutrition or gastroinintestinal disease may cause red-cell depletion of 2,3 diphosphoglyceraldehyde, and thus inhibit oxygen release at the cellular level. If this effect is coupled with metabolic alkalosis secondary to diuretic therapy, oxygen release to tissues will be even more impaired. At the same time, alkalosis produces cerebral vasoconstriction.

Finally, one must consider the effects of medications on brain function. A host of sedatives, tranquilizers, and antihypertensive drugs can depress cerebral function and accentuate the effects of cerebral ischemia. Antihypertensive agents may compound the sedative effect with orthostatic hypotension.

SYNDROME OF BASILAR ARTERY INSUFFICIENCY

Transient ischemic attacks involving the vertebral-basilar axis are more common than those involving the carotid distribution. In most cases, the patient has only one symptom—dizziness. This may be true vertigo, but is usually described as a feeling of light-headedness, unsteadiness, weakness, or visual blurring. Some patients actually have syncopal episodes, but syncope without dizziness is rare. Diplopia and dysarthria are other common symptoms during transient ischemic attacks of basilar origin. The other findings of basilar artery occlusion are found only in a small minority of patients. Crossed motor weakness, nystagmus, and severe cerebellar signs generally occur only with infarction of the brain stem and/or cerebellum. Thus, one usually finds little on neurologic examination during a transient attack. Many patients complain of almost continuous dizziness.

Since dizziness is a vague symptom that may be related to a host of extravascular factors, basilar artery insufficiency must be a diagnosis of last resort after an extensive medical work-up. If nystagmus, tinnitus, and unilateral hearing loss are present, one must think first of an acoustic neuroma. Suspicion of such a lesion grows if the corneal reflex is diminished or absent on the same side as the hearing loss. Roentgenograms of the acoustic foramen and CAT scanning are indicated for this constellation of findings. One must also look for middle-ear disease. All of the extracranial factors noted above must be considered in the differential diagnosis of basilar artery insufficiency.

When the diagnosis of symptomatic basilar artery insufficiency has been made, it is important to distinguish between extracranial and intracranial obstruction. In the majority of cases, symptoms are caused by occlusive disease distal to the basilar artery and its major branches. However, significant disease of one or both subclavian arteries is not uncommon, and may be principally responsible for ischemic symptoms. In the Joint Study of Extracranial Arterial Occlusion, the investigators found evidence of subclavian or innominate arterial occlusion or stenosis of 30% or more in 1114 of 6834 patients (17%).[9] Thus, the majority of patients with extracranial arterial disease have carotid rather than subclavian-vertebral lesions.

Subclavian Artery Disease

In any patient with symptoms of dizziness or cerebral ischemia, it is mandatory to measure the blood pressure in both upper extremities in the supine and standing positions. A difference in blood pressure of 30 mm Hg or more is highly significant, since a lumen must be two thirds occluded before any pressure gradient is found. If a difference in blood pressure is consistently present, the next step is careful palpation of the subclavian pulses in the supraclavicular fossae. In most cases, one can detect a difference in pulse volume or upstroke if the obstruction is in the proximal subclavian artery. Use of a Doppler apparatus may be helpful if palpation is difficult. Unfortunately, however, a gradient of 30 to 40 mm Hg can be missed by both digital and Doppler examination, especially if there is a great deal of adipose tissue overlying the arteries.

Auscultation of the subclavian artery may reveal a localized bruit in the supraclavicular fossa. These bruits are often missed because the physician auscultates along the carotid artery but forgets the supraclavicular fossa. When found, the bruits are often confused with carotid artery bruits. The examiner must auscultate carefully at the aortic area and then move the stethoscope slowly into the neck and laterally into the supraclavicular fossa. A subclavian bruit is one that becomes louder as the supraclavicular fossa is approached. If the patient has both carotid and subclavian artery bruits, it may be difficult to identify each one separately, but moving very slowly from the supraclavicular fossa to the neck may reveal first a diminution of the bruit and then increasing amplitude of the second bruit.

The presence of a weak subclavian pulse and low arm pressure are indicative of a significant stenosis of the proximal subclavian artery. Generally, it can be assumed that perfusion pressure through its first branch, the vertebral artery, is decreased. A bruit without any fall in distal pressure suggests the presence of arteriosclerotic disease that is not in itself hemodynamically significant. However, the presence of a bruit tends to correlate with the presence of more distal vertebral-basilar artery disease, and sometimes reflects a stenosis of the vertebral artery at its origin from the subclavian.

Bilateral subclavian bruits without a difference in blood pressure between the two arms may indicate relatively equal stenosis of both subclavian arteries. This possibility can be evaluated by checking the blood pressure in the lower extremities, provided they are free of occlusive arterial disease. Bilateral mild stenoses or one major stenosis plus a rudimentary or absent contralateral vertebral artery, can result in a significantly low basilar artery perfusion pressure and contribute significantly to the syndrome of basilar artery insufficiency.

Subclavian Steal Syndrome

If there is a stenosis in the innominate artery or one subclavian artery proximal to the origin of the vertebral artery, the patient may develop the subclavian steal syndrome. The pathophysiology of this disorder depends on inequality of perfusion pressures in the two vertebral arteries. Since fluid tends to flow from a high pressure to a low pressure system, a portion of the blood reaching the basilar artery from the vertebral artery with the higher perfusion pressure flows in a retrograde direction into the vertebral artery with the lower perfusing pressure, and then into the distal subclavian artery. In this way, blood flow intended for the brain is literally "stolen" by the arm with the subclavian stenosis. The likelihood of a steal syndrome depends on the severity of the subclavian artery stenosis and the degree of arteriosclerosis in the branch arteries distal to the basilar artery. A high peripheral resistance in the distal basilar system and a low resistance (pressure) in the subclavian artery beyond the stenosis favor retrograde flow. Generally, a steal syndrome requires at least a difference of 50 mm Hg in pressure between the two subclavian arteries. A severe steal syndrome may divert as much as 20% of the total cerebral blood flow to the arm.[10]

Symptoms of the subclavian steal syndrome are related to both the arm and the brain. Patients generally have intermittent claudication of the involved arm, often described as an achiness or fatigability on even minor exertion. At times, this symptom can be extremely disturbing, and the patient may unconsciously immobilize the extremity. The result may even be a severe shoulder-hand syndrome with marked limitation of motion at the shoulder joint. Cutaneous ischemia almost never occurs because of the excellent collateral circulation in the upper extremity and the slowness of the occlusive process.

Dizziness is the major neurological symptom associated with the subclavian steal syndrome. Patients complain of unsteadiness or lightheadedness, which may be paroxysmal or continuous. In the classic case, this dizziness is aggravated by exercise of the ischemic arm, and some patients may faint if the arm is moved vigorously for a few minutes. This occurs because vasodilatation of muscle arterioles lowers peripheral resistance distal to the stenosis, favoring further "stealing" of blood flow from the brain stem. Not all patients report this relationship. Along with dizziness, the patient may have focal neurologic symptoms such as diplopia and dysarthria, but rarely any motor signs.

Examination always reveals a decreased blood pressure and subclavian pulse in one arm, usually the left. Provocation of the neurological symptoms with exercise of the involved arm is strong evidence for the diagnosis, but failure to achieve this does not rule out the diagnosis. A definitive diagnosis cannot be made without aortic arch angiography. In addition to a proximal subclavian or innominate artery stenosis, retrograde flow through the stenotic vertebral subclavian axis must be demonstrated on sequential views. Recently, noninvasive measurements of the velocity of pulse propagation to the radial arteries have been found useful in predicting the presence of a subclavian steal syndrome.[11] A marked disparity in pulse propagation time through the two subclavian arteries is very suggestive of the diagnosis, but aortographic confirmation is still necessary if surgery is contemplated.

Subclavian steal syndrome is not rare. It was found in 168 of the 1117 cases of subclavian stenosis reported in the Joint Study of Extracranial Arterial Disease.[9] Its prognosis is remarkably good. Brain stem infarction almost never occurs, and the main danger is injury during dizzy spells. Effective surgical therapy is available, but it is never necessary on an emergency basis. Patients need not undergo surgery unless their symptoms are troublesome.

Surgical correction of the syndrome does not require an intrathoracic approach. Equalization of the blood pressure in the two arms corrects claudication and prevents "stealing" of blood flow. This can be accomplished through a carotid-subclavian bypass across the neck or an axillary-axillary bypass placed subcutaneously across the chest wall. The latter procedure can be performed under light anesthesia with minimal risk and without manipulation of the extracranial cerebral arteries.

TRANSIENT ISCHEMIC ATTACKS IN THE CAROTID CIRCULATION

In the carotid circulation, there are probably two mechanisms for the development of transient ischemic attacks. Ischemia on the basis of inadequate blood flow occurs with bilateral severe stenosis, or when systemic hypotension or a decreased cardiac output occurs. On the other hand, patients with unilateral stenosis usually have sufficient cerebral blood flow through extensive collateralization with the basilar and contralateral carotid circulation. In fact, many patients may gradually suffer total occlusion of a single carotid artery without ever having any symptoms.

The second and more common mechanism involves atheromatous and fibrin-platelet emboli from large atheromatous plaques. These plaques occur throughout the cerebral circulation. The area around the bifurcation of the common carotid into its external and internal branches is a frequent site for plaque formation, probably because turbulence is easily created at this point of angulation. The plaque may involve all three vessels or only the internal carotid artery. Since embolization is the principal mechanism for production of ischemia, the degree of luminal occlusion is not critical. A plaque that does not cause a fall in distal, distending pressure may still lead to transient ischemic attacks and cerebral infarction.

Symptoms of ischemic episodes due to carotid and middle cerebral artery disease may include hemiparesis, hemianesthesia, homonymous hemianopsia, and aphasias, depending on which vessels have received emboli. When small vessels are involved, the patient may have very focal symptoms such as transient weakness limited to a small area of one extremity, or a partial aphasia. If more than one small vessel is occluded, one may see a variety of limited symptoms representing dysfunction of widely separate areas of one side of the cerebral cortex or its subcortical pathways.

Internal carotid artery plaques can also microembolize to the retina, causing transient ipsilateral blindness or a variety of scotomas.

These so-called retinal strokes may occur repeatedly with or without other ischemic symptoms. Microemboli to the retina may also be asymptomatic. Routine funduscopic examination in arteriosclerotic individuals occasionally reveals a tiny plaque in a retinal arteriole.

The great majority of patients with carotid artery lesions are asymptomatic but often have a systolic bruit over the carotid artery in the midneck just behind and below the angle of the mandible. A bruit is most likely to appear when the stenosis approaches 50% of the lumen and is often not present over stenoses greater than 80%. Correlation between the presence of a carotid bruit and carotid artery disease is good. In an arteriosclerotic-prone population, 60% of patients with well-localized bruits have carotid artery disease. It has been estimated from several surveys that 1.8% to 4.4% [12,13] of people over the age of 45 have such a bruit.

Other physical signs of carotid artery disease include decreased or absent carotid and superficial temporal pulses, which may be found when the common carotid is occluded by a plaque, and asymmetry of pulsation in the medial, superior corner of the orbit. At this point, the internal and external carotid artery circulations anastomose through the supraorbital and frontal arteries. Normally, one can feel either no pulsation on either side or a weak, bilaterally equal pulse. If the internal carotid artery is occluded, flow may decrease, weakening the pulse on the affected side, or increase if increased flow occurs from external into internal carotid branches. Thus, asymmetry of these pulses suggests carotid artery disease severe enough to decrease distal perfusion pressure (at least 70% occlusion), but does not indicate which side is involved. Collateral circulation through the external carotid artery can be a pathway for microembolization from a totally occluded internal carotid to the ophthalmic or middle cerebral artery.[7]

A minority of patients with bruits will eventually have transient ischemic attacks, and an even smaller group will have a stroke secondary to the carotid lesion. In the Framingham study, only two of 245 subjects with carotid bruits had transient ischemic attacks, and ten had thrombotic strokes.[14] Most of the strokes occurred in another vascular area. In a study of 256 consecutive patients who had peripheral arterial surgery in the lower extremities, 60 had carotid bruits.[15] Twenty-one of these 60 patients (35%) developed symptomatic cerebrovascular disease during a two- to seven-year follow-up period, as compared to 16% of the patients without bruits. In a survey of a rural community in Georgia, strokes occurred in 13.9% of individuals with carotid bruits followed for a mean of six years, as compared to 3.4% of those without bruits.[13] Strokes appeared in 27.8% of men and 9.3% of women with bruits, and rose in incidence from 1.5% in the 45- to 54-year age group to 14.5% for those over 75. There was a poor correlation between the location of the bruit and the area of the stroke. In general, the majority of patients who have strokes have one or more preceding transient ischemic attacks.[16]

In contrast to these statistics, a surgical group reported a 26.8% incidence of transient ischemic attacks and a 17.4% incidence of stroke in asymptomatic patients with carotid bruits during a follow-up period of eight to ten years. They compared this outcome to a 4.5% incidence of transient ischemic attacks and a 2.3% incidence of strokes in asymptomatic patients who underwent carotid endarterectomy, and recommended this procedure for asymptomatic patients.[17] They and others reported a morbidity rate (neurological complications) of between 3% and 4%.

It is not easy to understand the discrepancies in outcome among various series. One factor may be the definition of an asymptomatic patient. Transient ischemic attacks may be very brief and are often manifested by rather mild symptoms such as momentary clumsiness, occasional dropping of objects, fleeting scotomas, or transient loss of memory or speech. Patients may not always recall these episodes or attribute any importance to them. Therefore, the clinician must take a careful and probing history at frequent intervals in order to identify almost all patients who are having transient ischemic attacks. If symptomatic patients are classified as asymptomatic, the risks of asymptomatic disease will appear higher than they really are. Taking the literature as a whole, we do not believe that there are sufficient data at this time to justify prophylactic carotid endarterectomy for asymptomatic individuals with audible bruits. However, these patients should be followed closely for the development of symptoms. (See Chapter 18 for a different opinion on this subject.)

NONINVASIVE TESTS FOR CAROTID ARTERY DISEASE

In recent years, batteries of noninvasive tests have been devised to diagnose and estimate the severity of internal carotid artery stenosis. These techniques depend on the distribution of internal carotid flow and its anastomoses with the external carotid system. There are three categories of tests: 1) analysis of the bruit, 2) Doppler determination of direction of flow and 3) indirect measurement of ophthalmic artery pressure.[18]

The first technique, phonoangiography, represents an extension of the principles of phonocardiography to a peripheral artery. A visual display of the frequency-amplitude pattern of the bruit is obtained. The longer the bruit, the more severe is the stenosis.

The second test involves the use of a directional Doppler flow meter, applied to the superior medial border of the orbit, which records the amplitude of pulse waves and the direction of flow through the supraorbital and frontal arteries. If blood flow is from the external to the internal carotid system, the patient has an internal carotid occlusion of at least 70%. The test can be repeated with manual compression of the temporal and maxillary branches of the external carotid artery. An abrupt decrease in pulse-wave amplitude during compression confirms the external carotid artery as the source of blood flow through the supraorbital and frontal arteries.

The third evaluation is concerned with ophthalmic artery blood pressure flow. This can be indirectly assessed with the use of a pneumoplethysmograph. A suction cup is placed on the sclera after the instillation of a local anesthetic. Through the application of a negative pressure, a vacuum is formed under the suction cup, which allows transmission of the ophthalmic artery pulsation to the recording device. Systolic blood pressure in the ophthalmic artery can be estimated from the magnitude of the negative pressure required to obtain a pulse. A vacuum pressure of 300 mm Hg corresponds to a systolic blood pressure of 110 mm Hg. Most devices cannot measure systolic pressures above 110 mm Hg, but the technique reliably detects levels below 110 mm Hg. Even if both ophthalmic arteries have pressures in excess of 110 mm Hg, unilateral stenosis can be detected by comparing amplitudes of the pulse waves from each eye. A low ophthalmic artery pressure indicates a stenosis of more than 70%

The accuracy of Doppler and oculoplethysmography techniques was evaluated in a comparative study of 72 patients who underwent cerebral arteriography because of clinical suspicion of carotid artery disease.[19] Using 60% stenosis by angiography as a true positive finding, the investigators found an accuracy rate of 97% for the Doppler test and 74% for ocular plethysmography. There were roughly the same number of false-positive and false-negative results.

The value of these noninvasive tests is still open to some question. Phonoangiography rarely detects an inaudible bruit, and the length of the bruit can usually be judged through careful auscultation. If a bruit is detected, Doppler recording and ocular plethysmography are not necessary for diagnosis of carotid artery disease; they merely assess the severity of the occlusion. Since there are no data to show that the likelihood of microemboli varies directly with the severity of the stenosis, these are of little value in deciding on therapy. Occasionally, these techniques demonstrate a stenosis in a patient without a bruit, but negative tests never totally rule out the diagnosis of carotid artery disease.

Doppler recording and ocular plethysmography are of value in evaluating a patient with a carotid bruit who has been selected for elective surgery. A patient with significant carotid stenosis may be at risk for cerebral infarction if intraoperative hypotension occurs. The need for surgery must be assessed more critically in such a patient and, perhaps, a carotid endarterectomy must first be considered. It is possible, however, that the risk of postoperative strokes in asymptomatic patients with carotid bruits has been overstated. In one study of 246 patients undergoing surgery for abdominal aortic aneurysms, no correlation was found between carotid bruits and the risk of cerebral infarction.[20]

TREATMENT OF PATIENTS WITH TRANSIENT ISCHEMIC ATTACKS IN THE CAROTID CIRCULATION

In evaluating patients with transient ischemic attacks of a cortical nature, it is important to consider the distribution of arteriosclerotic plaques that act as foci for embolization. The internal carotid artery is very frequently involved. In one study of 221 cases of completed strokes, arteriography demonstrated carotid occlusion in 68 and stenosis in 55, as compared to 42 anterior-cerebral and 28 middle-cerebral stenoses.[21] Controlled studies have shown that carotid endarterectomy decreases the incidence of strokes and improves longevity for patients with unilateral carotid artery disease and transient ischemc attacks.[22] Without surgery, 45% of these patients can be expected to have a major stroke within three years. Thus, one does not want to miss this diagnosis. The presence of a carotid bruit in a patient with transient ischemic attacks is a strong indication for cerebral arteriography.

Since 20% of patients with carotid artery disease do not have an audible bruit, and some of these patients have negative noninvasive studies, the option of performing cerebral angiography should be considered in some patients with transient ischemic attacks, even when a bruit is not heard. Factors in favor of performing arteriography in such a patients include:

1. Female sex,
2. Age under 65,
3. Frequent ischemic episodes, and
4. Episodes of unilateral blindness or scotomas.

Carotid Endarterectomy

Surgery should be strongly considered for patients with symptomatic, unilateral stenosis of the extracranial portion of the internal carotid artery. This is particularly true for patients who are having increasingly frequent attacks of weakness and/or sensory loss. If a patient has had only one or two attacks and then has been symptom-free for many months, a more conservative approach may be suitable, especially if the patient is elderly or debilitated. If a patient has no further episodes of ischemia for more than a year, the risk of stroke falls considerably. Treatment of patients who have only episodes of retinal ischemia is still somewhat controversial since some appear to remain free of major ischemic attacks for long periods of time.

Before considering endarterectomy, it is essential to determine that the symptoms are actually referable to the carotid lesion. Many patients with unilateral carotid stenosis complain only of dizziness, which is usually a symptom of basilar artery insufficiency and not an indication for carotid endarterectomy. Dizziness and syncope may be symptoms of bilateral carotid artery stenosis because of decreased total cerebral blood flow. Endarterectomy for bilateral lesions carries a significant morbidity rate but is indicated for patients who are severely symptomatic. In these cases, it is advisable to operate on the more severe occlusion first.

Medical Therapy

No subject in medicine has engendered more controversy than the medical therapy of transient ischemic attacks. Many investigators have advocated anticoagulation as a means of decreasing the frequency of transient ischemic attacks and preventing strokes.[23,24] A voluminous literature on this subject includes reports of efficacy and nonefficacy of warfarin and similar drugs in treating patients with cerebral ischemia. Studies showing a decreased incidence of strokes in anticoagulated patients have generally not been well-controlled. The precise role of anticoagulation is still not clear. Anticoagulation is not advisable for patients with uncontrolled hypertension because of an increased risk of intracerebral bleeding.

More recently, antiplatelet therapy has become standard for patients with transient ischemic attacks. In addition to a number of retrospective reports, the Canadian Cooperative Study of patients with transient ischemic attacks found that men treated with aspirin (1200 mg per day) had a significantly lower incidence of strokes and fewer transient ischemic attacks than men taking placebos.[25] Significant benefit was not apparent in women. The reason for this sex difference is not clear and has led some experts to question the results of the study. At present, many patients with a history of transient ischemic attacks are being treated with a combination of aspirin and dipyridamole or sulfinpyrazone. The overall efficacy of this therapy is not yet known. Many authorities advocate anticoagulation for women.

CEREBRAL EMBOLISM

The possibility of embolism into the cerebral circulation in any patient who suffers an acute episode of cerebral ischemia should never be overlooked. Particular attention should be given to this possibility in dealing with the following:

1. Patients under the age of 60,
2. Patients without hypertension or diabetes mellitus,
3. Patients with atrial fibrillation,
4. Multiple ischemic episodes with varying signs and symptoms, and
5. Neurologic signs involving both sides of the cerebral cortex, such as aphasia and left hemiparesis in a right-handed person.

One must be particularly careful in evaluating patients with atrial fibrillation. Although the great majority of patients with cerebrovascular disease have this arrhythmia because of chronic hypertension, occult mitral stenosis may be present even in very elderly patients. When obvious risk factors for cerebral arteriosclerosis are absent, bacterial endocarditis is also an important consideration, and blood cultures should be obtained even in afebrile patients. Other causes of embolism are discussed in the chapter dealing with acute arterial obstruction.

Recent work with CAT scans has demonstrated a significant rate of error in clinical distinction between infarct and hemorrhage. Moreover, many emboli produce hemorrhagic infarction.[26] Therefore, patients presumed to have emboli should not be anticoagulated without a prior CAT scan. If the infarct is hemorrhagic, anticoagulation should be delayed until signs of hemorrhage have disappeared.

MICROVASCULAR SURGERY

In recent years the development of the operating microscope has made possible anastomoses between smaller arteries (1 to 2 mm in size). These techniques have been applied to the treatment of intracranial occlusive arterial disease involving the internal carotid, middle cerebral, and vertebral arteries. Several groups have reported technical success with these procedures. In one series of patients operated on for frequent transient ischemic attacks, 110 shunts from the superficial temporal artery to the middle cerebral artery were performed with a 97% postoperative patency rate.[27] Twenty-two patients were given shunts from the occipital artery to the posterior inferior cerebellar artery with a 91% postoperative patency rate.

In another series, 40 patients had superficial-temporal to middle-cerebral artery shunts with a 97% postoperative patency rate.[28] Preoperatively, 6 had transient ischemic attacks; 22, mild infarctions; and 12, moderate infarctions. Operative mortality was zero. During a follow-up period up to 36 months, four patients died of heart disease, but no cerebral infarcts occurred. Three patients had one transient ischemic attack. Focal neurological signs remained unchanged in 21 patients and became less pronounced in the remaining 19.

Unfortunately, there are no controlled studies as yet to document the clinical efficacy of these procedures. If benefit is to accrue from microvascular surgery, it is more likely to be observed in patients with low-flow syndromes secondary to bilateral carotid artery disease and basilar artery insufficiency than in patients suffering from recurrent fibrin-platelet or atheromatous emboli. These procedures are still in the investigative stage.

SUMMARY

Cerebrovascular disease remains a confusing subject and controversy still exists concerning the value of noninvasive tests, indications for surgery, and the efficacy of medical therapy.[29] The use of anticoagulation for transient ischemic attacks is a case in point. Anticoagulation continues to enjoy popularity despite several studies suggesting that longevity is not increased, nor are strokes prevented.[30] Antiplatelet drugs certainly need further evaluation, and long-term epidemiologic studies have not yet delineated the *precise* indications for arterial surgery.

REFERENCES

1. Toole JF. Vascular diseases of brain and spinal cord. In Merrit HH (ed). *A Textbook of Neurology* ed 6. Philadelphia, Lea & Febiger, 1979, p 163.

2. Stallones RA. Epidemiology of cerebrovascular disease. A Review. *J Chron Dis* 18:859, 1965.

3. Eisenberg H, Morrison JT, Sullivan P, et al. Cerebrovascular accidents. Incidence and survival rates in a defined population, Middlesex County, Conn. *JAMA* 189:883, 1964.

4. Ladd AC. Cerebrovascular disease in an employed population. *J Chron Dis* 15:985, 1962.

5. Cutler JL. Cerebrovascular disease in an elderly population. *Circulation* 36:394, 1967.

6. Howells DPM. Arterial auscultation in a relatively atheroma-free population. *Lancet* 2:242, 1971.

7. Countee RW, Vijayanathan T. Intracranial embolization via external carotid artery: Report of a case with angiographic documentation. *Stroke* 11:465, 1980.

8. Walter PF, Reid SD Jr, Wenger NK. Transient cerebral ischemia due to arrhythmia. *Ann Intern Med* 72:471, 1970.

9. Fields WS, Lemark NA. Joint study of extracranial arterial obstruction. VII Subclavian Steal-A Review of 168 cases. *JAMA* 222:1139, 1972.

10. Reivich M, Holling HE, Roberts B, et al. Reversal of blood flow through the vertebral artery and its effects on cerebral circulation. *N Engl J Med* 265:878, 1961.

11. Berguer R, Higgins R, Nelson R. Non-invasive diagnosis of reversal of vertebral artery blood flow. *N Engl J Med* 302:1349, 1980.

12. Rhoads GG, Popper J, Yano K, Kagan A. Neck bruits and stroke in Hawaii Japanese men. (Abstract) *Circulation* (Suppl III) 49:50, 1974.

13. Heyman A, Wilkinson WE, Heyden S. Risk of stroke in asymptomatic persons with cervical arterial bruits. *N Engl J Med* 302:838, 1980.

14. Wolf PA, Kannel WB, McNamara GT, et al. Asymptomatic carotid bruit and risk of stroke: The Framingham study. *Stroke* 1:96, 1979.

15. Cooperman M, Martin EM Jr, Evans WE. Significance of asymptomatic carotid bruits. *Arch Surg* 113:1339, 1978.

16. Grindal AB, Toole JF. Surgical treatment of carotid and vertebral artery disease. *Ann Intern Med* 81:647, 1974.

17. Thompson JE, Patman RD, Talkington CM. Asymptomatic carotid bruit: Long-term outcome of patients having endarterectomy compared with unoperated controls. *Ann Surg* 188:308, 1978.

18. McDonald PT, Rich NM, Collins GJ, et al. Ocular pneumoplethysmography: Detection of carotid occlusive disease. *Ann Surg* 189:44, 1979.

19. McDonald PT, Rich NM, Collins GJ, et al. Doppler cerebrovascular examination, oculoplethysmography and ocular plethysmography. *Arch Surg* 113:1341, 1978.

20. Treiman RL, Foran RF, Shore EH, et al. Carotid bruit: Significance in patients undergoing abdominal aortic operation. *Arch Surg* 106:803, 1973.

21. Gurdjian ES, Lindner DW, Hardy WG, et al. "Completed stroke" due to occlusive vascular disease. *Neurology* 11:724, 1961.

22. Fields WS, Maslenikov V, Meyer JS, et al. Joint study of extracranial arterial occlusion. V. Progress report of prognosis following surgery or nonsurgical treatment for transient cerebral ischemic attacks and cervical carotid artery lesions. *JAMA* 211:1993, 1970.

23. Millikan CH, Siekert RG, Shick RM. Studies in cerebrovascular disease V. The use of anticoagulant drugs in the treatment of intermittent insufficiency of the internal carotid arterial system. *Mayo Clin Proc* 30:578, 1955.

24. Whisnant JP, Matsumoto N, Elveback LR. The effect of anticoagulant therapy on the prognosis of patients with transient cerebral ischemic attacks in a community. Rochester, Minn. 1955–1969. *Mayo Clin Proc* 48:844, 1973.

25. The Canadian Cooperative Study Group: A randomized trial of aspirin and sulfinpyrazone in threatened stroke. *N Engl J Med* 299:53, 1978.

26. Weissberg LA. Computed tomography in the diagnoses of intracranial disease. *Ann Intern Med* 91:87, 1979.

27. Sundt TM, Neurovascular microsurgery. *World J Surg* 3:53, 1979.

28. Lee MC, Ausman JI, Geiger JD, et al. Superficial temporal to middle cerebral artery anastomosis. Clinical outcome in patients with ischemia of infarction in internal carotid artery distribution. *Arch Neurol* 36:1, 1979.

29. Byer JA, Easton JD. Therapy of ischemic cerebrovascular disease. *Ann Intern Med* 93:742, 1980.

30. Pearce JMS, Gubbay SS, Walton J. Long-term anticoagulant therapy in transient cerebral ischemic attacks. *Lancet* 1:6, 1965.

13 Diabetic Neuropathy

Sandor A. Friedman

The peripheral neuropathy associated with diabetes mellitus is one of the most ubiquitous medical disorders. Of the eight to ten million patients in the United States with diabetes mellitus, approximately 50% have significant clinical evidence of neuropathy.[1] If one includes patients with very minor neurologic signs such as absent ankle reflexes and/or mild loss of vibratory sensation, the incidence rises much higher. Peripheral neuropathy is certainly the most common complication of diabetes and, in its more severe forms, can lead to a great number of disabling and sometimes puzzling syndromes. It can involve autonomic as well as somatic nerves.

Since many diabetic patients have both peripheral arterial disease and peripheral neuropathy, their clinical findings often represent a combination of the effects of both disorders. Autonomic neuropathy, when it affects the cardiovascular system, often aggravates the vascular problems of the diabetic patient. Other autonomic effects lead to symptoms that sometimes have to be differentiated clinically from vascular problems. Any clinician dealing with vascular problems must treat many diabetic patients and be fully aware of all the neurological ramifications of the disease. For the purpose of simplicity, one can classify specific neurological complications of diabetes mellitus into the following categories:

- Somatic polyneuritis
- Mononeuritis
- Autonomic neuropathy
- Miscellaneous disorders
  - Carpal tunnel syndrome
  - Myelopathy
  - Amyotrophy

SOMATIC POLYNEURITIS

By far the most common neurologic syndrome associated with diabetes mellitus is a symmetrical, distal peripheral neuropathy in a "stocking glove" distribution. It is primarily and usually only a sensory neuropathy. Although not all of diabetics have obvious signs of neuropathy, it can be considered an integral part of diabetes mellitus, almost as inevitable as the abnormal glucose tolerance. Several studies have shown that seemingly normal diabetics in every decade tend to have poorer sensation in the distal portions of their feet than age-matched nondiabetic individuals.[2] In one study, 88% of diabetic subjects had at least minimal evidence of peripheral nerve dysfunction.[3] Threshold for perception of vibratory sensation in the feet decreases with age but diminishes much more quickly in diabetic individuals.[4] Whereas total loss of vibratory sensation in the toes is a normal finding in individuals in the eighth decade, this sensory modality is absent in a large percentage of diabetics by the fifth and sixth decades. The same trend holds for loss of the ankle reflexes. Studies of nerve conduction velocity corroborate these clinical findings. At any given age, mean conduction velocity is lower in any group of diabetics than in normal individuals. If one measures sensory as well as motor nerve conduction time in the extremities, one finds abnormal results in a large sector of diabetic patients who have no significant sensory loss. Even many prediabetic individuals, whose glucose tolerance is abnormal only under stress, tend to have an increased vibratory threshold for their age and delayed sensory nerve conduction in the extremities. Diabetic neuropathy is probably the most common chronic neurologic disorder.

Pathogenesis

The reason for this distal nerve dysfunction is still the subject of conjecture. Many theories of pathogenesis have evolved during the last two decades, enjoyed transient popularity, and then have been replaced by still another hypothesis. Many rough correlations between the presence of diabetic neuropathy and various metabolic and vascular defects have been noted, but proof of a cause-and-effect relationship has never been forthcoming. It remains today a central enigma of diabetology and neurology. One interesting analogy is the comparison of diabetes mellitus and aging.[5] Almost every degenerative process occurs earlier and more frequently in diabetic individuals. Premature atherosclerosis is the prime and most serious manifestation of this principle. Other examples include osteoarthritis, calcific bursitis, resorption of the mandible with early loss of teeth, decreased hearing acuity,[6] cataract formation, and increased susceptibility to a variety of infections and malignancies. Cartilage taken from the knee of a 30-year-old diabetic, for example, often appears microscopically as though it had come from an individual in the seventh or eighth decade.[7] Even the glucose intolerance of diabetes can be seen as a marked exaggeration of aging since blood sugar levels rise with age in the normal population.[8]

Diabetic peripheral neuropathy can also be fitted into this concept of premature aging. Vibratory threshold in the feet rises progressively with age and is often absent in the later decades. Ankle reflexes are also lost with age. Although other sensory modalities remain clinically intact, nerve conduction velocity progressively diminishes after the age of 40.[9] More significant neurologic deficits might appear in a substantial proportion of the population if mean life span were long enough. Thus it is possible that the distal sensory loss of diabetic individuals may represent a kaleidoscope of a degenerative process which occurs very slowly in normal individuals as a natural part of the aging process. This theory, even if it is substantially correct, does not shed much light on the actual pathogenesis of the disorder. It does suggest, however, that the clue to understanding of the process may lie in finding an exaggeration of factors or defects that are present in smaller magnitude in normal individuals, rather than defects that are unique to people with diabetes mellitus.

For many years it was thought that polyneuropathy was a manifestation of diabetic microangiopathy involving the vasa nervora that nourish peripheral nerve fibers.[10] However, experimental and pathologic data have not supported this hypothesis.[11] It is generally agreed today that diabetic polyneuropathy is a metabolic disorder. The nature of this metabolic problem is still in question.

There has been much conjecture and debate about the role of glucose metabolism in the pathogenesis of the neuropathy. There have been several attempts to find a correlation between degree of control of hyperglycemia and severity of neuropathic changes. In one study, a transient increase in nerve conduction velocity was found after insulin therapy in a small group of previously uncontrolled diabetic patients with mild neuropathy.[12] Another group reported a positive correlation between blood sugar level and nerve conduction time in newly diagnosed, adult-onset diabetics.[13] Many clinicians have also noted digital paresthesias in uncontrolled diabetic patients that disappear with treatment of the glucose intolerance. On the other hand, well-established neurologic deficits are never reversible, and many patients with far advanced neuropathy have only mild glucose intolerance. Certainly, there is not sufficient evidence at this time to consider diabetic neuropathy a preventable disorder.

A number of metabolic products have been implicated in the pathogenesis of diabetic polyneuropathy. Because of higher blood sugar levels, there is increased utilization of glucose along the polyol pathway with consequent intracellular accumulation of sorbitol and fructose. Rats with experimental diabetes accumulate high concentrations of sorbitol and fructose in sciatic nerves, which decrease with insulin administration.[14] It has been theorized that these metabolites result in osmotic swelling and destruction of peripheral nerves.

Other investigators have found decreased levels of myoinositol in peripheral nerves in experimental diabetes and increased urinary excretion of myoinositol in diabetic patients.[15] This has been correlated with decreased nerve conduction velocity in experimental animals.

Clearly, we must still look upon diabetic neuropathy as a poorly understood degenerative process. The reason for the predominantly distal distribution of this lesion is also still speculative. The classical explanation has invoked a "dying-back process" in which the distal portions of the axon, being furthest from metabolic regulation by the body of the neuron, deteriorate first. An alternative theory involves the laws of probability. The longer the axon, the more prone it may be to a random injury somethere along its course. Any lesion along the length of the axon can interfere with transmission of impulses. Since the axons innervating the distal part of an extremity are the longest, they become the first to deteriorate. Computer simulation models have shown that randomly distributed lesions within peripheral nerves can account for the proximal-distal gradient of peripheral neuropathies.[1] This theory of random distribution may also help to explain why diabetic neuropathy involves the lower extremities earlier and more extensively than the shorter, upper extremities.

The incidence and severity of neuropathy are well related to duration of disease in juvenile-onset diabetes, but much better correlated with patient age in adult-onset diabetes. In general, most juvenile diabetics have some clinical evidence of peripheral nerve dysfunction after ten years of illness, and the great majority of all diabetics have at least mild neuropathy by the age of 60. There is no sex predilection for peripheral neuropathy.

A remarkable and unexplained phenomenon is the propensity of diabetes to involve sensory nerve fibers. Polyneuritis always begins as a sensory neuropathy and almost always remains a purely sensory lesion. Although motor nerve conduction velocity may be decreased, significant muscle weakness is quite uncommon. It is possible that this specificity is in part related to our clinical testing skills. Subtle changes in sensory threshold are much easier to find and document than early signs of motor weakness. Muscle strength is very variable within the normal population. However, this thought certainly does not explain how a diabetic patient with an almost totally anesthetized foot can have seemingly normal muscle function. It also does not explain why some other disease states, such as heavy metal poisoning, cause peripheral neuropathies with predominantly motor involvement.

Progression of diabetic polyneuropathy is quite variable. In most cases, sensory deficits worsen slowly and insidiously over several decades. Usually, the result is moderate deprivation of only some sensory modalities. However, nerve dysfunction can develop much more rapidly and result in serious deprivation within a few years. Between these two extremes, there is a whole spectrum of changes. Regardless of the rapidity of the process, the patient is usually unaware of what is happening.

Signs and Symptoms

Symptoms occur in a minority of cases of polyneuropathy before the late stages of sensory deprivation. Some patients report that their feet often "fall asleep," and others note uncomfortable paresthesias, but most have no idea that they are gradually losing their sensory abilities.

Occasionally, a patient has severe pain in the early stages of diabetic polyneuropathy. This pain usually involves both legs, is sharp and lancinating, and often radiates up and down the lower extremities. It may occur in paroxysms and closely resemble the pain of tabes dorsalis and trigeminal neuralgia. Walking and standing may aggravate the symptom, but it is most often unrelated to activity. Sensory loss is usually only mild or moderate when pain is present. As nerve dysfunction progresses, pain usually tends to abate and eventually disappear, but the patient may suffer greatly for several years.

In the late stages, patients are often aware of numbness in their feet. If proprioceptive sensation is seriously impaired, they may find themselves stumbling and falling. Significant sensory impairment in the more specialized fingers may lead to serious disability. There may be inability to perform fine motor functions. For example, tasks such as typing, sewing, and even buttoning a shirt may become virtually impossible because of inadequate sensory input.

As polyneuropathy gradually develops, loss of function usually follows a predictable sequence. Sensory loss always occurs first in the toes, and vibratory sensation is the first modality to be lost. Unfortunately, clinical testing of vibratory sensation is subjective and inexact. Using a tuning fork, the clinician measures vibratory threshold at only one frequency and generally compares the result to himself. If the clinician can feel the vibration when the patient cannot, the patient's vibratory sensation is generally considered impaired. The accuracy of this method depends to a large extent on the age difference between physician and patient. Often, clinical examination underestimates loss of vibratory sensation because it is not performed correctly. A patient with practically no vibratory sensation may mistake the pressure of the metal tuning fork for vibrations. It is essential to demonstrate the difference to the patient in an area of the body where he can clearly feel the vibrating of the tuning fork.

With the use of a biothesiometer, measurement of vibratory sensation is much more accurate and semiquantitative.[16] Measured vibratory stimuli over a whole range of amplitudes and at several different frequencies are applied to the feet or hands. Vibratory threshold can be estimated at each frequency and compared to the results in age-matched normal controls. With this technique, one can reliably diagnose diabetic peripheral neuropathy in its earliest clinical stage.

After vibratory sensation is involved, the next step is weakening and eventual loss of deep tendon reflexes. The ankle reflexes are lost first, followed in many cases by the patellar reflexes. Areflexia is not caused by muscle weakness; it is a reflection of sensory deprivation. Loss of deep pressure sensation interrupts the reflex arc while motor function is still normal.

Loss of distal vibratory sensation and ankle reflexes represents the full extent of diabetic polyneuropathy in most patients and is analogous to the changes seen in normal individuals two decades or more later in life. It is only when neuropathy extends beyond these modalities that it becomes hazardous to the patient. The slow insidious loss of pain sense in the foot begins in the toes and may extend proximally, in severe cases, as high as the thigh. Distal loss is usually very marked before the neuropathy extends above the foot. Position sense tends to be lost at about the same time as pain sensation but is usually confined to the toes. In very severe cases, the ankle joint may be involved, but never the knee. The last modality to be lost is light touch. At that stage, the foot is virtually autoanesthetized.

In the case of position and pain sensation, the inexperienced examiner often badly underestimates the degree of dysfunction. In fact, many patients with severe deficits due to diabetic neuropathy are erroneously labelled as normal. Position sense cannot be accurately assessed by vigorously flexing and extending the toes and asking the patient to determine the direction of movement. Even an individual with almost no proprioceptive sensation can recognize a strong thrust in an upward or downward direction. If the patient offers resistance to toe movement, he can also assess the direction with little or no sense of position. Thus it is important to relax the patient and to move each toe very slowly in an upward or downward direction. Normal individuals have a very keen sense of position and easily detect the direction of very small movements. With careful examination, one can find very early evidence of proprioceptive sensory loss.

Deficits in pain sensation are also often missed because of superficial examining techniques. One common technique is to begin checking pin sensation in the proximal portion of the extremity, move distally, and instruct the patient to inform the examiner of any change in intensity of the stimulus. It is remarkable how often a patient with very marked impairment of pin sensation notices no difference in intensity with this technique. One must give the patient a choice in order to evaluate pain sense properly. Beginning most distally, one should ask the patient to choose the sharper of two stimuli. If the patient cannot distinguish accurately between a relatively sharp and relatively dull stimulus (such as the point of a pen and the back of a pen), one moves proximally until coming to an area of normal sensation in order to map out the extent of neuropathy.

Diagnosis

Differential diagnosis of diabetic polyneuropathy is generally not difficult. The combination of abnormal glucose tolerance and "stocking-glove" sensory loss in the feet makes the diagnosis quite obvious in most cases. However, there are occasional problems in diagnosis. Uremic patients often have glucose intolerance and polyneuropathy that is indistinguishable clinically and biochemically from the abnormalities of diabetic patients with peripheral nerve dysfunction. Thus, without a previous history of diabetes mellitus, the diagnosis of diabetic neuropathy is extremely difficult to make in a patient with chronic renal failure. If glucose tolerance and peripheral nerve function improve significantly with dialysis, one can infer that renal failure is the principal cause of the abnormalities. However, even if dialysis has no effect, one cannot make a definite diagnosis of diabetic neuropathy.

If vibratory and position sense are severely blunted and pain sensation is normal, one must always consider the possible presence of damage to the posterior column of the spinal cord secondary to vitamin B_{12} deficiency or tabes dorsalis. In this situation, it is important to obtain a seriological test for syphilis and to rule out the presence of a macrocytic anemia. Finally, chronic alcoholism often leads to a predominantly sensory neuropathy that can simulate mild to moderate diabetic neuropathy.

Complications

Patients with significant deprivation of pain and position sense in their feet are at great risk of injury. Loss of proprioception alone can be hazardous. If proximal position sense is present, the patients may not be ataxic or fall, but they are unaware of the movements or location of their toes. They can easily place the distal portion of the foot onto a sharp or hard surface with sudden, unguided movements. When pain sensation is blunted, risk of trauma becomes much greater. Chronic low-grade insults to the foot can continue unrecognized for long periods of time. An improperly fitting shoe, for example, can gradually erode the skin around the instep or on a toe, and produce a deep ulcer that may become macerated and secondarily infected. The patient may first become aware of the lesion after developing calf pain, fever, and chills secondary to cellulitis and lymphangitis. Thermal insults may be very acute. It is not uncommon for patients with diabetic neuropathy to develop large, painless vesicles secondary to a burn inflicted by a warm bath or use of an electric blanket.

When the patient has arterial insufficiency as well as diabetic neuropathy, he is at double jeopardy. Chronic trauma is compounded by poor healing capacity, and metabolic demands quickly outstrip the circulatory capacity to deliver oxygen to tissue. The results are gangrene and nonhealing ulceration. Amputation rates are high with this combination of diseases.

Neurotrophic Ulcer

The most specific injury to result from diabetic polyneuropathy is the so-called neurotrophic ulcer (Figure 13-1). It occurs in patients with almost total loss of pain perception. Without subliminal appreciation of pressure on the foot, patients do not shift their weight regularly. This leads to direct trauma as well as ischemia because the pressure on the plantal surface exceeds arteriolar pressure.[17]

The neurotrophic ulcer is a painless area of skin breakdown on the plantar surface of the foot, usually in the metatarsal area. Most often, ulceration develops in the center of a thick callus that has accumulated over months or years. The ulcer is usually somewhat pale and well-demarcated. If untreated, it becomes easily infected, and infection

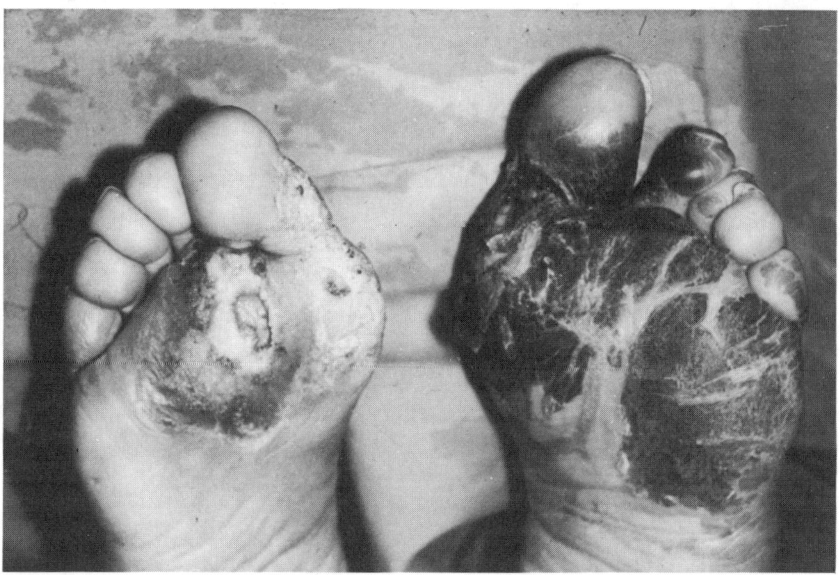

Figure 13-1 Typical plantar, neurotrophic ulcers. Dark areas represent iodine staining from tri-iodide solution.

may burrow deeply into the plantar fascia and even result in chronic osteomyelitis. Huge plantar ulcers and fascial abscesses may go undetected by the patient until swelling and cellulitis spread to the dorsum of the foot. This is not surprising since most people rarely look at the plantar surface of their feet. Once a plantar ulcer occurs, the area involved is prone to recurrence. Healing occurs with scarring and interruption of fascial planes so that the tensile strength of the subcutaneous tissue is never as strong as it originally was.

A nontender plantar ulcer almost always indicates the presence of diabetic neuropathy. The only other diseases associated with similar lesions are the neuropathy of leprosy and spinabifida. These three disorders share in common the ability to produce severe sensory deprivation for many decades. Most other illnesses associated with such severe neurologic deficits are not compatible with prolonged longevity. Even raised thick callus in the metatarsal area should raise the suspicion of diabetic neuropathy and prompt careful neurological examination of the feet.

Osteopathy

Bone disease is a frequent complication of severe polyneuropathy. Like plantar ulcers, this neuroosteoarthropathy occurs only when pain sensation is almost totally absent. It is the result of continuous trauma to the small bones of the foot and is analogous to the destructive arthropathy of knee and ankle (Charcot's joints) seen in patients with long-standing tabes dorsalis. In the latter disorder, these large joints are destroyed because of lack of protective proprioceptive reflexes. Diabetic neuropathy, in contrast, is a more distal process and, therefore, usually involves only the foot bones and occasionally the ankle, but never the knee. Instead of abnormal joint stretching as in tabes, diabetic neuropathy leads to direct pressure trauma on the bones of the feet. Any arthritic changes are caused by bone destruction on each side of the affected joint.

The metatarsal and phalangeal bones are most commonly involved in this diabetic osteopathy.[18] A variety of radiologic findings may develop and the lesions are always painless. A pathologic fracture of a metatarsal bone may be the first sign of osteopathy but, more often, the bones are gradually eroded. Loss or splintering of the heads of several metatarsal bones is often followed by gradual thinning of the necks of these bones (Figure 13-2). This latter lesion is sometimes called the "swan neck" deformity. In some cases, subluxation of metatarsophalangeal joints results from destruction of the metatarsal head.

The proximal phalanges are sometimes the only bones involved in the early stages of osteopathy. Destruction of the base of a phalanx may also occur in conjunction with damage to the corresponding metatarsal head. The characteristic lesion is thinning of the midportion of the phalanx, eventually producing an "hourglass" deformity (Figure 13-3). Subperiosteal new bone formation as a reparative process can often be seen in metatarsals and phalanges. In fact, the earliest radiologic sign of osteopathy is sometimes increased radiodensity and cortical thickening along the sides of one or two phalanges.

Metatarsophalangeal bone destruction is basically a benign process.[19] No matter how severe and widespread the radiologic changes appear, clinical problems do not usually arise. Walking is unimpaired and patients are totally asymptomatic. The only complication in very severe cases is a distortion of the skeletal architecture of the foot that focuses the pressures of standing on discrete areas and thus increases the potential for skin ulceration.

In a minority of cases, diabetic osteopathy involves the tarsal bones. This may occur in the absence of more distal lesions. When the distal small tarsal bones are involved, there is usually also damage to the bases of the adjoining metatarsals. In severe cases, the forefoot may take on a club-like shape, which makes the diagnosis of diabetic osteopathy obvious from inspection of the foot. From a skeletal point of view, those lesions also do not cause much clinical difficulty except for occasional erosion of skin. However, when the proximal tarsal

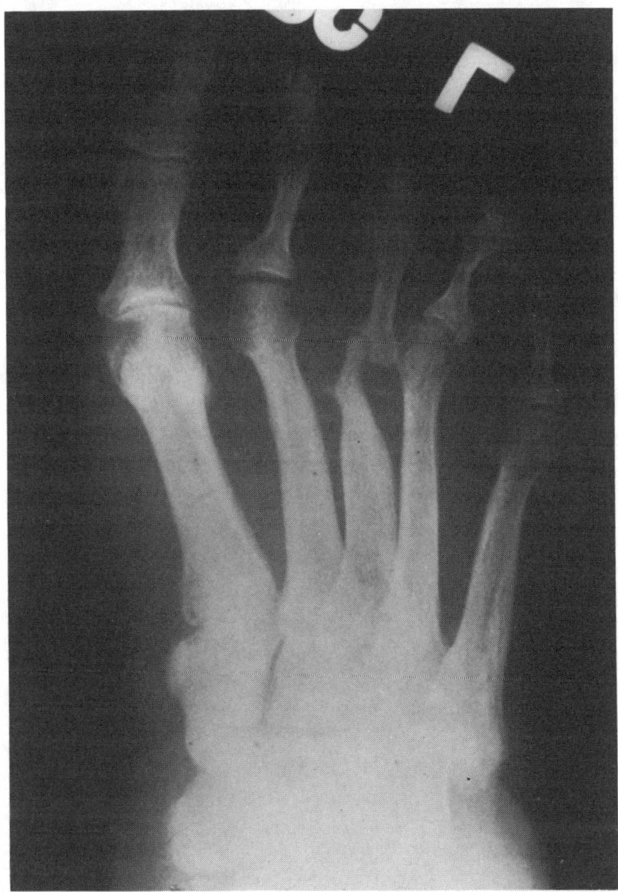

Figure 13-2 Diabetic osteopathy. Note the destruction of the third metatarsal head.

bones are involved, the viability of the ankle as a supporting structure is seriously threatened.[20] Marked destruction of the talus and calcaneous, sometimes associated with similar lesions in the distal fibula and tibia, may lead to collapse of the intricate ankle mortice and result in a totally useless ankle joint. Surgical repair is generally impossible, and the patient can no longer walk or support himself in an upright position.

Occasionally, diabetic osteopathy makes its first clinical appearance as a nonpainful arthritis. Warm, nontender swelling of the forefoot or ankle occurs as a synovial reaction to adjoining bony injury. An x-ray reveals extensive bone destruction in the area of swelling. Aspiration of fluid may reveal actual fragments of cartilage.

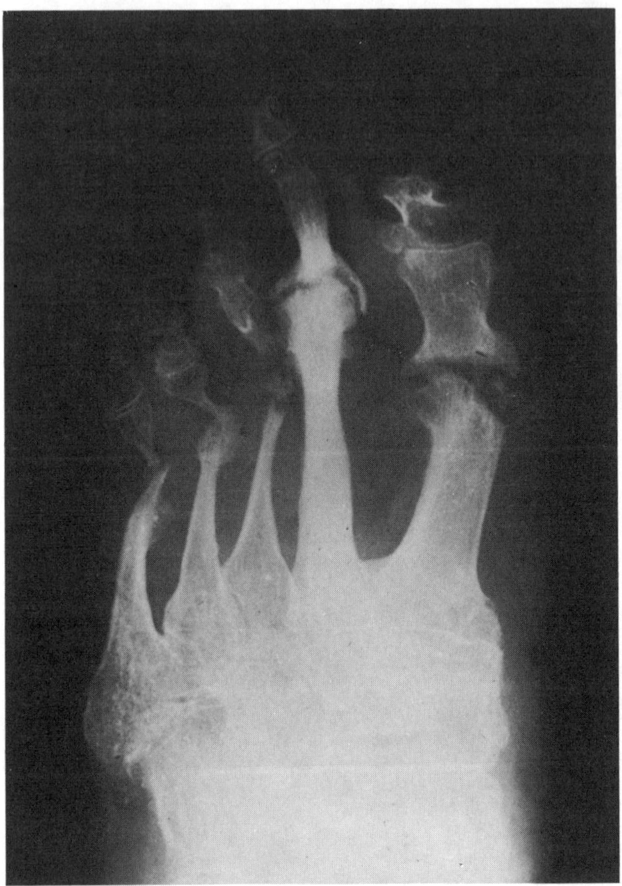

Figure 13-3 Advanced diabetic osteopathy of the metatarsophalangeal area. Note the "hourglass" configuration of the lateral proximal phalanges, thinning of metatarsal necks, and loss of joint architecture. Head of first metatarsal and base of first proximal phalanx are also involved.

It is of some interest that diabetic osteopathy rarely develops in an ischemic foot. Maintenance of adequate arterial circulation seems to be necessary for resorption of bone. In fact, many patients, during the stages of acute bone destruction, have a very warm, hyperemic foot almost suggestive of cellulitis.[19] Since pain and tenderness do not occur in these feet, it is sometimes difficult to distinguish clinically between osteopathy and cellulitis, and an x-ray of the foot is often necessary.

Since they share a similar pathogenesis, it is not surprising that plantar ulcers and osteopathy often coexist in patients with severe diabetic neuropathy. In this situation, difficulty often arises over the distinction between osteomyeltis and osteopathy. Suppuration in a plantar ulcer can burrow through fascia into bone and cause a severe osteomyelitis. On the other hand, ulceration and osteopathy both tend to occur in the area of greatest pressure, and thus a metatarsal ulcer may appear over a destroyed metatarsal head. It is radiologically impossible to distinguish between osteopathy and osteomyelitis if this metatarsal is the only bone involved. If there are multiple bone lesions in areas not adjoining the ulcer, bilateral lesions, or characteristic thinning of metatarsal necks, then it becomes easier to diagnose osteopathy. Clinically, one must look carefully at an infected ulcer and probe the lesion with a soft, sterile instrument. If osteomyelitis is present, there should be a sinus tract that extends directly to the bone. Finding no such tract, the physician should treat conservatively for a soft tissue infection.

Upper Extremity Involvement

Polyneuropathy of the upper extremities is usually quite mild, rarely leading to more than a moderate blunting of vibratory sensation. When it is severe, it can be quite handicapping. Loss of proprioceptive sensation interferes with coordinated activities of the fingers and may be a source of occupational disability.

Neuropathy is also associated with sclerodactyly of the distal portions of the fingers. The tightly bound skin superficially resembles early skin changes seen in patients with Raynaud's phenomenon, but can be distinguished from the latter by skin temperature. The diabetic with sclerodactyly tends to have vasodilation with warm fingers.

Treatment

At present, there is no way of preventing, reversing, or altering the natural course of diabetic neuropathy. One can only attempt to prevent the complications of this disorder. First and foremost, vigilant and diligent foot care is extremely important. This is particularly important for patients with arterial insufficiency. Patients must be clearly informed of their sensory deprivation and warned to inspect their feet regularly.

Since it is difficult to examine the plantar surface directly, a patient with neuropathy should be encouraged to use a small hand mirror in order to examine for callus, abrasions, or ulcerations. Any break in the skin should be immediately reported to the physician. The patient must learn to be compulsive about checking the temperature of bath or shower water with his arms. He must also be careful in choosing shoes.

When wearing new shoes for the first few days, he must look closely for any signs of pressure around the toes or instep of the foot. Simple instructions such as these can prevent serious morbidity and even loss of limb.

Regular podiatric care is another essential element of preventive maintenance of the feet. Not only should toe nails be trimmed regularly, but also pressure points must be cared for. Thick callus in the metatarsal area must be periodically planed down so that it does not become the nidus for a plantar ulcer. Areas of potential pressure against skin caused by corns, bony exostoses, or hammer toes must be carefully watched. If signs of pressure are present, the patient's shoe may have to be carefully molded to alleviate it.[21] Often, a latex shield can be placed around an area subject to pressure. The latex surrounds the area like a doughnut and absorbs the pressure from the shoe.

Plantar ulcers heal fastest if the patient stays off his feet. Continued standing and walking leads to more damage and eventual infection. An uncomplicated, early ulcer will often close almost completely with a few days of bed rest. If infection is present, it must be treated with lukewarm soaks and a local antibacterial agent. One very effective agent is tri-iodide solution (a saturated solution consisting of 500 mg potassium iodide and 500 mg iodine per 100 ml of water).[22] This mixture yields I_3 radicals, which penetrate into the wound and are highly bactericidal and fungicidal. The solution is applied as a "sandwich dressing." A gauze saturated with tri-iodide solution is placed between two pieces of dry gauze, and the combination is applied to the wound. If signs of surrounding cellulitis appear, systemic antibiotics are indicated. With extensive infection and plantar abscess, formal debridement and surgical drainage become necessary.

Once a plantar ulcer has developed, steps must be taken to prevent a recurrence. In the late stages of healing, the patient can be allowed to ambulate with the front part of the shoe cut off, if there is a metatarsal ulcer. The back is removed in the case of the less common heel ulcer. After complete healing and before full ambulation, an adjustment must be made in the patient's shoe in order to redistribute the weight away from the site of the lesion. This can be accomplished with the placement of a posterior bar on the outside of the shoe or the insertion of a latex mold inside the sole of the shoe.[21] This mold acts as a soft pocket for the involved area of the foot.

Bone lesions in the metatarsophalangeal region are best left alone unless there is a sinus tract from an infected ulcer. If true osteomyelitis is present, it is necessary to remove the diseased metatarsal bone and treat the patient with intravenous antibiotics for several weeks. Osteopathy, on the other hand, does not even call for restriction of any activities.

Tarsal involvement with osteopathy is a serious matter, but there is no satisfactory treatment. Some clinicians have suggested prolonged bedrest, but this stimulates more bone resorption. There is no evidence that bedrest leads to healing. Others have casted or even surgically pinned the ankle. Results have not been encouraging with any kind of therapy. If the ankle collapses completely, below-the-knee amputation is often the best treatment because it allows the patient to be fitted with a prosthetic limb.

AUTONOMIC NEUROPATHY

If relatively little is known about the basic pathogenesis of somatic diabetic neuropathy, even less is understood about the involvement of the autonomic nervous system. There are physiologic differences between autonomic and somatic nerve fibers, and it is possible that there are significant differences in the pathogenesis of their dysfunction. Autonomic axons appear to be much more resistant to the ravages of diabetes mellitus than somatic nerves because autonomic neuropathy is much less common than the "stocking glove" polyneuropathy of the extremities. Furthermore, autonomic neuropathy never appears in the complete absence of somatic nerve dysfunction. In most cases, rather far advanced changes are present in the feet before the first signs of autonomic neuropathy appear. At a minimum, vibratory sensation is blunted and ankle reflexes are weak or absent in patients with any evidence of autonomic neuropathy. These patients often have plantar ulcers and radiologic evidence of diabetic osteopathy.

Like somatic neuropathy, autonomic dysfunction appears to be primarily a disorder of sensory axons. It may be widespread or involve only one or two organ systems. Because of the multiplicity of functions that are controlled and regulated by the autonomic nervous system, diabetic autonomic neuropathy can produce a wide variety of troubling and confusing syndromes. Indeed, it can be one of the great masqueraders of internal medicine. The effects of this disorder are best summarized on a system-by-system basis.

Cardiovascular System

Except for iatrogenic causes, diabetic neuropathy is the most common etiology of orthostatic hypotension. As pointed out in a previous chapter, neuropathy-related hypotension can be recognized by a failure of the heart rate to increase as the blood pressure falls. Another characteristic finding associated with this type of postural hypotension is loss or blunting of the relationship between heart rate and respiration.[23] In normal individuals, heart rate decreases during inspiration. When this phenomenon is quite marked, it is called sinus arrhythmia. In most cases, this change is not easily recognized on physical examination, but an electrocardiogram demonstrates lengthening of the R-R interval during deep inspiration. In diabetic autonomic neuropathy, the R-R interval may remain almost constant.

Blood flow studies have demonstrated that patients with severe diabetic neuropathy can develop vasoconstriction in response to cold.[24] This indicates that alpha adrenergic motor fibers are intact. The defect, therefore, in postural hypotension is probably on the sensory side of the reflex arc and may involve the vagus nerves, since the effect of respiration on heart rate is also mediated through the vagi. There is also evidence of renal sympathectomy in diabetic neuropathy, which may lead to suboptimal renin levels when the patient assumes the upright position.[25]

Although only a small proportion of patients with neuropathy have symptomatic orthostatic hypotension, many others consistently have falls of 20 to 30 mm Hg in systolic blood pressure on rising from the lying to standing position. If these patients are treated for hypertension with autonomic blocking agents or are slightly volume-depleted with diuretics, they quickly become symptomatic.

Diabetic patients have a much higher incidence of silent myocardial infarcts than the normal population.[26] Autonomic neuropathy has been postulated as an explanation for this phenomenon. However, in many patients with silent infarcts, there is little or no evidence of peripheral neuropathy. Some investigators have suggested that bradyarrhythmias and supraventricular and ventricular escape rhythms may result from denervation of the heart.[27]

Treatment of symptomatic orthostatic hypotension is usually a simple matter. Discontinuation of any drugs that may be aggravating the situation and use of elastic support for the lower extremities usually suffice. In refractory cases, a small dose of a salt-retaining corticosteroid is often helpful.

Urinary Tract

Diabetic autonomic neuropathy is the most common cause of a neurogenic bladder. Again, the major defect is sensory. This sensory loss leads to detrusor muscle areflexia and a distended bladder.[28] Persistent overdistention of the bladder gradually stretches and further impairs detrusor contraction. This stretching causes narrowing of the bladder neck opening. The patient continues to be able to void until the bladder neck stenosis becomes very severe, but requires progressively more force to do so.

Patients with diabetic cystopathy develop painless bladder distension, which can lead to ureteral reflux and hydronephrosis. The first clinical clue may be painless dribbling, frequency, and nocturia secondary to overflow incontinence. In middle-aged men, it may be difficult to distinguish between prostatism and neurogenic bladder and, in many cases, both are actually present. The relative contribution of each to the symptoms can be assessed with a postvoiding film during intravenous pyelography, cystoscopy, and cystometric studies.

In the early stages, diabetic cystopathy can be managed with a scheduled, triple-voiding pattern and, if necessary, small doses of parasympathomimetic agents such as urecholine.[29] Moderately severe cases may respond to larger doses of these agents. Once there is severe bladder paralysis, surgical resection of the bladder neck may be necessary to obtain adequate urinary drainage. This procedure may produce retrograde ejaculation. The alternative is a permanent cystostomy. These procedures become necessary in the face of decreasing renal function or recurrent, debilitating urinary sepsis.[29]

Sexual Function

Genital neuropathy is a proven problem only in males. Retrograde ejaculation makes diabetic neuropathy a leading cause of male sterility. Impotence is an extremely difficult problem, which has significant effects not only for the patient but also his whole family.[30] Since many of these impotent patients are at an age when they would normally be in the prime of their sexual life, their sexual failure has a devastating impact on their own egos and causes frustration for themselves and their wives. Extramarital relationships and divorce are quite common in these families.

The pathogenesis of impotence is not entirely clear. Penile erection is a matter of filling the corpora cavernosum and corpus spongiosum with blood. This requires a good blood supply and vasodilatation of the feeding vessels. This vasodilatation is mediated by sacral parasympathetic and thoracolumbar sympathetic nerves.[31] It has been suggested in the past that diabetic impotence might be the result of small artery disease. However, the high incidence of impotence in patients with severe diabetic neuropathy and no evident arterial disease cannot be ignored.[32] It is possible that both factors play a role.

In some diabetics, psychological causes may be playing a major role. The debilitation and disability of diabetic neuropathy can understandably lead to severe depression. Psychologic factors should be suspected if the patient goes through alternating periods of successful sexual activity and impotence. With the use of sleep-tumescent studies, one can determine whether spontaneous nocturnal erections occur.[33] If there is spontaneous nocturnal activity, psychological and/or urologic counseling may be very helpful in reversing the patient's impotence.

If the impotence is organic, it is incurable. The only treatment available is a prosthetic device.[33] Removable prostheses are of value in some cases, but often do not result in satisfactory stimulation of the female partner. There have been marked improvements in recent years in penile implantation procedures. Good results have been reported with the use of an inflatable implant. The majority of patients with such an implant can ejaculate and report orgasm for themselves and their spouses. In one study, 33 of 36 patients with diabetic impotence reported orgasms, and 32 could ejaculate after the implantation procedure.[33] Thirty-four patients and 28 wives were happy with the results.

Some diabetologists have noted an increased incidence of sexual problems in their female patients.[34] It is possible but unproven that failure of these patients to reach orgasm may be a manifestation of diabetic neuropathy.

Gastrointestinal System

Involvement of the gastrointestinal tract occurs at many levels. Abnormal esophageal motility can be demonstrated in a significant proportion of patients with autonomic neuropathy, but dysphagia is rare. Patients with autonomic neuropathy must be evaluated for this symptom in the same fashion as all other individuals.

When the innervation of the stomach is involved, gastric atony and dilatation are quite common. An upper gastrointestinal series in these patients often reveals marked delays in emptying; the radiopaque material may remain in the stomach for many hours. Although this atony is ordinarily of no consequence, bedridden patients may easily aspirate. They must be fed with intermittent, small meals and kept upright for at least a few hours after each meal. Other patients suffer with the symptoms of reflux peptic esophagitis.

Vagal neuropathy plays a role in the increased incidence of achlorhydria and atrophic gastritis seen in patients with diabetes mellitus. These changes decrease the likelihood of peptic ulcer, but increase the incidence of gastric carcinoma.[35]

Impaired and disordered small bowel motility leads to the most common symptom associated with gastrointestinal neuropathy—nocturnal diarrhea.[36] This can be a very distressing symptom, responding only partially to opiates. If motility is severely involved, chronic, continuous diarrhea and even a mild malabsorption syndrome may appear. Some patients have intermittent periods of severe diarrhea that may be due to bacterial overgrowth. Treatment with broad spectrum antibiotics is often useful in terminating these episodes. Other patients with impaired motility suffer from severe constipation.

Pupil

There may be changes in pupillary function secondary to involvement of the parasympathetic fibers of the oculomotor nerve. With the use of a pupillograph, it has been shown that the pupils of patients with severe diabetic neuropathy tend to have a delayed response to a standard light stimulus.[37] The Argyll-Robertson pupil, characteristic of tertiary lues, also occurs in patients with diabetic neuropathy. These changes have no clinical significance.

DIABETIC MONONEURITIS

A relatively unusual lesion in diabetes mellitus is dysfunction of a discrete peripheral nerve. Instead of "stocking-glove" sensory loss, there is loss of function of specific structures. This kind of neuropathy is not etiologically related to polyneuropathy. There is strong histologic evidence to implicate microvascular disease in the pathogenesis of mononeuropathy. Necrosis of the axon with retrograde degeneration can be seen in microscopic sections of an involved nerve, and subintimal thickening of the walls of vasa nervora and capillaries is apparent. The entire histology is compatible with ischemic necrosis of the nerve.[38]

The clinical course of this neuropathy is consistent with an acute vascular accident. Symptoms usually appear quite suddenly, followed by gradual improvement. Prognosis is excellent as total recovery is the rule, usually within three to six months. The oculomotor nerve is most commonly involved followed by the abducens. Rarely, mononeuropathy occurs outside of the cranial area and involves a sensory nerve such as the lateral cutaneous nerve of the thigh.

With third-nerve involvement, medial, upward, and downward gaze is impaired, and severe diplopia occurs. However, the pupillary reaction, which is impaired in autonomic neuropathy, is usually spared. An intact light reflex is helpful in differentiating diabetic mononeuritis from an intracranial mass lesion such as a posterior communicating artery aneurysm. The reason for pupillary sparing is related to the course of the oculomotor nerve through the cavernous sinus. The fibers innervating the pupil are located in the periphery of the nerve bundle and manage to obtain adequate oxygen supplies from venous blood flowing through the cavernous sinus.

OTHER NEUROLOGIC SYNDROMES

A variety of other neurologic lesions are seen in patients with diabetes mellitus. Carpal tunnel syndrome, although not a specific lesion, occurs more commonly in diabetic than nondiabetic individuals. One must always rule out infiltrative disease such as sarcoidosis, myxedema, and amyloidosis before assuming that it is related to diabetes mellitus. The syndrome is that of distal median nerve neuropathy. Clinical signs include sensory loss in the lateral one and one-half fingers, lateral interosseous weakness and atrophy, difficulty with opposing movements of the thumb, and atrophy of the thenar eminence. It can also cause a great deal of pain in the involved fingers. The diagnosis is confirmed by finding decreased median nerve conduction velocity with normal ulnar conduction—the converse of findings with thoracic outlet syndrome and cervical spine disease. Occasionally, injection of steroids into the carpal tunnel is helpful in ameliorating symptoms, but significant neurologic deficits usually require surgical release of the median nerve from compressing connective tissue bands. Rarely, patients with diabetic polyneuropathy have an extensor plantar response, suggesting myelopathy. These same patients usually have decreased deep tendon reflexes, creating a combination of findings seen in very few other conditions. The main disorder to consider in differential diagnosis is subacute combined degeneration of the spinal cord secondary to vitamin B_{12} deficiency.

Diabetic amyotrophy is a rare disorder involving the pelvic musculature.[39] Occurring mostly in older men, this syndrome consists of severe and rapid atrophy of pelvic and proximal thigh muscles associated with leg pain. Since weight loss is often prominent, amyotrophy is easily confused with polymyositis secondary to a malignancy. Cerebrospinal fluid protein levels are usually very high. Muscle biopsies show atrophy, and some patients have regained muscle strength after many months.

SUMMARY

Diabetic neuropathy encompasses a wide spectrum of lesions. In its most common form, it leads to insidious sensory deprivation of the feet and lower extremities, and can become disabling. It aggravates the problems imposed by arterial insufficiency. Autonomic neuropathy can cause a wide variety of confusing and seemingly unrelated syndromes.

REFERENCES

1. Waxman SG. Pathophysiology of nerve conduction: Relation to diabetic neuropathy. *Ann Intern Med* 92:297, 1980.
2. Steiness I. Vibratory perception in diabetes. *Acta Med Scand* 158:327, 1957.
3. Friedman SA, Simmons EM. Diabetic peripheral neuropathy: Clinical manifestations. *Geriatrics* 22:141, 1967.
4. Collens WS, Zilensky JD, Boas LC. Impaired vibratory sense in diabetes. *Am J Med* 1:638, 1946.
5. Shagan BP. Is diabetes a model for aging? *Med Clin North Am* 60:1209, 1976.
6. Friedman SA, Schulman RH, Weiss S. Hearing and diabetic neuropathy. *Arch Intern Med* 135:573, 1975.
7. Hamlin CR, Kohn RR, Luschin JH. Apparent accelerated aging of human collagen in diabetes mellitus. *Diabetes* 24:902, 1975.
8. Andres R. Aging and diabetes. *Med Clin North Am* 55:835, 1971.
9. Norris AH, Shock NW, Wagman FH. Age changes in the maximum conduction velocity of motor fibers of human ulnar nerves. *J Appl Physiol* 5:589, 1953.
10. Fagerberg SE. Studies on the pathogenesis of diabetic neuropathy. *Acta Med Scand* 154:145, 1956.
11. Sharma AK, Thomas PK. Peripheral nerve structure and function in experimental diabetes. *J Neurol Sci* 23:1, 1974.
12. Gregersen G. Diabetic neuropathy: Influence of age, sex, metabolic control, and duration of diabetes on motor conduction velocity. *Neurology* 17:972, 1967.
13. Graf RJ, Halter JB, Halar E, et al. Nerve conduction abnormalities in untreated maturity-onset diabetes: Relationship to levels of fasting plasma glucose and glycosylated hemoglobin. *Ann Intern Med* 90:298, 1979.
14. Stewart MA, Sherman WR, Kurien MM, et al. Polyol accumulations in nervous tissue of rats with experimental diabetes and galactosemia. *J Neurochem* 14:1057, 1967.
15. Winegrad AI, Greene DA. Diabetic polyneuropathy: The importance of insulin deficiency, hyperglycemia and alterations in myoinositol metabolism in its pathogenesis. *N Eng J Med* 295:1416, 1976.
16. Mirsky IA, Futterman P, Brohkahn RH. The quantitative measurement of vibratory perception in subjects with and without diabetes mellitus. *J Lab Clin Med* 41:221, 1953.
17. Bauman JH, Girling JP, Brand PW. Plantar pressures and trophic ulceration: An evaluation of foot wear. *J Bone Joint Surg* (Am) 45:652, 1963.
18. Friedman SA, Rakow RB. Osseous lesions of the foot in diabetic neuropathy. *Diabetes* 20:302, 1971.
19. Sinha S, Choodappa MD, Munichoodappa S, et al. Neuro-arthropathy (Charcot joints) in diabetes mellitus (clinical study of 101 cases). *Medicine* 51:191, 1972.

20. Shagan BP, Friedman SA, Allesandri R. Diabetic osteopathy: Report of a relentlessly progressive case, with clinico-pathologic correlations. *J Am Geriatr Soc* 21:561, 1973.

21. Friedman SA, Rakow RB. Methods to avoid pressure on foot ulcers. *Arch Phys Med Rehabil* 51:304, 1970.

22. Collens WS. Conservative management of gangrene in the diabetic patient. *JAMA* 181:692, 1962.

23. Watkins PJ, MacKay JD. Cardiac denervation in diabetic neuropathy. *Ann Intern Med* 92 (Part 2):304, 1980.

24. Friedman SA, Freidberg P, Colton J. Vasomotor tone in diabetic neuropathy. *Ann Intern Med* 77:353, 1972.

25. Christlieb AR. Renin-angiotensin-aldosterone system in diabetes mellitus. *Diabetes* 25:820, 1976.

26. Faerman I, Faccio E, Miller J, et al. Autonomic neuropathy and painless myocardial infarction in diabetic patients: Histologic evidence of their relationship. *Diabetes* 26:1147, 1977.

27. Ewing PJ, Campbell IW, Clarke BF. Assessment of cardiovascular effects in diabetic autonomic neuropathy and prognostic implications. *Ann Intern Med* 92 (Part 2):308, 1980.

28. Ellenberg M. Development of urinary bladder dysfunction in diabetes mellitus. *Ann Intern Med* 92 (Part 2):321, 1980.

29. Frimedt-Moller C, Mortensen S. Treatment of diabetic cystopathy. *Ann Intern Med* 92 (Part 2):327, 1980.

30. Ellenberg M. Sexual function in diabetic patients. *Ann Intern Med* 92 (Part 2):331, 1980.

31. DeGroat WC, Boeth AM. Physiology of male sexual function. *Ann Intern Med* 92 (Part 2):329, 1980.

32. Karacan I. Diagnosis of erectile impotence in diabetes mellitus. *Ann Intern Med* 92 (Part 2):334, 1980.

33. Scott FB, Fishman IJ, Light JK. An inflatable penile prosthesis for treatment of diabetic impotence. *Ann Intern Med* 92 (Part 2):340, 1980.

34. Sacerdote A, Bleicher SJ. Sexual dysfunction in diabetes mellitus. (Letter to Editor) *Ann Intern Med* 93:147, 1980.

35. Dotevall C. Incidence of peptic ulcer in diabetes mellitus. *Acta Med Scand* 164:463, 1959.

36. Colby AO. Neurologic disorders of diabetes mellitus. *Diabetes* 14:424, 1965.

37. Friedman SA, Feinberg R, Podolak E, et al. Pupillary abnormalities in diabetic neuropathy, *Ann Intern Med* 67:977, 1967.

38. Dreyfus PM, Hakim S, Adams RD. Diabetic ophthalmoplegia. *Arch Neurol Psychiatr* 77:337, 1957.

39. Diabetic amyotrophy (Annotation). *Lancet* 2:287, 1963.

14 Vasculitis: An Overview

Harry Bienenstock

Since the original description of periarteritis nodosa by Kussmaul and Maier[1] in 1966, the concept of vasculitis has undergone significant changes as to etiology, pathogenesis, and treatment. In most reviews of vasculitis, the classification of Zeek[2] in 1952 is cited as a major contribution in organizing a potpourri of entities into reasonably distinct groupings. More recently, Christian, Gilliam, and Fauci[3,4] have employed clinical and morphological classifications to describe syndromes in which vasculitis is a prominent feature.

A particularly lucid description of the clinical approach to systemic vasculitis by Fan et al[6] summarizes much of the clinical information relating to vasculitis. They derive diagnostic, therapeutic and prognostic information from the major sites of vascular inflammation and the size of the vessels involved.

This chapter will focus on unique clinical, morphological, and laboratory features of syndromes associated with vasculitis and describe generally accepted approaches to the treatment of this disparate group of conditions.

Zeek's original classification of necrotizing angiitis has served as a framework to which others have added in light of the evolution in our understanding of the spectrum of vasculitis. She divided necrotizing angiitis into five categories:

1) Hypersensitivity angiitis, an acute systemic illness involving the arterioles, venules, capillaries and small arteries of the skin, heart, lungs, and kidneys.
2) Allergic granulomatous angiitis, an illness of several months' to years' duration involving arteries of variable size, often associated with asthma and other allergic states.
3) Rheumatic arteritis, affects small arteries and veins of the heart, lungs, and other organs in fulminating rheumatic fever.
4) Periarteritis nodosa, a necrotizing arteritis of small and medium sized muscular-type arteries near hila of viscera, in striated muscles and near peripheral nerves. The vascular lesions are of various ages and often involve vascular bifurcations.
5) Temporal arteritis, a disease of temporal and other cranial arteries, in which the vascular lesions are characterized by the presence of multinucleated giant cells.

In the ensuing years, this classification has been expanded upon and refined. Christian[3] classified vasculitis into two main categories: those conditions characterized by necrotizing vasculitis, and those in which necrotizing vasculitis is occasionally noted. Gilliam and Smiley[4] modified Zeek's criteria to include allergic granulomatosis of Churg and Strauss[7] and Wegener's granulomatosis. They relate each clinical syndrome to the size and anatomical distribution of involved vessels. Hence, it is noted that leukocytoclastic angiitis is principally a dermal vasculitis while giant cell arteritis never involves the skin or subcutaneous tissue.

It will become apparent that there is considerable overlap of many of the clinical and anatomical features of each of the subcategories of disease. Nevertheless, the classification serves as a useful tool in understanding the spectrum of vasculitis.

In this chapter, a modification of Gilliam and Smiley's model has been utilized to classify necrotizing vasculitis (Table 14-1).

HYPERSENSITIVITY VASCULITIS (Leukocytoclastic Angiitis)

Leukocytoclastic angiitis describes a vasculitis that most frequently affects small vessels, especially the postcapillary venules of

Table 14-1
Classification of Necrotizing Vasculitis

Hypersensitivity vasculitis (leukocytoclastic angiitis)
- a. Henoch-Schönlein purpura
- b. Chronic urticaria (hypocomplementic vasculitis)
- c. Essential mixed cryoglobulinemia
- d. Vasculitis associated with other primary diseases:
    - Rheumatic diseases
    - Malignancy
    - Infection

Wegener's granulomatosis

Allergic granulomatosis (Churg-Strauss angiitis)

Polyarteritis Nodosa
- a. Classic type
- b. Associated with hepatitis B antigen
- c. Drug associated
- d. In serous otitis media

Giant cell arteritis
- a. Temporal arteritis
- b. Takayasu's arteritis

the epidermis.[4,6,8] On histologic examination, vascular endothelial and muscle cells are often destroyed and the nuclei of polymorphonuclear leukocytes are left bare and surrounded by "nuclear dust." IgM, IgG and complement components may be seen in, and adjacent to, vessel walls by immunofluorescent staining methods.[9,10] Although leukocytoclastic angiitis is characteristically associated with the dermal manifestations of vasculitis, it may be present in a variety of conditions in which visceral involvement is the result of inflammation of larger vessels.

Leukocytoclastic angiitis has been reported in association with a variety of conditions[6] including infections,[11] liver diseases,[12] and malignancy.[13,14]

Henoch-Schönlein Purpura

Henoch-Schönlein purpura is a generalized leukocytoclastic angiitis that most often presents with fever, purpura, arthritis and abdominal pain.[15,16] It occurs most frequently in children between the ages of four and eight years,[17] and is preceded by an upper respiratory infection in up to 90% of cases. Palpable purpura, the characteristic lesion of this condition, usually involves the skin of the lower extremities (Figure 14-1). This rash may also appear as an urticarial eruption, hemorrhagic bullae, or superficial ulcers. Intermittent, colicky abdominal pain is the most common gastrointestinal symptom. Others may present with intussusception,[18] hemorrhage, intestinal perforation, or protein-losing enteropathy. Perforation of the bowel is a rare complication. The arthritis is transient, nondeforming, and usually affects the knees and ankles. Renal disease occurs in about 40% of the patients.[15] Most patients have a mild self-limited form of renal disease, characterized by hematuria and proteinuria. The renal lesion on light microscopy shows focal glomerulonephritis. A small percentage of patients develop a rapidly progressive glomerulonephritis with hematuria, proteinuria, hypertension, and oliguria, which may lead to chronic renal failure.[19]

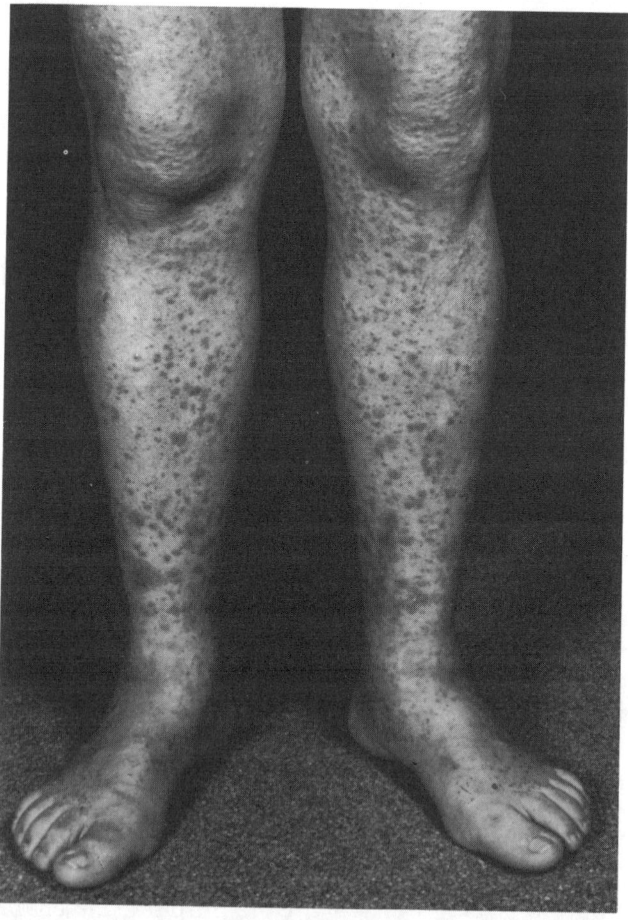

Figure 14-1 Purpuric lesions in the lower extremities in Henoch-Schönlein purpura.

The disease primarily affects small arterioles and capillaries. Deposits of IgA may be present in dermal vessels and in the glomerular mesangium alone or in association with IgG, IgM, and complement.[20] It has been postulated that IgA deposits in vessels may be related to the respiratory infections that often precede this condition.[4] Symptoms usually abate within one month. There is a tendency for the presenting symptoms to recur, often at six- to eight-week intervals.

Treatment with steroids may ameliorate gastrointestinal symptoms but has little effect on other manifestations.[6] In patients with renal failure, treatment with steroids should be individualized depending on the clinical course and findings on renal biopsy.

Chronic Urticaria (Hypocomplementemic Vasculitis)

Chronic urticaria, originally described by McDuffie in 1973,[21] is a form of cutaneous vasculitis characterized by fever, arthritis, abdominal pain, and recurring episodes of erythematous urticarial skin lesions associated with marked hypocomplementemia.[32,23] Skin biopsy specimens show the presence of a leukocytoclastic angiitis. Congenital deficiencies of C1Q and C2 and activation of the alternate complement pathway have been reported.[23] The clinical course is usually prolonged.

Essential Mixed Cryoglobulinemia

Essential mixed cryoglobulinemia, a syndrome characterized by purpura, arthralgia, anemia, hyperglobulinemia, and glomerulonephritis,[24-26] is yet another condition in which the underlying lesion is predominantly a leukocytoclastic vasculitis. Prior to 1958, over half the reported cases of cryoglobulinemia were in patients with myeloma or lymphatic leukemia.[27] In 1962, LoSpalluto and co-workers[24] described a patient with renal tubular acidosis and a cryoglobulin composed of IgG and IgM with rheumatoid factor activity. In 1966, Meltzer and Franklin[25,26] reported the presence of mixed cryoglobulins in which rheumatoid activity was present in the IgM fraction. Patients with the syndrome may have severe renal disease, usually proliferative glomerulonephritis.

In a study (1960–1978) of forty patients with the systemic complex of arthralgia, purpura, and renal disease, the average age of onset of disease was 50.7 years with a range of 21 to 72. There was no sex or racial preference.

Palpable purpura is seen in almost all patients and is a frequent presenting feature. Purpuric lesions appear more frequently in the winter, are characteristically nonpruritic and more frequently involve the lower extremities and lower trunk. Symptom-free periods vary from days to months, when periodic showers of petechiae again may appear. The histologic appearance of the skin is consistent with a leukocytoclastic angiitis.

Raynaud's phenomenon and arthralgias in the absence of arthritis may be present in the early stages of this condition. Significant renal disease is present in over 50% of patients and is characterized clinically by diastolic hypertension, edema and/or renal failure. Red blood cells in the urine, pyuria, and red blood cell casts may be early signs of renal disease. Azotemia is generally a later manifestation of renal involvement. A significantly elevated diastolic blood pressure and renal failure are associated with a poor prognosis. On microscopic examination of kidney tissue, immune reactants are seen along glomerular basement membrane and in vessel walls. Most of the mixed cryoglobulins contain IgG and IgM. The IgM fraction invariably exhibits rheumatoid factor activity.

Liver involvement has been frequently described in this condition. Hepatomegaly, splenomegaly, and abnormal liver function tests have been reported in as high as 70% of patients.[27] Biopsy specimens show a range of findings from normal architecture to chronic active hepatitis and frank cirrhosis. The presence of hepatitis B surface antigen has been described in a small number of patients.

Anemia is found in approximately one third of patients with mixed cryoglobulinemia. Leukopenia is uncommon but may be noted when patients are being treated with cytotoxic drugs. The cryoglobulin concentration has been reported as high as 400 mg%.[6] The sedimentation rate is elevated and the latex fixation test for rheumatoid factor is positive in almost all patients with the disease. A striking depression of C4 levels in the serum has been reported.[27]

Vasculitis Associated with Rheumatic Diseases

Necrotizing arteritis may occur in the course of a variety of rheumatic diseases,[4,6,28] including rheumatoid arthritis,[29,30] systemic lupus erythematosus,[31] scleroderma, mixed connective tissue disease, and childhood dermatomyositis. Signs of vasculitis may range from a mild, superficial, dermal vasculitis involving arterioles and venules to necrotizing vasculitis of small and medium sized arteries that may result in peripheral gangrene or infarction of visceral organs.

Rheumatoid arthritis The vasculitis associated with rheumatoid arthritis[30] characteristically involves medium and small sized vessels and is seen more frequently in patients with seropositive disease.

The clinical expression of superficial dermal vasculitis in rheumatoid arthritis includes livido reticularis (Figure 14-2) and infarctions of the nailbed.[6] When the deeper layers of the skin and larger vessels are involved, chronic leg ulcers (Figure 14-3) and peripheral gangrene may occur. Neuropathy, both motor and sensory, may develop as a result of vasculitis of the vasa nervora of peripheral nerves.[30] Mesenteric arteritis with intestinal infarction has been reported.[32]

The histologic features of vasculitis in rheumatoid arthritis are often indistinguishable from polyarteritis nodosa. Commonly, there

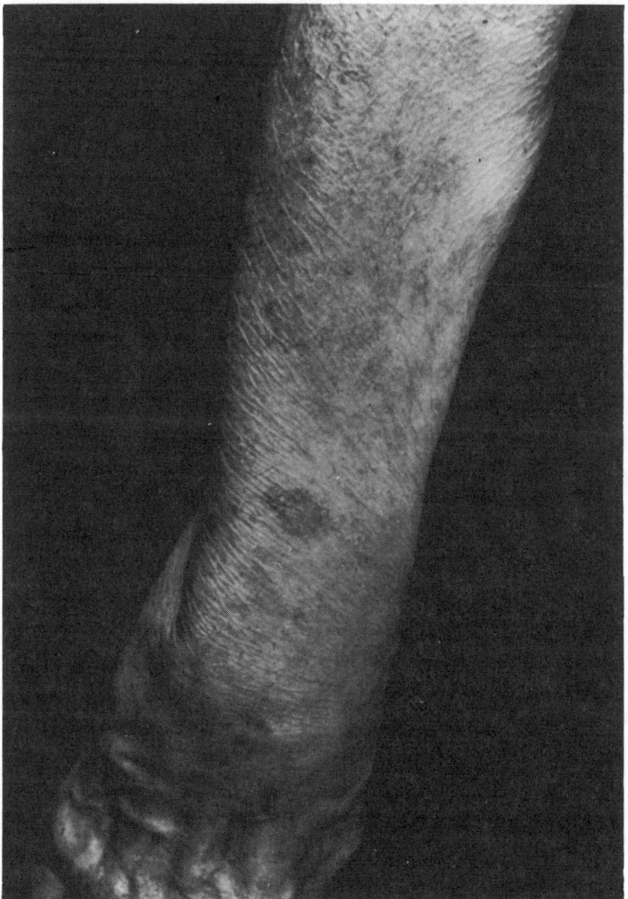

Figure 14-2 Livido reticularis in rheumatoid arthritis.

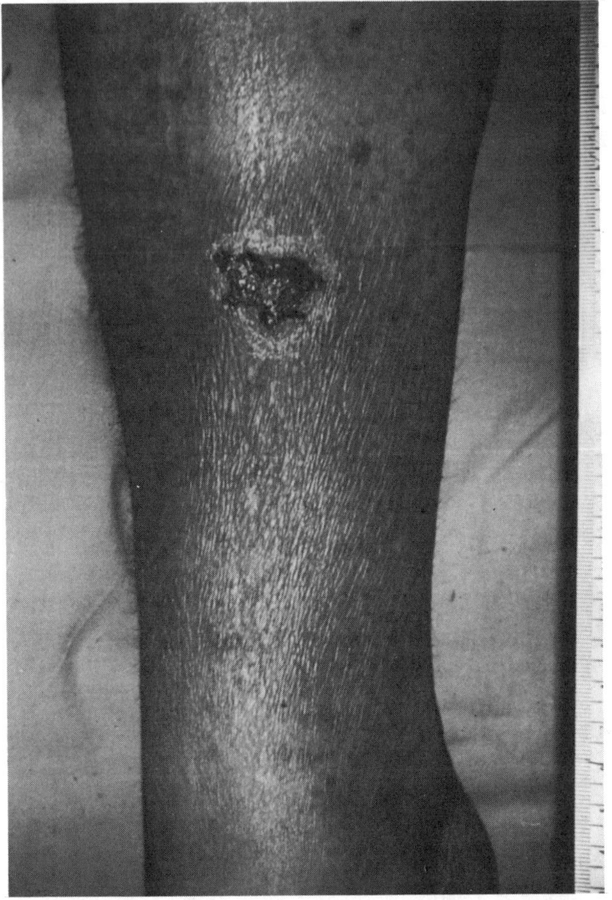

Figure 14-3 Chronic leg ulcer and skin lesions of superficial vasculitis in rheumatoid arthritis.

is necrotizing arteritis with involvement of all vessel layers and an infiltrate of lymphocytes and plasma cells. Less frequently, obliterative endarteritis is seen.

Systemic lupus erythematosus About 20% of patients with systemic lupus erythematosus develop dermal vasculitis[33] manifested clinically as livido reticularis[34] papular lesions, cutaneous infarctions, and subcutaneous nodes.[35] In addition, small and medium sized vessel disease may manifest itself as peripheral gangrene and/or ulcers, especially of the lower extremities. Patients may also present with syndromes associated with infarction of the bowel secondary to mesenteric arteritis. Other large and medium sized vessels may be involved, leading to a variety of ischemic syndromes in the central nervous system, extremities, and elsewhere.

Vascular involvement in lupus erythematosus is characterized histologically by fibrinoid deposits in the vessel walls. Immunofluorescent studies of dermal skin may show IgG, IgM and complement deposits within the vessel walls. In systemic lupus erythematosus, these vessel wall changes may be present in areas of uninvolved skin. Deposition of immunoglobulins and complement components also may be seen at the dermal epidermal junction.

Treatment of Hypersensitivity Vasculitis

The treatment of leukocytoclastic angiitis varies with the underlying disease and with the clinical expression of the vascular lesion. Patients who present with livido reticularis, superficial ulcers of the skin, or maculopapular lesions require no specific treatment for vasculitis, and therapy should be directed to the underlying disease.

The course of Henoch-Schönlein purpura is usually benign and patients may be treated with salicylates and, on rare occasions, with small doses of corticosteroids.

The lesions in chronic urticaria with hypocomplementemia may respond to the use of moderate to high doses of corticosteroids for short periods of time. No satisfactory treatment regimen has been reported, however, for the recurrent eruptions seen in this condition.

Therapy for mixed cryoglobulinemia will vary with the extent of visceral disease, especially when renal involvement is present. The efficacy of drugs such as corticosteroids and immunosuppressive agents is unclear. Plasmapheresis and penicillamine both have been used in the treatment of this condition without significant clinical improvement or change in the cryocrit.[27] High dosages of corticosteroids alone or in combination with immunosuppressive drugs have been used in the treatment of patients with renal disease with varying results. Reports of prolonged survival in some instances without using steroids or immunosuppressive agents have raised questions concerning the efficacy of current methods of treatment.

Treatment of superficial dermal vasculitis in patients with rheumatic diseases should be directed to the underlying disease. When larger vessels that supply the visceral organs and extremities are involved, treatment with moderate to high doses of corticosteroids and/or cytotoxic agents, ie, azothiaprine or cyclophosphamide, should be considered.[6,30]

WEGENER'S GRANULOMATOSIS

Wegener[36] initially described a condition characterized by necrotizing granulomata and vasculitis of the upper and lower respiratory tracts, systemic vasculitis, and focal glomerulonephritis. In 1966, Carrington and Liebow[37] proposed a concept of limited Wegener's granulomatosis in which the lung was involved in the absence of renal disease. This group of diseases is probably best viewed as a part of a spectrum of conditions in which there is a necrotizing granulomatous vasculitis of small arteries and veins. In the milder forms of the disease, the upper airway and/or ear, nose, and throat are involved. Progressive, unremitting vasculitis involving the upper and lower airways, lung, and kidney is seen in severely affected individuals. The condition is most commonly encountered in middle-aged men. Patients present with fever, weight loss, upper respiratory tract infections, and inflammation of the nasal mucosa, which may lead to septal perforation. Nasal granulomata with mucosal ulceration and saddle nose deformity are not unusual.[38] Secondary infection, most commonly with *Staphylococcus aureus,* is a common complication.

Ophthalmic disease is common[5,39] and may manifest as keratoconjunctivitis, granulomatous sclerouveitis and scleromalacia perforans, and lacrimal duct obstruction. Otitis media with secondary bacterial infection is seen in about 35% of cases. Involvement of the middle ear may lead to varying degrees of hearing loss and labyrinthitis with vertigo.

The lung is the organ most commonly involved histologically. Occasionally, patients may present with bronchitis and pneumonia. In most instances, however, there are no pulmonary symptoms initially. Invariably, secondary infection takes place with development of fever and purulent sputum. X-rays may show solitary or multiple unilateral or bilateral nodules, which often cavitate.[40]

The initial clinical findings in patients with renal involvement may be few. In time, an abnormal urinary sediment with proteinuria and red cell casts, followed by progressive azotemia, is seen. Other organ system involvement includes the heart, where coronary vasculitis and pericarditis may occur, and the nervous system by direct extension from the sinuses into the brain and meninges by granulomatous lesions, or by the development of mononeuritis multiplex or cranial neuritis. In 40% to 50% of patients, a dermal vasculitis may occur. About half of the patients complain of polyarthralgia but true arthritis is not a common feature.

There are no specific laboratory findings. Patients often present with a mild anemia and leukocytosis and elevation of the sedimentation rate. Serum complement levels are usually normal or slightly increased.

The diagnosis is arrived at by biopsy of the nasopharynx, lung, or kidney. The characteristic histologic findings are those of a necrotizing vasculitis with adjacent necrotizing granulomatous involvement of the small arteries and veins. The cellular infiltrate tends to be predominantly mononuclear, and eosinophilia is not a feature of this disease.[6]

On renal biopsy, necrotizing glomerulonephritis is seen (Figure 14-4). Subendothelial deposits of electron dense material and immune reactants such as IgG and complement have been described.[41] It is uncertain whether immune complexes play a role in the pathogenesis of Wegener's granulomatosis.

Variants of Wegener's granulomatosis include: limited Wegener's granulomatosis,[38] lymphomatoid granulomatosis,[42] and lethal midline granuloma.[43] Limited Wegener's granulomatosis involves only the lung or the upper midline respiratory tract. Lethal midline granuloma also involves the upper respiratory tract but tends to be more severe than the classic disease. It usually does not affect the lungs or kidney, and differs from Wegener's granulomatosis in that there is no evidence of necrotizing vasculitis.

Lymphomatoid granulomatosis is characterized by an angiotrophic and angiodestructive infiltration of the lungs by lymphocytoid and plasmacytoid cells.[42] These cells are polymorphic in nature and are made up of normal-appearing lymphoid cells and atypical lymphocytoid

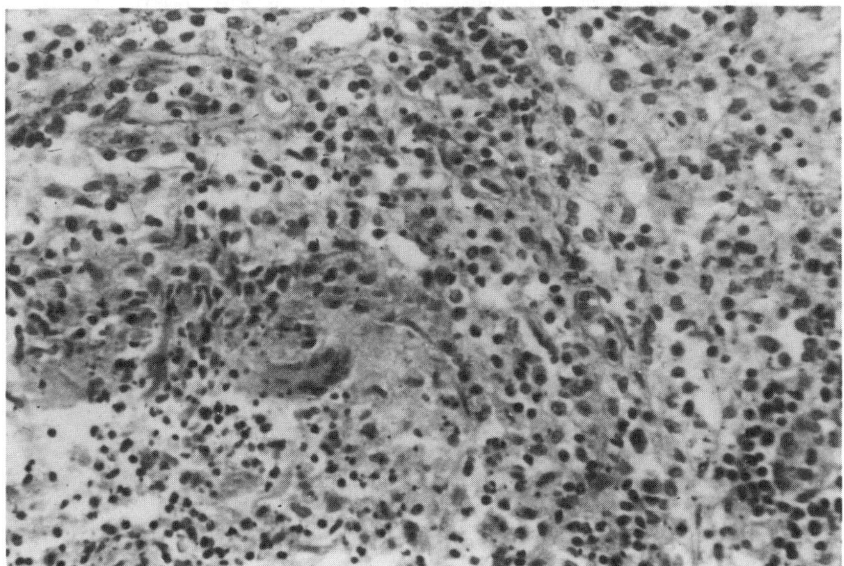

Figure 14-4 Granuloma with giant cells in the interstitium of the kidney in Wegener's granulomatosis.

and plasmacytoid cells with varying numbers of mitotic figures. The histologic appearance is that of a lymphoproliferative disease. Granulomas are less numerous than in Wegener's granulomatosis. The disease does not involve the upper respiratory tract or sinuses. In the lung, however, multiple nodules of varying sizes that tend to cavitate are seen. The disease may also affect the skin, kidney, and central nervous system. Unlike Wegener's granulomatosis, leukopenia may be a feature of the disease, and the sedimentation rate may be normal in some patients during the active phase of the disease. If untreated, the disease usually progresses rapidly, often with pulmonary or central nervous system disease complications.

Treatment

There has been a significant improvement in the mortality rates for all forms of granulomatous angiitis in the past decade. Until recently, Wegener's granulomatosis and lymphomatoid granulomatosis as well as their variants frequently pursued a progressive downhill course. Corticosteroids would often ameliorate the disease for varying periods of time. The mean one-year survival for untreated Wegener's granulomatosis has been reported to be 18% with only 10% survival at two years.[44] The use of corticosteroids improves mean survival rates to 12½ months but does not significantly alter the long term prognosis. With the advent of therapy combining corticosteroids with cytotoxic drugs, there has been a significant improvement in survival statistics. Dramatic long-term improvement has been achieved with cyclophosphamide alone or, in more severe cases, with cyclophosphamide combined with high dosage corticosteroid therapy.[45]

In Wegener's granulomatosis, the treatment of choice is cyclophosphamide orally or intravenously in a dose of 4 mg/kg per day for three days followed by 1 to 2 mg/kg per day as a single morning dose and thereafter in combination with prednisone 60 mg/day in divided doses for the first two to three weeks, with subsequent reduction of corticosteroid dosage depending upon the clinical response. Careful attention should be paid to the complete blood counts and the urinalyses in monitoring cyclophosphamide treatment. Peripheral blood counts, urinalysis, and periodic chest x-rays and sinus films are useful tools to follow disease activity. Treatment with cyclophosphamide should continue for at least a year after the disease has become completely controlled as judged by clinical and laboratory parameters.[6] At that time gradual reduction of dosage may be undertaken, with careful evaluation for signs of recurrent disease activity.

ALLERGIC GRANULOMATOUS ANGIITIS

In 1951, Churg and Strauss[7] described allergic granulomatous angiitis, a condition often associated with asthma and other allergic diseases. The arterial lesions are similar to those seen in polyarteritis nodosa except for the presence of a large number of eosinophils in the acute lesions and vascular and extravascular granulomas. Patients with this condition often have an allergic background. The paranasal sinuses are infected in a majority of patients, and in almost all instances there is lung involvement. On roentgen examination, pulmonary disease is expressed by the presence of fleeting, patchy infiltrates that come and go. Renal disease is less common than in polyarteritis nodosa. Genitourinary involvement has been reported in about 10% of patients.[46]

The pathologic findings in allergic granulomatosis consist of necrotizing vasculitis and perivascular eosinophilic nodules adjacent to both veins and arteries.[6,46] The blood count often shows a leukocytosis, occasionally with marked eosinophilia as high as 80% to 90%. The sedimentation rate is invariably elevated. The diagnosis is most frequently established by obtaining a peripheral skin and muscle biopsy or, if necessary, an open lung biopsy.

In patients with allergic granulomatosis (Churg-Strauss vasculitis) treatment should begin with prednisone in a dose of 60 mg/day in divided doses. In the absence of significant improvement or in patients with life-threatening disease, cyclophosphamide should also be administered. The dose should be 1 to 2 mg/kg/body weight/day with adjustments of the dosage based on the leukocyte count. The latter should be maintained above 3000/ml^3 with a total neutrophil count of 1000 to 5000 ml.[5] Azothiaprine also has been successful in the treatment of allergic granulomatosis.[6] It is given in a dose of 1.5 to 3 mg/day and may be employed in less severely involved patients.

POLYARTERITIS NODOSA

Polyarteritis nodosa is a disease of unknown etiology, which is characterized by segmental necrotizing vasculitis of small and medium sized muscular arteries (Figure 14-5).[1,2] The lesions show a predeliction for the bifurcations of arteries and spread distally to involve arterioles and, occasionally circumferentially, adjacent veins. The disease is more common in men and may occur at any age although it usually appears in the third to the sixth decade. Clinically there is an insidious onset of fever, malaise, anorexia, weakness, and weight loss. Ar-

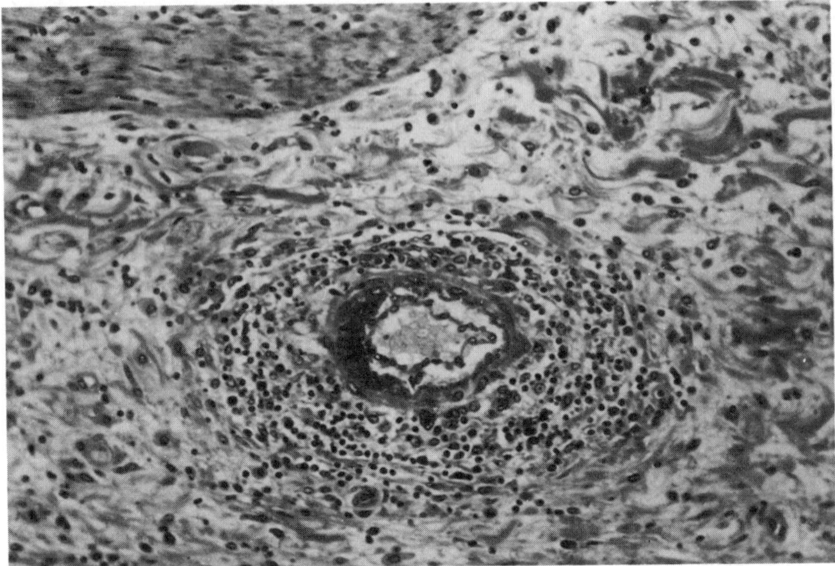

Figure 14-5 Medium sized artery showing cellular infiltrate and fibrinoid necrosis in polyarteritis nodosa.

thralgias and myalgias, hypertension, and peripheral neuropathy are commonly reported features of this disease. Less frequently, patients have some form of cutaneous involvement, which may include subcutaneous nodules along the course of superficial arteries, subcutaneous hemorrhages resulting from bleeding aneurysms, and occasionally gangrene (Figure 14-6). Infarction of viscera, subclinical liver disease secondary to chronic active hepatitis in patients with hepatitis B antigenemia, clinically apparent liver disease related to vasculitis, and involvement of the genitourinary tract are other features of classical polyarteritis nodosa.[5] The lung and spleen are usually uninvolved.

Renal disease is present in the majority of patients with polyarteritis nodosa. This is primarily a vasculitis affecting the arcuate arterial system. Hypertension is a prominent feature with the urinary sediment often mildly abnormal at the onset. As the disease progresses, patients may develop hematuria, significant proteinuria, casts, and progressive azotemia.

Involvement of the peripheral nervous system can be both sensory and/or motor. It is caused by an arteritis of the vasa nervora. Patients may develop foot drop as a result of involvement of the peroneal nerve, or sensory abnormalities such as nocturnal paresthesias. Mononeuritis multiplex[6] may occur in polyarteritis nodosa but also has been reported in a variety of rheumatic diseases, including rheumatoid arthritis and systemic lupus erythematosus. Pericarditis and myocarditis have been reported in polyarteritis as has coronary arteritis. Clinically apparent myocardial infarction is, however, unusual. Abdominal pain as a result of vascular infarction may present as cholecystitis, while right upper quadrant tenderness may be secondary to vasculitis of the hepatic capsule, necrotizing pancreatitis, or bowel infarction secondary to mesenteric vasculitis.

Association with Hepatitis B_s Antigenemia

Hepatitis B infection may result in two distinct clinical presentations. The first, a self-limited acute form of hepatitis manifested by urticaria, polyarthritis, and hypocomplementemia, has been related etiologically to hepatitis B_s antigenemia and to anti-HB_s antibody production. A second group, also HB_s positive, pursues a more chronic course. The association of hepatitis B antigenemia and a necrotizing arteritis indistinguishable from polyarteritis nodosa has been the subject of many recent reports.[47–49] Signs and symptoms of vasculitis may precede, appear concurrently, or follow clinical hepatitis, or may be associated with only minor liver test abnormalities. The vasculitis is clinically indistinguishable from HB_s negative polyarteritis. Circulating immune complexes involving HB_s antigen may be involved in the pathogenesis of polyarteritis nodosa.

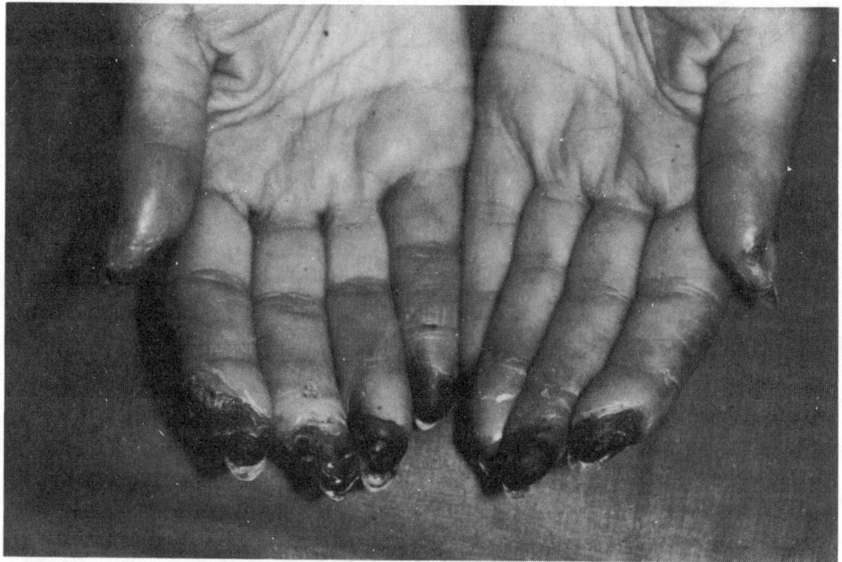

Figure 14-6 Gangrene of the tips of the fingers in polyarteritis nodosa.

Drug Associated Polyarteritis

Citron[50] and associates have reported necrotizing angiitis indistinguishable from periarteritis nodosa in six women and eight men who had used narcotic stimulants, hallucinogens, and depressants. Vascular changes of necrotizing arteritis including arterial aneurysm and sacculations were seen in the kidney, liver, pancreas, and small bowel when selective angiography was performed. No single etiological agent was established, but methamphetamine appeared to be the common denominator alone or in combination with heroin or d-lysergic acid diethylamide. HB infection was not excluded in this drug abuse group.

Polyarteritis in Association with Serious Otitis Media

Sergent and Christian[51] reported seven patients with acute serous otitis media who subsequently developed polyarteritis nodosa. They suggested that a virus may have triggered the onset of polyarteritis nodosa in these patients.

Laboratory Findings

Patients with polyarteritis nodosa frequently have a polymorphonuclear leukocytosis, elevated sedimentation rate, and a normochromic normocytic anemia. Hypocomplementemia is present in from 20% to 70% of patients, most frequently in those patients with HB_s antigenemia.[49] Peripheral eosinophilia is uncommon and its presence should suggest the possibility of allergic granulomatosis. Aneurysms at bifurcations of medium sized arteries may be demonstrated by angiography in about 80% of patients (Figures 14-7A,B).[52] In some patients in whom aneurysms are not seen, stenosis, elongation, tortuosity, or diminished number of patent arteries may be helpful findings that point to the diagnosis. Such aneurysms may be seen in other connective tissue disorders, ie, systemic lupus erythematosus, allergic granulomatosis and infection. Nerve or muscle involvement may be verified by the use of electromyography, which may locate an area from which a skin and muscle biopsy should be taken.

Treatment

The treatment of polyarteritis nodosa is similar to that described for allergic granulomatosis. Use of corticosteroids alone[53] or in combination with an immunosuppressive drug, ie, azothiaprine or cyclophosphamide, significantly increases the five year survival.[54] In a study[55] of 60 patients with polyarteritis with multi-system arteritis, 8 of 64 received only supportive therapy, 34 received corticosteroids alone, and 22 received both corticosteroids and immunosuppressive agents. Survival rates at five years were 12%, 53%, and 80% respectively ($P < 0.05$). These data suggest that overall survival was significantly increased by the addition of an immunosuppressive agent to corticosteroid therapy.

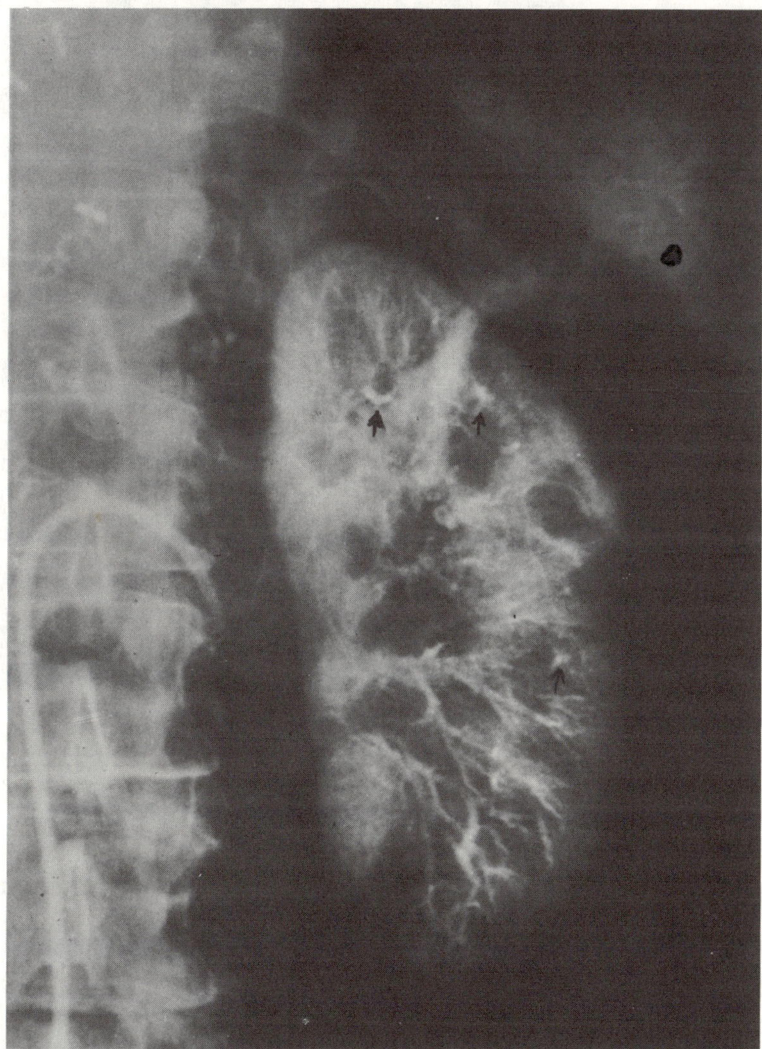

Figure 14-7A Arrows show aneurysms in small intraparenchymal vessels.

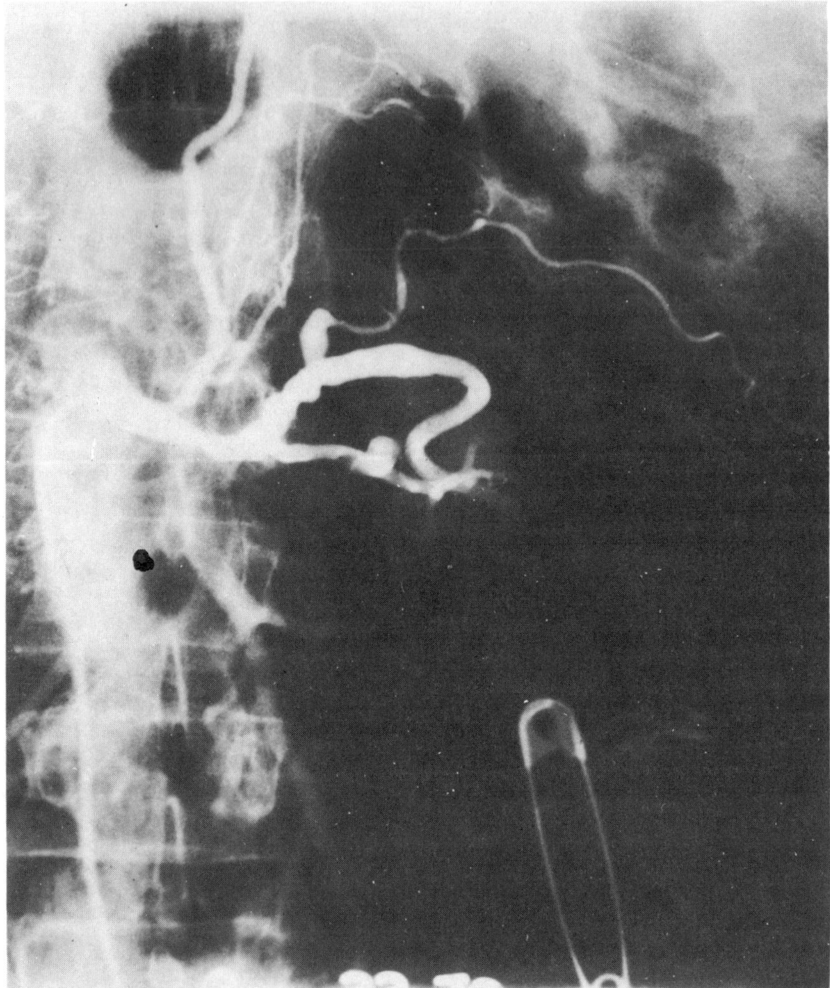

Figure 14-7B Lesions are seen in arcuate vessels.

GIANT CELL ARTERITIS

The concept of giant cell arteritis (GCA) has undergone a significant evolution since the original description in 1890 by Hutchinson.[56] In 1932 Horton et al[57] described patients who presented with headache and jaw complications. The first description of blindness in a patient with giant cell arteritis was in 1938.[58] Barker[59] recognized that mild clinical manifestations of an underlying vasculitis involving large arteries may present with a syndrome known as polymyalgia rheumatica, or with symptoms resulting from involvement of the aorta or any of its large branches. This concept has been expanded further so as to divide patients into two major groups: an elderly group of patients in whom polymyalgia rheumatica, or signs of temporal arteritis, are the major clinical presentations; and a second group, most commonly seen in younger women with constitutional symptoms and involvement of the aorta in its branches, known as Takayasu's arteritis.

The etiology of giant cell arteritis is unknown. There have been occasional reports of patients developing GCA following drug exposure.[60,61] No clearcut association between an infectious agent and this disease has ever been reported. There is no evidence of an association of HLA type with the disease. Liang et al[62] have described deposition of immunoglobulins adjacent to the internal elastic lamina in temporal arteries of 7 to 15 patients with giant cell arteritis, and suggested that these deposits might be antibodies to antigens in the arterial wall or that they may result from a passive deposition of immune complexes on the arterial wall.

Temporal Arteritis

The most extensive epidemiologic study of temporal arteritis was carried out by Huston[63] and associates who surveyed the population of Olmstead County, Minnesota. They identified 42 patients with temporal arteritis during a 25-year period. The average annual incidence per 100,000 population aged 50 or older was noted to rise from 5.1 in 1950–1959 to 17.4 in 1970–1974. A prevalence of 133 per 100,000 population over the age of 50 was found. The increased prevalence of temporal arteritis in the latter years of the study probably was the result of greater general recognition of the disease. The authors found that temporal arteritis had no significant effect on survival. Ostberg found temporal arteritis in 1.7% of 889 postmortem cases in which sections of temporal arteries and aorta were performed. Temporal arteritis is a disease of the elderly with the age of onset ranging from the mid-forties to ninety. In Hamilton's[64] series, 12% of patients were less than 60 years old. Patients under the age of 50 have been the subject of occasional reports.

Clinical findings The clinical manifestations of temporal arteritis include: the insidious onset of mild aches and pains, and the development of a complex of ophthalmologic and neurologic symptoms as a result of occlusions of large vessels.

Polymyalgia rheumatica (PMR) is a complex of symptoms characterized by morning stiffness, aching in the neck and shoulder and pelvic girdle, and accompanied by constitutional symptoms, ie, malaise, fever, and weight loss. The sedimentation rate is invariably elevated above 50 mm/hr (Westergren). There is little or no evidence of muscle atrophy or true muscle weakness. Polymyalgia is present in from 41% to 62% of patients with giant cell arteritis.[65] Conversely, aproximately 15% to 78% of patients with clinical constellations of symptoms consistent with polymyalgia rheumatica were found to have giant cell arteritis.

Patients with polymyalgia respond dramatically to small to moderate doses of prednisone over a short period of time. Symptoms of PMR may precede, accompany, or follow symptoms or signs of vasculitis. The diagnosis may be easily overlooked for long periods of time because of the vague nature of the clinical complaints. Elderly patients may describe aching and fatigue, a mild flu-like illness, and low grade fever, in the absence of objective clinical signs. Often these patients are labelled as malingerers or "crocks" and are sent to a variety of subspeciality clinics for evaluation or, at times, are labelled as having depression and referred for psychiatric help. Visual symptoms and headache are uncommon in the absence of vasculitis. Two thirds of patients experience some morning stiffness or paresthesias. Joint pain is a common symptom but frank arthritis is rare. Joint scintograms were found to be abnormal in 24 of 25 patients with polymyalgia rheumatica.[66] Abnormal uptake in the joints of patients with polymyalgia rheumatica did not differ from that of biopsy-proven giant cell arteritis. PMR is more common in women and has rarely been reported in blacks. No generic predisposition to this disease has been defined.

Headache, a frequent early manifestation of temporal arteritis, has been reported in from 36% to 100% of patients with temporal arteritis. The headache is usually located over the distribution of the temporal arteries. Scalp tenderness with paroxysms of discomfort initiated by brushing of the hair or resting the head on the pillow suggests the diagnosis. Tender nodules or trigger points on the scalp have been described. The location and type of pain may be ill-defined and vague. Sudden or gradual onset of headache in an elderly patient should suggest the possibility of an underlying vasculitis.

Neuro-ophthalmic manifestations A catastrophic complication of temporal arteritis is the sudden onset of blindness that occurs in approximately 10% of patients with temporal arteritis. Blindness is most frequent in the first weeks of the disease, and usually occurs during the first year of illness.[67] Early signs such as ptosis, diplopia, transient blurring of vision, and photophobia usually precede loss of vision. Once blindness has occurred, vision is rarely regained. Funduscopic examination may reveal ischemic optic neuritis characterized by a swollen or pale disc, the presence of cotton wool patches, or small hemorrhages in the retina. It is imperative that elderly patients with polymyalgia rheumatica, who develop ocular symptoms or signs of ocular ischemia, be immediately treated for temporal arteritis prior to obtaining histologic evidence of temporal arteritis by biopsy. In the absence of giant cell arteritis the incidence of blindness is less than 1% in patients with *pure* polymyalgia rheumatica.

Diplopia has been reported as an early sign of temporal arteritis by Lockshin.[68] Prompt therapy resulted in remission of symptoms and preservation of vision. Diplopia is found in approximately 10% to 15% of patients with temporal arteritis. When present in elderly persons, it should lead to a search for other manifestations of the disease.

Jaw claudication, considered a classical sign of giant cell arteritis, has been described in one third of patients. It is the result of narrowing or obliteration of the temporal, maxillary, or facial arteries. Other findings include: loss of taste, trismus, dysphagia, and gangrene of the tongue.

Since neuropsychiatric manifestations of temporal arteritis usually are vague, the diagnosis should be considered in patients who present with anxiety, memory loss, and a variety of *functional* complaints.

Laboratory findings The sedimentation rate is invariably elevated in both giant cell arteritis and polymyalgia rheumatica.[65] Usually values range from 60 to 100 mm/hr (Westergren) but have been reported as high as 160 mm in some patients. On rare occasions, patients with biopsy-proven giant cell arteritis or characteristic polymyalgia rheumatica have been found to have sedimentation rates in the near normal or normal range. The frequent association of an elevated sedimentation rate with both polymyalgia rheumatica and temporal arteritis should not deter the clinician from considering other conditions in which the sedimentation rate is elevated.

There may be a mild normocytic, normochromic anemia, low serum iron concentration and normal iron-binding capacity. Bone marrow iron stores are usually normal. The anemia does not respond to iron therapy. The leukocyte and platelet counts usually are within the normal range, although a slight thrombocytosis may occur. An increase in globulins and fibrinogen and a decrease in albumin concentration may be present in some patients with polymyalgia rheumatica or giant cell arteritis. Haptoglobin levels may also be increased. There are no specific serologic markers for polymyalgia or giant cell arteritis. Tests for rheumatoid factor, antinuclear antibodies, serum complement and ASLO titers are usually normal. Mildly abnormal liver function tests have been reported by a number of observers, both in polymyalgia rheumatica and giant cell arteritis. High levels of serum glutamic oxalic transaminase and serum alkaline phosphatase, prolonged prothrombin times and increased bromsulphalein retention have been reported. Muscle enzymes, ie, aldolase and creatine phosphokinase, and the urinary creatine excretion are within the normal range. With rare exceptions, the electromyograms are normal.

Renal abnormalities have been reported in a few patients who have presented with mild proteinuria, hematuria, and red cell casts.

Temporal artery angiograms may show irregularity of the intimal surface of the artery in patients with temporal arteritis. These studies are of little diagnostic value in determining the presence of temporal arteritis, as other studies[69] have shown that in most instances narrowing and alterations of the intimal blood vessels are the result of arteriosclerotic plaques rather than vasculitis.

Temporal artery biopsy Biopsy of the temporal artery is indicated in patients with visual loss or field defects, amaurosis fugax, diplopia, ptosis, ophthalmoplegia, or a tender area over a scalp vessel. The clinician may be more hesitant to perform a biopsy in patients with *pure* polymyalgia rheumatica. Biopsy confirmation is recommended in all patients suspected of having giant cell arteritis. Because of the segmental distribution of giant cell arteritis, a specimen 3 to 6 cm in length should be taken from the side in which there are signs and symptoms of disease.[70] If clinical signs of temporal arteritis are very prominent and the initial biopsy is negative, a biopsy of the contralateral artery has been recommended by some.

Pathological findings The temporal artery or one of its branches is usually selected as the site of biopsy, although histologic signs consistent with giant cell arteritis have been reported in almost all large and medium sized arteries of the body.[71,72] On gross examination, lesions may vary from small aneurysmal dilatations to complete obliteration of the lumen of the vessel. The histologic findings during the acute stage are those of necrosis of the arterial wall with granulomatous inflammation characterized variably by histiocytes, giant cells, lymphocytes, and plasma cells (Figures 14-8A, B). There is fragmentation and necrosis of the internal elastic lamina. Multi-nuclear giant cells, when present, are seen best on the medial side. Often there are zones of inflammation with intervening segments of uninvolved vessel. Intimal thickening and luminal obstruction may be present.

In addition to the temporal artery, the aortic arch and any of its branches may be involved. There may be intermittent claudication in the upper extremities, bruits over the affected arteries, and decreased or absent pulses in the neck or arms. The subclavian steal syndrome and frozen shoulder have also been reported. Temporal arteritis of large vessels of lower extremities has also been reported and may present as intermittent claudication.[72]

Treatment Temporal arteritis should be treated with doses of prednisone in the range of 40 to 60 mg/day. When visual signs or symp-

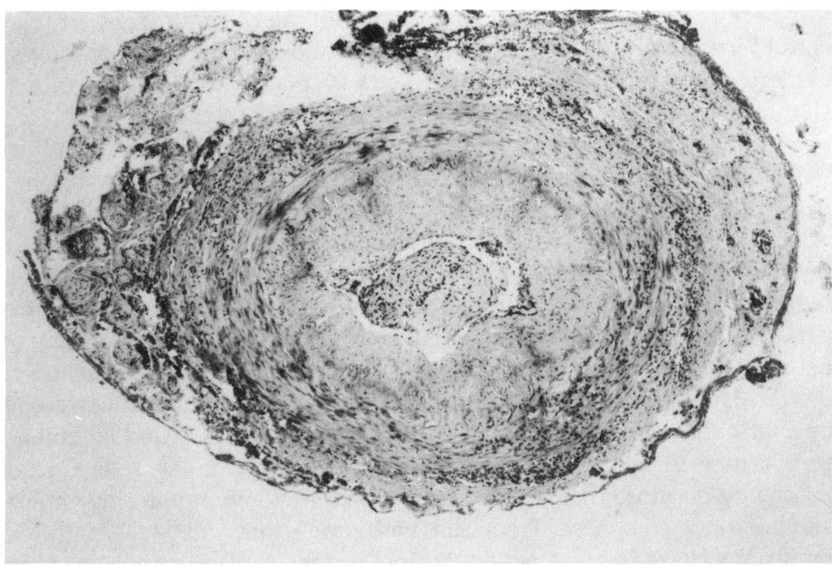

Figure 14-8A Section of temporal artery showing thickening of all layers, and a cellular infiltrate adjacent to the disrupted internal elastic membrane.

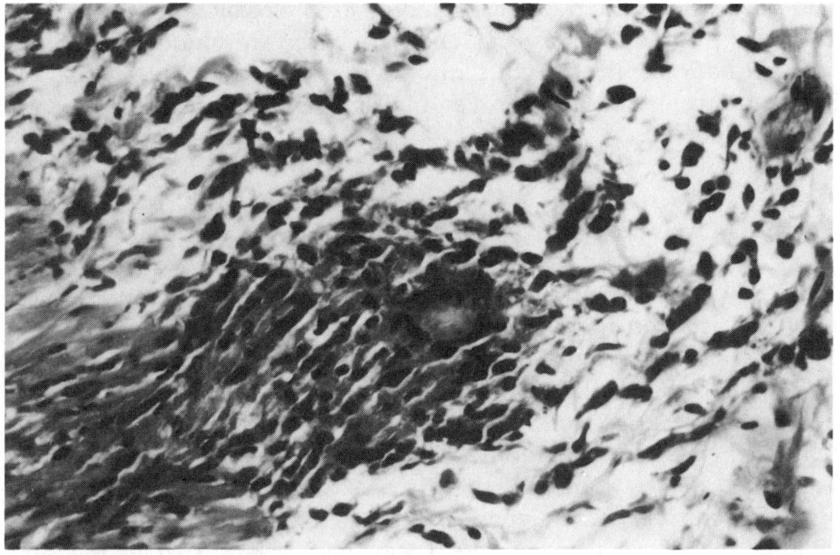

Figure 14-8B High power view of temporal artery showing cellular infiltrate and giant cells.

toms are present, treatment with 60 to 100 mg of prednisone per day should be instituted immediately. One should not wait for biopsy evidence of arteritis. If the diagnosis is suspected clinically, a biopsy should be performed and treatment instituted immediately thereafter.

Usually, conticosteroid treatment will not alter the histologic findings within the first 24 hours of treatment. It may be necessary to continue treatment with moderately high doses of prednisone for extended periods of time. Patients often require a daily maintenance dose of 60 to 80 mg of prednisone for a month or longer or until manifestations of the disease regress. The rate at which the dose of corticosteroids is reduced will depend on the clinical response. Monitoring the sedimentation rate may be helpful in deciding when to initiate a program of gradual reduction of dosage. Hunder and Allen[65] suggest that the initial level of corticosteroids be continued until all symptoms and signs have subsided and laboratory tests return to normal. This may be followed by weekly reduction of dosage by no more than 10% of the daily dose while monitoring clinical and laboratory response. Treatment with prednisone can be discontinued within one year in most patients. Most instances of relapse seem to be related to inadequate suppression of the continuous inflammatory process rather than spontaneous exacerbations.[63]

Patients who present with *pure* polymyalgia, without evidence of vasculitis, may be treated with moderate to low doses of corticosteroids in the range of 10 to 15 mg of prednisone per day. The dose of steroid is gradually tapered, again using the patient's clinical response and the sedimentation rate as a guide. Often a reduction of as little as 2.5 mg of prednisone may result in a rise in the sedimentation rate and reexacerbation of the patient's initial symptoms. Alternate day therapy with corticosteroids have proven ineffective in treating patients with polymyalgia.

Takayasu's Arteritis

Takayasu's arteritis[73-75] is much less commonly encountered than temporal arteritis. It is a chronic, obstructive, inflammatory arteritis of the aorta and its branches, as well as the pulmonary arteries.[6] It occurs in young women with a peak incidence in the third decade and has been described much more frequently in the Orient. It is, however, neither racially nor geographically restricted. Described originally by Takayasu and by Omesha, the disease's early literature originated almost exclusively from Japan.[75] Another name used to describe this condition is *pulseless disease.* The disease should be suspected in young women who present with absent pulses, numbness or claudication, discrepancies in the pulse volume in the upper and lower extremities, and signs of involvement of the bifurcation of the aorta. Hypertension in Takayasu's disease may be the result of blunting of the carotid sinus and aortic reflexes, stenosis of the aorta above the renal arteries, or partial to complete occlusion of the renal arteries by disease in the contiguous aorta.[75] Aortic insufficiency occurs in 5% to 8% of patients.

Neurological manifestations include dizziness, headache, and syncope. Transient blindness, diplopia, hemiparesis and paraparesis have been described. Strokes occur in up to 10% of patients. A prepulseless phase of the systemic disease has been reported by Roberts et al.[76]

Laboratory findings The sedimentation rate is invariably elevated. Other laboratory findings are similar to those noted in temporal arteritis. These include a moderate anemia, low serum iron, occasional thrombocytosis and elevation of the plasma fibrinogen. A Japanese study has shown an increased incidence of HLA-B5 in patients with Takayasu's arteritis when compared to controls.[77]

Radiological examination of the chest invariably shows left ventricular hypertrophy. The aortic arch is dilated and the contour of the thoracic aorta is distorted. Notching of the ribs is unusual. Right ventricular hypertrophy may occur in the presence of pulmonary artery involvement. The most specific diagnostic test for Takayasu's arteritis is angiographic study of the aorta and its branches.[6] The aorta is rigid and elongated and narrowed with poststenotic fusiform dilatation.[78,79]

On histologic examination, a panarteritis with inflammatory mononuclear cell infiltration, intimal proliferation, and fibrosis in all three layers of the vessel wall results in marked destruction of the internal elastic lamina. This frequently leads to aneurysmal dilatation. Although the aortic arch most frequently is affected, any level of the aorta may be involved, from the aortic arch distally to the bifurcation.

Treatment Various agents have been employed in the treatment of Takayasu's arteritis. These include anticoagulants, vasodilators, salicylates, antimicrobial and cytotoxic drugs. Most commonly, patients are treated with corticosteroids in dosages from 30 to 60 mg/day initially followed by gradual reduction in steroid dosage. One must watch for clinical and laboratory evidence of rebound. There is no evidence that life expectancy in Takayasu's arteritis is altered significantly by treatment with corticosteroid therapy. Arterial surgery should be considered only when medical therapy has been unsuccessful.

REFERENCES

1. Kussmaul A, Maier R. Ueber eine bishir nicht beschriebene eigenthumliche Arterioenerkrankung (periarteritis nodosa) die mit morbus Brightii und rapid fortschreitender allgemeiner muskellahmung einhergeht. *Disch Arch Klin Med* 1:484, 1866.

2. Zeek PM. Periarteritis nodosa, a critical review. *Am J Clin Pathol* 22:777, 1952.

3. Christian CL, Sergent JS. Vasculitis syndromes: Clinical and experimental models. *Am J Med* 61:385, 1976.

4. Gilliam JN, Smiley JD. Cutaneous necrotizing vasculitis and related disorders. *Ann Allergy* 37:328, 1976.

5. Fauci AS: The spectrum of vasculitis: Clinical, pathologic, immunologic, and therapeutic considerations. *Ann Intern Med* 89(1):660, 1978.

6. Fan PT, Davis FA, Somer T, et al. A clinical approach to systemic vasculitis. *Semin Arthritis Rheum* 9:248, 1980.

7. Churg J, Strauss L. Allergic granulomatosis, allergic angiitis, and periarteritis nodosa. *Am J Pathol* 27:277, 1951.

8. Sams WM Jr, Thorne ER, Small P, et al. Leukocytoclastic vasculitis. *Arch Dermatol* 112:219, 1976.

9. Braverman IM, Yen A. Demonstration of immune complexes in spontaneous and histamine-induced lesions and in normal skin of patients with leukocytoclastic angiitis. *J Invest Dermatol* 64:105, 1975.

10. Schroeter AL, Copeman OWM, Jordon RE, et al. Immunofluorescence of cutaneous vasculitis associated with systemic disease. *Arch Dermatol* 104:254, 1971.

11. Horwitz LD, Silber R. Subacute bacterial endocarditis presenting as purpura. *Arch Intern Med* 120:483, 1967.

12. Hellstrom HR, Perez-Stable EC. Retroperitoneal fibrosis with disseminated vasculitis and intrahepatic sclerosing cholangitis. *Am J Med* 40:184, 1966.

13. Sams WM. Harville DD, Winklemann RK. Necrotizing vasculitis associated with lethal reticuloendothelial diseases. *Br J Dermatol* 80:555, 1968.

14. Brody JL, Samitz HH. Cutaneous signs of cryoparaproteinemia: Control with burst alkeran and prednisone. *Am J Med* 55:211, 1973.

15. Cream JJ, Gumpel JM, Peachey RDG. Schönlein-Henoch purpura in the adult: A study of 77 adults with anaphylactoid or Schönlein-Henoch purpura. *QJ Med* 39:461, 1970.

16. Bywaters EGL, Isdale I, Kempton JJ. Schönlein-Henoch purpura. *QJ Med* 26:161, 1957.

17. Answell BM. Henoch-Schönlein purpura with particular reference to the prognosis of the renal lesion. *Br J Dermatol* 82:211, 1970.

18. Lindenaver SM, Tank ES. Surgical aspects of Henoch-Schönlein's purpura. *Surgery* 6:982, 1966.

19. Ballard HS. Renal manifestations of the Henoch-Schönlein syndrome in adults. *Am J Med* 49:328, 1970.

20. Baart de La Faille-Kuyper EH, Kater L, Kooiker CJ, et al. IgA deposits in cutaneous blood vessel walls and mesangium in Henoch-Schönlein syndrome. *Lancet* 21:892, 1973.

21. McDuffie FC, Sams WM Jr, Maldonado JE, et al. Hypocomplementemia with cutaneous vasculitis and arthritis: Possible immune complex syndrome. *Mayo Clin Proc* 48:340, 1973.

22. Miller DA, Freeman GL, Akers WA. Chronic urticaria: A Clinical study of 50 patients. *Am J Med* 44:68, 1968.

23. Mathison DA, Arroyave CM, Bhat KN, et al. Hypocomplementemia in chronic idiopathic urticaria. *Ann Intern Med* 86:534, 1977.

24. LoSpalluto J, Dorward B, Miller W Jr, et al. Cryoglobulinemia based on interaction between a gamma macroglobulin and 7S gamma globulin. *Am J Med* 32: 142, 1962.

25. Meltzer M, Franklin EC. Cryoglobulinemia: A study of twenty-nine patients: I. IgG and IgM cryoglobulins and factors affecting cryoprecipitability. *Am J Med* 40:828, 1966.

26. Meltzer M, Franklin EC, Ellias K, et al. Cryoglobulinemia—a clinical and laboratory study. II. Cryoglobulins with rheumatoid factor activity. *Am J Med* 40: 837, 1966.

27. Gorevic PD, Kassab HJ, Levo Y, et al. Mixed Cryoglobulinemia: Clinical aspects and long-term follow-up of forty patients. *Am J Med* 69:287, 1980.

28. Lightfoot RW. The vasculitis syndromes in McCarthy DJ (ed). *Arthritis and Allied Conditions,* ed 9. Philadelphia, Lea & Febiger, 1979, p. 723.

29. Ansell BM, Loewe G. Rheumatoid arthritis: General features. *Clin Rheum Dis* 3:385, 1977.

30. Decker JL, Plotz PH. Extra-articular rheumatoid diseases, in McCarthy DJ (ed). *Arthritis and Allied Conditions,* ed 9. Philadelphia, Lea & Febiger, 1979, p 470.

31. Dubois EL. *Lupus Erythematosus,* ed 2. Los Angeles, University Southern California, 1974, p 414.

32. Bienenstock H, Minick CR, Rogoff B. Mesenteric arteritis and intestinal infarction in rheumatoid disease. *Arch Intern Med* 119:359, 1967.

33. Mentz G, Fraga A. Arteritis in systemic lupus erythematosus. *Arch Intern Med* 116:55, 1965.

34. Golden RL. Livido reticularis in systemic lupus erythematosus. *Arch Dermatol* 87:67, 1963.

35. Rudusky BM. Recurrent Osler's nodes in systemic lupus erythematosus. *Angiology* 20:33, 1969.

36. Wegener F. Uber generalisierte, septische Gefasserkarnkungen. *Verl Dtsch Ges Pathol* 29:202, 1936.

37. Carrington CB, Liebow AA. Limited forms of angiitis and granulomatosis of Wegener's type. *Am J Med* 41:497, 1966.

38. Wolff SM, Fauci AS, Horn RG, et al. Wegener's granulomatosis. *Ann Intern Med* 81:513, 1974.

39. Haynes BF, Fishman ML. Fauci AS, et al. The ocular manifestations of Wegener's granulomatosis. *Am J Med* 63:131, 1977.

40. Israel HL, Patchefsky AS. Wegener's granulomatosis of lung: Diagnosis and treatment: Experience with twelve cases. *Ann Intern Med* 74:881, 1971.

41. Horn RG, Fauci AS, Rosenthal AS, et al. Renal biopsy pathology in Wegener's granulomatosis. *Am J Pathol* 74:423, 1974.

42. Israel HL, Patchefsky AS, Saldana MJ. Wegener's granulomatosis, lymphomatoid granulomatosis, and benign lymphocytic angiitis and granulomatosis of the lung: Recognition and treatment. *Ann Intern Med* 87:691, 1977.

43. McDonald TJ, DeRemee RA, Harrison EG et al. The protean clinical features of polymorphic reticulosis (lethal midline granuloma). *Laryngoscope* 9:936, 1975.

44. Walton EW. Giant cell granuloma of the respiratory tract (Wegener's granulomatosis). *Br Med J* 2:265, 1958.

45. Fauci AS, Wolff SM. Wegener's granulomatosis: Studies in eighteen patients and a review of the literature. *Medicine* 52:535, 1973.

46. Chumbley LC, Harrison EG Jr, DeRemee RA. Allergic granulomatosis and angiitis (Churg-Strauss syndrome): Report and analysis of 30 cases. *Mayo Clin Proc* 52:477, 1977.

47. Gocke DJ, Morgan KN, Lockshin M, et al. Association between polyarteritis and Australia antigen. *Lancet* 2:1149, 1970.

48. Sergent JS, Lockshin MD, Christian CL, et al. Vasculitis with hepatitis B antigenemia: Long-term observations in nine patients. *Medicine* 55:1, 1976.

49. Duffy J, Lidsky MD, Sharp JT, et al. Polyarthritis, polyarteritis and hepatitis B. *Medicine* 55:19, 1976.

50. Citron BP, Halpern M, McCarron M, et al. Necrotizing angiitis associated with drug abuse. *N Engl J Med* 283:1003, 1970.

51. Sergent JS, Christian CL. Necrotizing vasculitis after acute serous otitis media. *Ann Intern Med* 81:195, 1974.

52. Travers RL, Allison DJ, Brettle RP, et al. Polyarteritis nodosa: A clinical and angiographic analysis of 17 cases. *Semin Arthritis Rheum* 8:184, 1979.

53. Frohnert PP, Sheps SG. Long term follow up study of periarteritis nodosa. *Am J Med* 43:8, 1967.

54. Fauci AS, Katz P, Haynes BF, et al. Cyclophosphamide therapy of severe systemic necrotizing vasculitis. *N Engl J Med* 301:235, 1979.

55. Leib ES, Restivo C, Paulus HE. Immunosuppressive and corticosteroid therapy of polyarteritis nodosa. *Am J Med* 67:941, 1979.

56. Hutchinson J. Diseases of the arteries. On a peculiar form of thrombotic arteritis of the aged which is sometimes productive of gangrene. *Arch Surg* (London) 1:323, 1889.

57. Horton BT, Magath TB, Brown GE. An undescribed form of arteritis of the temporal vessels. *Proc Staff Meet Mayo Clin* 7:700, 1932.

58. Jennings GH. Arteritis of the temporal vessels. *Lancet* 1:424, 1938.

59. Barber HS. Myalgic syndrome with constitutional effects: Polymyalgia rheumatica. *Ann Rheum Dis* 16:230, 1957.

60. Lee DK, Andrews JM. Temporal arteritis developing in the course of sulfonamide therapy. *JAMA* 200:720, 1967.

61. Bailey RR, Neale TJ, Lynn KL: Allopurinol-associated arteritis (letter to the editor). *Lancet* 2:907, 1976.

62. Liang GC, Simkin PA, Mannik M. Immunoglobulins in-temporal arteritis: An immunofluorescent study. *Ann Intern Med* 81:19, 1974.

63. Huston KA, Hunder GG, Kennedy RH, et al. Temporal arteritis: A 25 year epidemiologic, clinical and pathologic study. *Ann Intern Med* 88:162, 1978.

64. Hamilton CR, Shelley WM, Tumulty PA. Giant cell arteritis: including temporal arteritis and polymyalgia rheumatica. *Medicine* (Baltimore) 50:1, 1971.

65. Hunder GG, Allen GL. Giant cell arteritis: A review. *Bull Rheum Dis* 29:980, 1978.

66. O'Duffy D, Wahner HW, Hunder GG. Joint imaging in polymyalgia rheumatica. *Mayo Clin Proc* 51:519, 1976.

67. Cohen DN, Damaske MM. Temporal arteritis: A spectrum of ophthalmic complications. *Ann Ophthalmol* 7:1045, 1975.

68. Lockshin MD. Diplopia as early sign of temporal arteritis: Report of two cases. *Arthritis Rheum* 13:419, 1970.

69. Horwitz HM, Pepe PF, Johnsrude IS, et al. Temporal arteriography and immunofluorescence and diagnostic tools in temporal arteritis. *J Rheumatol* 4:76, 1977.

70. Goodman BJ. Temporal arteritis. *Am J Med* 67:839, 1979.

71. Wilkinson IMS, Russel RWR. Arteries of the head and neck in giant cell arteritis: A pathological study to show the pattern of arterial involvement. *Arch Neurol* 27:378, 1972.

72. Klein RG, Hunder GG, Stanson AW, et al. Large artery involvement in giant cell (temporal) arteritis. *Ann Intern Med* 83:806, 1975.

73. Strachan RW. The natural history of Takayasu's arteriopathy. *QJ Med* 33:57, 1964.

74. Ishikawa K. Natural history and classification of occlusive thromboaortopathy (Takayasu's disease). *Circulation* 57:27, 1978.

75. Bonventre MV. Takayasu's disease: Revisited. *NY State J Med* 1960: 1974.

76. Roberts WC, MacGregor RR, DeBlanc HJ, et al. The prepulseless phase of pulseless disease, or pulseless disease with pulses: A newly recognized cause of cardiac disease, monoclonal gammopathy and "fever of unknown origin." *Am J Med* 46:313, 1969.

77. Naito S, Arakawa K, Saito S, et al. Takayasu's disease: Association with HLA-B5. *Tissue Antigens* 12:143, 1978.

78. Paloheimo JA. Obstructive arteritis of Takayasu's type: Clinical, roentgenological and laboratory studies on thirty-six patients. *Acta Med Scand* (suppl) 468:7, 1967.

79. Lande A, Gross A. Total aortography in the diagnosis of Takayasu's arteritis. *Am J Roentgenol Rad Ther Med* 116:165, 1972.

15 Pathogenesis, Prevention and Treatment of Arterial and Venous Thrombosis

Shafkat Hussain
Joel M. Schwartz

The magnitude of the clinical challenge posed by occlusion of the arterial and venous limbs of the circulation is clearly illustrated with a few statistics. Arterial thromboembolism is a major factor in mortality due to acute myocardial infarction, stroke, and renal disease, which are the first, third, and fourth most frequent causes of death in the United States.[1] Venous thrombosis is the cause for the hospitalization of approximately 300,000 Americans annually, of whom more than 50,000 die, often as the result of pulmonary embolism.[2] Pulmonary embolism has been estimated to occur in over 500,000 Americans each year, and to be fatal in over 100,000.[3]

Over a century ago, Virchow enunciated a concept which to this day has formed the framework for study of the pathogenesis of thrombosis. Thrombosis was considered to result from changes in the blood flow.[4]

A thrombus is a mass of cellular material held together by a fibrin network, which occludes a blood vessel. The relative proportion of cells and fibrin may vary considerably according to the conditions of development of the thrombus as well as its age. Venous thrombi, formed under conditions of relatively slow blood flow, resemble blood clots in vitro. The major components are red cells and fibrin. Platelets are caught up in the process as well, indicated by the shortened half-life of platelets *and* fibrinogen, but each is corrected by heparin.[5] Arterial thrombi, on the other hand, develop in areas of rapid blood flow. They consist mainly of platelets. Fibrinogen half-life is normal and the accelerated turnover of platelets is corrected by antiplatelet drugs but not by heparin.[5] Initiation of arterial thrombosis is primarily related not to stasis, but to interactions between platelets and abnormal vessel surfaces.[6,7]

In recent years there has been an explosion of new facts and concepts concerning hemostasis. Major improvement in our understanding of the physiology and biochemistry of platelet function and of the dynamics of clot formation and lysis has, in turn, shed new light on the pathogenesis of the occlusive thrombus. This chapter will review: 1) the role of platelets in hemostasis and atherogenesis, 2) the pathogenesis of thrombus formation at various sites in the circulation and 3) the rationale and the forms of therapy now available for the prevention and treatment of arterial and venous thromboembolism.

PLATELETS AND NORMAL HEMOSTASIS

Normal Platelet Functions

Clarification of the normal functions of platelets is central to the assignment of a role to platelets in the pathogenesis of thrombosis and atherosclerosis. Normal platelets play key roles in maintaining the integrity of blood vessels, restoring the continuity of interrupted vessel linings (primary hemostasis), and in blood coagulation (secondary hemostasis). These subjects have been extensively reviewed.[8-11]

Absence of platelets leads to hemorrhage from cutaneous and submucosal capillaries; the transfusion of platelets quickly corrects this tendency to the formation of petechiae and ecchymoses. The mechanisms whereby platelets control the fragility and permeability of normal blood vessels are poorly understood.

The initial response of platelets to interruption of endothelial continuity is known as primary hemostasis. Platelets adhere to subendothelial microfibrils, basement membrane, and collagen. Adherence "stimulates" the platelet membrane, exposing platelet factor 3, and triggers a series of biochemical sequences which culminate in the secretion of several components previously stored in platelet granules. One of these substances is adenosine diphosphate (ADP). Upon release, it aggregates platelets in the immediate environment by a direct effect upon their membranes. Aggregated platelets in turn release further ADP. Other biologically active substances released from the activiated platelets include catecholamines, serotonin, platelet factor 4 (a heparin neutralizing protein), certain lysosomal enzymes, and a factor involved in the promotion of smooth muscle proliferation and growth.[12] We shall return to this platelet growth factor in our discussion of atherogenesis.

Primary hemostasis merges into secondary hemostasis with the contribution of factor 3 exposed in the platelet surface by contact with collagen, and of additional coagulant factors induced in the membrane by collagen and ADP.[13] These membrane properties catalyze the activation of circulating procoagulants of the intrinsic coagulation pathway. The end product of this pathway is thrombin, which is elaborated in close proximity to the platelet, and is itself a powerful platelet aggregant. It releases ADP from platelet granules, stimulates the oxidation of arachidonic acid, and exerts yet another aggregating and releasing effect unrelated either to ADP or to prostaglandins. Thrombin also converts fibrinogen to fibrin monomer. The monomers polymerize to fibrin strands, which strengthen the platelet plug formed at the site of endothelial injury.

Prostaglandins and Hemostasis

The aggregation of platelets at the site of endothelial injury as well as inhibition of this process is profoundly influenced by the metabolism of arachidonic acid[14] released from membrane phospholipids by the action of phospholipase A2 (Figure 15-1). Phospholipase A2 in platelet membrane is activated by collagen, by ADP and epinephrine released from platelets, and by thrombin elaborated in the immediate vicinity. (The activation of phospholipase in the endothelium is presumably triggered by similar processes.)[15,16] Arachidonic acid moieties are rapidly metabolized via the cyclooxygenase pathway to the labile endoperoxide prostaglandins (PG) G2 and H2; this step is inhibited by aspirin[17] and sulfinpyrazone.[18] An enzyme called thromboxane (TX) synthetase, present in platelet microsomes, catalyzes the synthesis from PGG2 and PGH2 of TXA2, a vasoconstrictor and potent inducer of platelet aggregation and release. On the other hand, PGG2 and PGH2 formed in endothelial cells, or diffusing from platelets and taken up by endothelial cells,[19] are converted by prostacyclin (PGI2) synthetase to PGI2, a vasodilator and potent inhibitor of platelet aggregation and release. TXA2 aggregates platelets directly and by causing the release of ADP.[20] Prostacyclin may inhibit aggregation by

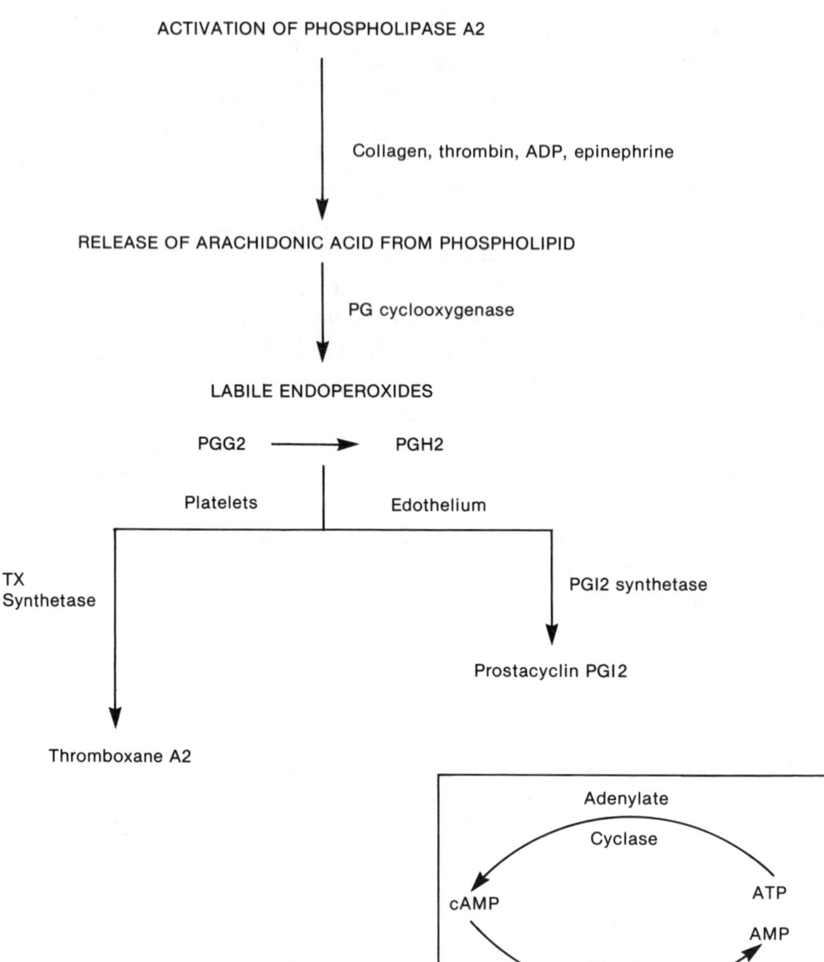

Figure 15-1 Prostaglandin metabolism in platelets and endothelium.

Arachidonic acid is released from the lipid bilayers of platelet and arterial membranes. Prostaglandin (PG) cyclooxygenase is present both in platelets and endothelium; it is blocked by aspirin and sulfinpyrazone. Prostacyclin (PGI2) synthetase in endothelium converts labile endoperoxides to PG12, whereas thromboxane (TX) synthetase in platelets converts the same substrates to TXA2.

PGI2 stimulates platelet adenylate cyclase to form cyclic AMP (cAMP). Dipyridamole inhibits the catabolism of cAMP by blocking platelet phosphodiesterase.

TXA2, PGG2, PGH2, and the activators of membrane phospholipase A2 promote platelet release and aggregation. PGI2, cAMP, and inhibitors of cyclooxygenase and phosphodiesterase enzymes inhibit these reactions.

stimulating adenylate cyclase and the synthesis of cyclic AMP (cAMP),[14] which inhibits aggregation.[21] The catabolism of cAMP by phosphodiesterase is inhibited by dipyridamole.[22]

The fate of the platelet-fibrin plug formed at the site of endothelial injury is determined, in part, by a balance between proaggregatory TXA2 formation from platelets and antiaggregatory prostacyclin formation from the blood vessel wall.[20] The concentration of proaggregatory elements within blood vessel walls increases from subendothelium to adventita, whereas the concentration of prostacyclin synthetase progressively decreases from intima outward.[14] Therefore, extensive damage to the intima destroys the ability to generate prostacyclin even as it exposes microfibrils and collagen, which stimulate platelet phospholipase and the synthesis of TXA2.

The integrity of the platelet-fibrin plug and the possibility of its enlargement to form an occlusive thrombus are influenced by additional factors: platelet function and counts, local concentrations of non-prostaglandins which stimulate platelet release, plasma levels of circulating procoagulants and inhibitors, the force of the blood flow which can detach pieces and cause them to embolize, and by the processes of phagocytosis, fibrinolysis, and atherogenesis.

PLATELETS AND ARTERIAL DISEASE

Platelets and Atherogenesis

The pathogenesis of atherosclerosis has recently been reviewed.[23] Repair of the intima of an artery which has been traumatized involves the initial formation of a platelet thrombus as described above. The size of the platelet thrombus will reflect the exposure of different proaggregatory elements within the vessel wall. Basement membrane present beneath the internal elastic membrane has relatively low activity in the initiation of the platelet release reaction; collagen of the arterial media has high activity.[24] Repair of the injured artery occurs via migration of smooth muscle cells of the media through gaps in the internal elastic membrane under the influence of a growth factor released from the alpha granules of platelets.[12,23] The smooth muscle cells proliferate in their new location between the endothelium and the internal elastic membrane. They produce collagen fibers with high release-inducer potential characteristic of collagen in the arterial media.[24] A new endothelium arises by overgrowth from the sides of the lesion. Repeated injury at the same site, eg, at a bifurcation in the arterial tree, will bring platelets into contact with the highly reactive collagen now present in the subendothelium, and will cause a much enhanced series of platelet and smooth muscle reactions. Repeated injury can lead to the incorporation of lipid and the formation of an atherosclerotic plaque.

Platelet Reactivity in Thrombotic Arterial Disorders

Although platelets are important in the pathogenesis of experimental thrombosis and atherosclerosis, there is as yet no definite evidence that "hyperactive" platelets exist in vivo or that they predispose to these lesions. Nevertheless, a number of in vitro and in vivo tests of platelet function have been applied in the attempt to demonstrate increased platelet reactivity. Among these are measurements of aggregability, membrane coagulant activites, in vivo survival and turnover, circulating platelet aggregates, and release of specific granular components.

Enhanced platelet aggregation with ADP, epinephrine, or collagen has been reported in patients with: 1) diabetes mellitus[25] and deteriorating retinopathy,[26] 2) type II hyperlipoproteinemia,[27] and 3) angina pectoris.[28] Platelet hyperaggregability in diabetes may be related to enhanced formation of prostaglandin in vitro upon exposure to these reagents.[29] Platelet aggregation is generally quantified with the use of an aggregometer, which measures the change in optical density of platelet-rich plasma under constant temperature and continuous agitation after the addition of different concentrations of aggregating agents.[30]

Spontaneous platelet aggregation occurs in some patients with 1) myeloproliferative disorders and thrombocytosis,[31,32] 2) diabetes mellitus,[33] 3) transient cerebral ischemia,[34] and 4) angina pectoris.[34] Treatment with aspirin has reversed both the digital ischemia and the spontaneous aggregation of platelets in several patients with essential thrombocythemia.[31]

Recent studies by Walsh suggest that platelets exposed to collagen activate factor XII and platelets exposed to ADP activate factor XI.[13] These coagulant activities in the platelet membrane are increased in patients with postoperative venous thrombosis of the legs and in patients with attacks of transient cerebral ischemia.[35,36] The nature of the relationship between these activities and thromboembolism is unknown.

A test which purports to detect circulating platelet aggregates in vivo has been described by Wu and Hoak.[37] The presence of aggregates is inferred from a difference in the platelet count of blood drawn into edetic acid (EDTA) and blood drawn into EDTA-formalin. Abnormal test values have been found in patients with essential thrombocythemia, transient cerebral ischemia, angina pectoris, myocardial infarction, and acute occlusion of peripheral arteries.[32,37,38] The abnormal test result was reversed in some patients with attacks of cerebral ischemia by treatment with aspirin and dipyridamole.[38]

Reduced survival of chromium 51-labeled platelets and increased platelet turnover have been associated with an increased risk of thromboembolism in several disorders: arterial thrombosis, homocystinuria, rheumatic valvular disease, prosthetic heart valves, ischemic heart disease, and arteriovenous shunts.[5,39,40] The increased risk of thromboembolism in these consumptive disorders of platelets presumably results from the compensatory delivery to the circulation of young platelets capable of increased reactivity when they contact an abnormal surface.[41,42] Treatment with dipyridamole corrected platelet survival and dramatically reduced the frequency of arterial fibromuscular lesions and the incidence of thrombosis in experimental homocystinuria.[43]

Attempts have been made to measure components of the platelet release reaction circulating in the plasma, eg, platelet factor 4 and platelet-specific beta thromboglobulin released from granules (along with platelet growth factor) by thrombin or collagen. Radioimmunoassay of platelet factor 4 in plasma has indicated increased levels in patients with stable coronary artery disease,[44] exercise-induced angina,[45] and acute myocardial infarction.[46,47] Increases in specific beta thromboglobulin have been recorded in acute, proximal deep vein thrombosis,[48] acute pulmonary embolism,[48] and renal vein thrombosis associated with the nephrotic syndrome.[49]

THERAPY WITH ANTIPLATELET DRUGS

Mechanisms of Drug Activity

Many compounds are potentially useful in the prevention of arterial thrombosis by virtue of their ability to inhibit various platelet functions in vitro. Three of these have been widely used clinically: aspirin, sulfinpyrazone, and dipyridamole. We shall now discuss the mechanisms of action of these drugs and the therapeutic benefits derived from their use.

Aspirin acetylates cyclooxygenase and alters its binding affinity for arachidonic acid[11,50] (Figure 15-1). The inhibition of platelet cyclooxygenase is irreversible and impairs the synthesis of TXA2 for the duration of the platelet life (7 to 10 days). The bleeding time of patients who have ingested therapeutic doses of aspirin is prolonged, and their acetylated platelets fail to undergo a release reaction upon the addition of epinephrine, collagen, or ADP.[51,52] Unlike platelets which essentially have no protein-synthesizing capacity, nucleated endothelial cells retain the capacity to synthesize cyclooxygenase.[53] Thus the effects of aspirin upon the endothelial synthesis of prostacyclin can be transient if aspirin is given at spaced intervals. Furthermore, several authors have reported differential sensitivity of cyclooxygenase in endothelium as compared to platelets, raising the possibility that small doses of aspirin which suppress platelet synthesis of TXA2 may spare endothelial synthesis of prostacyclin.[53,54]

Sulfinpyrazone interferes with adhesion of platelets to the subendothelium.[55] Doses of the drug sufficient to prolong the shortened platelet survival in patients with recurrent venous thromboembolism do not interfere with platelet aggregation (induced by ADP, collagen, or thrombin) in vitro.[56,57] This has given rise to speculation that the drug may act primarily on the vessel wall rather than on the platelet. However, inhibition of platelet cyclooxygenase (Figure 15-1) and platelet release can be demonstrated upon direct addition of the drug to platelets.[18]

The precise mechanism for the antiplatelet effect of dipyridamole is uncertain. It seems likely that its antiplatelet action results from inhibition of platelet phosphodiesterase[22] (Figure 15-1). The resulting elevation of cyclic AMP levels in platelets inhibits aggregation. Inhibition of phosphodiesterase by dipyridamole potentiates the effect of circulating prostacyclin upon platelets.

Clinical Usefulness of Antiplatelet Drugs

The clinical relevance of antiplatelet drugs used singly and in combination is currently under investigation in many conditions.

Coronary artery disease Aspirin and sulfinpyrazone are the antiplatelet drugs used most frequently to prevent cardiac deaths in patients who are recovering from an acute myocardial infarction. The Anturane Reinfarction Trial Research Group study of sulfinpyrazone (200 mg, four times daily) demonstrated significant reduction in sudden death and in overall mortality (though not in reinfarction) in patients entered on protocol within a month of the acute cardiac damage.[58] The protective effect of sulfinpyrazone was limited to the first seven months of study. Clinical trials with aspirin have shown a similar trend,[59,60] but the reductions in mortality have not been significant, perhaps because entry into the studies after an acute infarct was often delayed for many months. There are anecdotal reports[61,62] but no well-designed studies which indicate that antiplatelet drugs will prevent primary infarcts of the heart.

Cerebral vascular disease The Canadian Cooperative Study Group demonstrated effectiveness for aspirin (325 mg, four times daily) but not sulfinpyrazone in reducing the incidence of stroke and death in patients who had suffered one or more transient attacks of cerebral or retinal ischemia in the previous three months.[63] The favorable outcome was significant in males but not in female patients. Aspirin reduced the risk of stroke or death in men by 48%. A similar study done in the United States showed a trend toward reduced transient ischemic attacks, stroke, and death in patients who took aspirin, but the results did not reach statistical significance.[64]

Prosthetic heart valves Aspirin or dipyridamole combined with oral warfarin has been more effective than oral anticoagulants alone in reducing the incidence of embolism in patients with prosthetic heart valves.[65,66] Although antiplatelet drugs may normalize the reduced platelet survival seen in some of these patients, clinical efficacy has not been proved for these agents when used without oral anticoagulants.

Rheumatic heart disease Shortened platelet survival has been demonstrated in patients with rheumatic mitral disease and thromboembolism but not in patients without this complication.[67] The platelet survival improved and the frequency of thromboembolism decreased when the patients were treated with sulfinpyrazone.[68]

Arteriovenous shunts Aspirin (160 mg per day)[69] and sulfinpyrazone[70] each reduced the incidence of arteriovenous shunt thrombosis in patients undergoing hemodialysis for chronic renal failure.

In summary, aspirin has been found to be beneficial in patients with transient cerebral ischemia, and sulfinpyrazone has benefited patients with mitral stenosis and thromboembolism, and patients who are recovering from a very recent infarct of the heart. Aspirin and sulfinpyrazone are each effective in reducing the frequency of thrombosis in arteriovenous shunts of patients undergoing hemodialysis. Aspirin or dipyridamole combined with oral anticoagulants were more effective than oral anticoagulants alone in preventing systemic embolism from prosthetic heart valves. Aspirin abolished symptoms in patients with digital ischemia, thrombocytosis, and spontaneous platelet aggregation.

PATHOGENESIS OF VENOUS THROMBOSIS

Retarded Blood Flow

Venous thrombi are usually formed in regions of slow or disturbed blood flow. They begin as small deposits in valve cusp pockets or in venous sinuses of the deep leg veins.[71] There is controversy as to the relative importance of platelets and of fibrin formation in the initiation of venous thrombosis,[72,73] but there is general agreement that the growing thrombus is a red clot composed of red blood cells interspersed with fibrin. The increased incidence of venous thrombosis in patients with congestive heart failure, immobility, or paralyzed limbs attests to the importance of stasis in the development of venous occlusion. However, data in both animals and man suggest that retarded blood flow alone may not be sufficient to initiate intravascular coagulation, and that some alteration of the circulating constituents of the blood may also be required.[74]

The altered state of the blood which favors the formation of venous thrombi has been referred to as the hypercoagulable state. Among the changes described which may contribute to hypercoagulability are increased concentration of normal and activated clotting factors, decreased levels of circulating inhibitors, impaired function of the fibrinolytic system, and the presence of hyperactive platelets.[75,76] Nevertheless, there is as yet no evidence that any one change or combination of changes cited above can of itself account for the formation of venous thrombi. Assuming, however, that one or several of these factors may indeed have a role either in the initiation or propagation of venous thrombosis, stasis will surely facilitate the process by protecting thrombogenic elements from dispersion, from neutralization by natural inhibitors, and from clearance by the liver.[74] Stasis may additionally contribute to the formation of thrombin by damaging the venous valve cusps which are avascular and, therefore, wholly dependent on luminal blood for their oxygen and nutrition.[77]

Possible Alterations in the Coagulability of Blood

Elevated concentration of factors I, V, and VIII have been reported in pregnancy,[78] in women taking contraceptive drugs,[79] and in patients with recent thrombosis.[80] Since these factors are acute phase reactants, the increase in their concentration has been considered a nonspecific response to extensive vascular occlusion, inflammation, or some associated disease rather than an indication of impending venous thrombosis.

Mucin produced by adenocarcinomas[81] or tissue factors released into the circulation during surgery, childbirth, or trauma can activate the coagulation pathways and cause disseminated thrombosis of the microcirculation. Venous thrombosis and disseminated intravascular coagulation have been reported after the administration of concentrated preparations of factors II, VII, IX, and X (Konyne, Proplex), particularly in postoperative patients and in patients with liver disease.[82,83] The preparations contain activated forms of the clotting factors.

Activated clotting and fibrinolytic factors are normally inhibited by naturally occurring protease inhibitors such as antithrombin III (AT III), alpha-2 macroglobulin, alpha-1 antitrypsin, and C1 esterase inactivator. AT III is the main inhibitor of activated factors XII, XI, IX, X, and II (thrombin),[84] whereas alpha-2 macroglobulin and alpha-1 antitrypsin are the main inhibitors of plasmin.[85] Increased incidence of venous thrombosis has been reported in hereditary deficiency of AT III,[86,87] and in postoperative women who had used oral contraceptives preoperatively and had acquired low levels of AT III.[88]

Fibrin clots are normally split into soluble products by plasmin, a proteolytic enzyme generated form plasminogen by the action of humoral or tissue activators. Decreased fibrinolytic activity in plasma, due either to decreased plasminogen activator or increased antiplasmin activity, has been found in pregnancy,[89] women who take oral contraceptives,[90] postoperative states,[91] malignancy,[92] and obesity.[93] The same conditions, of course, are associated with increased incidence of venous thrombosis.

The role of platelets in the formation of the hemostatic plug and in the pathogenesis of arterial thrombi is well recognized. Several laboratory and clinical observations suggest a role for platelets in venous thrombosis as well: 1) Walsh and his associates observed increased platelet coagulant activities in postoperative patients who subsequently developed deep vein thrombosis and in patients with acute thrombosis of the retinal vein[35,94]; 2) unusually severe and frequent venous thrombosis has occurred following surgery, particularly splenectomy, in patients with essential thrombocythemia and other myeloproliferative disorders.[95,96]

The association of venous thrombosis and certain laboratory findings suggest that the following measurements may be important when evaluating patients with venous thrombosis: 1) plasma levels of AT III, alpha-1 antitrypsin, alpha-2 macroglobulin, and plasminogen activator, 2) platelet coagulant activities, 3) tests for fibrin monomer or fibrinopeptides A and B, which reflect activation of the clotting pathways and the generation of thrombin, and 4) tests for degradation products of fibrin, which reflect secondary activation of fibrinolysis. However, it should again be emphasized that none of these activities in the blood has been conclusively shown to bear a causal relationship to venous thromboembolism. Thus, alterations in plasma levels of inhibitors, components, or products of the coagulation and fibrinolytic pathways—as currently tested—may occur in patients with diseases other than intravascular thrombosis. Furthermore, evidence is lacking that correction of a blood change presumed to predispose to thrombosis has actually reduced the frequency of venous thromboembolism.

PREVENTION OF VENOUS THROMBOSIS

Scanning studies of the legs utilizing ^{125}I-labeled fibrinogen have indicated that calf vein thrombosis is a common event in hospitalized patients.[97] The incidence in patients with myocardial infarction has been reported to be about 20%,[98,99] and in patients with stroke about 60%.[100] In patients over the age of 40 years undergoing major abdominal surgery, almost 30% developed calf vein thrombosis.[99,101] A still higher incidence has been found in patients following hip, prostate, or oncologic surgery. One third of these calf thrombi extended into proximal veins of the thigh, and one half of proximal vein thrombi embolized to the lungs.[107] These observations underscore the importance of prophylactic therapy for venous thrombosis. Several approaches to the prevention of venous thrombosis are currently in use: 1) anticoagulation with oral coumarin derivatives, 2) anticoagulation with full doses of intravenous heparin or low doses of subcutaneous heparin, 3) stimulation of blood flow in the legs by mechanical means, and 4) therapy with antiplatelet drugs.

Oral Anticoagulants

There is convincing evidence from many studies that therapy with oral anticoagulants is effective in preventing venous thrombosis. However, the increased risk of bleeding and the need for frequent monitoring has discouraged their use.[99]

Heparin in Full Doses

Full therapeutic doses of intravanous heparin followed by treatment with oral anticoagulants has reduced the frequency of venous thrombosis in patients with myocardial infarction.[108-110] Such therapy is generally restricted to patients without contraindications to anticoagulation such as a bleeding diathesis, active peptic ulcer disease, severe hypertension, a recently completed stroke, or liver and kidney dysfunction.

Low Dose Heparin

Recent developments in understanding the mechanism of action of heparin have provided a pharmacologic basis for this approach.[84,111] In brief, the anticoagulant action of heparin depends on the presence in plasma of an alpha-2 globulin known as AT III which inhibits several activated coagulation factors and, in particular, activated factor X (Xa) and thrombin. Heparin binds to AT III and alters its conformation. In so doing, heparin accelerates the reaction between AT III and the activated factors. The primary physiologic target of AT III is Xa, neutralization of which apparently helps to keep blood in the fluid state. Because the coagulation cascade represents a series of amplification steps, a smaller amount of heparin will be required to neutralize an intermediate product of the coagulation pathway (Xa) than is required to neutralize the final product (thrombin). By the same token, a lower dose of heparin will prevent thrombosis by neutralizing Xa than is required to turn off an established thrombotic process that has already generated large amounts of thrombin. The antithrombotic action of heparin may relate not only to its role as an inhibitor of the coagulation sequence, but also to its ability to adhere to the endothelium and increase the negative electrical potential of the vascular wall. The supranegative charge conferred by heparin may inhibit the accumulation of platelets.[77]

Many studies have demonstrated the effectiveness of small doses of subcutaneous heparin in preventing venous thrombosis in the legs and thighs of high-risk patients.[99,101,112,113] Persuasive evidence that low dose heparin prevents venous thrombosis and major pulmonary embolism in the surgical patient comes from the International Multicenter Trial.[101] This study involved more than 4000 patients who were over 40 years of age and undergoing major elective surgery. It showed significant reduction of the incidence of calf vein thrombosis (68% decline) as well as a decrease in total and fatal pulmonary embolism in the heparin-treated as compared to the control group. Bleeding was not a significant problem. Subcutaneous heparin was given in doses of 5000 units two hours prior to surgery and every eight hours thereafter for seven or more days. Patients convalescing from myocardial infarction are also protected from venous (but not mural) thrombosis by this method.[99,113,114]

Low dose heparin does not adequately protect patients who are recovering from hip or prostate surgery.[99,102-106] In the case of the patient with hip surgery, the process of venous thrombosis may establish itself preoperatively at the time of initial trauma[115]; if this were so, *prophylactic* doses of heparin would not be appropriate. Furthermore, the extensive bleeding inherent in certain forms of hip surgery implies extensive local release of platelet factor 4 (heparin-neutralizing activity) which may neutralize small doses of heparin and render the prophylaxis ineffective.[116,117] Another factor which promotes thrombosis in these patients is the extreme immobility that is common postoperatively.

Methods Which Increase Blood Flow in the Legs

Early mobilization following surgery and physiotherapy are simple procedures designed to overcome stasis in the legs and thereby reduce the incidence of venous thrombosis; their value is unproven. More complex methods of calf muscle stimulation using electrical and pneumatic means during and after surgery have proven safe and effective prophylactics against venous thrombosis.[118-120]

Antiplatelet Drugs

The use of aspirin for the prevention of venous thrombosis has given equivocal results.[121,122] This outcome is hardly surprising in view of the limited role of platelets in initiating and propagating the venous clot.

Dextrans are glucose polymers whose antithrombotic effects have been attributed to: 1) expansion of the blood volume which decreases blood viscosity, 2) surface-coating properties thought to reduce the interactions between endothelium and formed elements of the blood,[123] 3) induced platelet dysfunction[124] and, 4) copolymerization of dextran with fibrin monomer to produce an altered clot with increased susceptibility to fibrinolysis.[125] The efficacy of dextran 70 (mean molecular weight of 70,000) in preventing venous thrombosis has been demonstrated in controlled studies of surgical patients.[126-128] Side effects include volume expansion, allergic reaction, oliguria, and bleeding. The side effects, expense, and the need for repeated intravenous infusion has made dextran less than an ideal prophylactic agent in spite of the demonstrated efficacy.

The Council on Thrombosis of the American Heart Association has recommended low dose heparin as primary prophylaxis for all patients over the age of 40 years who undergo abdominal or thoracic surgery and who have no hemostatic defect or other contraindication to anticoagulation.[129] Low dose heparin therapy is not recommended in patients undergoing hip surgery because it is much less effective as a prophylactic and because the operative results may be jeopardized by a relatively minimal wound hematoma. The optimal preventive regimen for patients who require hip surgery has not yet been defined. Platelet suppression beginning before surgery and oral anticoagulation beginning one to two days after surgery, are under study.[99]

TREATMENT OF ACUTE VENOUS THROMBOEMBOLISM

Anticoagulant Therapy of Acute Pulmonary Embolism

A few patients have massive pulmonary embolism, which blocks the main pulmonary artery or the bifurcation; these patients usually die before effective therapy can be given. However, most patients survive the initial pulmonary embolism because of the large reserve in the pulmonary circulation. The immediate need in this group is to stop propagation of the thrombus in the lungs and at its source in the large veins of the thighs or pelvis. The rapid administration of a bolus of intravenous heparin and the maintenance of heparin anticoagulation for a number of days thereafter aims to neutralize preformed thrombin and frustrate the generation of more thrombin. In this way the closing off of additional pulmonary vessels is prevented and a fatal outcome is averted.

More heparin is needed to activate AT III so that it can neutralize preformed thrombin than is required to prevent thrombin formation (by neutralizing factor Xa).[84,111] Whereas the usual dose for prophylaxis is 10,000 to 15,000 international units per day subcutaneously, approximately 30,000 units per day intravenously are used for treatment of the acute thrombotic process. Lower doses are indicated in the elderly, particularly elderly women, where the risk of hemorrhage is greater.[130,131] Other factors which increase the risk of hemorrhage include diastolic hypertension; active peptic ulceration; abnormal hemostasis prior to therapy (eg, low platelet count, coagulation factor deficiency, uremia, or history of recent aspirin use); a history of recent surgery, invasive vascular procedures, or intramuscular injections; and coexisting renal or hepatic insufficiency.[132] The incidence of major bleeding episodes reported in patients treated with intermittent intravenous injections of heparin has ranged between 25% and 50% in the high risk group and between 7% and 15% in the others.[133] The administration of heparin by continuous intravenous infusion avoids the periods of blood incoagulability that regularly follow bolus injections and is significantly safer with respect to bleeding complications.[132]

Following three to six days of heparin therapy, oral anticoagulation with coumarin derivatives is begun, allowing an overlap of three to five days. The oral anticoagulants are generally continued for three to six months, but may be continued for longer periods if major risk factors persist, eg, deep venous insufficiency, prolonged immobility, obesity, or refractory heart failure. Recurrent pulmonary emboli, especially if associated with pulmonary hypertension, require long-term anticoagulation.

Anticoagulant Therapy of Fresh Deep Venous Thrombosis

The extraordinary risk of pulmonary embolism from an active thrombotic process in the popliteal, femoral, or iliac veins mandates immediate therapy with heparin. Acute thrombosis in the veins of the calf, whether clinically apparent or detected by ^{125}I-labeled fibrinogen scanning, may be treated supportively and should be carefully monitored for proximal extension.

The pharmacologic rationale of the anticoagulant therapy of fresh deep venous thrombosis and the methods of administration and control of heparin and coumarin are the same as for pulmonary embolism. The relative safety of continuous infusions with respect to bleeding and the apparently equal effectiveness in preventing recurrent thromboembolism recommend this procedure as the method of choice.[132] After an initial dose of 70 units/kg, heparin is infused at a constant rate of 1000 units per hour (range 500 to 1500 units per hour) with adjustments as required to maintain the activated partial thromboplastin time at 1.5 to 2 times control. Once the acute inflammation is suppressed and no proximal embolism has ensued (about two to six days), the patient may be treated with warfarin, 10 to 15 mg per day, allowing an overlap of three to five days before discontinuing the heparin. Some physicians continue the warfarin only until the patient has completely recovered and is fully ambulatory (about six weeks), whereas others treat for three to six months, depending on the size of the initial deep vein thrombus. Recurrent deep vein thrombosis requires long-term anticoagulation therapy and, where possible, correction of recognized as well as potentially important risk factors.

The major complication of warfarin treatment is bleeding, which is not likely to be severe provided that the prothrombin time is maintained between 1.5 and 2.5 times control. Oral anticoagulants interact with many drugs,[134,135] so that drugs must be introduced or withdrawn cautiously and with repeated testing of the prothrombin time during the first 10 to 14 days. The most dramatic nonbleeding side effect of warfarin is skin necrosis, which may develop between the third and tenth day of treatment.[136]

Thrombolytic Therapy with Streptokinase and Urokinase

Anticoagulation therapy for pulmonary embolism and deep venous thrombosis prevents life-threatening propagation of the clots which have traveled to the lungs, and of the source thrombi in the deep veins. Unless the endogenous fibrinolytic system in the veins and the pulmonary arteries clears the vessels of their fibrin clots, these clots undergo variable degrees of fibrous organization which can reduce the size of the pulmonary vascular bed and the competence of the deep venous valves. Failure of complete lysis by the endogenous system is particularly likely when the clots are large. Pulmonary hypertension following exercise or even at rest, or postphlebitic deep venous incompetence and insufficiency, with the attendant risks of recurrent episodes of thrombophlebitis and pulmonary embolism, may then ensue.

Thrombolytic therapy with streptokinase or urokinase accelerates the disappearance of acute pulmonary emboli,[137,138] decreasing pulmonary hypertension within six hours[139] and restoring the patency of the pulmonary microcirculation at one year.[140] In contrast, therapy with heparin has no capacity to lyse emboli. Indeed, patients who were randomized to treatment with heparin in the control arms of the studies cited above showed no reduction in pulmonary pressure or improvement in pulmonary capillary blood volume during the timeframes which were observed. In acute proximal deep vein thrombosis, thrombolytic therapy causes substantial or complete lysis in about one-half the patients, and results in much higher preservation of functional venous valves (confirmed venographically at three to five months) than does treatment with heparin alone.[141] The potential economic impact of intact and functioning venous valves is enormous. O'Donnell and his colleagues recently estimated the cost per patients of a severe postphlebitic syndrome at $40,000 over a period of ten years.[142]

In spite of the documented efficacy of thrombolytic agents in the therapy of pulmonary embolism and deep venous thrombosis, acceptance of this therapy by the medical community has been less than enthusiastic. The apparent reluctance to use thrombolytic agents stems in part from fear of serious bleeding and partly from lack of reliable data concerning the frequency of the postphlebitic syndrome and the frequency and clinical significance of the pulmonary hypertension which follow treatment with anticoagulants alone.

Much of the bleeding associated with the original trials of streptokinase and urokinase occurred from sites of venous cutdown and arterial puncture. Excessive surface bleeding of this nature can be eliminated by avoiding unnecessary vascular invasion and manipulation, by utilizing the arm rather than the thigh for pulmonary angiography, and by carefully compressing all sites of arterial and venous puncture. Even when this is done, the incidence of hemorrhage serious enough to require blood transfusion or interruption of therapy (eg, bleeding into the head, retroperitoneum, muscles, urinary, or gastrointestinal tracts) is 5% to 9% in low-risk patients treated with thrombolytic agents plus heparin, compared to 4% in patients treated with heparin alone.[143] Candidates for thrombolytic therapy must be screened carefully. For optimal treatment results, the clinical duration of the acute thrombosis should be less than seven days. Patients with active internal bleeding and those who have suffered a stroke or other active intracranial process within the previous two months must be rejected. Relatively major contraindications to thrombolytic therapy include a history of major surgery, organ biopsy, or invasion of a non-compressible vessel within the previous ten days; recent internal bleeding or serious trauma; and severe arterial hypertension (systolic pressure greater than 200 mm Hg, diastolic pressure greater than 110 mm Hg).[144]

Schrier[145] has recently called attention to widely divergent estimates of the frequency of the postphlebitic syndrome reported for patients with deep venous thrombosis who are treated with heparin alone: 11% in one review,[146] 40% to 80% in another.[147] He emphasized the need for prospective studies of the prevalence and clinical importance of hypertensive sequelae which occur as a result of thromboembolism in the pulmonary and venous circulations. Baseline information of this kind is required to assess intelligently the risk-to-benefit ratios of the thrombolytic methods which are currently available and of the modalities and regimens which will become available in the future.

Streptokinase, a product of the β hemolytic streptococcus, is antigenic in man. Individual patients differ in the streptococcal resistance of their plasma, which must be overcome in order to form the streptokinase-plasminogen complex that converts plasminogen to plasmin. Urokinase, concentrated from human urine or harvested from in vitro cultures of human embryonic kidney cells, activates plasminogen directly. The plasmin generated within fibrin clots after penetration of the drugs produces therapeutic thrombolysis.

Treatment of acute pulmonary embolism with one course of streptokinase (24 hours) costs about $230 and of urokinase (12 hours), about $2100.[148] The Food and Drug Administration has recommended streptokinase for primary lysis of acute deep vein thrombosis. Dissolution of the clot may be monitored serially with impedance plethysmography, and often requires 72 or more hours of streptokinase infusion.[141] Guidelines for the use of thrombolytic agents, including eligibility requirements, dosages, and laboratory monitoring, and for the tandem initiation of anticoagulation with heparin, have recently been published.[149,150]

REFERENCES

1. Wessler S. Prevention and treatment of thrombosis. *Adv Intern Med* 22:187, 1977.

2. National Heart, Blood Vessel, Lung, and Blood Program, National Heart and Lung Institute Summary, National Heart and Lung Institute—National Institutes of Health, Department of Health, Education and Welfare, Vol 1, 1973, p 10.

3. Dalen JE, Alpert JS. Natural history of pulmonary embolism. In Sasahara AA, Sonneblick EH, Lesch M. (eds). *Pulmonary Emboli* New York, Grune & Stratton, 1975, p 77.

4. Virchow R. *Gesammette Abhandlungen Zur Wissenschaftlichen Medicin,* Frankfurt: Meidinger Sohn M. Comp., 1856, p 158 ff. Cited by Brinkhous, KM. The problem in perspective. In Sherry S, Brinkhous KH, Genton E, et al (eds). *Thrombosis* Washington, National Academy of Sciences; 1969, p 335.

5. Harker LA, Slichter SJ. Arterial and venous thromboembolism: Kinetic characterisation and evaluation of therapy. *Thromb Diath Haemorrh* 31:188, 1974.

6. Chandler AB. The anatomy of a thrombus. In Sherry S, Brinkhous M, Genton E, et al (eds). *Thrombosis.* Washington, National Academy of Sciences, 1969, p 279.

7. Didisheim P, Fuster V. Action and clinical status of platelet suppressive agents. *Semin Hematol* 15:55, 1978.

8. Marcus AJ. Platelet function. *N Engl J Med* 280:1213-1220, 1278-1284, 1330-1335, 1969.

9. Marcus AJ. The role of lipids in platelet function with particular reference to the arachidonic acid pathway. *J Lipid Res* 19:793, 1978.

10. Weiss H. Platelet physiology and abnormalities of platelet function. *N Engl J Med* 293:531-540, 580-588, 1975.

11. Sixma JJ, Wester J. The hemostatic plug. *Semin Hematol* 14:265, 1977.

12. Ross R, Glomset JA. Atherosclerosis and the arterial smooth muscle cell: Proliferation of smooth muscle is a key event in the genesis of the lesions of atherosclerosis. *Science* 180:1332, 1973.

13. Walsh PN. Platelet coagulant activities and hemostasis: A hypothesis. *Blood* 43:597, 1974.

14. Moncada S, Vane JR. Arachidonic acid metabolites and the interactions between platelets and blood-vessel walls. *N Engl J Med* 300:1142, 1979.

15. Weksler BB, Leye W, Jaffe EA. Stimulation of endothelial cell prostacyclin production of thrombin, trypsin and the ionophore A23187. *J Clin Invest* 62:923, 1978.

16. Whiting J, Salata K, Bailey JM. Aspirin: An unexpected side effect on prostacyclin synthesis in cultured vascular smooth muscle cells. *Science* 210:663, 1980.

17. Roth GJ, Stanford N, Marjerus RW. Acetylation of prostanglandin synthase by aspirin. *Proc Natl Acad Sci USA* 72:3073, 1975.

18. McDonald JWD, Ali M, Nagi GR, et al. Inhibition of platelet prostaglandin synthetase and platelet release reaction by sulfinpyrazone. *Blood* 46:10, 1975.

19. Marcus AJ, Weksler BB, Jaffe EA, et al. Synthesis of prostacyclin from platelet-derived endoperoxides by cultured human endothelial cells. *J Clin Invest* 66:979, 1980.

20. Gerrard JM, White JG. Prostaglandins and thromboxanes: "Middlemen" modulating platelet function in hemostasis and thrombosis. *Prog Hemost Thromb* 4:87, 1978.

21. Zucker MB. Unpublished observation cited in: Marcus AJ, Zucker MB: *The Physiology of Blood Platelets* New York, Grune & Statton, 1965, p 53.

22. Mills DCB, Smith JB. The influence on platelet aggregation of drugs that affect the accumulation of adenosine 3′,5′—cyclic monophosphate in platelets. *Biochem J* 121:185, 1971.

23. Ross R, Glomset JA. The pathogenesis of atherosclerosis. *N Engl J Med* 295:369–377, 420–425, 1976.

24. Michaeli D, Orloff KG. Molecular consideration of platelet adhesion. *Prog Hemost Thromb* 3:29, 1976.

25. Sagel J, Colwell JA, Crook L, et al. Increased platelet aggregation in early diabetes mellitus. *Ann Intern Med* 82:733, 1975.

26. Heath H, Brigden WD, Canever JV, et al. Platelet adhesiveness and aggregation in relation to diabetic retinopathy. *Diabetologia* 7:308, 1971.

27. Carvalho ACA, Colman RW, Lees RS. Platelet function in hyperlipoproteinemia. *N Engl J Med* 290:434, 1974.

28. Frishman WH, Weksler B, Christodouleu JP, et al. Reversal of abnormal platelet aggregability and change in exercise tolerance in patients with angina pectoris following oral propranolol. *Circulation* 50:887, 1974.

29. Halushka PV, Lurie D, Colwell JA. Increased synthesis of prostaglandin-E-like material by platelets from patients with diabetes mellitus. *N Engl J Med* 297:1306, 1977.

30. Born GVR, Cross MJ. The aggregation of blood platelets. *J Physiol* (Lond) 168:178, 1963.

31. Preston PE, Emmanual IG, Winfield DA, et al. Essential thrombocythemia and peripheral gangrene. *Br Med J* 3:548, 1974.

32. Wu KK. Platelet hyperaggregability and thrombosis in patients with thrombocythemia. *Ann Intern Med* 88:7, 1978.

33. O'Malley BC, Timperly WR, Ward JD, et al. Platelet abnormalities in diabetic peripheral neuropathy. *Lancet* 2:1274, 1975.

34. Wu KK, Hoak JC. Spontaneous platelet aggregation in arterial insufficiency. Mechanism and implications. *Thromb Haemost* 35:702, 1976.

35. Walsh PN. Role of platelets in the pathogenesis of venous thrombosis. In Frantantoni J, Wessler S (eds). *Prophylactic Therapy of Deep Vein Thrombosis and Pulmonary Embolism.* Washington, U.S. GPO (DHEW Publication No. NH 76-886), 1975, p 60.

36. Walsh PN, Pareti FI, Corbett JJ. Platelet coagulant activities and serum lipids in transient cerebral ischemia. *N Engl J Med* 295:854, 1974.

37. Wu KK, Hoak JC. A new method for the quantitative detection of platelet aggregates in patients with arterial insufficiency. *Lancet* 2:924, 1974.

38. Wu KK, Hoak JC. Increased platelet aggregates in patients with transient ischemic attacks. *Stroke* 6:521, 1975.

39. Harker LA, Slichter SJ, Scott CR, et al. Hemocystinemia. Vascular injury and arterial thrombosis. *N Engl J Med* 291:537, 1974.

40. Harker LA. Platelet survival time: Its measurement and use. *Prog Hemost Thromb* 4:321, 1978.

41. Garg SK, Lackner H, Karpatkin S. The increased percentage of megathrombocytes in various clinical disorders. *Ann Intern Med* 77:361, 1972.

42. Mustard JF, Packham MA. Platelets and diabetes mellitus. *N Engl J Med* 297:1345, 1977.

43. Harker L, Ross K, Slichter J, et al. Homocystine induced arteriosclerosis. The role of endothelial cell injury and platelet response in its genesis. *J Clin Invest* 58:731, 1976.

44. Ellis JB, Krentz LS, Levine SP. Increased plasma platelet factor 4 (PF4) in patients with coronary artery disease. (Abstract) Supplements to *Circulation* 57 and 58, (suppl II):II-116, 1978.

45. Green LH, Seroppian E, Handin RI. Platelet activation during exercise induced myocardial ischemia. *N Engl J Med* 302:193, 1980.

46. Handin RI, McDonough M, Lesch M. Elevation of platelet factor 4 in acute myocardial infarction: Measurement by radioimmunoassay. *J Lab Clin Med* 91:340, 1978.

47. Marouf AA, Workman EF, White GCII. Elevation of high affinity platelet factor 4 (HA-PF4) in hypercoagulable states. (Abstract) Supplements to *Circulation* 57 and 58 (suppl II):II-116, 1978.

48. Ludlam Ca, Bolton AE, Moore S, et al. New rapid method for diagnosis of deep vein thrombosis. *Lancet* 2:259, 1975.

49. Adler AJ, Lundin AP, Feinroth MV, et al. β-thromboglobulin levels in nephrotic syndrome. *Am J Med* 69:551, 1980.

50. Roth GJ, Majerus PW. The mechanism of the effect of aspirin on human platelets. I. Acetylation of a particular protein fraction. *J Clin Invest* 56:624, 1975.

51. Weiss JH, Aledort LM. Impaired platelet/connective tissue reaction in man after aspirin ingestion. *Lancet* 2:495, 1967.

52. Weiss HJ. The pharmacology of platlet inhibition. *Prog Hemost Thromb* 1:191, 1973.

53. Kelton JC, Hirsch J, Buchanan MR. Thrombogenic effects of high dose aspirin in rabbits. Relationship to inhibition of vessel wall synthesis of prostaglandin I2-like activity. *J Clin Invest* 62:892, 1978.

54. Benziger NL, Dillender MJ, Majerus PW. Cultured human skin fibroblast and arterial cells produce a labile platelet—inhibitor prostaglandin. *Biochem Biophys Res Commun* 78:294, 1977.

55. Harker LA, Wall RT, Harlan JM, et al. Sulfinpyrazone prevention of homocystine induced endothelial cell injury and arteriosclerosis. *Clin Res* 26:554A, 1978.

56. Marcus JF, Packham MA. Factors influencing platelet function: Adhesion, release and aggregation. *Pharmacol Rev* 22:97, 1970.

57. Mustard JF, Kinlough-Rathbone RL, Jenkins CSP, et al. Modification of platelet function. *Ann NY Acad Sci* 201:343, 1972.

58. The Anturane Reinfarction Trial Research Group. Sulfinpyrazone in the prevention of sudden death after myocardial infarction. *N Engl J Med* 302:250, 1980.

59. Elwood PC, Sweetnam PM. Aspirin and secondary mortality after myocaridal infarction. *Lancet* 2:1313, 1979.

60. Klint CR. CDPA study. *Thromb Haemost* 35:49, 1976.

61. Wood L. Aspirin and myocardial infarction. *Lancet* 2:1021, 1972.

62. Boston Collaborative Study Surveillance Group. Regular aspirin intake and acute myocardial infarction. *Br Med J* 1:440, 1974.

63. The Canadian Cooperative Study Group. A randomised trial of aspirin and sulfinpyrazone in threatened stroke. *N Engl J Med* 299:53, 1978.

64. Fields WS, Lemak NA, Frankowski RF, et al. Controlled trial of aspirin in cerebral ischemia. *Stroke* 8:301, 1977.

65. Sullivan JM, Harken DE, Gorlin R. Pharmacologic control of complications of cardiac valve replacement. *N Engl J Med* 284:1391, 1971.

66. Altman R, Boulton F, Rouvier J, et al. Aspirin and prophylaxis of thromboembolic complications in patients with substitute heart valves. *J Thorac Cardiovasc Surg* 72:127, 1976.

67. Steele PP, Weilby HS, Davies H, et al. Platelet survival in patients with rheumatic heart disease. *N Engl J Med* 290:537, 1974.

68. Steele PP, Rainwater JO, Genton E. Favorable effects of sulfinpyrazone on thromboembolism in patients with rheumatic heart disease. *Clin Res* 27:205A, 1979.

69. Harter HR, Burch JW, Majerus RW, et al. Prevention of thrombosis in patients on hemodialysis by low dose aspirin. *N Engl J Med* 301:577, 1979.

70. Kaegi A, Pineo GF, Shimizu A, et al. Arteriovenous-shunt thrombosis. Prevention by sulfinpyrazone. *N Engl J Med* 290:304, 1974.

71. Sevitt S. Venous thrombosis in injured patients (with some observation on pathogenesis). In Sherry S, Brinkhous KM, Genton E, et al (eds). *Thrombosis.* Washington, National Academy of Sciences; 1969, p 29.

72. Sevitt S. Organization of valve pocket thrombi and the anomalies of double thrombi and valve cusp involvement. *Br J Surg* 61:641, 1974.

73. Paterson JC. The pathology of venous thrombi. In Sherry S, Brinkhous KM, Genton E, et al (eds). *Thrombosis.* Washington, National Academy of Sciences, 1969, p 321.

74. Wessler S. The role of stasis in thrombosis. In Sherry S, Brinhous KM, Genton E, et al (eds). *Thrombosis.* Washington, National Academy of Sciences; 1969, p 461.

75. Hirsh J. Hypercoagulability. *Semin Hematol* 14:409, 1977.

76. Sixma JJ. Techniques for diagnosing prethrombotic states. A review. *Thromb Haemost* 40:252, 1978.

77. Jacques LB. Heparin: An old drug with a new paradigm. *Science* 206:528, 1979.

78. Gjonnaess H, Fagerhol MK. Studies on coagulation and fibrinolysis in pregnancy. *Acta Obstet Gynecol Scand* 54:363, 1975.

79. Poller L, Thomson JM, Thomas W. Oestrogen-progestrogen oral contraception and blood clotting. A long term follow up. *Br Med J* 4:648, 1971.

80. Penick GD, Dejanov II, Reddick RL, et al. Predisposition to intravascular coagulation. *Thromb Diath Haemorrh* (suppl) 21:543, 1966.

81. Pineo GF, Brain MC, Gallus AS, et al. Tumors, mucus production and hypercoagulability. *Ann NY Acad Sci* 230:262, 1974.

82. Blatt RM, Lundblad RL, Kingdon HS, et al. Thrombogenic materials in prothrombin complex concentrates. *Ann Intern Med* 81:766, 1974.

83. Preston FE, Winfield DA, Malia RG, et al. Serial changes in the coagulation system following clotting factor concentrate infusion. *Thromb Diath Haemorrh* 34:475, 1975.

84. Rosenberg RD. Actions and interactions of antithrombin and heparin. *N Engl J Med* 292:146, 1975.

85. Harpel PC, Rosenberg RD. α_2 macroglobulin and antithrombin-heparin cofactor: Modulators of hemostatic and inflammatory reaction, *Prog Hemost Thromb* 3:145, 1976.

86. Egeberg O. Inherited antithrombin deficiency causing thrombophilia. *Thromb Diath Haemorrh* 13:516, 1965.

87. Marciniak E, Farley CH, DeSimone PA. Familial thrombosis due to antithrombin III deficiency. *Blood* 43:219, 1974.

88. Sagar S, Stamatakis JD, Thomas DP, et al. Oral contraceptives, antithrombin III activity and postoperative deep vein thrombosis. *Lancet* 1:509, 1976.

89. Astedt B. Significance of placenta in depression of fibrinolytic activity during pregnancy. *J Obstet Gynaecol Br Common* 79:205, 1972.

90. Astedt B, Isacson S, Nillson IM, et al. Thrombosis and oral contraceptives. Possible predisposition. *Br Med J* 4:631, 1973.

91. Yagge J. Changes in blood coagulation and fibrinolysis during the postoperative period. *Am J Surg* 119:225, 1970.

92. Rennie JAN, Ogston D. Fibrinolytic activity in malignant disease. *J Clin Pathol* 28:872, 1975.

93. Grace CS. The fibrinolytic enzyme system in obesity. The effects of venous occlusion and in vitro activation of surface contact. *Clin Sci* 34:497, 1968.

94. Walsh PN, Goldberg RE, Tax RL, et al. Platelet coagulant activities and retinal vein thrombosis. *Thromb Haemost* 38:399, 1977.

95. Gunz FW. Hemorrhagic thrombocythemia; a critical review. *Blood* 15:706, 1960.

96. Hirsh J, Dacie JV. Persistent post-splenectomy thrombocytosis and thromboembolism. A consequence of continuing anemia. *Br J Haematol* 7:44, 1966.

97. Gallus AS, Hirsh J, Hull R, et al. Diagnosis of venous thromboembolism. *Semin Thromb Hemostas* 2:203, 1976.

98. Maurer BJ, Wray R, Schillingford JP. Frequency of venous thrombosis after myocardial infarction. *Lancet* 2:1385, 1971.

99. Gallus AS, Hirsh J. Prevention of venous thromboembolism. *Semin Thromb Hemostas* 2:232, 1976.

100. Warlow C, Ogston D, Douglas AS. Venous thrombosis following strokes. *Lancet* 1:1305, 1972.

101. International Multicenter Trial. Prevention of fatal postoperative pulmonary embolism by low doses of heparin. *Lancet* 2:45, 1975.

102. Field ES, Micolaides AN, Kakkar VV, et al. Deep vein thrombosis in patients with fractures of the femoral neck. *Br J Surg* 59:377, 1972.

103. Hampson WGJ, Harris FC, Lucas HK, et al. Failure of low dose heparin to prevent deep vein thrombosis after hip replacement arthroplasty. *Lancet* 2:795, 1974.

104. Morris GK, Henry APJ, Preston BJ. Prevention of deep vein thrombosis by low dose heparin in patients undergoing total hip replacement. *Lancet* 2:797, 1974.

105. Mayo ME, Habil T, Browse NL. The incidence of deep vein thrombosis after prostatectomy. *Br J Urol* 43:738, 1971.

106. Nicolaides AN, Field ES, Kakkar VV, et al. Prostatectomy and deep vein thrombosis. *Br J Surg* 59:487, 1972.

107. Kakkar V, Howe C, Flanc C, et al. Natural history of postoperative deep vein thrombosis. *Lancet* 2:230, 1969.

108. Wright IS, Marple CD, Beck DF. Report of the committee for the evaluation of anticoagulants in the treatment of coronary thrombosis with myocardial infarction. *Am Heart J* 36:801, 1948.

109. Handley AJ, Emerson PA, Fleming PR. Heparin in the prevention of deep vein thrombosis after myocardial infarction. *Br Med J* 2:436, 1972.

110. Wray R, Maurer B, Schillingford J. Prophylactic anticoagulant therapy in the prevention of calf vein thrombosis after myocardial infarction. *N Engl J Med* 288:815, 1973.

111. Rosenberg RD. Heparin action. *Circulation* 44:603, 1974.

112. Nicolaides AN, Dupont PA, Desais S, et al. Small doses of subcutaneous heparin in preventing deep vein thrombosis after major surgery. *Lancet* 2:890, 1972.

113. Warlow C, Terry G, Kenmure ACF, et al. A double-blind trial of low doses of subcutaneous heparin in the prevention of deep vein thrombosis after myocardial infarction. *Lancet* 2:934, 1973.

114. McGehee W, Hirsh J. Antithrombotic Therapy. Education Program of the American Society of Hematology, 1980, p 61.

115. Heatley RV, Hughes LE, Morgan A, et al. Preoperative or postoperative deep-vein thrombosis? *Lancet* 1:437, 1976.

116. Sagar S, Stamatakis JD, Higgins AF, et al. Efficacy of low-dose heparin in the prevention of extensive deep vein thrombosis in patients undergoing total hip replacement arthroplasty. *Lancet* 1:1151, 1976.

117. Walsh PN. Platelets, heparin and blood coagulation. In Kakkar VV, Thomas DP (eds). *Heparin, Chemistry and Clinical Usage.* London, Academic Press, 1976, p 125.

118. Nicolaides AN, Kakkar VV, Field ES, et al. Optimal electrical stimulus for prevention of deep vein thrombosis. *Br Med J* 3:756, 1972.

119. Hills NH, Pflug JJ, Jeyasingh K, et al. Prevention of deep vein thrombosis by intermittent pneumatic compression of calf. *Br Med J* 1:131, 1972.

120. Roberts VC, Cotton LT. Prevention of postoperative deep vein thrombosis in patients with malignant disease. *Br Med J* 1:358, 1974.

121. Medical Research Council (Report of the Steering Committee). Effect of aspirin on postoperative venous thrombosis. *Lancet* 2:441, 1972.

122. Harris W, Salzman EW, Athanasoulis CA, et al. Aspirin prophylaxis of venous thromboembolism after total hip replacement. *N Engl J Med* 297:1246, 1977.

123. Ponder E, Ponder RV. Age and molecular weight of dextrans, their coating effects, and their interactions with serum albumin. *Nature* 190:277, 1961.

124. Weiss H. The effect of clinical dextran on platelet aggregation, adhesion and ADP release in man: In vivo and in vitro studies. *J Lab Clin Med* 69:37, 1967.

125. Wallenbeck IAM, Tangen O. On the lysis of fibrin formed in the presence of dextran and other macromolecules. *Thromb Res* 6:75, 1975.

126. Data JL, Nies AS. Dextran 40. *Ann Int Med* 81:500, 1974.

127. Carter AE, Eban R. The prevention of postoperative deep vein thrombosis with dextran 70. *Br J Surg* 60:681, 1973.

128. Atik M. Dextran 40 and dextran 70: A review. *Arch Surg* 94:664, 1967.

129. American Heart Association. Prevention of venous thromboembolism in surgical patients by low-dose heparin. Special report prepared by the Council on Thrombosis. *Circulation* 55:423A, 1977.

130. Jick H, Slone D, Borda IT, et al. Efficacy and toxicity of heparin in relation to age and sex. *N Engl J Med* 279:284, 1968.

131. Vieweg WVR, Piscatelli RL, House JJ, et al. Complications of intravenous administration of heparin in elderly women. *JAMA* 213:1303, 1970.

132. Salzman EW, Deykin D, Shapiro RM, et al. Management of heparin therapy: controlled prospective trial. *N Engl J Med* 292:1046, 1975.

133. Thomas DP. Heparin in the prophylaxis and treatment of venous thromboembolism. *Semin Hematol* 15:1, 1978.

134. Koch-Weser J, Sellers EM. Drug interaction with coumarin anticoagulants. *N Engl J Med* 285:487–498, 547–588, 1971.

135. O'Reilly RA. The pharmacodynamics of the oral anticoagulant drugs. *Prog Hemost Thromb* 2:175, 1974.

136. Romanucci D, Jackovic LG, Smedberg K. Anticoagulants and hemorrhagic breast necrosis: A case report. *Angiology* 25:612, 1974.

137. The urokinase pulmonary embolism trial: A national cooperative study. *Circulation suppl* 47:II-1, 1973.

138. Urokinase-streptokinase embolism trial: Phase 2 results: A cooperative study. *JAMA* 229:1606, 1974.

139. Murray JA, Blackman JR. Rate of resolution of pulmonary emboli treated with urokinase (Abstr). *Circulation suppl* 43 and 44:II-56, 1971.

140. Sharma GVRK, Burleson VA, Sasahara AA. Effect of thrombolytic therapy on pulmonary capillary blood volume in patients with pulmonary embolism. *N Engl J Med* 303:842, 1980.

141. Elliot MS, Immelman EJ, Jeffrey R, et al. A comparative randomized trial of heparin versus streptokinase in the treatment of acute proximal venous thrombosis: An interim report of a prospective trial. *Br J Surg* 66:838, 1979.

142. O'Donnell TF, Browse NC, Burnand KG, et al. The socioeconomic effects of an ilio-femoral thrombosis. *J Surg Res* 22:483, 1977.

143. Marder VJ. Are we using fibrinolytic agents often enough? (editorial). *Ann Intern Med* 93:136, 1980.

144. A National Institutes of Health consensus development conference. Thrombolytic therapy in thrombosis. *Ann Intern Med* 93:141, 1980.

145. Schrier SL. Thrombolytic therapy (editorial). *Ann Intern Med* 93:629, 1980.

146. Verstraete M. Biochemical and clinical aspects of thrombolysis. *Semin Hematol* 15:35, 1978.

147. Kistner RL, Sparkuhl MD. Surgery in acute and chronic venous disease. *Surgery* 85:31, 1979.

148. Sherry S. Personal communication. October 1980.

149. Bell WR, Meed AG. Guidelines for the use of thrombolytic agents. *N Engl J Med* 301:1266, 1979.

150. Marder VJ. The use of thrombolytic agents: Choice of patients, drug administration, laboratory monitoring. *Ann Intern Med* 90:802, 1979.

16 Noninvasive Diagnosis of Vascular Disease

Edward H. Smith

The addition of ultrasound and computed tomography to the diagnostic armamentarium has revolutionized the radiologic diagnostic approach in most areas of medicine. This is especially true in neuro-diagnosis, the staging of malignancies, the evaluation of renal transplants, to name just a few. In many instances these noninvasive, or relatively noninvasive, techniques have greatly streamlined the diagnostic workup and have obviated the need for more hazardous procedures, including angiography and exploratory surgery.

In the area of vascular disease, these new modalities have proven to be quite useful, but arteriography has remained the diagnostic method of choice in most instances.

This chapter will illustrate the application of these modalities to the diagnosis of vascular disease.

ULTRASOUND

Ultrasound consists of mechanical pressure waves, which propagate through a medium as particle oscillations with a frequency, as applied to medical diagnosis, in the order of 1 to 10 MHz. Because a sound beam is sensitive to differences in acoustic impedance, ultrasonography can detect boundaries between structures of similar radiologic density. At these acoustical boundaries or interfaces, a portion of the sound beam is reflected back to the transducer, which functions both as a transmitter and receiver. The reflected echoes are converted to electrical impulses, which in turn coalesce to form an image that can be recorded.[1]

At the present time, there are no known adverse effects from ultrasound at the energy levels used in medical diagnosis. No special preparation of the patient is needed and only minimal patient cooperation is required. Since the ultrasound beam cannot penetrate gas, the application of ultrasound to abnormalities of the lungs is extremely limited. Similarly, abdominal ileus may markedly interfere with satisfactory completion of the examination. Scanning over bony structures, as well as marked obesity, may contribute to a suboptimal examination.

Equipment and Technique

Up until recently, the majority of examinations have been performed with an articulated arm scanner, in which the transducer, attached to a rod system, is manually moved over the desired plane of interrogation, with the transducer in contact with the skin surface. This produces a static image, which is then photographed. More recently, dynamic scanners have become available. These may be either electronic or mechanical and produce dynamic images analogous to fluoroscopy so that moving structures, such as a pulsating vessel, may be imaged in "real time." Dynamic scanning allows imaging in an infinite number of planes, greatly facilitating three-dimensional conceptualization as well as significantly reducing examination time and dependence upon operator skill.

Abdominal Aortic Aneurysm

Ultrasound examination should be the first diagnostic examination when an abdominal aortic aneurysm is suspected.[2,3] Very often, especially in elderly women with lax abdominal musculature, the abdominal aorta is quite anterior and easily palpable and an aneurysm is often diagnosed. Ultrasound examination quickly reveals the aorta to be superficially situated and normal in diameter, ie, up to 3 cm in diameter[4] (Figure 16-1). One can also visualize the branches of the abdominal aorta including the celiac axis (Figures 16-2, 16-3), the superior mesenteric artery (Figure 16-3), and the renal artery (Figure

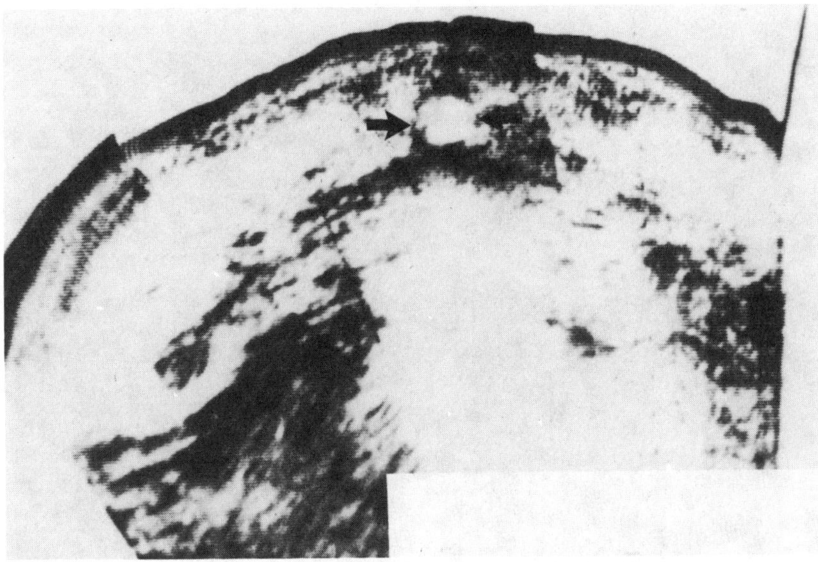

A

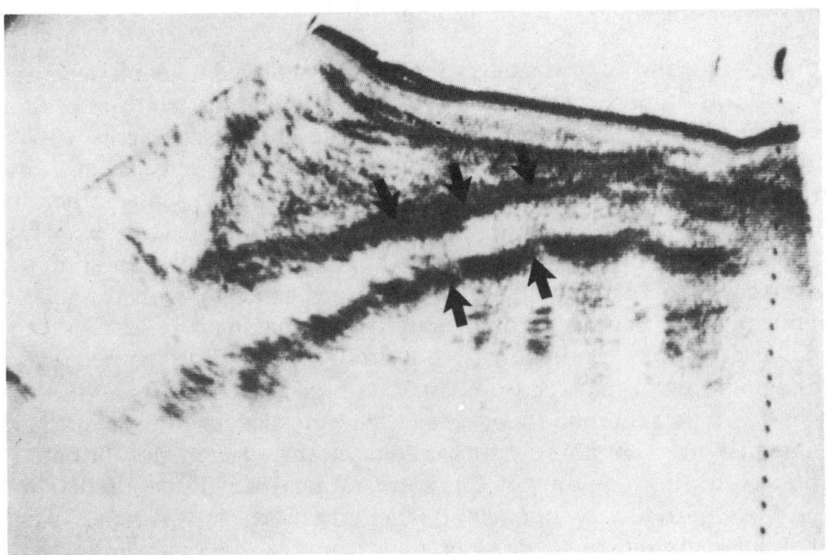

B

Figures 16-1A,B Transverse and sagittal scans revealing a normal-sized aorta (arrows) very superficially located.

16-4). Occasionally, a mass surrounding or adjacent to the aorta simulates an aneurysm clinically. Again, ultrasound examination will readily distinguish between the two conditions (Figure 16-5).

An aortic aneurysm is essentially a fluid-filled structure, sur-

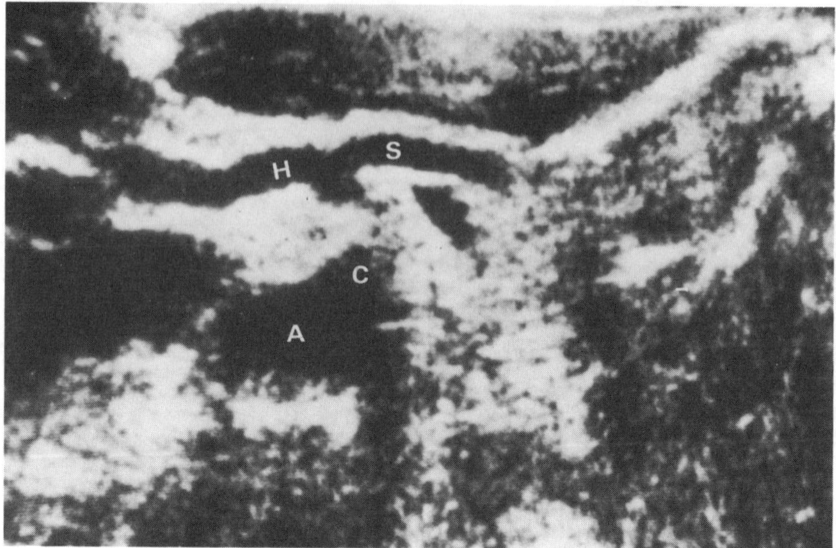

Figure 16-2 Transverse scan through abdominal aorta (A) with celiac axis (C). H = Hepatic artery, S = splenic artery.

rounded by solid organs and is therefore readily detectable (Figure 16-6). Occasionally, angiography will fail to reveal the true size of the aneurysm due to clot within the wall of the aneurysm (Figure 16-7). Ultrasound examination can often distinguish the patent lumen from thrombus (Figures 16-8, 16-9). It is a matter of opinion as to whether or not arteriography should be perfomed after an aneurysm is detected by ultrasound.[2,3] Some surgeons require angiographic documentation of the extent of involvement, while others are satisfied with the ultrasound imaging. With high quality dynamic imaging, the level of the renal arteries may be demonstrated, probably avoiding the necessity for angiography in many instances.

It is important not to overestimate the size of the aneurysm erroneously by obtaining transverse sections, which are oriented obliquely to the long axis of the aorta rather than perpendicular to it. This is particularly important when the aorta is tortuous. With dynamic scanning, the course of the aorta can be easily followed, essentially eliminating this problem.

Complications of aortic aneurysm surgery can also be evaluated with ultrasound. Figure 16-10 demonstrates the ultrasound findings in a patient with an aortic "Y" graft surrounded on both sides of the midline by a fluid collection. The clinical impression was partial dehiscence of the graft with hemorrhage. Under ultrasound guidance,

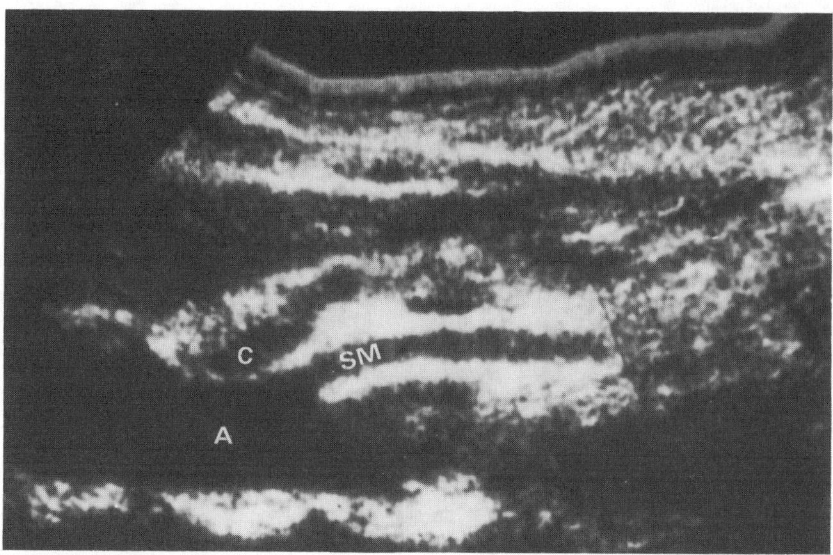

Figure 16-3A Sagittal scan through aorta (A), celiac axis (C), and superior mesenteric artery (SM).

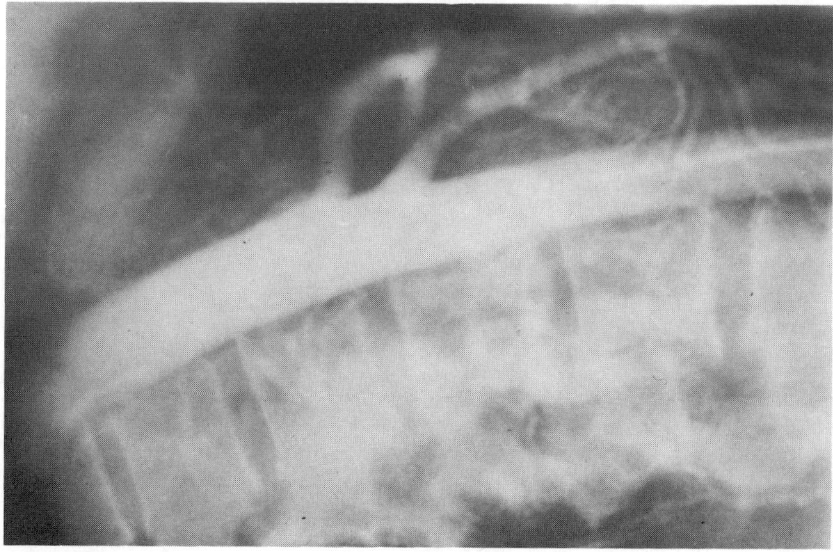

Figure 16-3B Lateral abdominal aortogram revealing celiac axis and superior mesenteric artery.

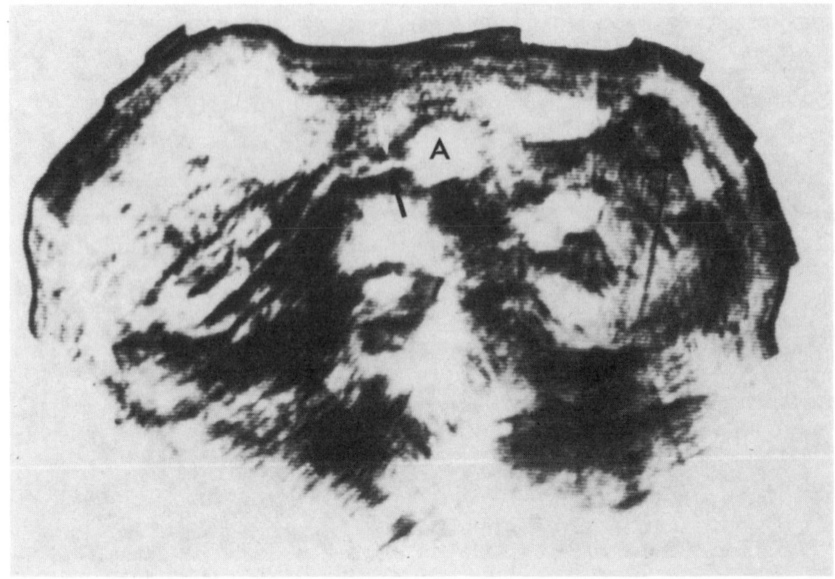

Figure 16-4 Transverse section through abdominal aorta (A) and right renal artery (arrows).

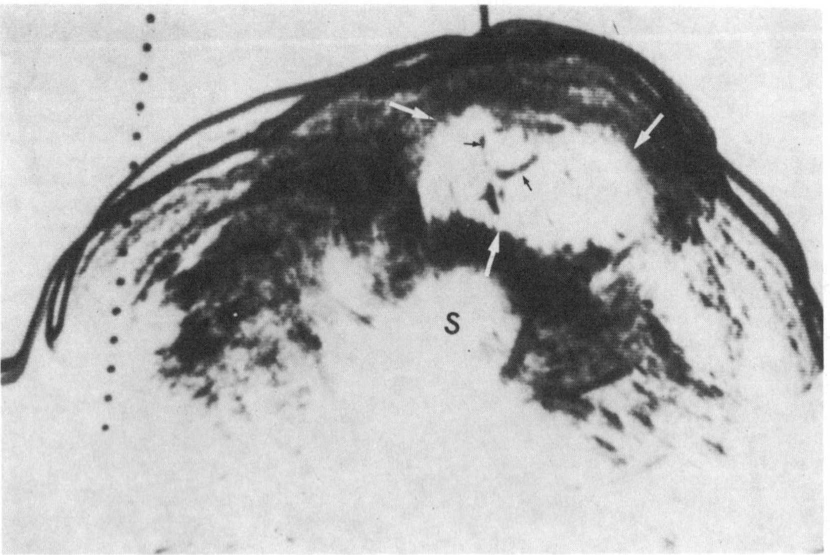

Figure 16-5 Transverse ultrasound scan showing normal caliber aorta (black arrows) separated from spine (S) by large echo poor lymphomatous mass (white arrows).

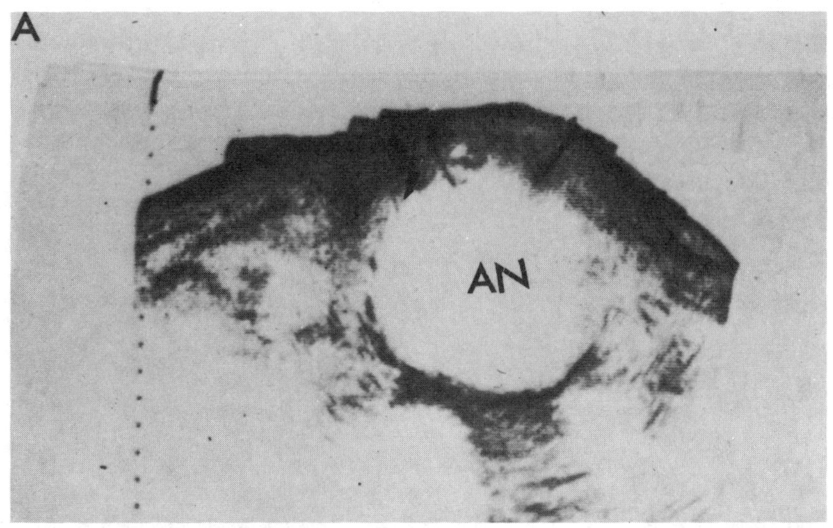

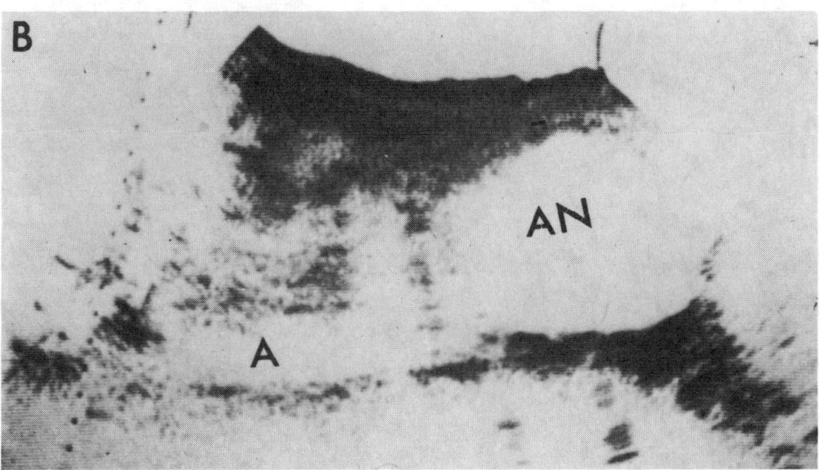

Figures 16-6A,B Transverse and sagittal ultrasound scans through sacular abdominal aortic aneurysm. Centimeter marker to left. A = normal caliber proximal aorta, AN = aneurysm.

fine needle aspiration of the fluid collection revealed a seroma and further surgery was avoided. Aortic rupture with hematoma formation will have a similar appearance.[5] Dissecting aneurysms cannot be visualized consistently, but ultrasound examination may demonstrate an interface within an aneurysm. In some instances, ultrasound studies may be diagnostic when angiography has been normal.[6]

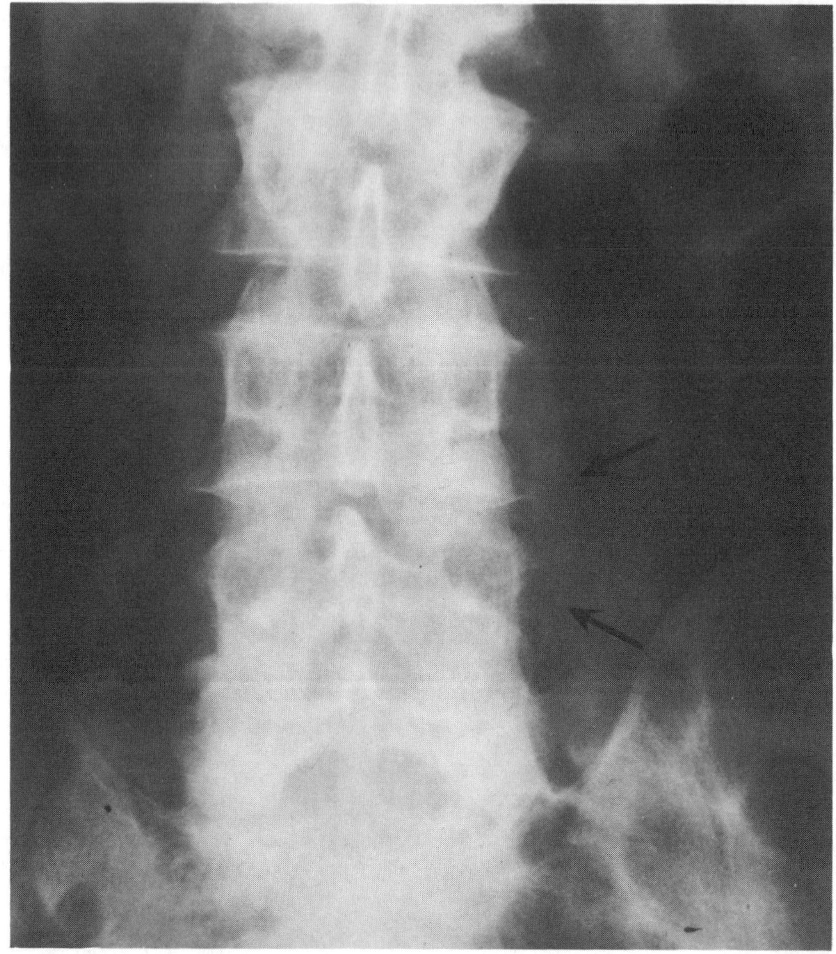

Figure 16-7A Plain film of the abdomen reveals curvilinear calcification to the left of the lumbar spine (arrows).

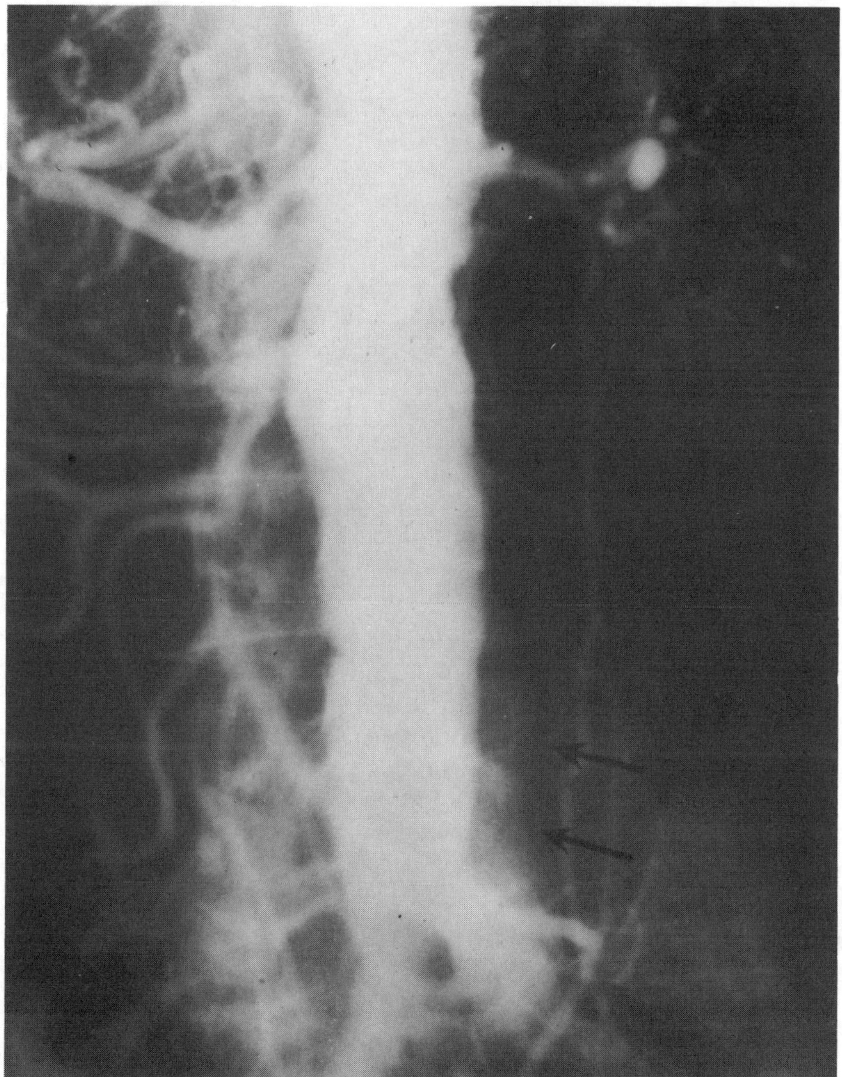

Figure 16-7B Aortogram reveals what appears to be a normal-sized aortic lumen. Note the calcification (arrows) to be situated well lateral of the contrast-filled portion of the lumen. Also note lack of filling of the lumbar arteries on the left.

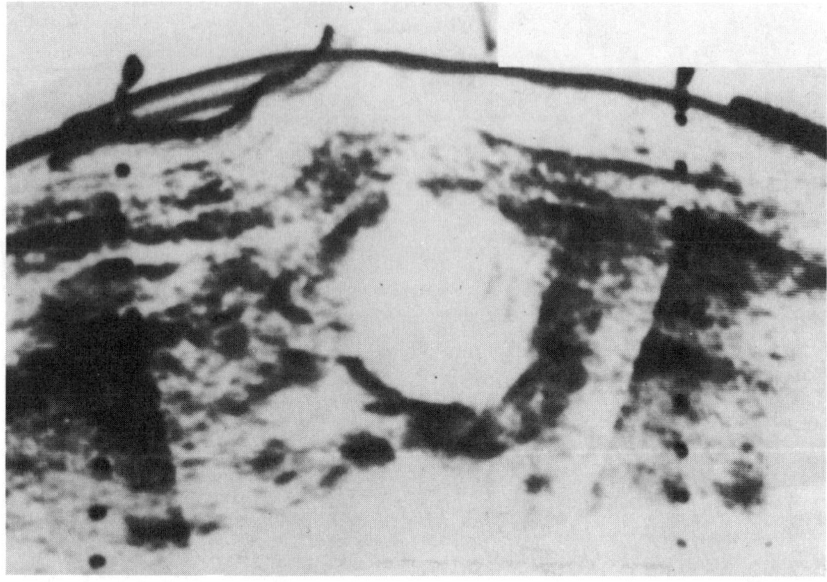

C

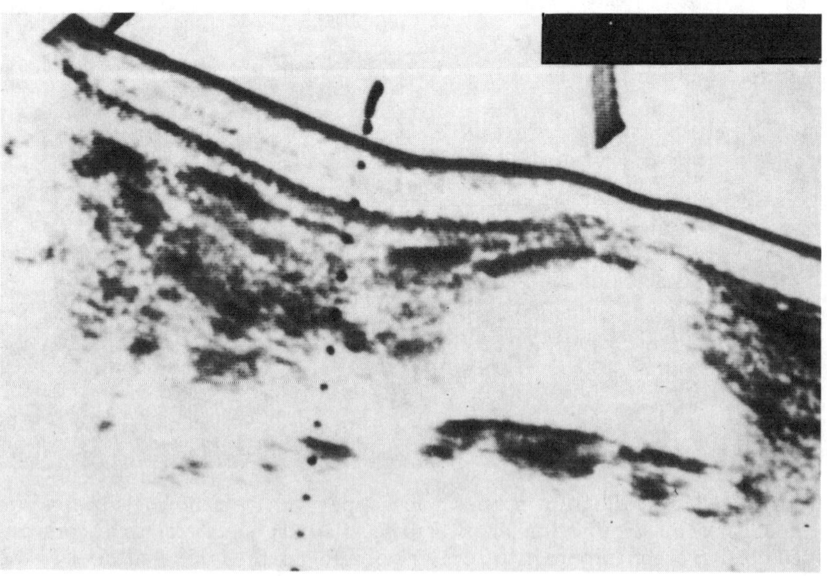

D

Figure 16-7C,D Transverse and sagittal section through abdominal aortic aneurysm in same patient measuring approximately 5 cm in diameter.

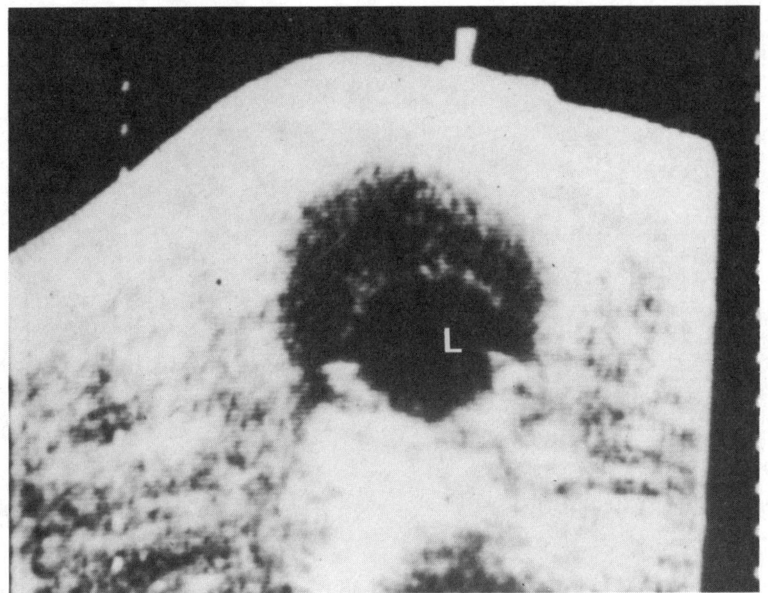

Figure 16-8 Transverse scan through aortic aneurysm with patent lumen (L) surrounded by crescentic-shaped echogenic structure superolaterally representing clot.

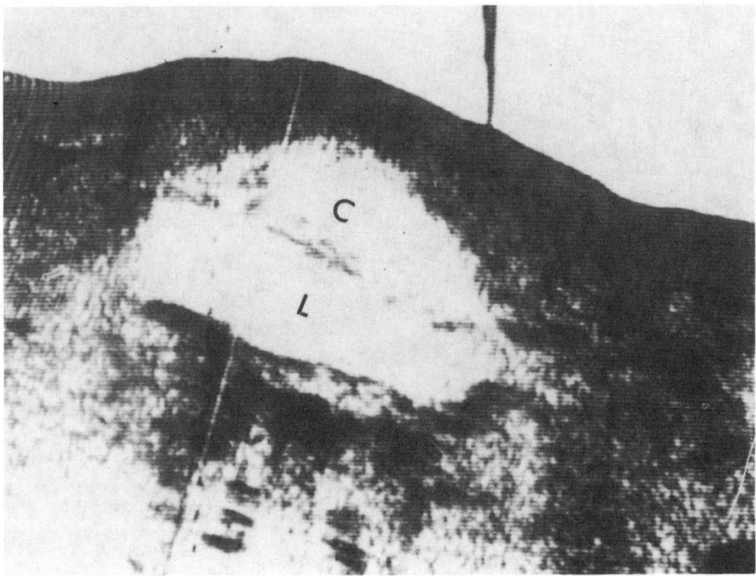

Figure 16-9 Sagittal scan through aneurysm with patent lumen (L) with clot in superior portion of aneurysm (C).

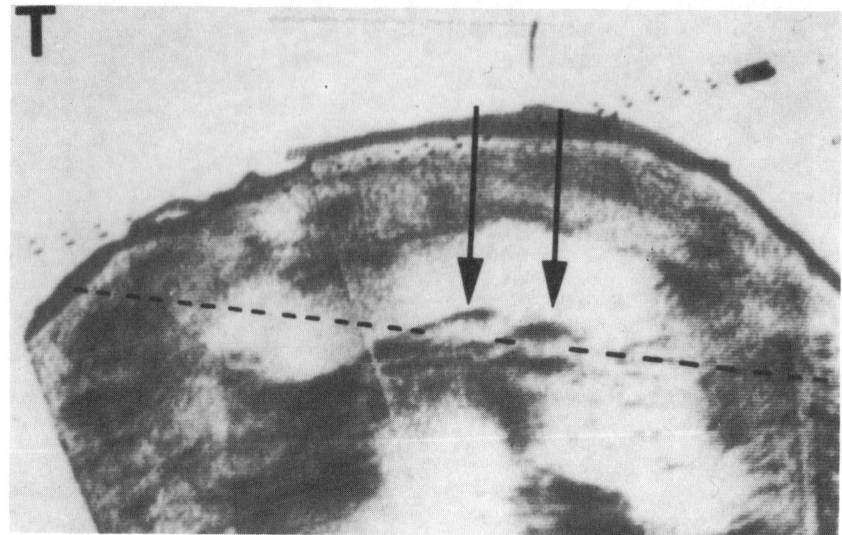

Figure 16-10A (T) transverse scan through aortic "Y" graft with surrounding echo poor area. Arrows point to the limbs of the aortic "Y" graft.

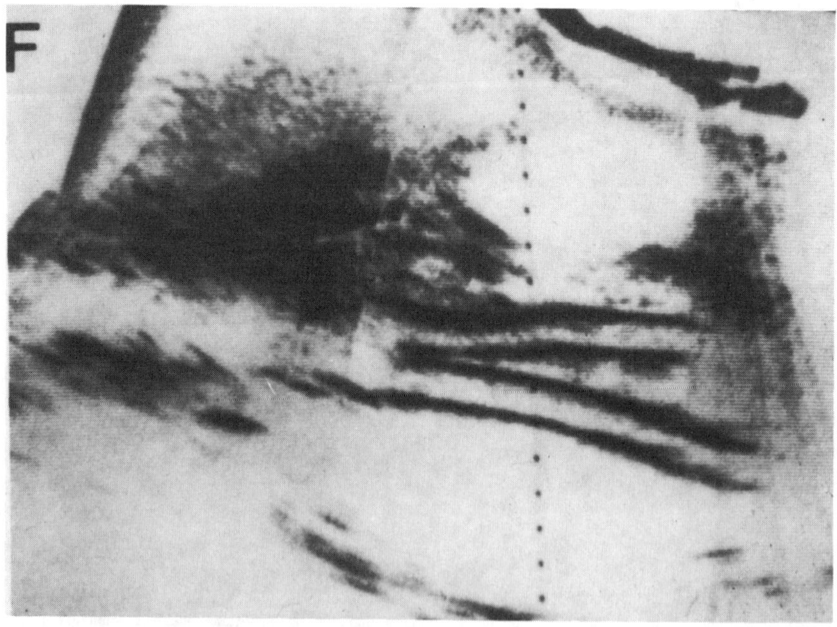

Figure 16-10B Frontal scan (F) through place indicated by dotted line in transverse section. The aortic "Y" graft is clearly seen surrounded by echo poor structure on either side.

Peripheral Arteries

Ultrasound examination of the iliac arteries is usually less satisfactory due to overlying small intestinal bowel gas. The more peripheral vessels, ie, the femoral and popliteal arteries, can be visualized fairly easily especially with dynamic scanners. Popliteal artery aneurysms, since they are superficially located, usually are readily identified[7] (Figure 16-11).

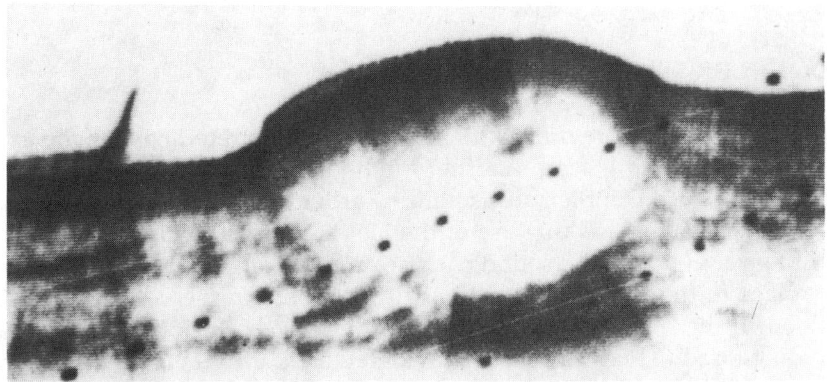

A

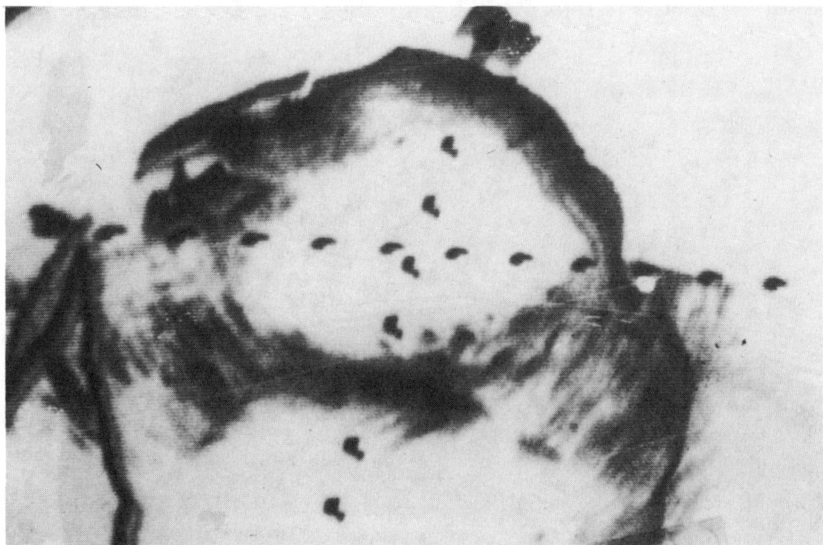

B

Figure 16-11A,B Sagittal and transverse ultrasound scan through popliteal artery aneurysm. Dots represent cm markers.

Inferior Vena Cava

The inferior vena cava is routinely visualized on abdominal examination (Figure 16-12). With dynamic scanning, its characteristic pulsations can be identified and distention during the Valsalva maneuver can be seen; with congestive heart failure, these will be diminished or absent.

Thrombus within the inferior vena cava can be visualized as an echogenic mass within the lumen (Figure 16-13).

DOPPLER ULTRASOUND

The methods previously mentioned and illustrated have made use of the ultrasound B scan. Another method of investigation of vascular disease is with Doppler ultrasound.[8] Earlier Doppler methods used a continuous signal making use of the Doppler effect, which is the shift of the frequency of the sound back-scattered from moving acoustic interfaces in the blood. This shift is proportional to the velocity of the blood. If there is no shift, there is no flow, and occlusion of the vessel is diagnosed. This ultrasonic flow detector is useful in localizing an arterial or venous obstruction, in the determination of the patency of arteries distal to an obstruction, as well as in the evaluation of the results of operative treatment. Continuous wave Doppler technique is

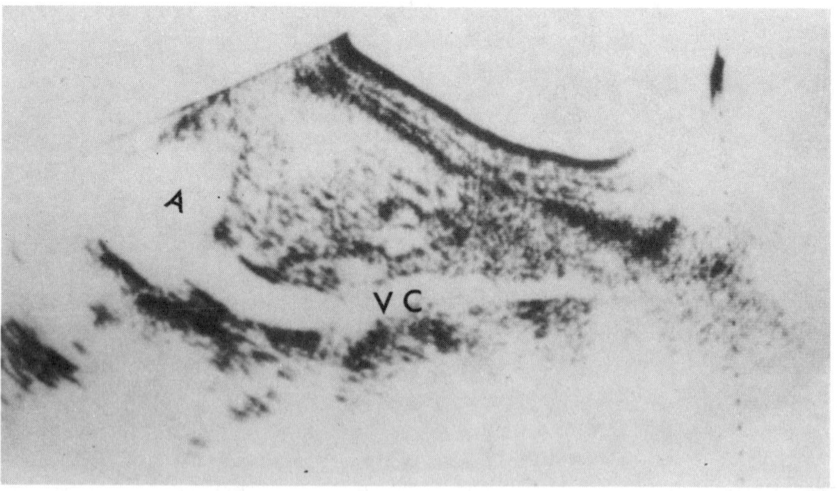

Figure 16-12 Sagittal scan through inferior vena cava (VC), entering right atrium (A). Array of dots are 1 cm apart.

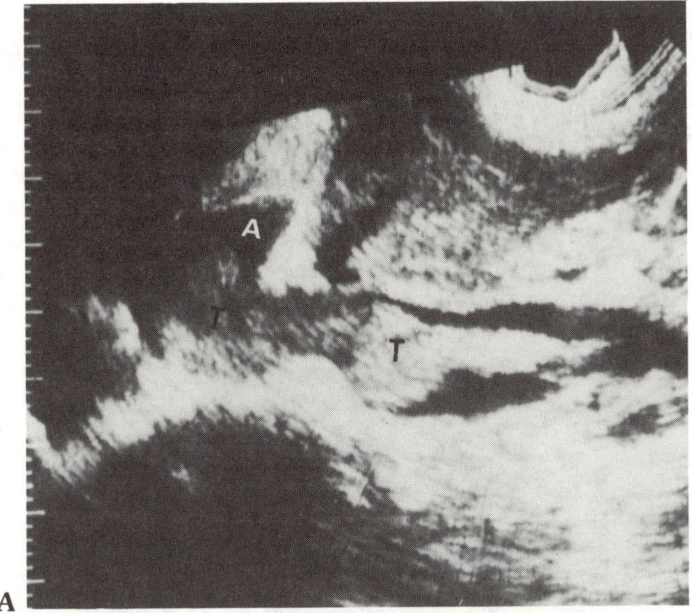

A

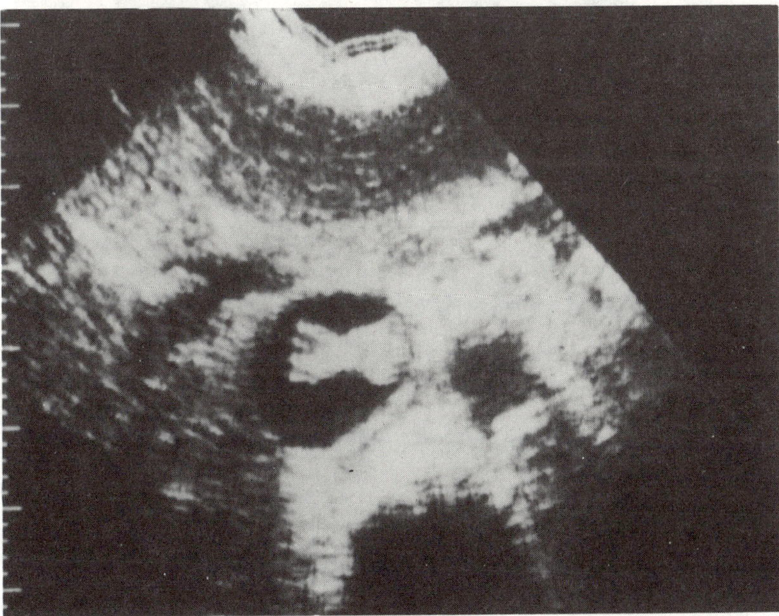

B

Figure 16-13A,B Sagittal and transverse scans through inferior vena cava in patient with renal carcinoma with tumor thrombus within inferior vena cava extending into right atrium. T = tumor thrombus.

limited by lack of precise arterial dimensions, and appears to be clinically useful where the major question is the presence or absence of a flow signal.

Pulsed Doppler techniques, as opposed to continuous Doppler methods, permit detection of blood flow at selected locations in the blood stream.[9] This allows the assessment of the caliber of a blood vessel and an indication of flow velocity at various locations across the vessels. Thus, both an image and an audio signal are produced. This method has been used to detect lesions in the extracranial carotid arteries in a number of clinical trials (Figures 16-14, 16-15).

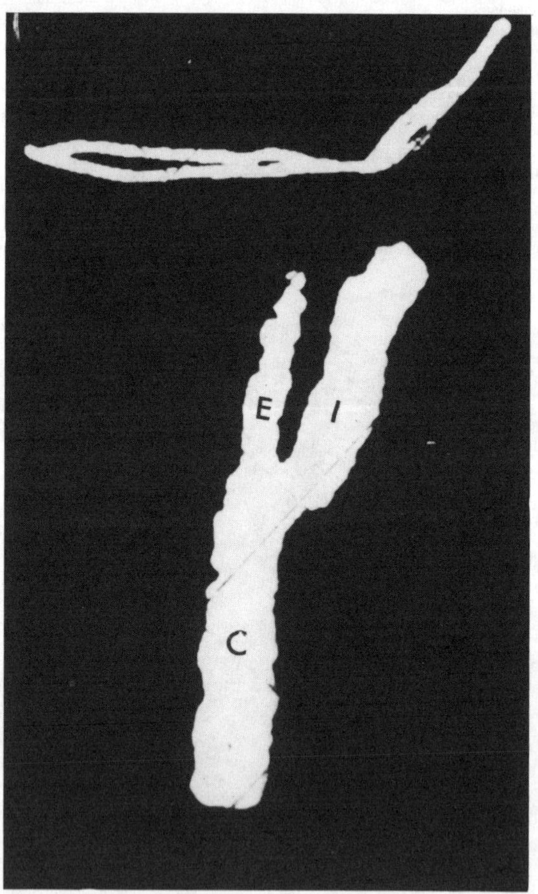

Figure 16-14A Pulsed Doppler image of normal carotid artery and bifurcation. C = common carotid artery, E = external carotid artery, I = internal carotid artery. The white line at the top represents the level of the mandible for orientation purposes. (Courtesy of Dr Bruce S. Cutler, University of Massachusetts Medical Center, Worcester, MA.)

In one such study, normal and occluded internal carotid arteries were diagnosed with 75% and 87% accuracy, respectively. Precise quantification of lesions with either less than, or greater than 50% stenosis, was less successful. Specificity was 84% and sensitivity 89%. Overall accuracy was 85%. Ulcerated atherosclerotic lesions were diagnosed in only 10 of 23 patients, or 43%. A major limitation is this inability to detect ulcerated atherosclerotic lesions, which are not associated with hemodynamically significant stenoses.[10] However, new developments in the field, namely duplex instruments, which combine simultaneous Doppler with high resolution, high frequency B

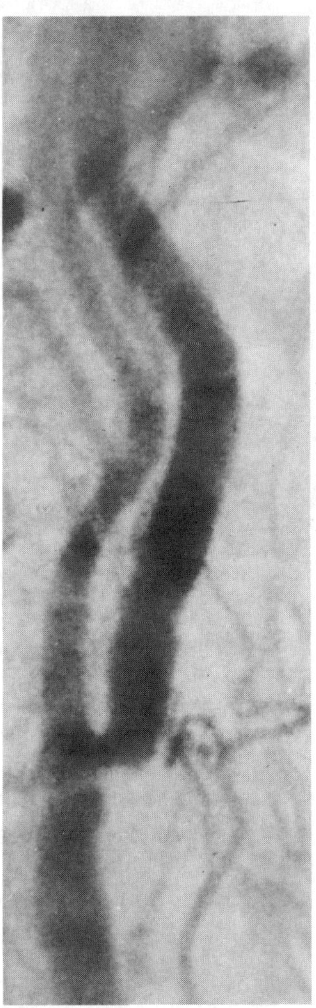

Figure 16-14B Normal carotid angiogram on same patient (14A).

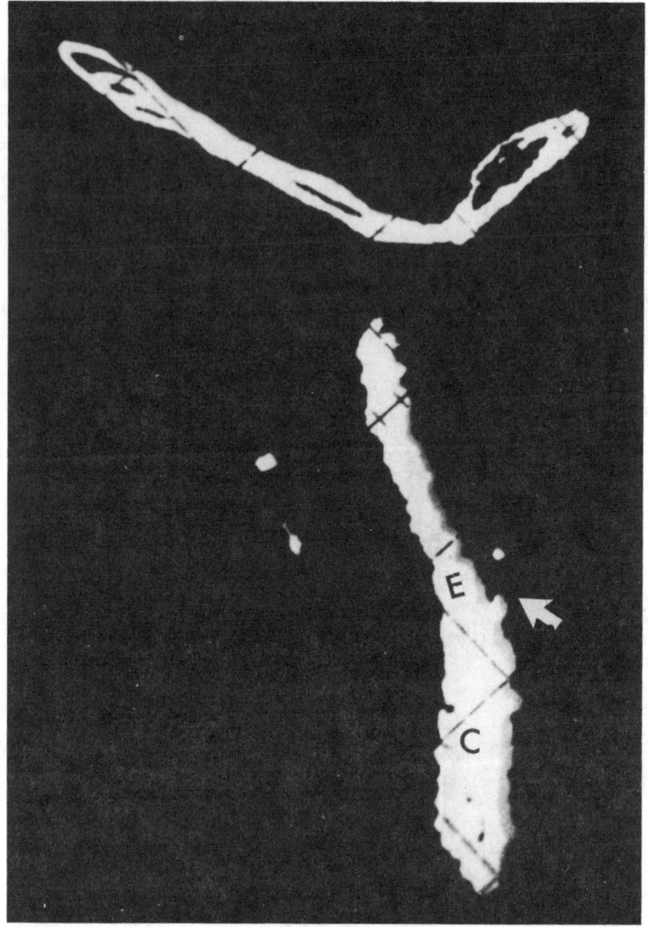

Figure 16-15A Pulsed Doppler image of occluded internal carotid artery (arrow). C = common carotid artery, E = external carotid artery. Mandible delineated above for a reference. (Courtesy of Dr Bruce S. Cutler, University of Massachusetts Medical Center, Worcester, MA.)

scanning, are most promising.[11,12] This technique allows accurate visualization of the vessel as well as amplitude and direction of blood flow. Experience with this instrument is limited, but it appears to represent a significant advance (Figure 16-16).

NUCLEAR FLOW STUDIES

A radionuclide flow study, in which a computer collects the counts over an area within a varying period of time and displays the informa-

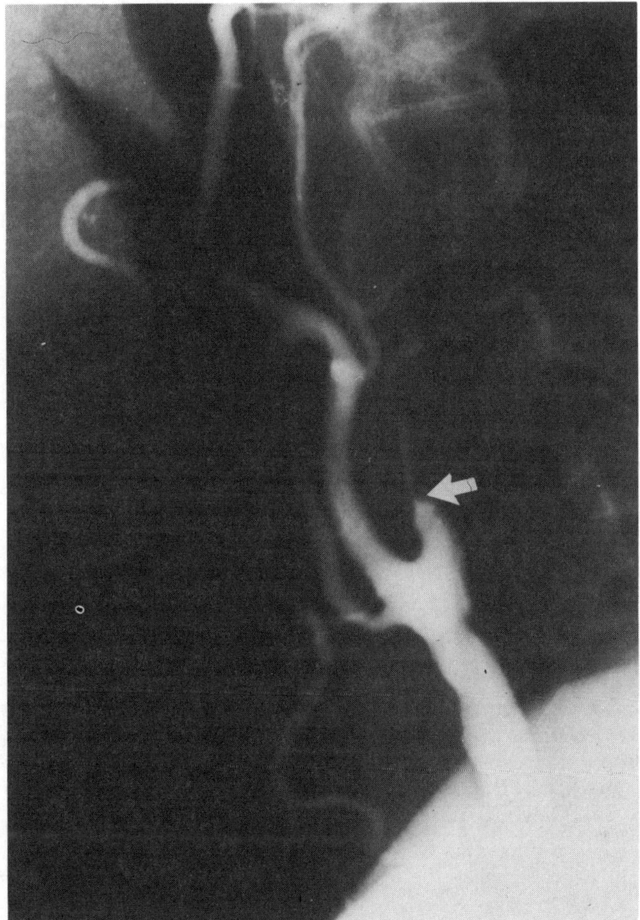

Figure 16-15B Carotid angiogram on same patient confirming occlusion of the internal carotid artery (arrows).

tion obtained in a dynamic fashion, is another method of detecting vascular occlusion.[13] Although resolution is inadequate to detect subtle abnormalities, large aneurysms or major occlusions can be detected (Figure 16-17, 16-18). This method may supplement the ultrasound examination by providing information regarding flow, bleeding, fistula information, etc.[14]

COMPUTED TOMOGRAPHY

Computed tomography is the newest modality to arrive on the scene and it is having a major impact on the field of diagnostic

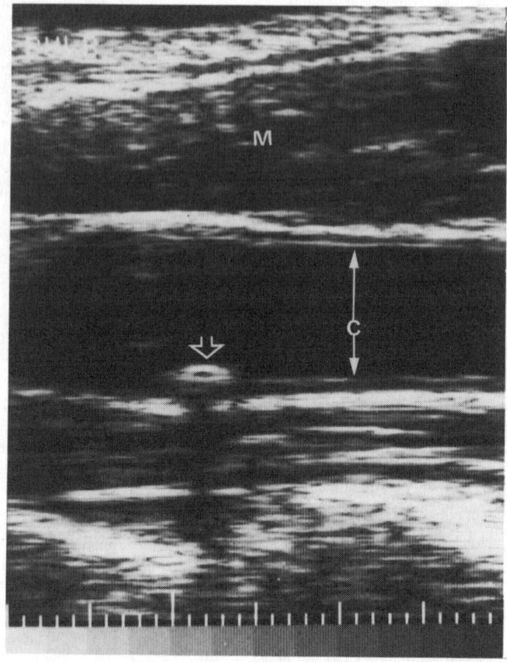

Figure 16-16A High resolution B scan of the neck demonstrating the carotid lumen (C) with the arrows pointing to what appears to be the intima. Hollow arrowhead points to an intimal plaque with shadowing. (M) represents superficial musculature of the neck. (Courtesy of Dr George Leopold, University of California, San Diego, CA.)

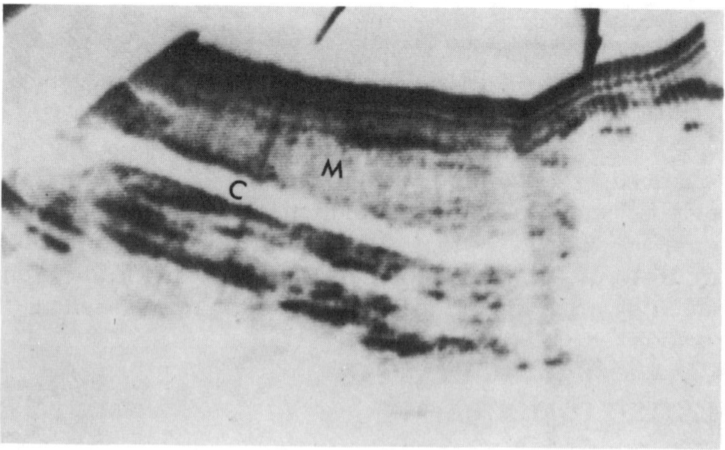

Figure 16-16B Conventional B scan of the neck for comparison. M = anterior musculature, C = carotid lumen.

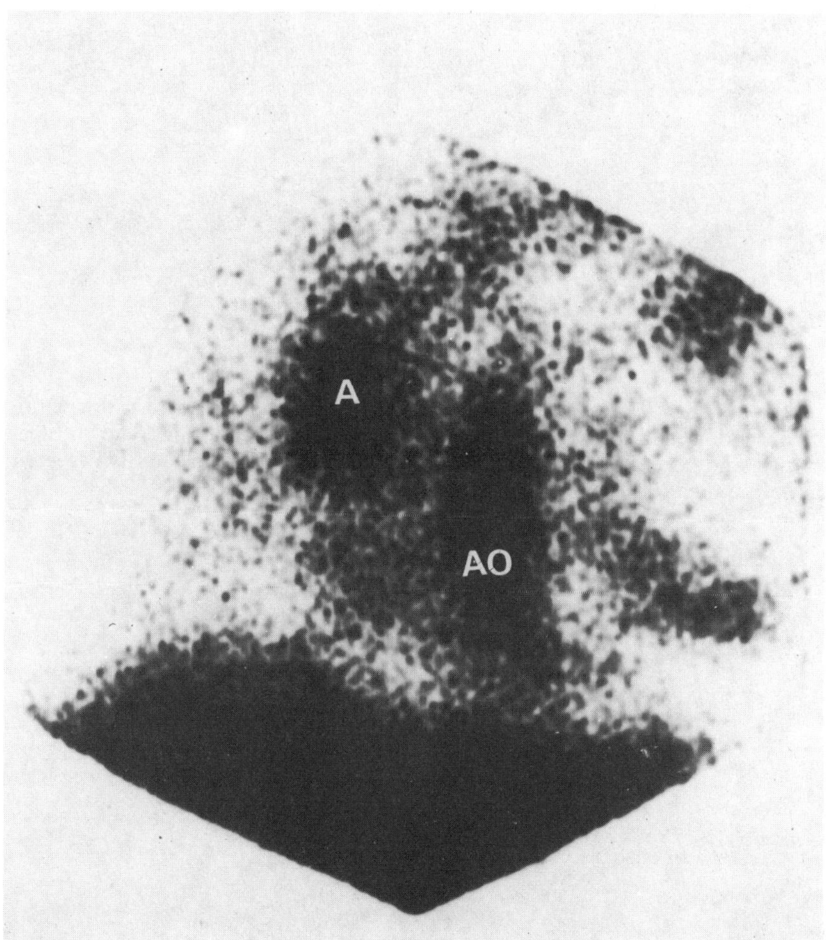

Figure 16-17 Single image from nuclide flow study revealing aneurysm of ascending aorta measuring approximately 5 cm in diameter. A = aneurysm, AO = normal descending thoracic aorta. (Courtesy Dr Paul W. Doherty, University of Massachusetts Medical Center, Worcester, MA.)

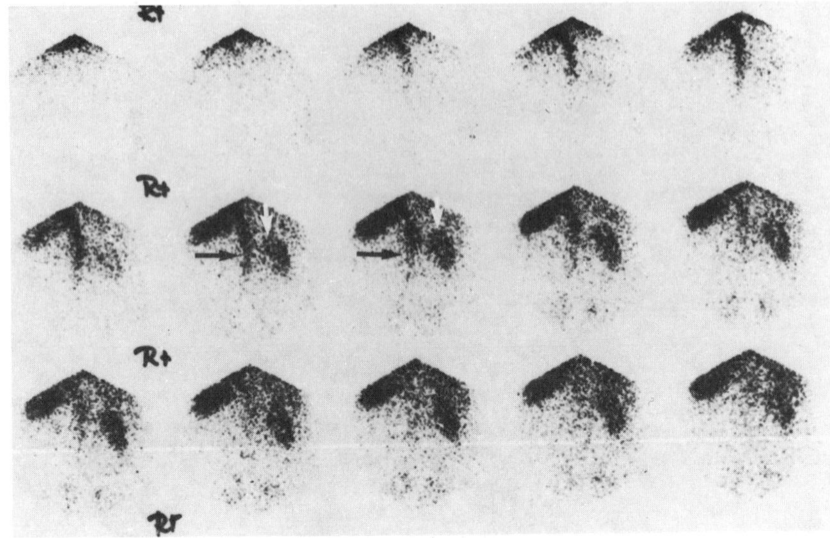

Figure 16-18A Series of images from a nuclear medicine dynamic flow study of the abdominal aorta revealing activity within the abdominal aorta (black arrows) and perfusion of the right kidney (white arrows). No activity is seen in the left kidney indicating obstruction of the right renal artery.

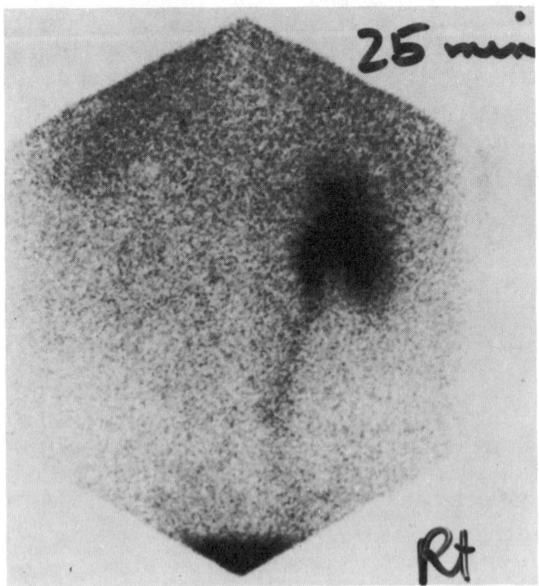

Figure 16-18B Delayed excretory phase of same study revealing activity within the right kidney and ureter. No activity is seen on the left.

radiology. Multiple x-ray sources rotate about the patient. Very sensitive detectors are connected to a dedicated computer, which measures the attenuation of the x-ray beam by the cross section of the body being interrogated. A shade of gray is assigned to a minute volume (Pixel) of tissue according to its degree of attenuation of the x-ray beam, and an image is thus constructed. Very small differences in density can be appreciated and extraordinarily detailed images are produced.

The latest generation scanners create a high resolution cross-sectional image in five seconds or less, and have the further capability of allowing rapid sequential images of the same section. Intravenous administration of radiographic contrast material is easily detected in the major vessels of the body and an aortic aneurysm is readily apparent (Figure 16-19).[15] Complications, ie, hematoma, dissection, may be detected (Figure 16-20).[16,17] Thrombus is detected as an area of diminshed density within the contrast-filled lumen (Figure 16-21).[18] Whereas, the earlier scanners were capable of producing only transverse cross-sectional images, the newer instruments permit sagittal reconstruction, so that an abnormality can be imaged in two planes. An advantage over ultrasound is that CT is not limited by air or bone so that thoracic aneurysms may be easily visualized (Figure 16-22).

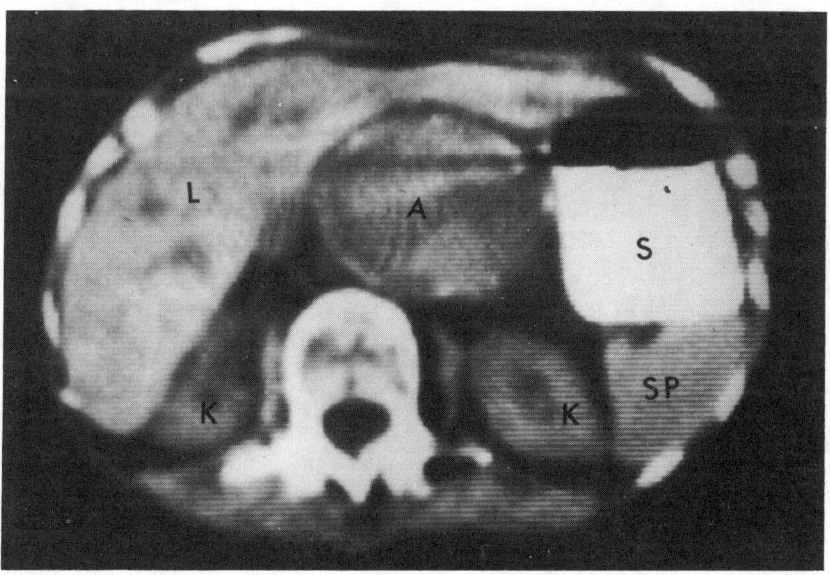

Figure 16-19 CT scan through abdominal aortic aneurysm. A = aortic aneurysm, L = liver, S = barium filled stomach, K = kidney, SP = spleen tip. Wall of aneurysm is partially calcified.

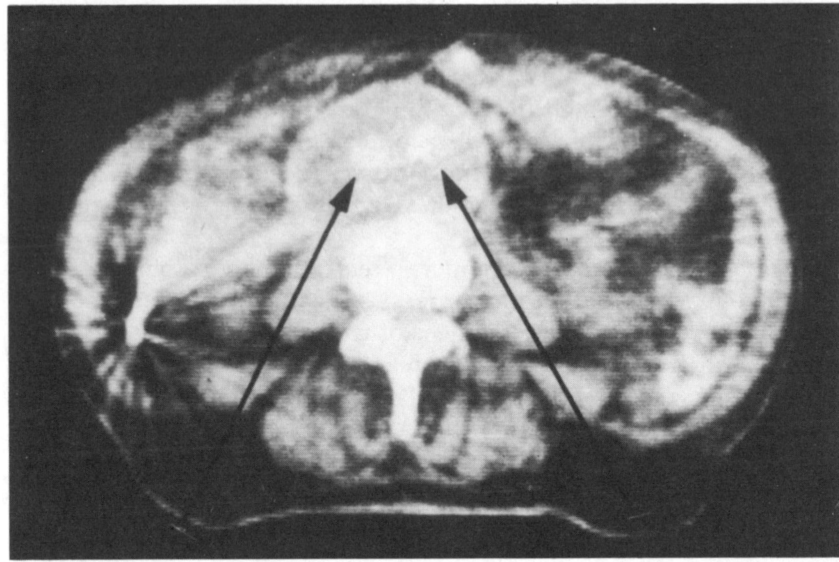

Figure 16-20 Arrows point to contrast-filled limbs of aortic "Y" graft surrounded by hematoma with contrast enhanced rim. Compare to ultrasound study in a similar case (Figure 16-10).

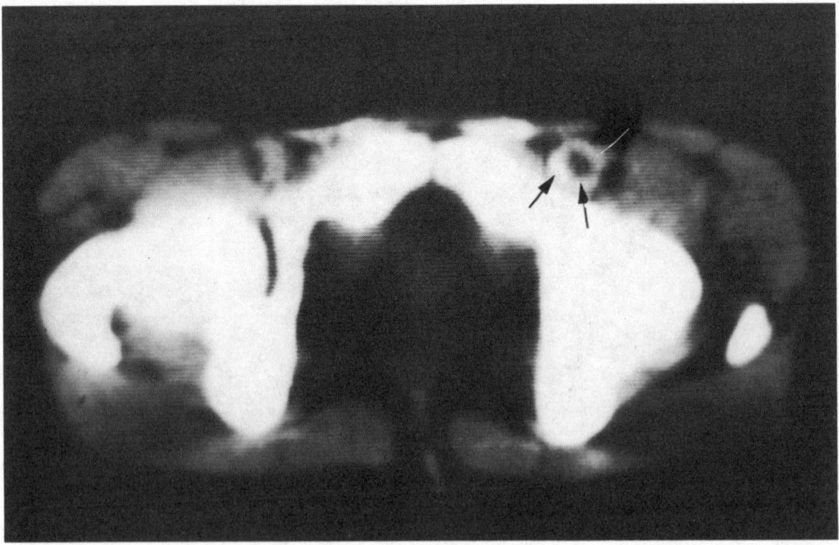

Figure 16-21 CT Scan in patient with thrombus in left femoral artery (arrows). Thrombus is represented by filling defect in contrast-filled lumen.

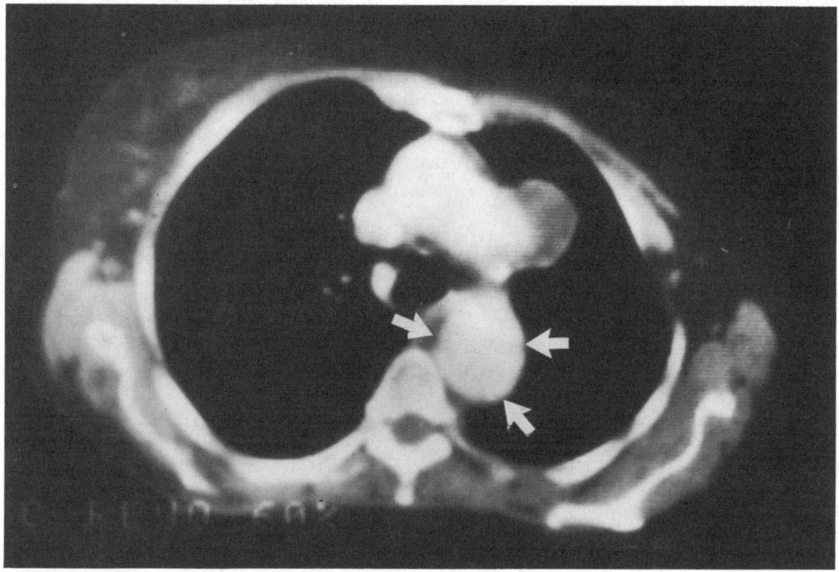

Figure 16-22 CT scan. Aneurysm descending thoracic aorta (arrows) after intravenous contrast administration.

Since ultrasound examination is cheaper, simpler, and more rapid, it would appear that this modality should be the method of choice for the initial examination. However, if the examination is nondiagnostic because of bowel gas, obesity, location of the lesion in the thorax, or simply because the lesion is too small to be imaged, then CT scanning would be the next logical step.

REFERENCES

1. Holm HH. Abdominal ultrasound. In *Basic Physics of Diagnostic Ultrasound,* ed 2. Munksgaard, 1980, pp 21–34.

2. Karp W, Eklof BO. Ultrasonography and angiography in the diagnosis of abdominal aortic aneurysm. *Acta Radiol Diagnosis* 19:955–960, 1978.

3. Wheeler WE, Beachley MC, Ranniger K. Angiography and ultrasonography: A comparative study of abdominal arotic aneurysms. *AJR* 126:95–100, 1976.

4. Leopold GR. Ultrasonic abdominal arotography. *Radiology* 96:9–14, 1970.

5. McGregor JC, Pollock JG, Anton HC. Ultrasonography and possible ruptured abdominal aortic aneurysms. *Br Med J* 3:78–79, 1975.

6. Bresnihan ER, Keates PG. Ultrasound and dissection of the abdominal aorta. *Clin Radiology* 31:105–108, 1980.

7. Neiman HL, Yao JST, Silver TM. Gray-scale ultrasound diagnosis of peripheral arterial aneurysms. *Radiology* 130:413–416, 1979.

8. Mozersky DJ, Hokanson DE, Baker DW, et al.Ultrasonic arteriography. *Arch Sur* 103:663–667, 1971.

9. Felix WR Jr, Sigel B, Gibson RJ, et al. Pulsed Doppler ultrasound detection of flow disturbances in arteriosclerosis, *J Clin Ultrasound* 4:275–282, 1976.

10. Berry SM, O'Donnell JA, Hobson RW. Capabilities and Limitations of Pulsed Doppler Sonography in Carotid Imaging. *J Clin Ultrasound* 8:405–412, 1980.

11. Barber FE, Baker DW, Strandness DE Jr, et al. *Duplex Scanner II for Simultaneous Imaging of Artery Tissues and Flow.* Ultrasonic Symposium Proceedings, Milwaukee, WI, IEEE Catalogue #74CHO 896-ISU, 1974.

12. Yeh E, Meade RC. Pulsed Doppler studies in B-mode ultrasound scanning. *Radiology* 122: 521–522, 1977.

13. Bergan JJ, Yao JST, Henkin RE, et al. Radionuclide Aortography in detection of arterial aneurysms. *Arch Surgery* 109:80, 1974.

14. Bunko H, Seto H, Tonami N, et al. Detection of active bleeding from ruptured aortic aneurysm by emergency radionuclide angiography. *Clin Nuc Med* 3:276–277, 1978.

15. Egan TJ. Computed tomography in the diagnosis of aortic aneurysm dissection or traumatic injury. *Radiology* 136:141–146, 1980.

16. Larde D, Belloir C, Vasile N, et al. Computed tomography of aortic dissection. *Radiology* 136:147–151, 1980.

17. Bergman AB, Neiman HL. Computed tomography in the detection of retroperitoneal hemorrhage after translumbar aortography. *AJR* 131:831–833, 1978.

18. Marks WM, Korobkin M, Callen PW, et al. CT diagnosis of tumor thrombosis of the renal vein and inferior vena cava. *AJR* 131:843–846, 1978.

17 Invasive Radiology of Arterial Disease

David A. Phillips

New technology and clinical skills have established the angiographic procedure as a creditable means of diagnosing and treating certain vascular problems. In the hands of well-trained vascular radiologists, major complications are minimal.[1-3] Patient discomfort is minimized through the judicious use of analgesics and modern, less toxic contrast agents. Most procedures can be performed safely in less than one hour, and nearly all can be done within two and one-half hours or less.

The procedure entails puncture of a major size artery (femoral, brachial or abdominal aorta), with an 18-gauge or smaller needle, threading an appropriate size wire (guidewire) through the needle into the abdominal aorta. The needle is removed over the guidewire, while firm pressure is applied at the site of the arterial puncture. A catheter is passed over the guidewire and positioned in the appropriate vessel. A bolus of contrast is mechanically injected over a period of a few seconds, while rapid sequence filming takes place. The filming sequence should extend long enough to provide sufficient information concerning the anatomic state and blood flow within the vessels under scrutiny.

CONGENITAL ARTERIAL DISEASE

Congenital arterial disease can involve any vessel within the body. Angiography is especially useful in assessing the extent of vascular pathology and determining if surgical correction of the anomaly is feasible. Only a selected few of the more common congenital arterial abnormalities will be discussed in this brief text.

Arteriovenous Fistulas

Arteriovenous fistulas may cause congestive heart failure, degeneration of vessel walls, aneurysm formation, abnormal limb growth patterns, and numerous other complications.[4-6] Their anatomy,

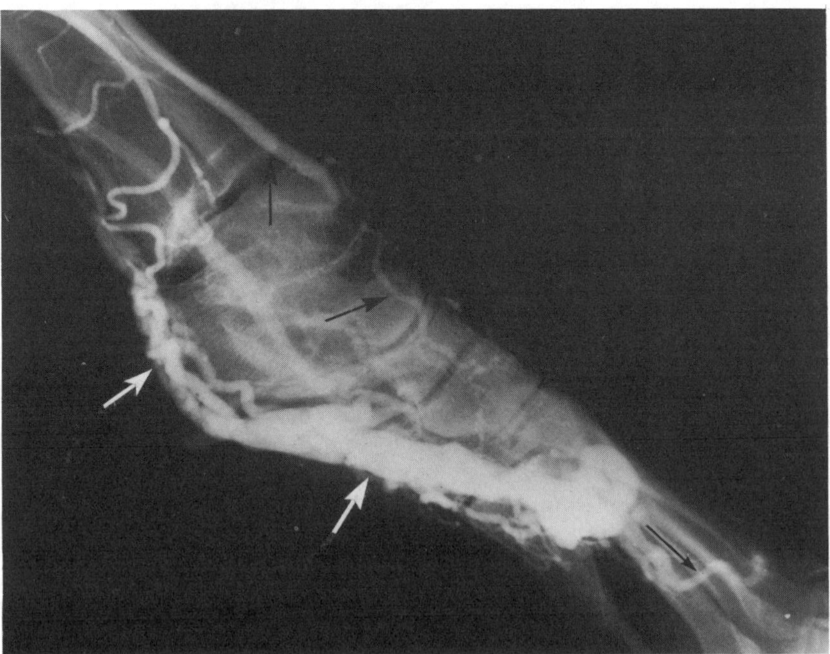

Figure 17-1 Arteriovenous fistula of the foot. Note: 1) simultaneous opacification of arteries (black arrows) and veins (white arrows), indicating shunting of arterial blood flow, 2) large veins and arteries.

pathophysiology, and clinical presentation have been described.[6-9] An example of an arteriovenous fistula of the foot is shown in Figure 17-1. Angiographically, they are characterized by early venous appearance, large arteries, and veins. The veins are usually larger. The course of the vessels may be tortuous. Vessel obstruction, narrowing, or marginal irregularities are atypical and, when seen, the diagnosis of a malignancy should be entertained. Surgery for these lesions has met with varying success.[10,11] In selected cases, embolization through a selectively placed arterial catheter, using gelfoam or metallic particles, has been successful in closing off the fistula.[5]

Coarctation

Coarctation of the aorta results from a congenital narrowing or occlusion of the aorta, usually just below the left subclavian artery (more than 95%).[12] However, abdominal aortic coarctations have been reported as well.[13] Other associated congenital anomalies occur. Bicuspid aortic valves have been found in 46% of infants with coarctation of the aorta, but are seldom hemodynamically significant.[14] Isolated coarctation of the aorta occurs more frequently in males than in females, with an incidence ratio of three to one (3:1). Fifty percent of patients will develop congestive heart failure within the first three weeks of life; in the other 50%, signs and symptoms will not appear until childhood or adult life.[12] Aortography will delineate the site and severity of the coarctation, the collateral circulation, the presence of a patent ductus arteriosus, and sites of origin of brachiocephalic vessels. Figure 17-2 is an example of coarctation of the aorta in an adult. Characteristic findings on a plain chest film have been described to suggest the diagnosis of coarctation of the thoracic aorta.[15]

ARTERIOSCLEROSIS

Severe arteriosclerosis of the aorta and its branches may cause luminal dilatation and/or luminal obstruction. In the aorta, per se, dilatation is far more common and aneurysm may occur in its transverse, descending thoracic and abdominal portions. Obstruction, resulting from atherosclerosis, affects only its branches and abdominal portions.[16] Visualization of the aorta and its branches, angiographically, is the most accurate means of determining the extent of involvement of the atherosclerosis. At the time of angiography, pressure measurements may be taken across stenotic lesions to assess their clinical significance. Figures 17-3, 17-4, 17-5, 17-6, 17-7 are examples of atherosclerotic lesions assessed angiographically.

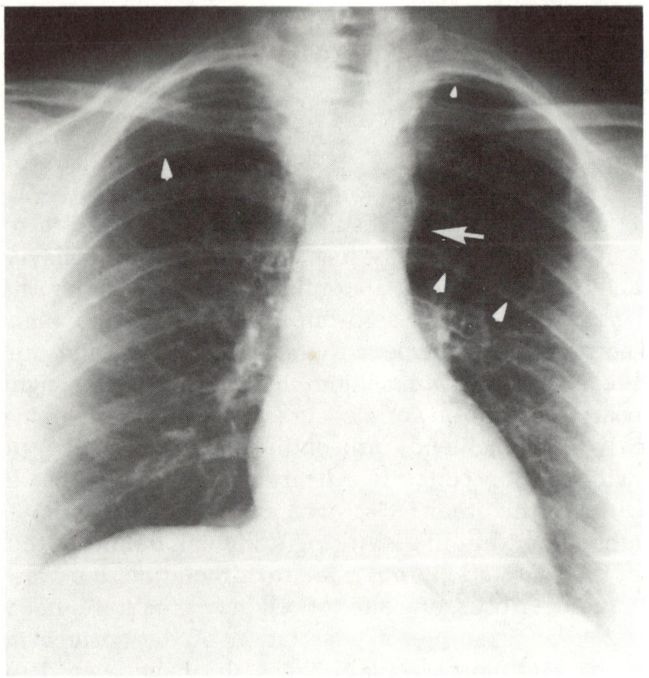

A

Figure 17-2 Coarctation of the aorta. **A** Posterior-anterior chest. Note: 1) so-called 3 sign of aorta (white arrow), caused by prominence of descending thoracic aorta, above and below coarcted area, 2) posterior rib notching (small white arrows). **B** Lateral chest. Note: shows stenosed descending thoracic aorta (black arrow). **C** Thoracic aortogram (left anterior oblique). Note: 1) site of coarctation (large white arrow), with dilatation of descending thoracic aorta distal to the coarctation, 2) enlarged left subclavian artery (curved black arrow), 3) enlarged left internal mammary artery (black arrow), 4) numerous arterial collaterals (white arrows).

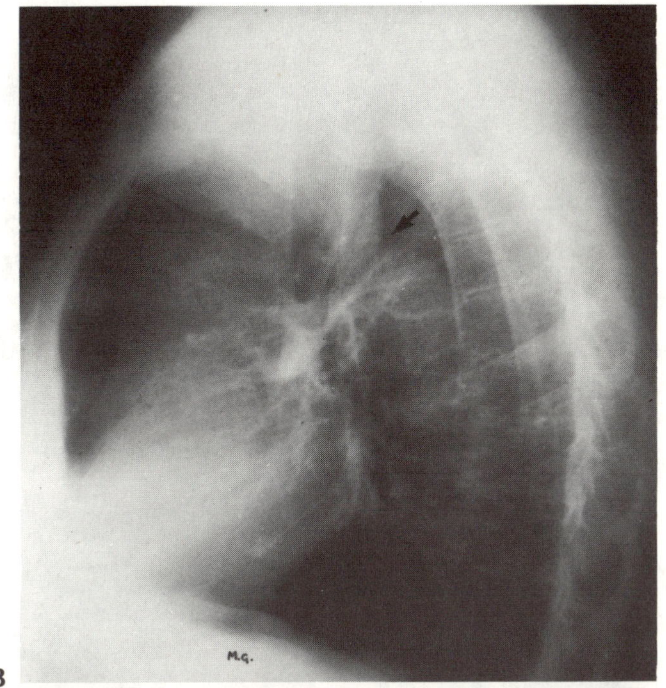

B

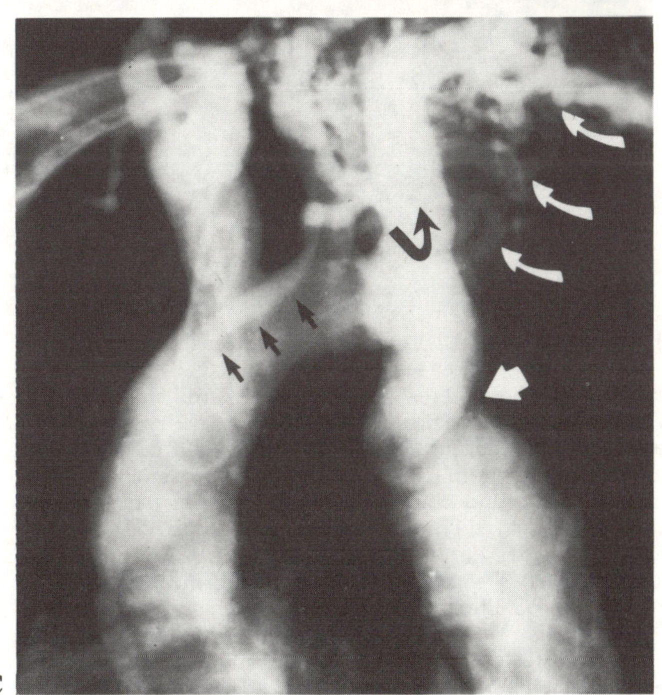

C

A

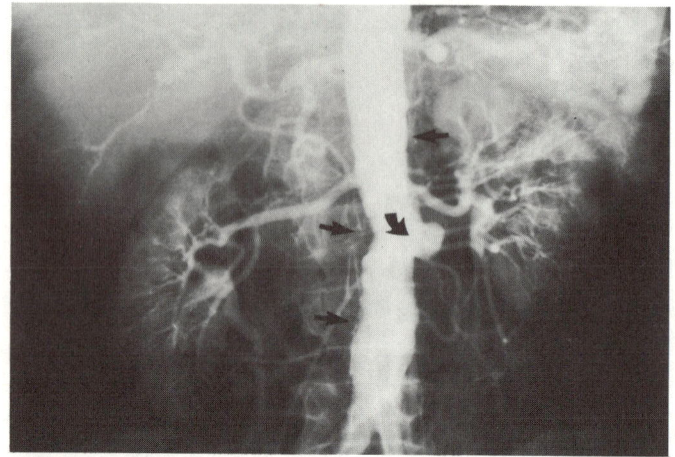

B

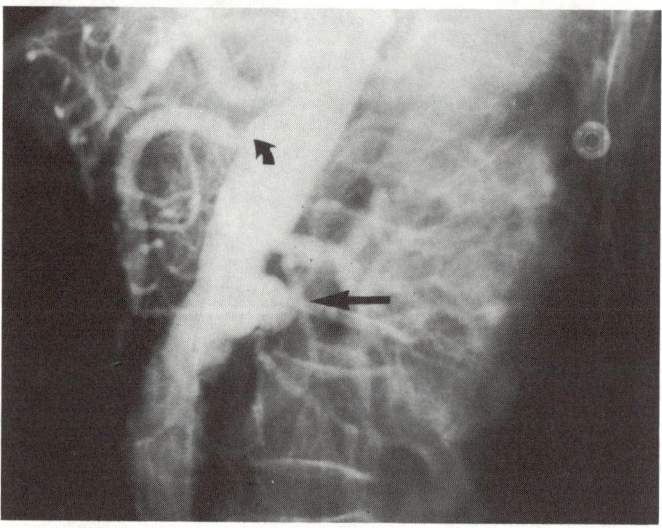

Figure 17-3 **A** Abdominal aortogram (anterior-posterior view). Note: 1) small saccular aneurysm just below left renal artery (curved arrow), 2) irregularity of aortic lumen suggesting atherosclerotic process (straight arrows). **B** Lateral abdominal aortogram. Note: 1) posterior location of aneurysm (straight arrow), 2) plaque at origin of superior mesenteric artery (curved arrow). **C** Anterior-posterior pelvic arteriogram. Note: mild luminal irregularities in both common iliacs, internal iliacs, and common femoral arteries (straight arrows, small curved arrows, and large curved arrows, respectively). **D** Anterior-posterior superficial femoral (SFA) arteriogram. Note: 1) localized marked stenosis midportion of right SFA, 2) several plaques in midportion of left SFA (arrows). **E** Anterior-posterior popliteal arteriogram. Note: marked stenosis in proximal portion of left anterior tibial artery (arrow). **F** Anterior-posterior arteriogram of distal extremity arteries. Note: good visualization of the anterior tibial and posterior tibial arteries in both lower limbs.

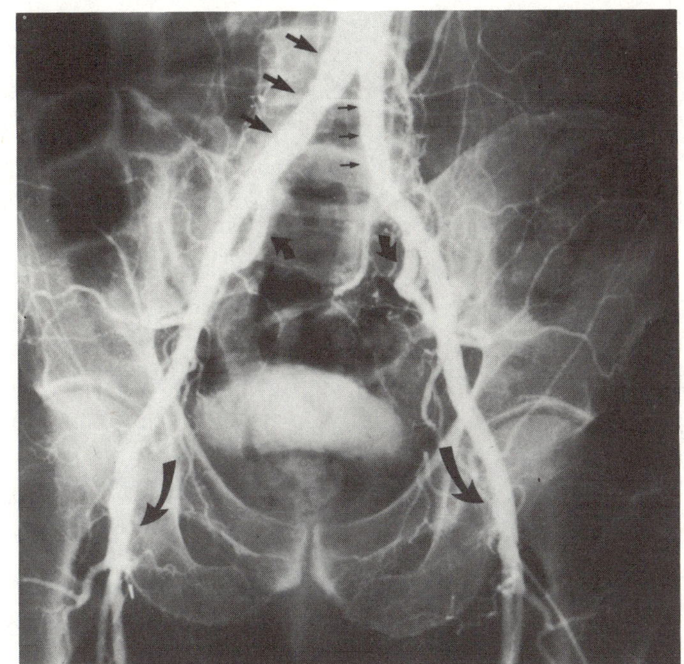
C

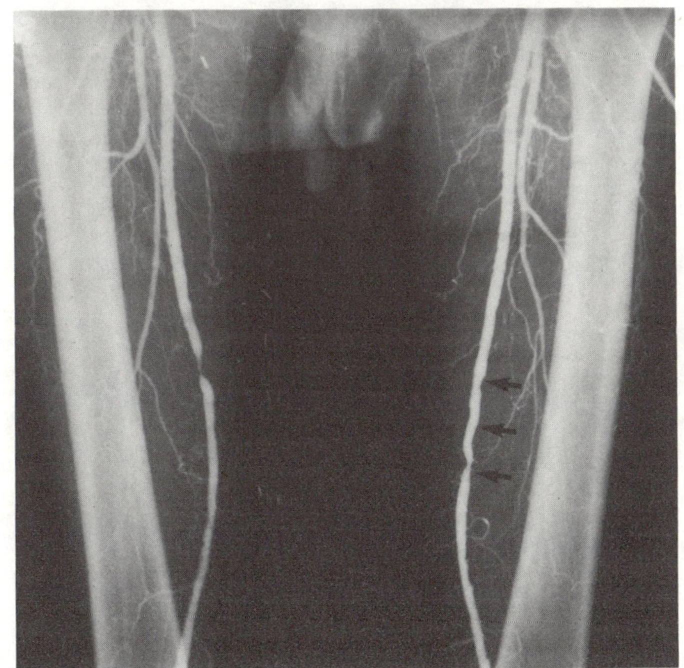
D

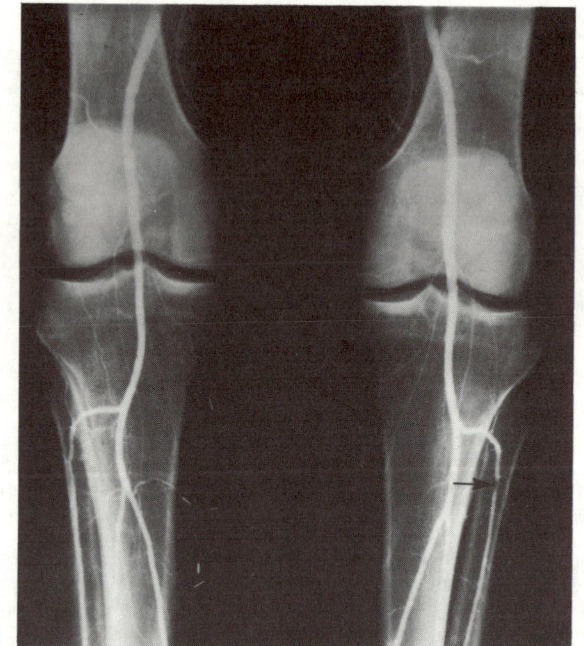

E

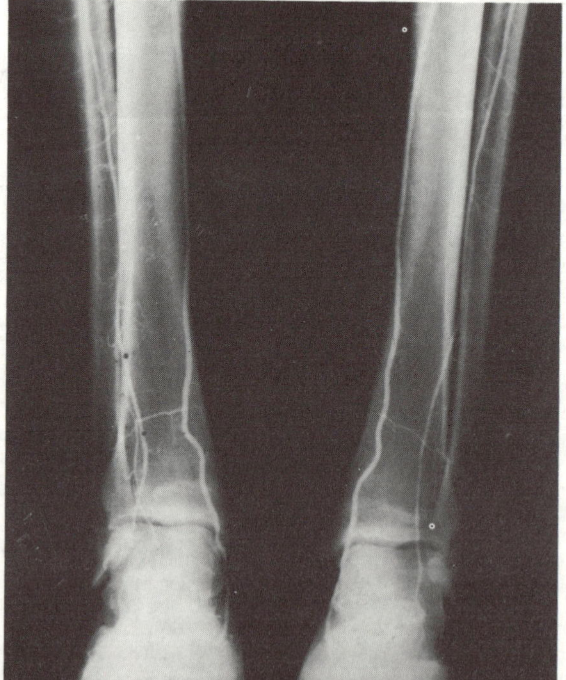

F

Figure 17-3—*Continued*

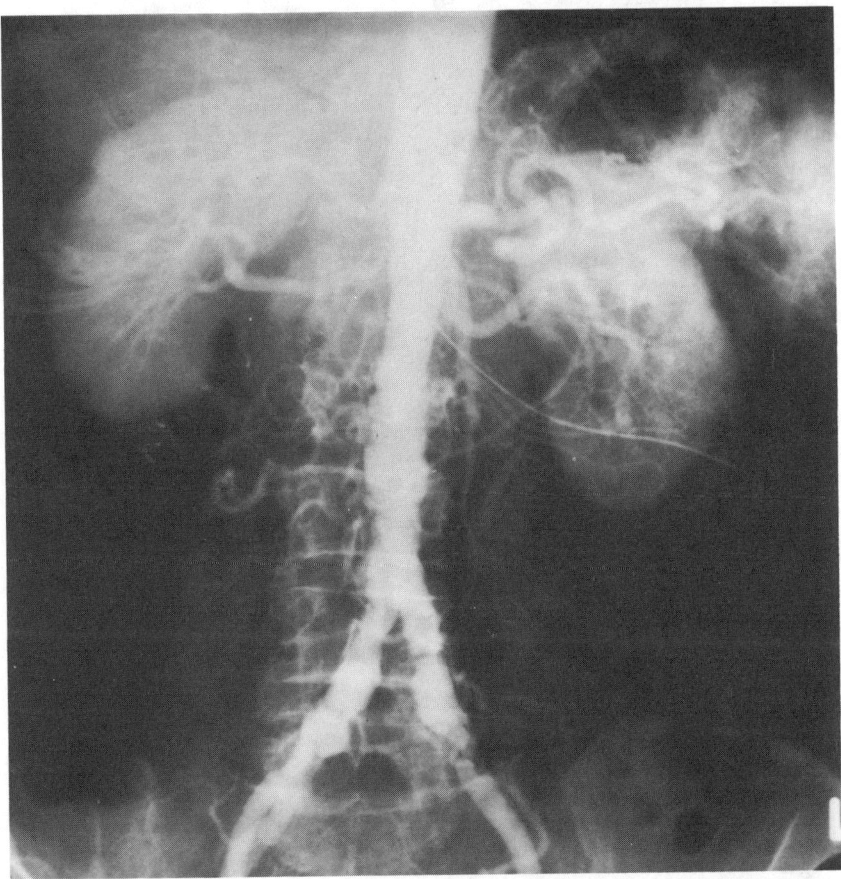

Figure 17-4 Anterior-posterior abdominal aortogram. Note: marked atherosclerotic plaques in abdominal aorta and both common iliac arteries.

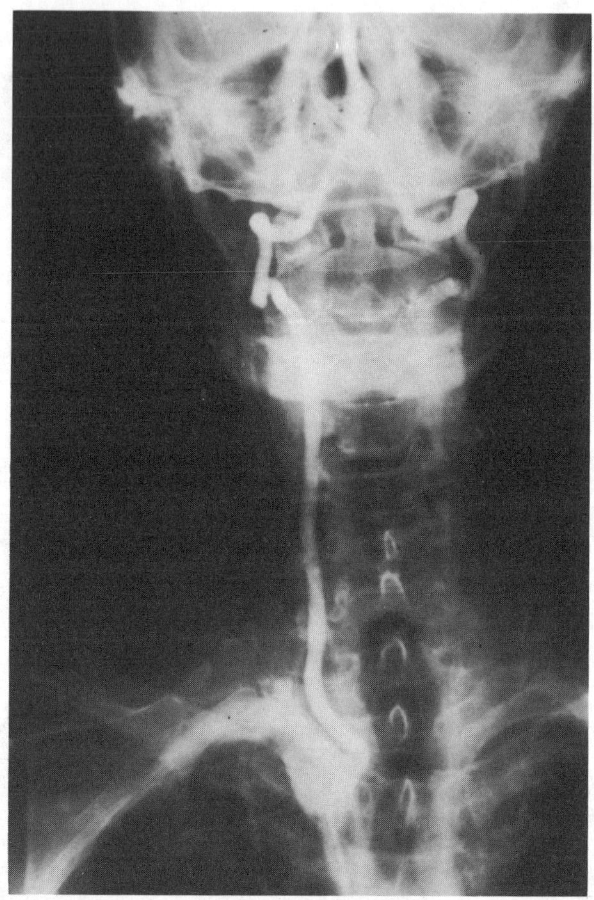

Figure 17-5 Left subclavian artery steal secondary to atherosclerotic thrombosis. **A** Selective right vertebral artery injection. Note: 1) good filling of the right vertebral artery and beginning filling of the left vertebral artery with contrast, 2) blood flow is antegrade in the right vertebral and retrograde in the left vertebral. **B** Note: good filling of the left vertebral artery and beginning filling of the left subclavian artery (arrow) with contrast. **C** Note: good filling of left subclavian artery with contrast, revealing its site of occlusion (arrow).

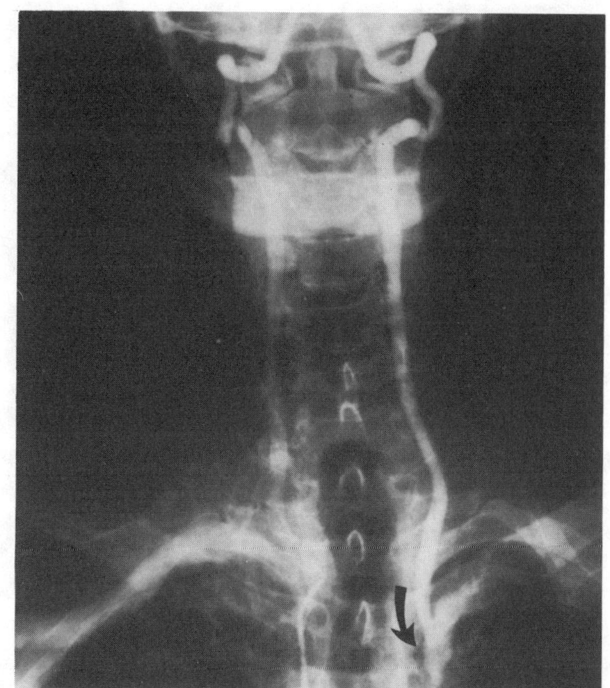

B

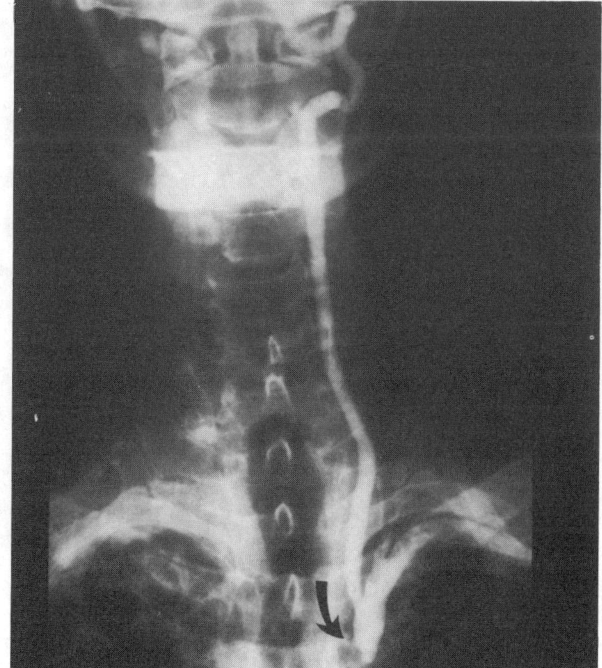

C

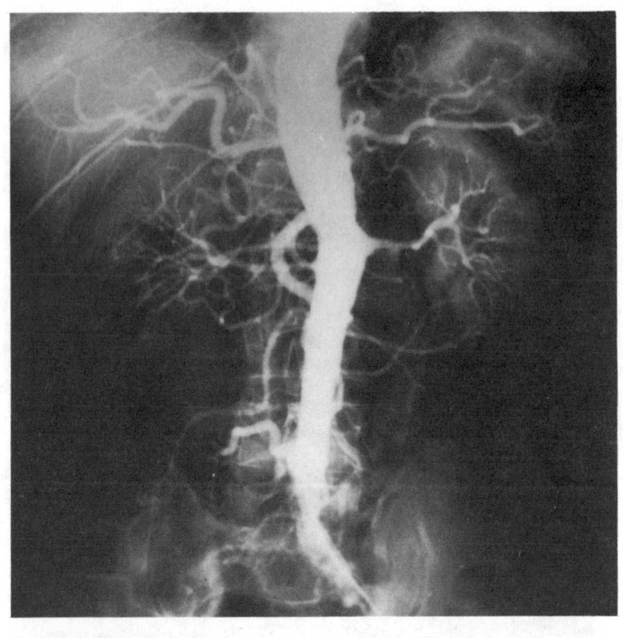

A

B

Figure 17-6 Atherosclerotic disease. **A** Anterior-posterior abdominal aortogram. Note: left renal artery stenosis (arrow) secondary to atherosclerosis. **B** Anterior-posterior pelvic arteriogram (same patient). Note: 1) occluded right common iliac artery, 2) generous formation of pelvic collaterals on right side.

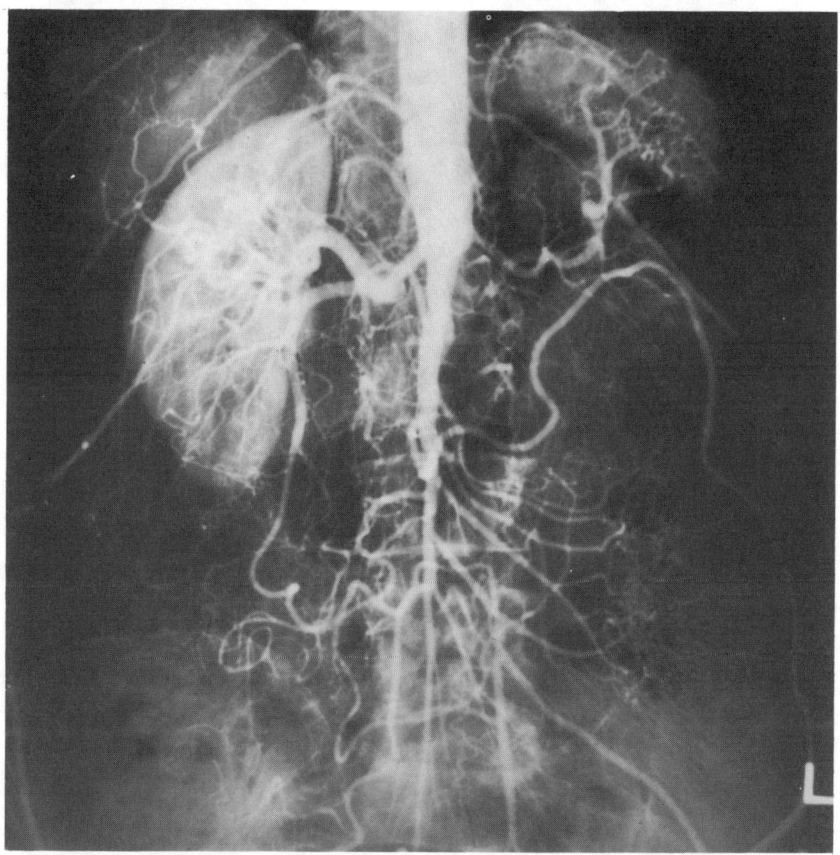

A

Figure 17-7 Atherosclerotic disease. **A** Anterior-posterior abdominal aortogram. Note: 1) abdominal aorta occluded just below renal arteries, 2) intercostal and visceral artery collaterals to the pelvis and distal extremities. **B** Lateral abdominal aortogram. Note: the celiac axes and superior mesenteric artery are patent. **C** Anterior-posterior pelvic arteriogram. Note: blood flow via intercostal collaterals (primarily) to the ileo-femoral circumflex arteries (curved arrows) and into the common femoral arteries (straight arrows). This patient had a six-month history of buttock claudication and weakness in both legs.

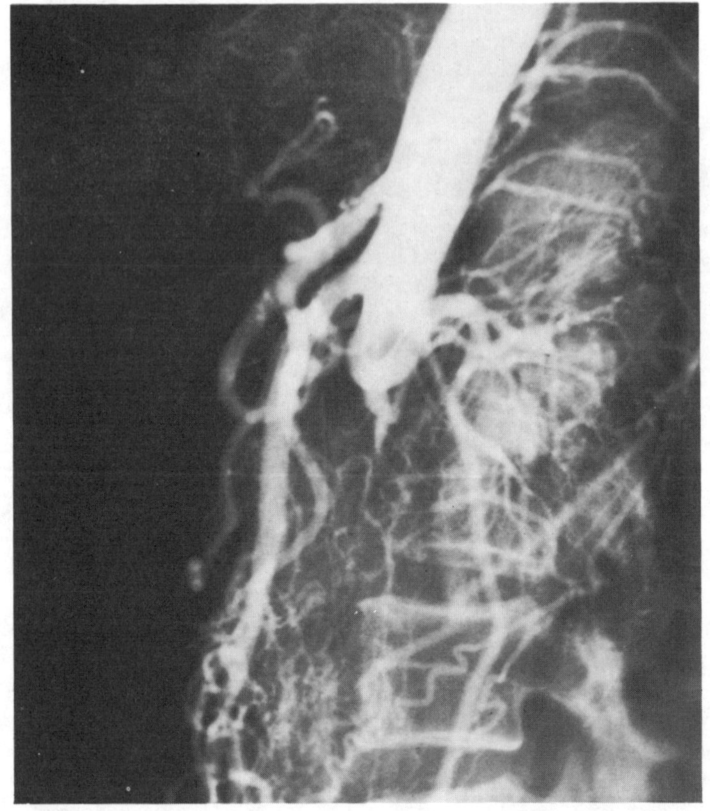

B

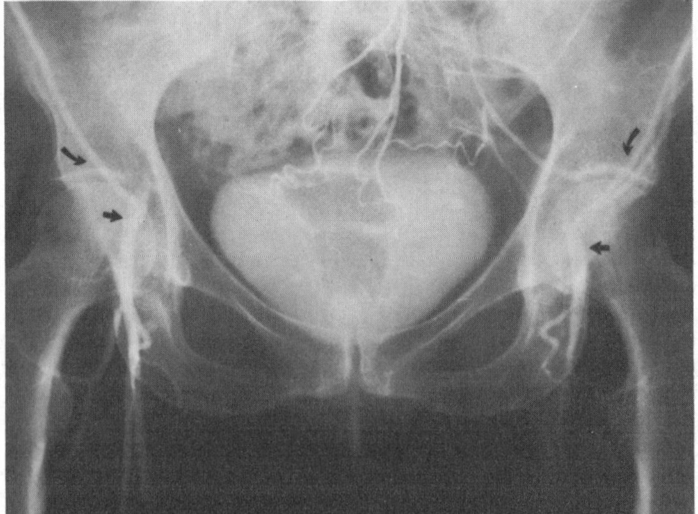

C

Figure 17-7—*Continued*

ANEURYSMS OF THE AORTA

The aorta may become dilated as a result of increased pressure, such as in the case of essential hypertension, or proximal to a narrowed area, as in coarctation. Situations, such as aortic regurgitation and patent ductus arteriosus, which result in volume overload, may lead to dilatation as well. In both of these conditions, the ascending aorta and arch are usually dilated. Turbulent flow distal to a stenosis may lead to dilatation; ie, dilatation of the ascending aorta secondary to aortic valve stenosis.

An aneurysm is an abnormal local dilatation of a vessel, resulting from weakness of its wall. True aneurysms involve all three layers of the aortic wall. Aneurysms are classified as: fusiform, involving the full circumference of the vessel wall; or saccular, involving only a portion of the circumference, thus communicating with the vessel lumen by a relatively narrow neck.[17]

Arteriosclerotic Aneurysms

Aneurysms of arteriosclerotic origin involve the abdominal aorta (Figures 17-8, 17-9) more often than the thoracic aorta, and are more common in elderly males. It has been reported that 20% occur in the thoracic, and 80% in the abdominal portion.[18] They usually occur below the level of the renal arteries.[19]

Arteriosclerotic aneurysms of the thoracic aorta usually involve the distal part of the arch, just below the origin of the left subclavian artery (Figure 17-10). The next most common site is the lower descending portion, and aneurysms in this location extend below the diaphragm into the abdominal portion, producing the so-called *thoraco-abdominal aneurysm* (Figure 17-11). Angiographically, arteriosclerotic aneurysms are usually described as being more fusiform than saccular. It has been reported that as much as 80% of the time, there is laminated mural thrombus. This may result in the lumen appearing normal in caliber on the aortogram, even in the presence of a large aneurysm.[20] In such a case, calcification of the aortic outer wall, widely separated from the apparent luminal margin and displacement of visceral arteries around the aneurysm suggest its presence (Figure 17-12). Rupture is considered the most serious complication in an arteriosclerotic aneurysm. Most abdominal aortic aneurysms rupture retroperitoneally; when this occurs, leakage initially may be slow. The danger of rupture is considered to be greatly increased when the diameter of the aorta reaches 6 to 7 cm. Intraperitoneal rupture is rare.[20] However, when it does occur, it is generally fatal. Rupture into the gastrointestinal tract and other adjacent structures has been reported.[21] Aortography can demonstrate an early leakage. A retrograde femoral approach is most commonly performed, the axillary approach being reserved for those instances in which an attempt at passage of the catheter via the femoral approach fails.

Luetic Aneurysms

Luetic aneurysms predominantly involve the ascending aorta, although they may occur in any portion of the thoracic or abdominal aorta. Dilatation of the aorta is usually maximum in the mid-ascending aorta, gradually tapering distally (Figures 17-13, 17-14). The normal diameter of the ascending thoracic aorta has been reported in the range of 16 to 38 mm.[22] Dilatation tends to be accompanied by tortuosity of the

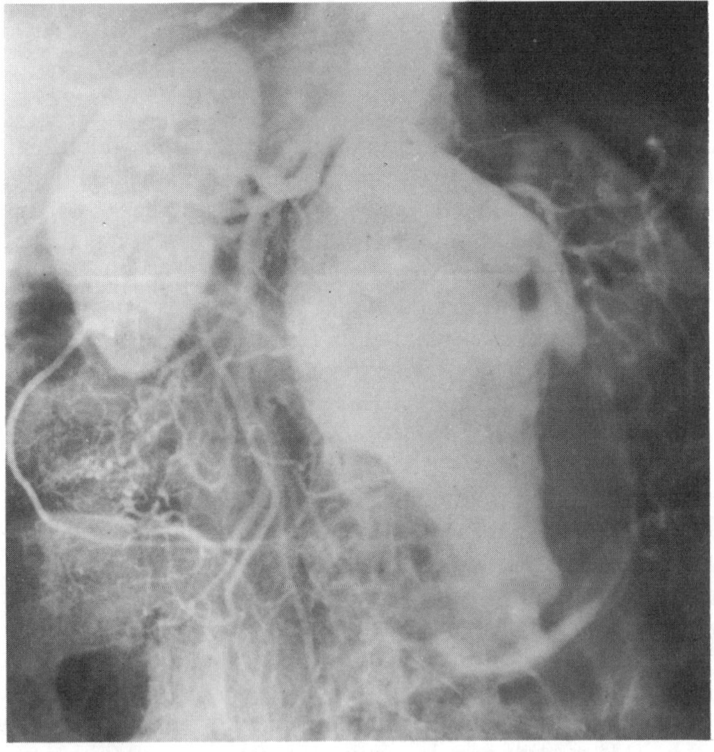

Figure 17-8 **A** Anterior-posterior abdominal aortogram. Note: huge abdominal aortic aneurysm originating just below the renal arteries. **B** Lateral abdominal aortogram (late phase). Note: mark anterior bulging of aneurysm. **C** Anterior-posterior view of aneurysm (late phase). Note: mark wall thickening (space between facing black arrows).

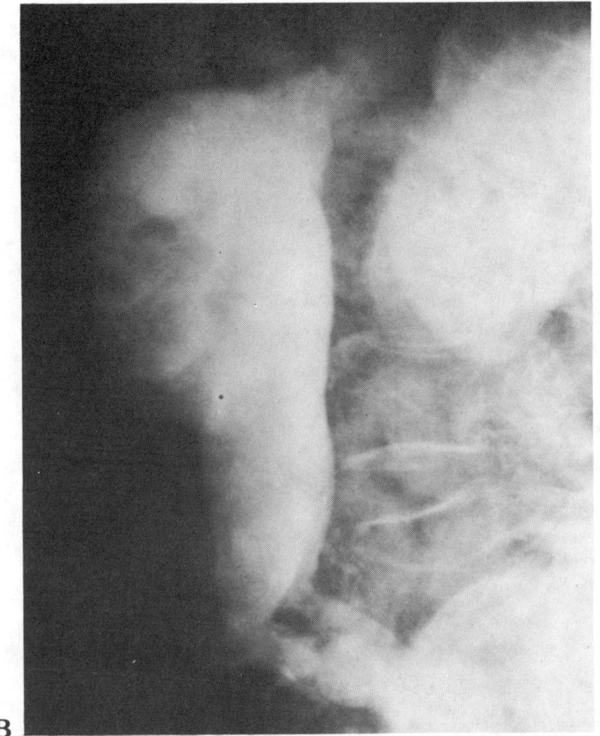

B

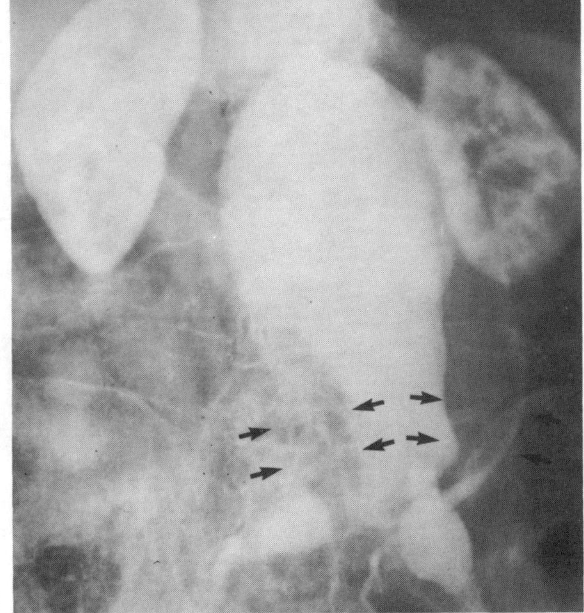

C

A 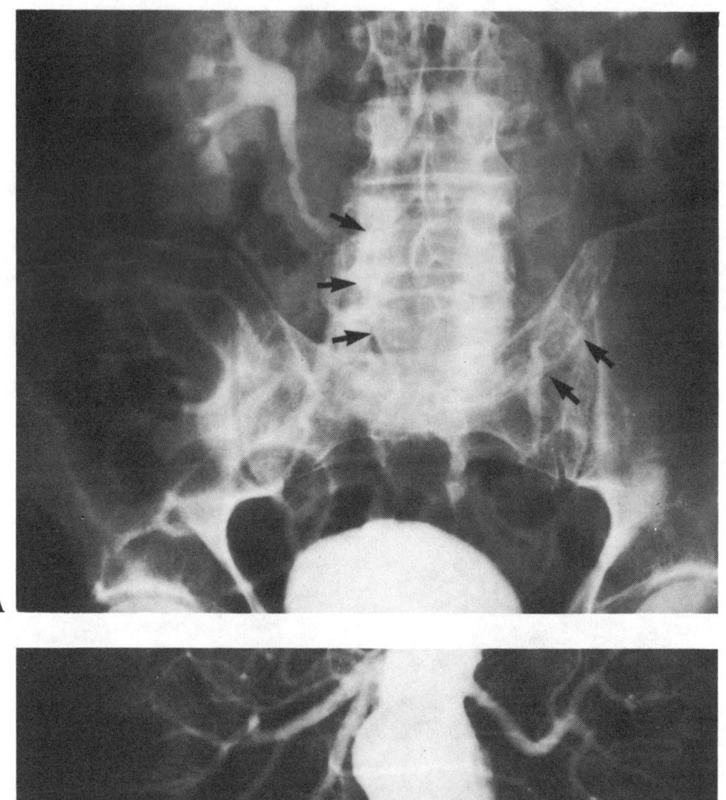

B 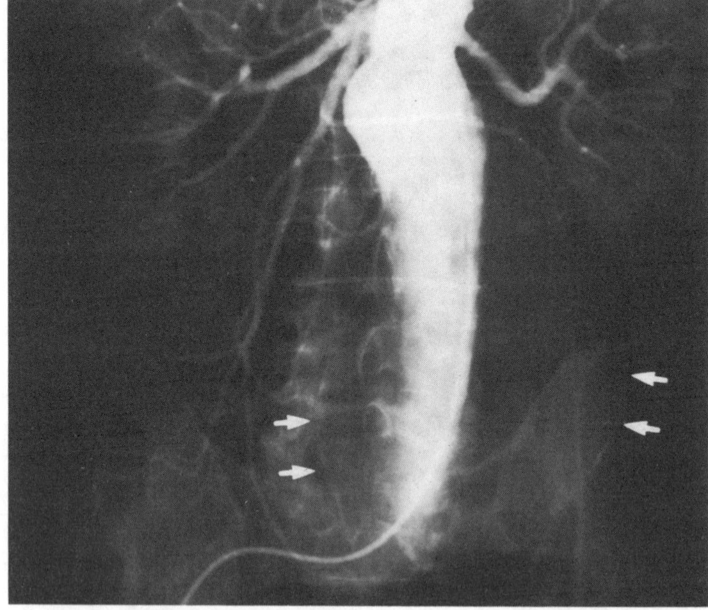

Figure 17-9 **A** Plain film of the abdominal aorta. Note: calcification in wall of aneurysm (arrows). **B** Anterior-posterior abdominal aortogram. Note: 1) minimal dilatation of the abdominal aorta just below renals, 2) marked wall thickening (arrows). **C** Anterior-posterior pelvic arteriogram. Note: aneurysm extends to bifurcation of abdominal aorta (arrows).

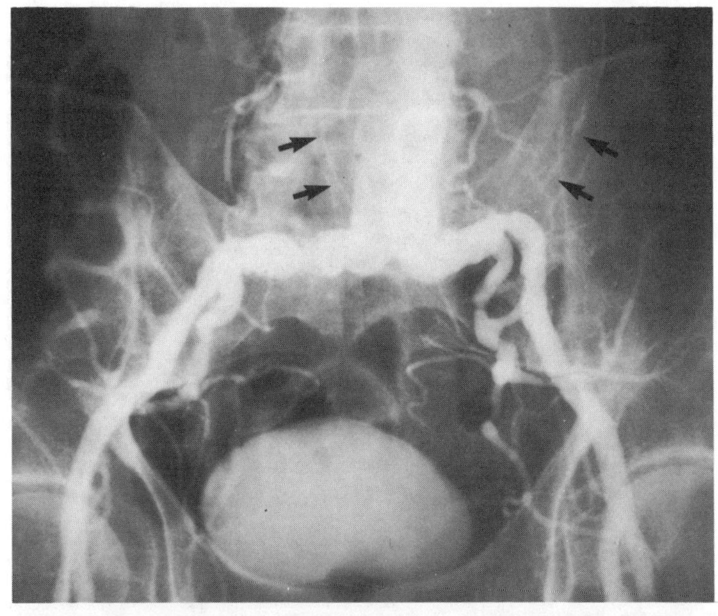

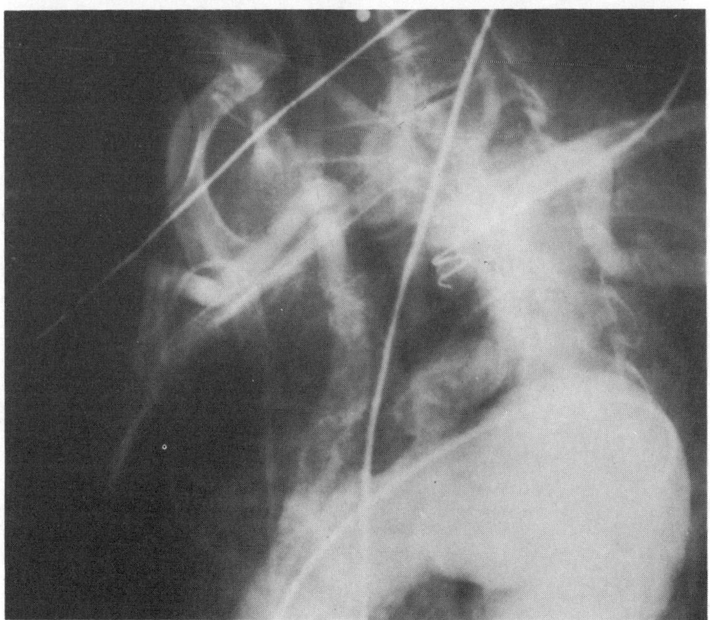

Figure 17-10 Thoracic aortogram (left anterior oblique view). Note: 1) aneurysm originating just distal to origin of left subclavian artery, 2) aneurysm at origin of left subclavian artery. Patient had severe three-vessel coronary artery disease and peripheral vascular disease. Aneurysm thought to be on the basis of atherosclerosis.

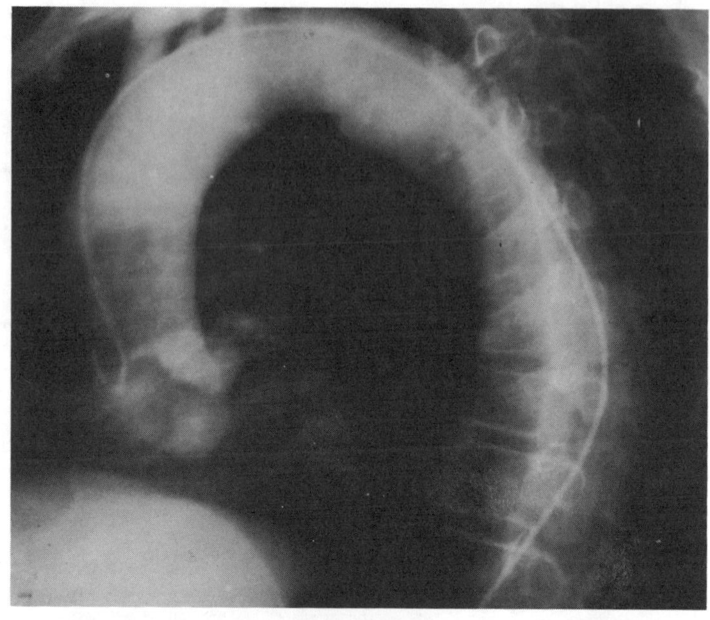

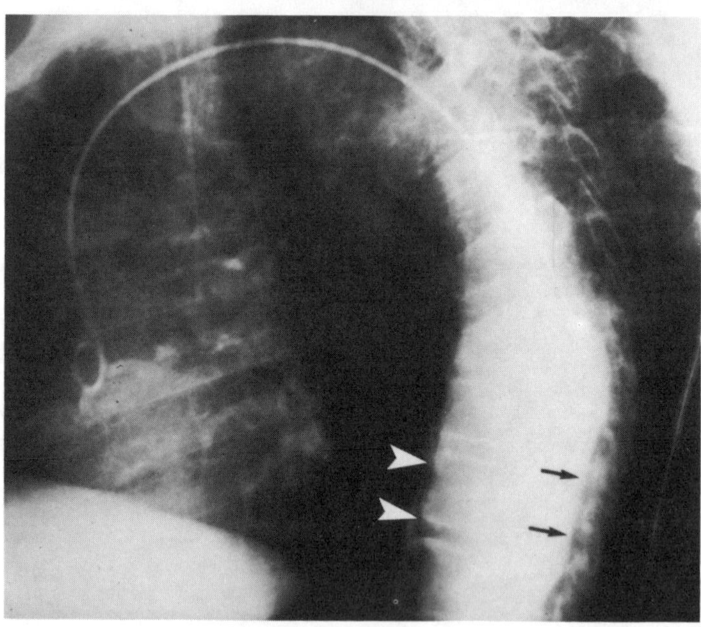

Figure 17-11 **A** Right anterior oblique thoracic aortogram. Note: normal-appearing ascending aorta. **B** Descending thoracic aorta aneurysm. Note: 1) descending aorta has atherosclerotic aneurysm (large arrows), which extends into the abdominal aorta, 2) thickening of aneurysm wall, presumably secondary to plaque formation (small arrows).

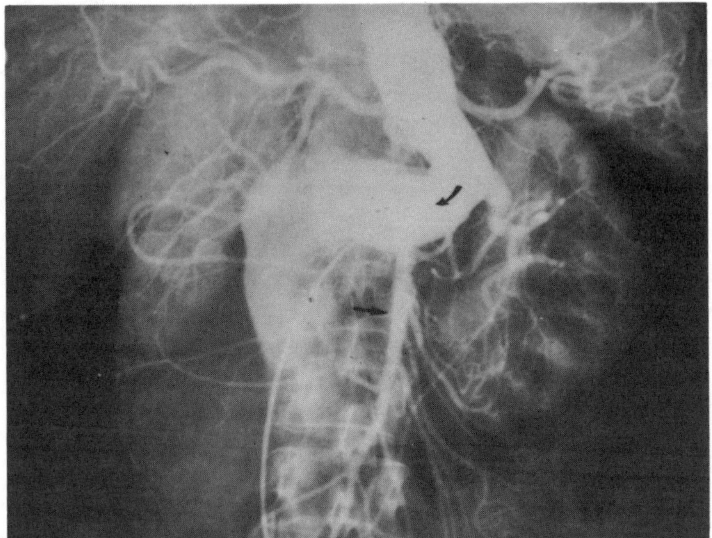

A

B

Figure 17-12 **A** Anterior-posterior abdominal aortogram. Note: 1) large abdominal aortic aneurysm, 2) abdominal aorta, just below renal arteries, curves sharply toward the right side (curved arrow), 3) the superior mesenteric artery is displaced slightly toward the left side (straight arrow). **B** Late phase of abdominal aortogram. Note: 1) column of contrast (intralumen) in aorta appears relatively normal in size, 2) the transverse diameter of the contrast column (at the level of the two facing small arrows) is 2.5 cm; whereas, the transverse diameter of the abdominal aorta (where the two large arrows outline the calcified wall) is 10.4 cm, 3) the right kidney is shifted superiorly, and the left kidney inferiorly.

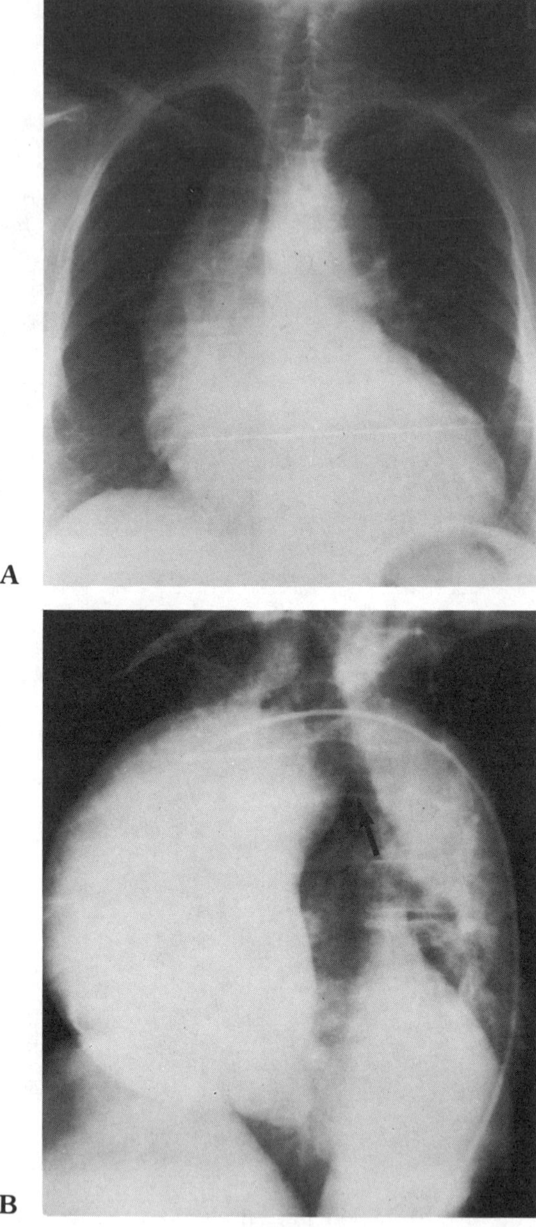

Figure 17-13 **A** Posterior-anterior chest—syphilitic thoracic aortic aneurysm. Note: 1) large ascending aorta, 2) enlarged heart. **B** Left anterior oblique thoracic aortogram. Note: 1) dilated ascending aorta, which gradually tapers just beyond the great neck vessels (arrow), 2) asymmetry of coronary sinuses. Postmortem examination revealed no involvement of them with aneurysm.

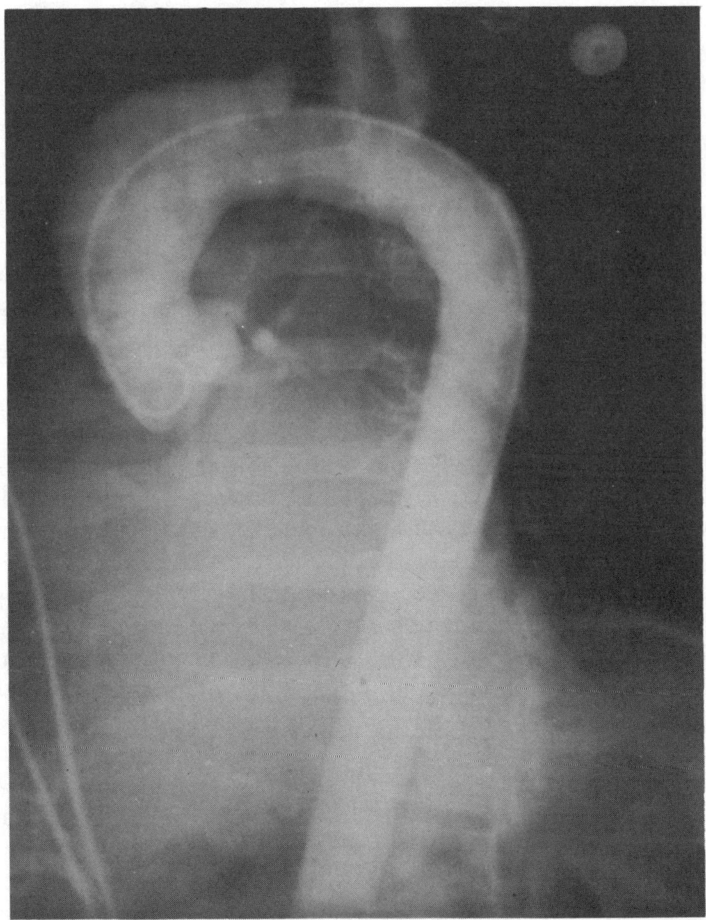

Figure 17-14 Syphilitic thoracic aortic aneurysm. Note: 1) left anterior oblique thoracic aortogram, 2) dilated ascending aorta, with gradual tapering to a normal size at the great neck vessels, 3) normal coronary sinuses.

aorta. There may also be extensive calcification in the intima, primarily in the ascending aorta. The absence of calcification does not exclude syphilis; but, the incidence of intimal calcification in patients with syphilitic aneurysms has been reported in the range of 27% to 40%.[22,23] Luetic aneurysms may be either fusiform of saccular. Aortic sinus aneurysms caused by syphilis may occur, but the sinuses of Valsalva are usually spared (a fact that is useful in distinguishing luetic aneurysms from those caused by cystic medial necrosis of the aorta). Aortic regurgitation is commonly associated with syphilitic involvement of the aortic valve, with folding and separation of the commissure.[24]

When syphilitic aneurysms involve the abdominal aorta, they usually occur between the diaphragm and the renal artery. The superior mesenteric artery and celiac trunk are likely to arise from the aneurysmal sac in such aneurysms.[25]

Cystic Medial Necrosis Aneurysms

Cystic medial necrosis is characterized microscopically by medial degeneration of the elastic tissue of the aorta and grossly by fusiform dilatation. Cystic medial necrosis involves predominately the ascending portion of the aorta and is often part of Marfan's syndrome, although cystic medial necrosis frequently exists without the stigmata of Marfan's disease.[26] It is usually accompanied by annular dilatation of the aortic valve and aortic regurgitation.[27] It may be complicated by dissection in patients, either with or without Marfan's features.[28] It has been reported in at least one series as being the most common cause of aneurysmal dilatation of the ascending aorta.[29] The lesions appear to involve the aortic sinuses alone in the early state, with gradual progression to involve the ascending portion of the thoracic aorta. Aortic sinus dilatation alone may be quite extensive before becoming apparent on the chest radiograph, since the sinuses are hidden by the cardiovascular silhouette. The majority of cases, however, show dilatation of the ascending aorta and, in the presence of aortic insufficiency, there may be dilatation of the left ventricle as well. Calcification of the aorta is rare. Characteristically, one expects to see symmetrical dilatation of the ascending aorta, especially the aortic sinuses on aortography. Higher in the ascending aorta, the aneurysmal dilatation of cystic medial necrosis generally tapers to an almost normal caliber in the arch.

Ultrasonography and computerized tomography may be more accurate in determining the size of an aneurysm. However, these modalities at present are not as good as angiography in determining flow dynamics and the extent of involvement of other structures by the aneurysm.

Pseudoaneurysms

Pseudoaneurysms of the artery are distinguished from true aneurysms in that, instead of the dilated segment of the artery containing the three layers of the vessel wall, a perforation of the intima and media exists, creating an incapsulated hematoma in the periadventitial tissues of the artery. Pseudoaneurysms most commonly are traumatic

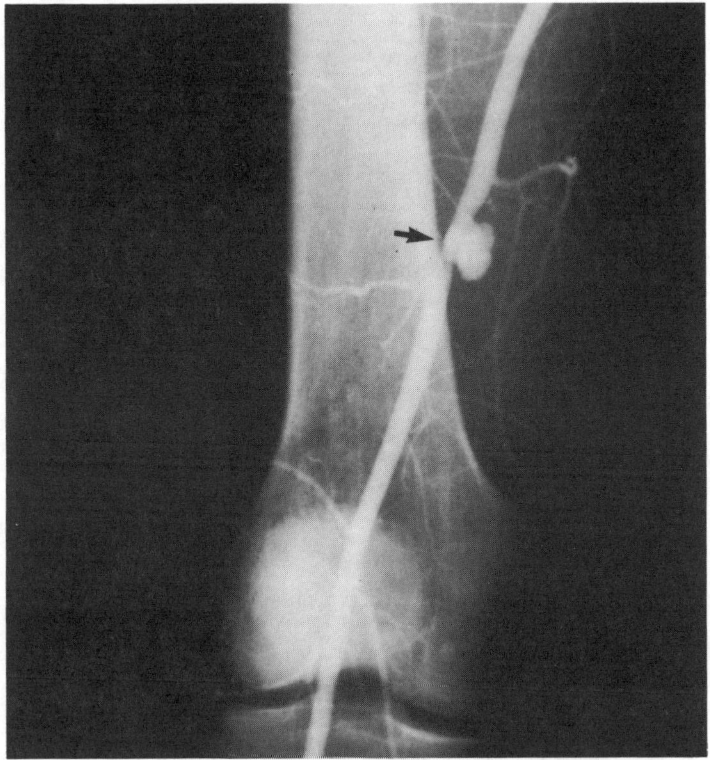

Figure 17-15 Superficial femoral artery pseudoaneurysm, secondary to gunshot wound to thigh (arrow).

in origin (Figure 17-15); they may occur in any artery, and are occasionally secondary to complications of vascular surgery or angiography (Figure 17-16). Mycotic aneurysms are produced by inflammatory involvement of the aortic wall, usually resulting from sepsis (Figure 17-17). Since these aneurysms are not covered by three layers of the aortic wall, they represent a type of pseudoaneurysm.

AORTIC DISSECTIONS

Aortic dissections are not uncommon occurrences. Men more commonly than women are affected, and the incidence is highest in the fifth to seventh decades of life. In the majority of cases (approximately 60% of the time), the dissection occurs within 2 to 3 cm of the aortic valve, and the dissection spreads up through the ascending aorta, frequently going around the arch and down the thoracic aorta. The next

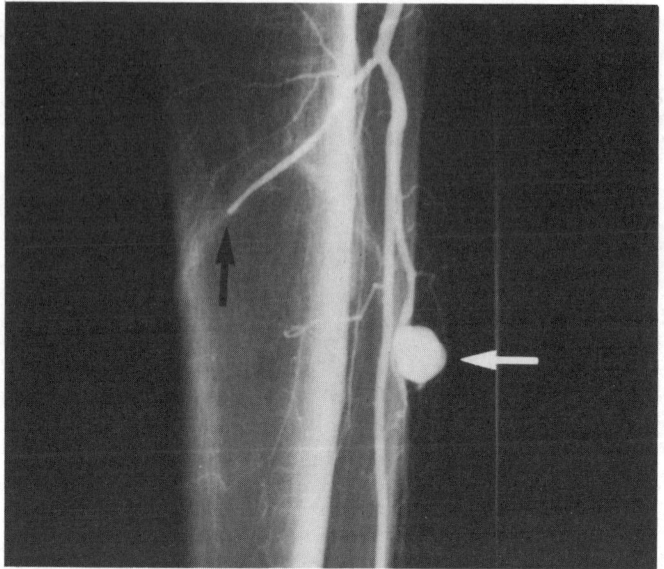

Figure 17-16 Pseudoaneurysm of peroneal artery (white arrow). Patient had peroneal artery probed during popliteal artery embolectomy one month prior to this arteriogram. Note: occluded anterior tibial (black arrow).

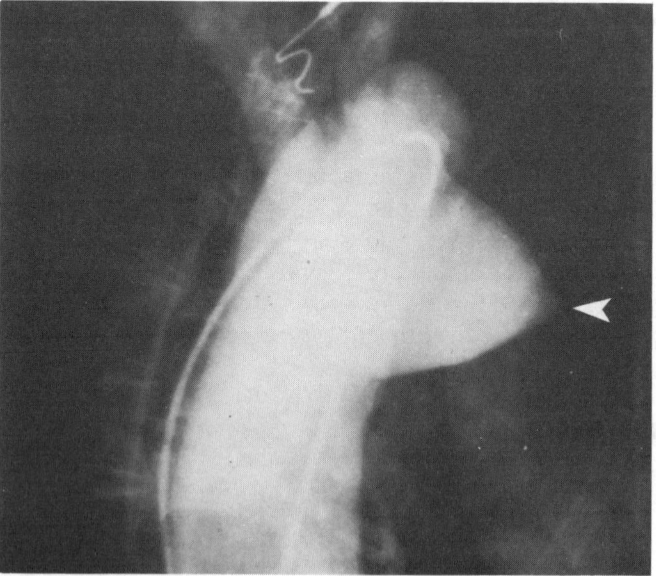

Figure 17-17 Mycotic aneurysm of thoracic aorta (arrow). Note: right anterior oblique projection. Patient had sepsis secondary to bacterial endocarditis.

most common dissection (about 25%) begins with an intimal tear within a few centimeters distal to the origin of the left subclavian artery, and the dissection extends down the descending thoracic aorta.

There have been several attempts by clinicians to classify aortic dissections, none of which seems to satisfy all situations.[30,31] The most popular classification however, is an anatomic one put forth by Debakey.[32] He classified thoracic aortic dissections into three types, according to the origin of the tear and the degree of extension. Type I begins in the ascending aorta and extends beyond the neck vessels of the arch (Figure 17-18). Type II begins in the ascending aorta and stops at or before the neck vessels (Figure 17-19); and Type III begins after the neck vessels (usually just below the left subclavian artery) and extends distally (Figure 17-20). Types I and III may extend to involve the abdominal aorta and iliac vessels. Types I and II may extend proximally to involve the coronary sinuses or pericardial sac. Aortic regurgitation may result from Types I and II dissections.

The pathogenesis of aortic dissections is of considerable interest. The essential underlying lesion is a degenerative state of the aortic media, whereas the initiating event is hemorrhage into the degenerate tissue. When the disease develops in subjects under 40 years of age, the degenerative change is of a florid character and constitutes the condition known as mucoid medial degeneration (Erdheim's disease).[33] In these cases, the blood pressure is usually within normal limits. When a dissecting aneurysm develops in subjects over 50 years of age, the medial degeneration (though similar in character) is often patchy and much less severe; and a higher proportion of the older patients are hypertensive. It has been suggested, if systemic hypertension were eliminated, aortic dissection would almost disappear.[34]

The dissection, which is secondary to hemorrhage deep within the media, usually produces a second lumen (false lumen) with a potential for carrying blood. This false lumen is usually situated between the inner two thirds of the media and intima, and the outer one third of the media and adventitia. The most useful sign on a plain chest film is an obvious increase in mediastinal width on a good posteroanterior film (Figure 17-21). However, the chest x-ray in a small number of cases may not show evidence of aortic widening. Other signs, such as local dilatation of the thoracic aorta and abdominal aorta, are less reliable.

Aortography is indicated for definitive diagnosis, particularly if surgery is contemplated. Biplane thoracic aortography, via the femoral or axillary approach, is the usual method of study. To make the diagnosis of aortic dissection, one of three major angiographic criteria should be present: 1) identification of entry site (tear site) of contrast into the dissection (false lumen); 2) identification of the intimal flap

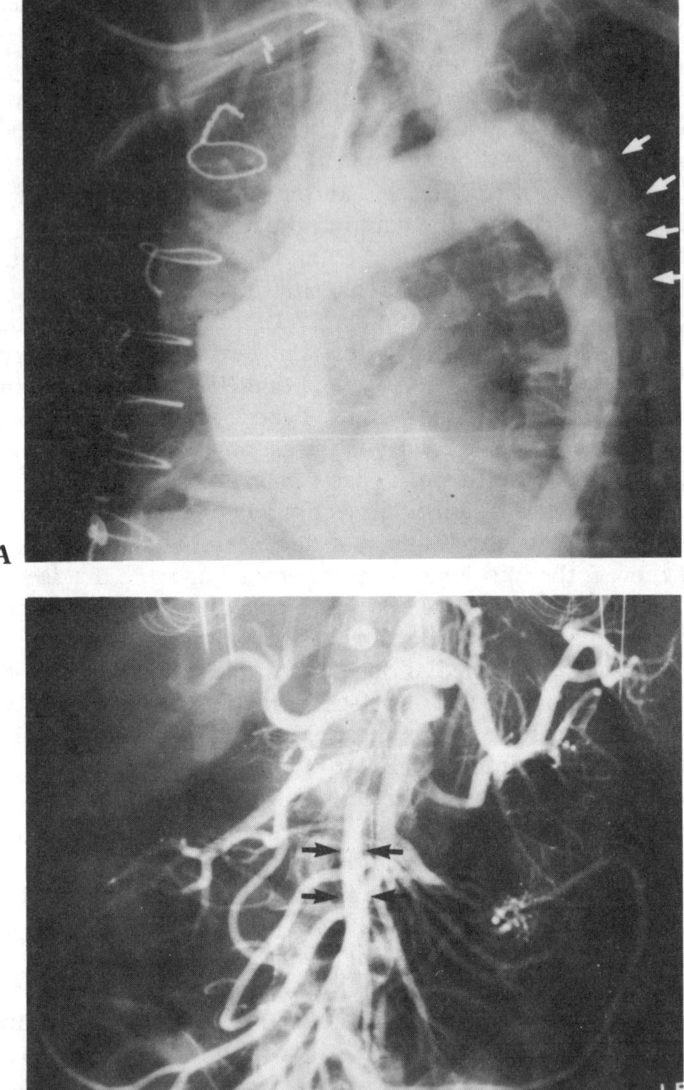

Figure 17-18 **A** Type I thoracic aortic dissection. Note: 1) lucent band across ascending aorta just above the coronary cusp, 2) gouge defect along the outer margin of the ascending thoracic aorta, just proximal to the innominate artery, 3) mark narrowing of the contrast column, 4) contrast has begun to appear in the false lumen (arrows). **B** Anterior-posterior abdominal aortogram (same patient). Note: 1) narrowed contrast column in abdominal aorta, 2) all major branches of the abdominal aorta are patent. **C** Lateral abdominal aortogram (same patient). Note: renál arteries patent, in spite of marked narrowing of the abdominal aorta at their level.

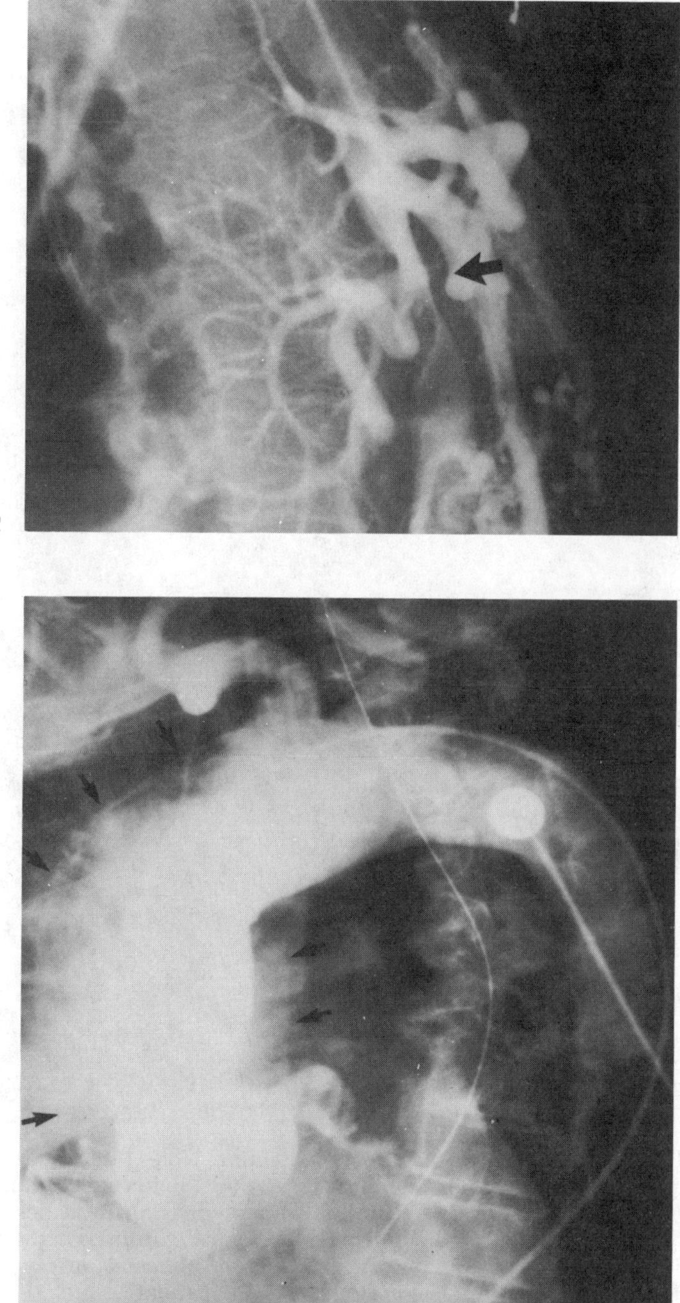

Figure 17-19 Type II thoracic aortic dissection. Note: 1) contrast filling the false lumen (arrows), 2) normal-looking descending aorta.

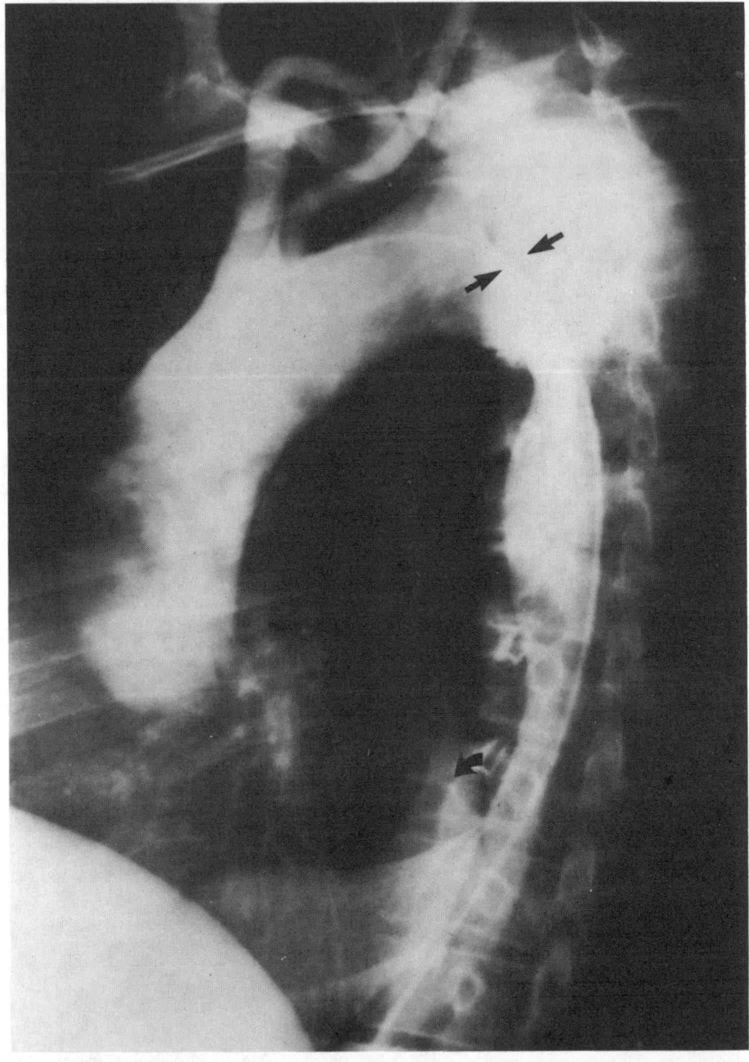

A

Figure 17-20 **A** Type III thoracic aortic dissection. Note: 1) lucent defect (intimal flap) in contrast column, beginning just below the left subclavian artery (arrows), 2) contrast filling false lumen, 3) markedly narrowed descending thoracic aorta, 4) catheter in true lumen, resting far away from posterior wall of descending thoracic aorta, 5) contrast entering an intercostal artery (curved arrow). **B** Late phase of thoracic aortogram (same patient). Note: 1) contrast

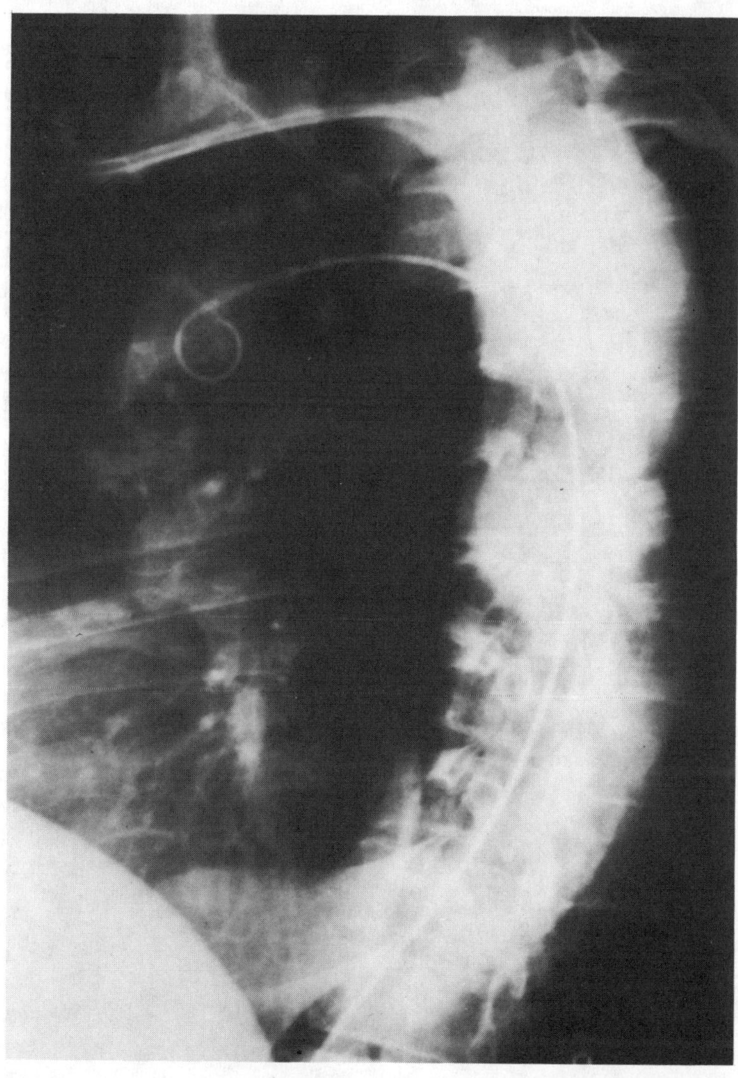

B

now filling the false lumen, 2) note absence of contrast entering any intercostal arteries. **C** Anterior-posterior abdominal aortogram (same patient). Note: 1) dissection involves the abdominal aorta, causing it to narrow, 2) the celiac axes, SMA, and both renal arteries are patent. **D** Anterior-posterior pelvic arteriogram (same patient). Note: dissection extends to right pelvic arteries, causing occlusion at the level of the proximal external iliac artery.

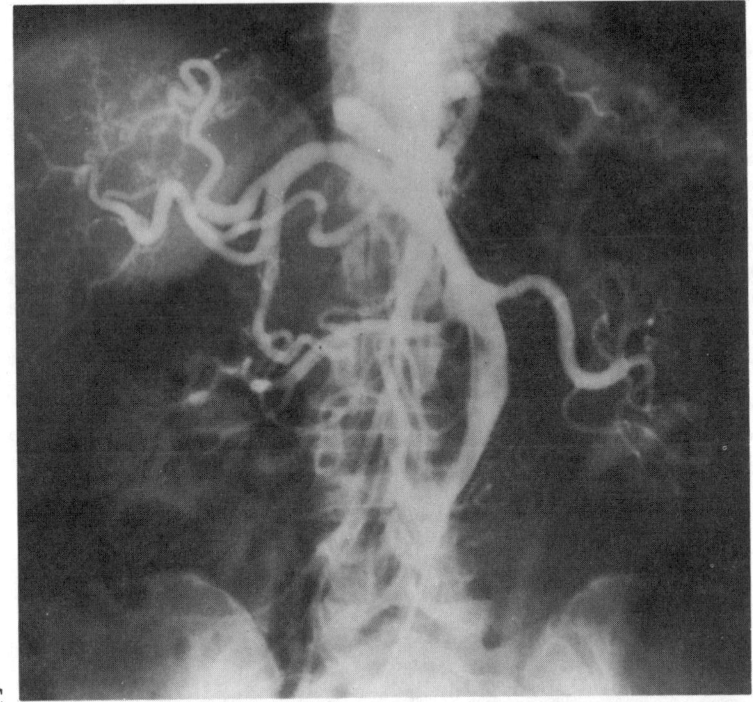

C

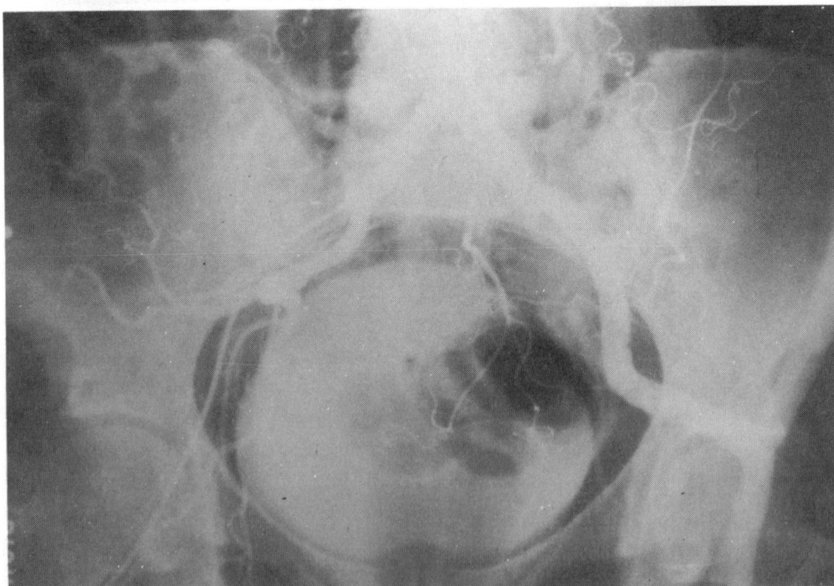

D

Figure 17-20—*Continued*

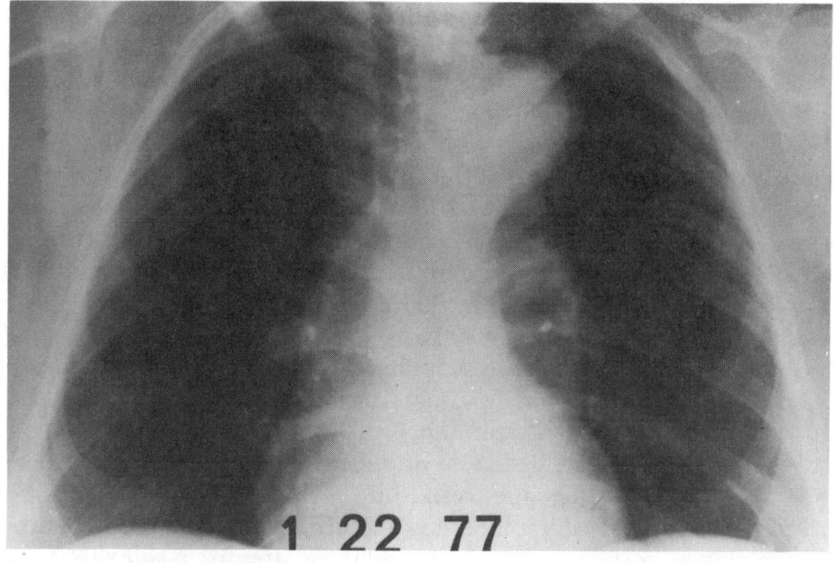

A

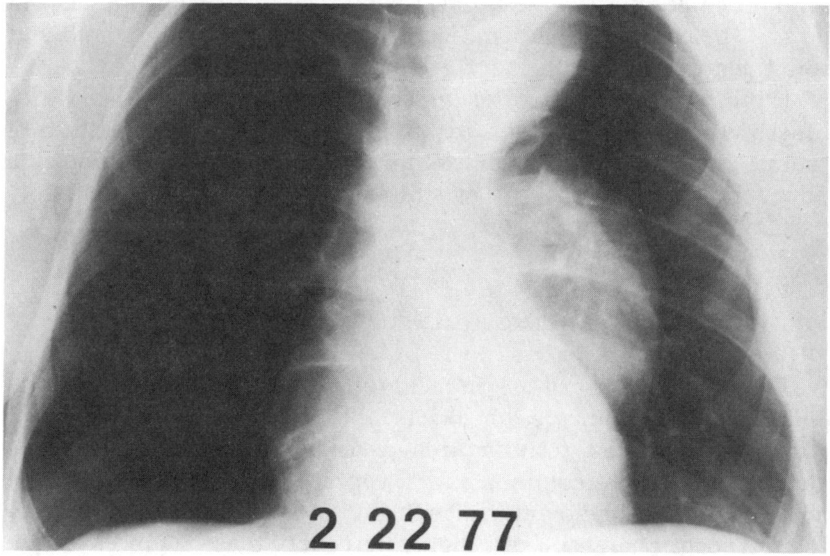

B

Figure 17-21 **A** Posterior-anterior chest film (of patient in Figure 17-20), one month before entering hospital. Note: the aortic arch is prominent, and the descending aorta is dilated and tortuous. **B** Posterior-anterior chest film (of patient in Figure 17-20), at the time of entering the hospital. Patient complaining of having an episode of excruciating left thoracic back pain, which began under the scapula and radiated downward to her groin.

(usually consisting of intima and inner two thirds of media); and 3) identification of the false lumen.

The intimal flap characteristically appears as a vertical or spiralling filling defect within the contrast column of the aorta (Figure 17-20A). The false lumen is usually identified by seeing contrast enter it, or by delayed appearance of the contrast in a section of the aorta not previously identified (Figure 17-20B). Opacification of the false lumen is usually slower than that of the true, indicating slower blood flow in the false lumen. When the communication between the two lumina is very large, however, then there will be very nearly equal flow. Hence, opacification of both lumina may be equal. There may not be free flow throughout the length of the false lumen, because of partial thrombosis and hematoma formation. In other instances, depending upon the amount of time having transpired before angiography, the false lumen may not be demonstrated because of thrombosis at the site of rupture. Diagnosis of dissecting aneurysm in such cases, on angiographic criteria alone, is virtually impossible and ultrasonography and/or computerized tomography may be indicated in an attempt to show the true and false lumina. Secondary angiographic signs are helpful, ie, failure to fill the major neck vessels, intercostals, or other major branches of the aorta below the diaphragm. A significant separation of the catheter from the outer wall of the aorta is very suggestive of dissection.

Primary abdominal aortic dissections are rare and, in most instances when they do occur, are usually secondary to some form of trauma.[35-37] Figure 17-22 is an example of abdominal aortic dissection secondary to placement of an intraaortic balloon for circulatory assistance in a patient postsurgery for coronary artery disease.

Traumatic Rupture of the Aorta

Traumatic rupture of the thoracic aorta, or its great neck vessels, is quite prevalent in our present society. It is usually secondary to blunt trauma to the thorax, resulting in a shearing force on the aorta or its branches. The more common site of rupture is at the isthmus of the thoracic aorta, just below the left subclavian artery; however, the rupture can occur at any site.[38-40] Eighty percent of these ruptures lead to massive hemorrhage, with death occurring before definitive surgical therapy can be implemented. For the 20% that do not die, there may be no symptoms or they may present with a bruit over the upper anterior or posterior thorax. A history of dizziness or loss of consciousness may be elicited. The patients may be hypotensive or have hypertension of the upper extremities. A chest film may show a widened mediastinum and/or apical pleural shadow secondary to hemorrhage into the medi-

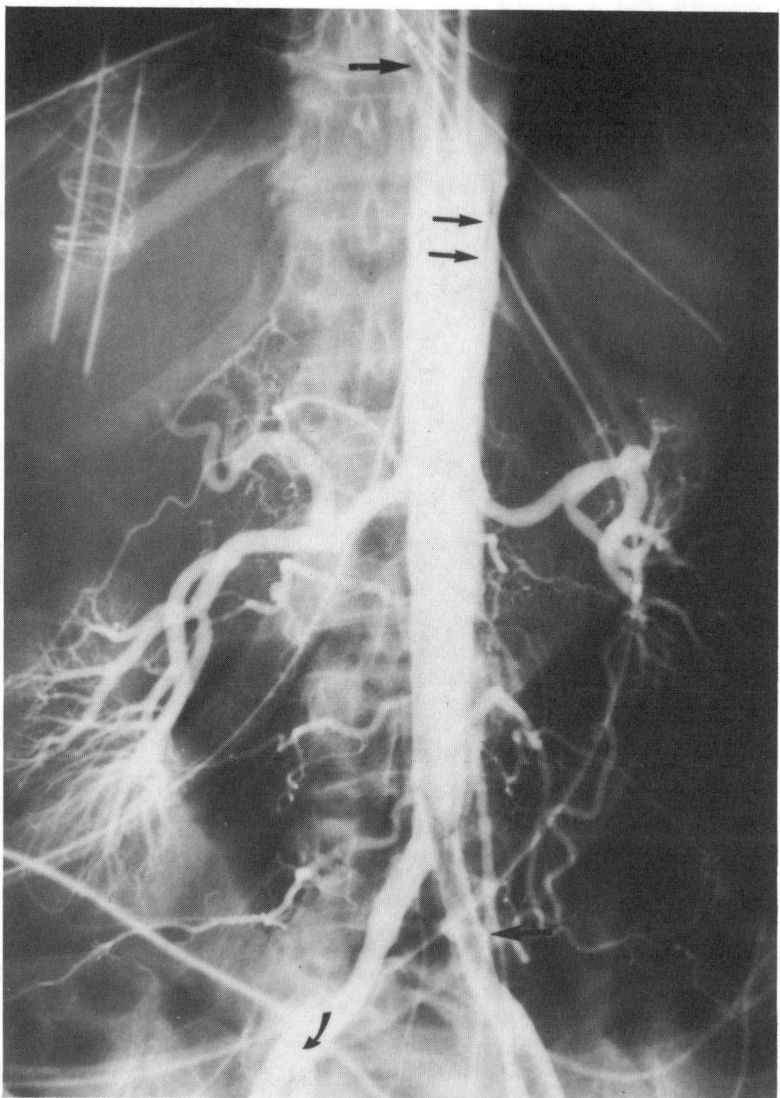

A

Figure 17-22 **A** Anterior-posterior abdominal aortogram. Sixty-four-year-old female, placed on intraaortic balloon counterpulsation at time of cardiac surgery. Immediately postsurgery, patient became hypotensive and oliguric. Note: 1) 14-french catheter in left iliac vessel and abdominal aorta (large arrow), 2) vertical filling defect (intimal flap) along left lateral border of contrast column, above the left renal artery (small arrows), 3) another intimal flap in right common iliac artery (curved arrow). **B** Lateral aortogram (same patient). Note: 1) filling defect at origin of superior mesenteric artery (large arrow), 2) occluded celiac axes (small arrow).

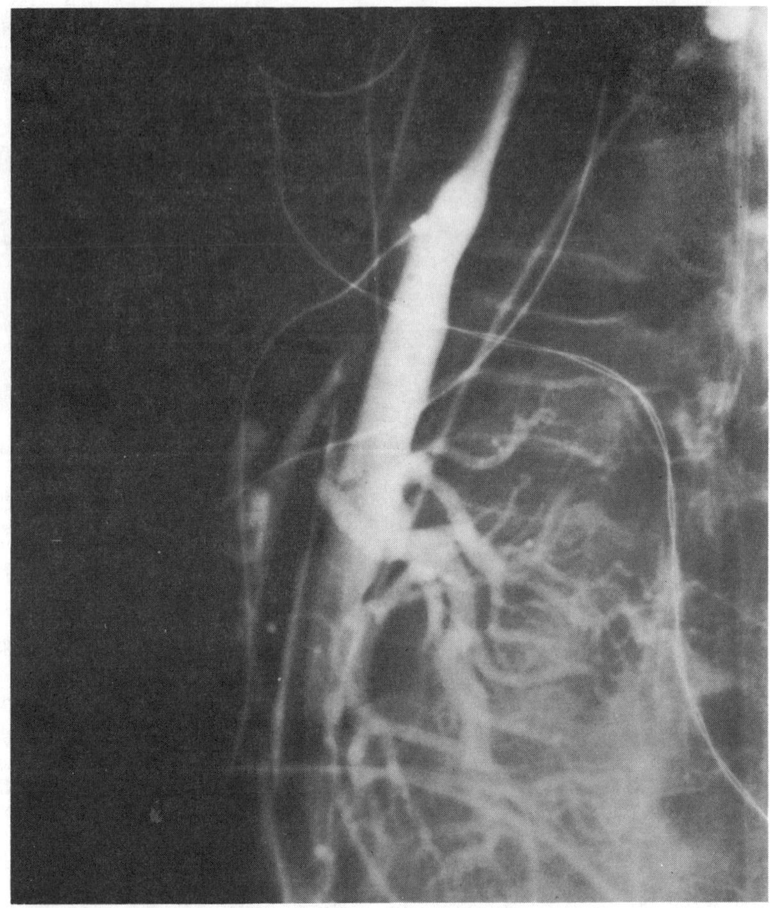

Figure 17-22—*Continued*

astinum or apical extrapleural space. The patient may have difficulty ventilating, and pulmonic infiltrates may be apparent. At angiography, a localized collection of contrast and/or vascular flap may be present at the site of rupture (Figures 17-23, 17-24). The aorta should be viewed in at least two planes before excluding a rupture. Rupture of the abdominal aorta secondary to trauma is not as frequent as thoracic aortic rupture; however, it has been reported.[41]

Renovascular Hypertension and Thrombosis

Arteriography is essential in determining renovascular causes of hypertension such as atherosclerosis, fibromuscular dysplasia, and

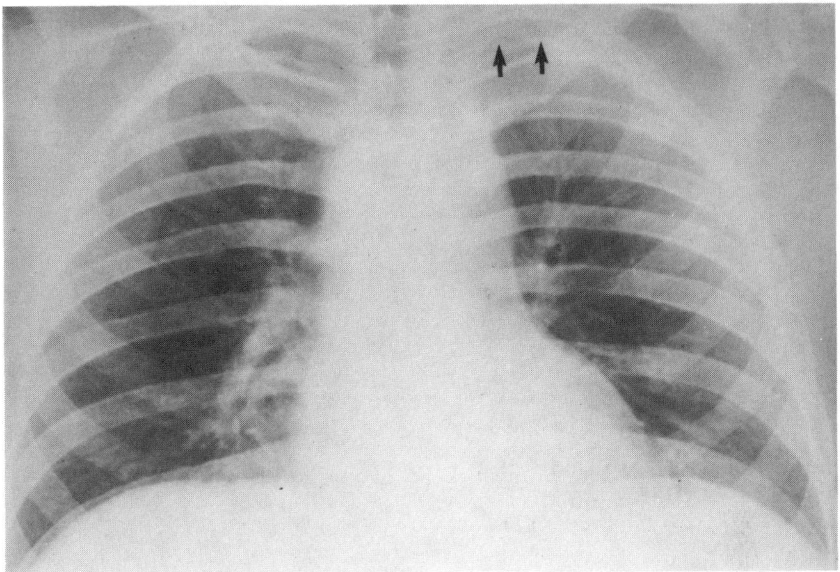

A

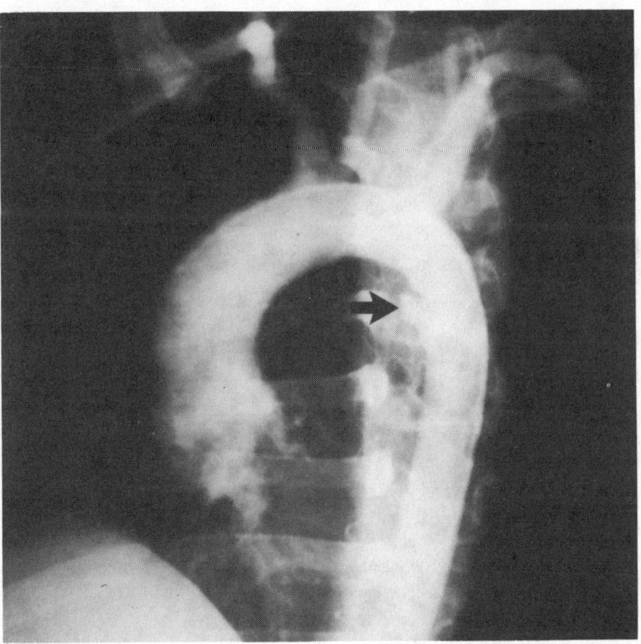

B

Figure 17-23 **A** Posterior-anterior chest. Note: 1) widen mediastinum, 2) left apical extrapleural cap (vertical arrows). **B** Thoracic aortogram left anterior oblique. Note: extraluminal collection of contrast at anterior border of descending thoracic aorta, just below subclavian artery (level of isthmus—see arrow).

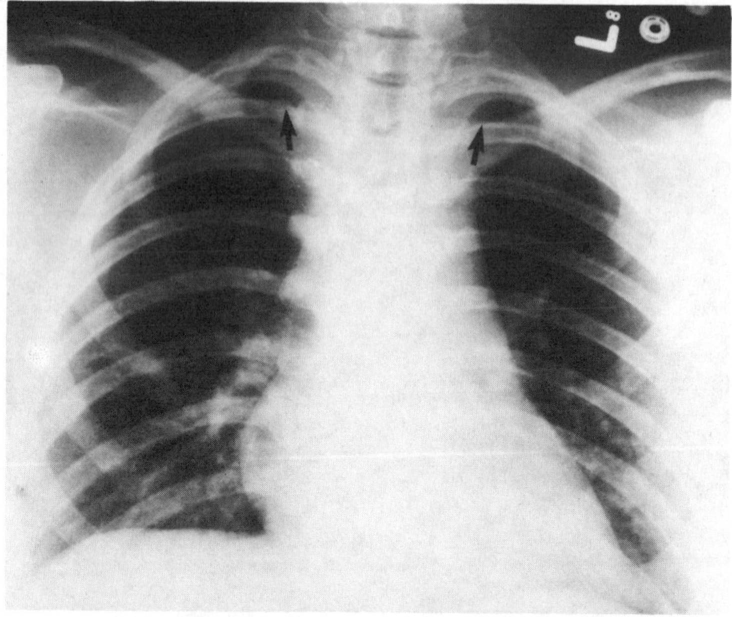

A

B

Figure 17-24 **A** Posterior-anterior chest. Note: 1) wide mediastinum, 2) bilateral apical extrapleural caps (arrows). **B** Thoracic aortogram (posterior-anterior). Note: dilated right innominate artery at the site of fracture (arrowheads).

rarely the vasculitidies. Angiographically, renal stenosis secondary to atherosclerosis is characteristically located at the origin or proximal one third of the main renal artery, and may present as short or diffuse segmental narrowings. Renal artery stenosis secondary to atherosclerosis is the most common cause of renovascular hypertension (Figure 17-25). Fibromuscular disease, as a cause of renovascular hypertension, is more common in young adult women.[42] The renal arteries may be bilaterally involved and involvement of other vessels, such as the mesenteric and cephalic arteries, may occur (Figure 17-26). Characteristically, this disease entity may appear angiographically as saccular aneurysms (*string of beads*) located primarily in the middle to distal one third of the main renal artery (Figure 17-27). However, occasional focal or tubularlike stenoses in the middle to distal one third of the main renal artery may make the diagnosis on angiographic criteria alone impossible.

VASCULITIDIES

The vasculitidies are many. They are defined in this chapter as representing necrotizing inflammation of blood vessels.

Most forms of vasculitis are thought to be caused by immunologic phenomena. This belief is supported by clinical observations and animal experiments.[43-57] Necrotizing inflammation of blood vessels is a common finding in experimentally induced immune-complex diseases. Vasculitis is a known manifestation of human serum sickness and has a frequent association with several known immune-complex diseases.[45] In systemic lupus erythematosus, antibodies to DNA and complement components have been identified in vascular lesions. Also, in mixed cryoglobulinemia 1gG, antibodies to 1gG and complement components have been seen in involved vessels.[46] In some patients with polyarteritis, the hepatitis-associated antigen has been implicated as the causal agent with the finding of antigen, immunoglobulins, and complement in the lesion.[47]

The characteristic angiographic findings in only the more common vasculitidies will be discussed in this chapter.

Periarteritis Nodosa

In periarteritis nodosa (polyarteritis nodosa), the necrotizing inflammatory process involves medium and small arteries and their adjacent veins, occasionally arterioles and venules, but not capillaries. Its distribution is usually segmental and there is a predilection for the

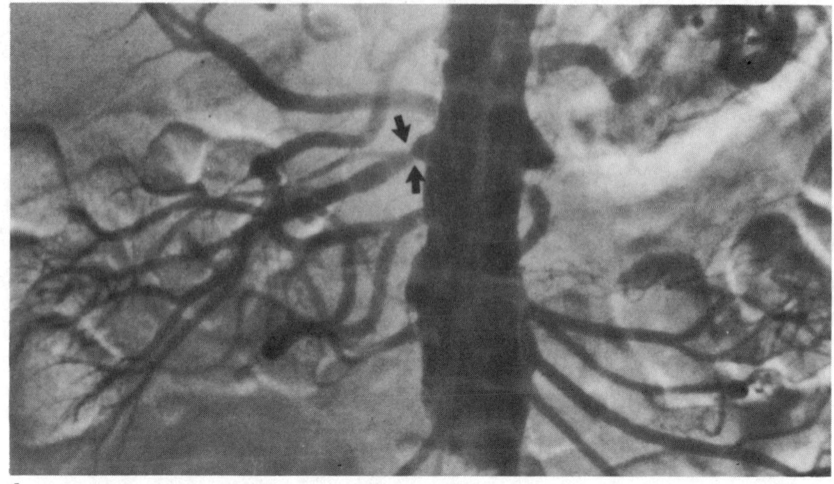

A

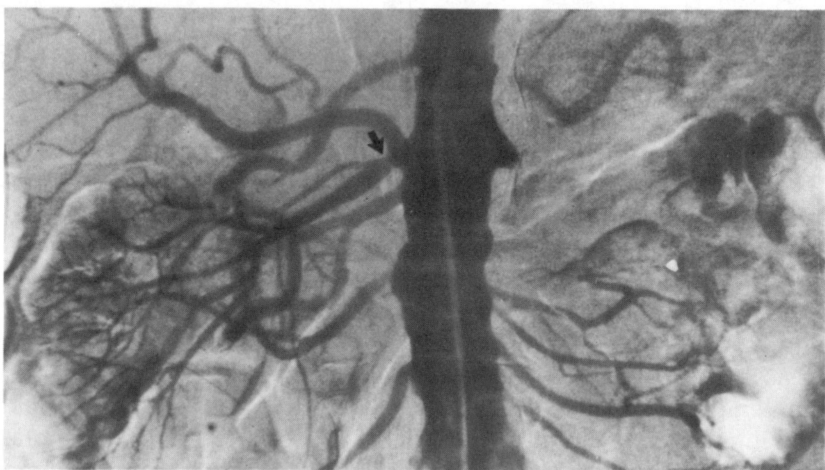

B

Figure 17-25 **A** Eighty-four-year-old male with carcinoma of the lung, chronic hypertension, and recent onset of renal failure (lab). Note: 1) abdominal aortogram shows totally occluded left renal artery, 2) stenosed right renal artery in its proximal one-third (arrows), 3) this patient had a percutaneous transluminal angioplasty (PTA) procedure performed on the right renal artery (see text on Percutaneous Transluminal Angioplasty), 4) he experienced two days of acute renal failure and then began to have a diuresis, 5) his blood pressure returned to normal off medications, 6) his creatinine stabilized at 2 mg and he was discharged from the hospital within two weeks with a sense of well being. **B** Repeat abdominal aortogram post PTA shows relief of the stenosis (arrow). A 6-french catheter, placed across the stenosis (pre and post PTA), showed mean systolic pressures of 50 and 90, respectively. Mean aortic pressure was 140.

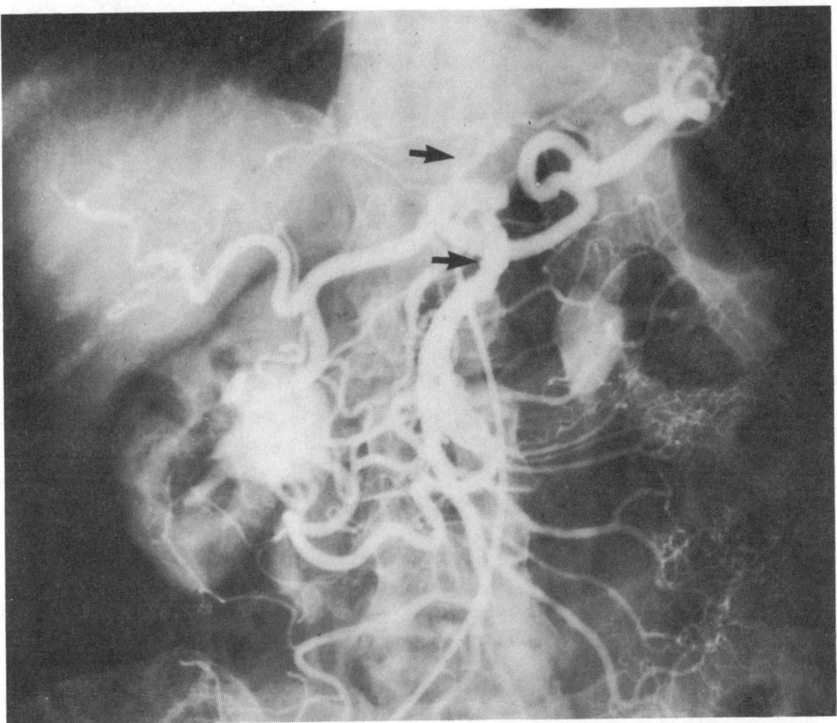

Figure 17-26 Fibrous dysplasia of superior mesenteric and left gastric arteries (37-year-old female). Note: beaded appearance in proximal portion of those arteries (arrows).

bifurcation of arteries. Small aneurysms may form, some of which may rupture. Acute lesions show predominately polymorphonuclear (neutrophiles) leukocytes infiltrating the vessel walls and perivascular areas[48]; whereas, chronic lesions show mononuclear cell infiltration primarily and partial healing. During the active state of the disease, chronic and acute lesions may be present.

Angiography is useful in documenting the diagnosis of periarteritis nodosa and its extent. Characteristically, aneurysms at branch points of arteries occur in kidneys, mesentery, liver, pancreas, and elsewhere during the acute phase of the disease (Figure 17-28). In late states of the disease, narrowing and thrombosis of arteries predominate in the same area.

Takayasu's Arteritis

Takayasu's arteritis is a primary arteritis of undetermined etiology that affects the aorta, the proximal (neck) portions of its major

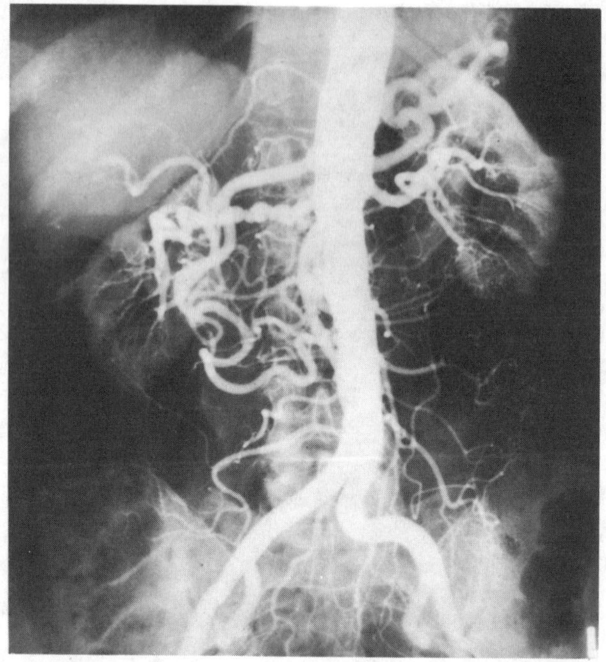

A

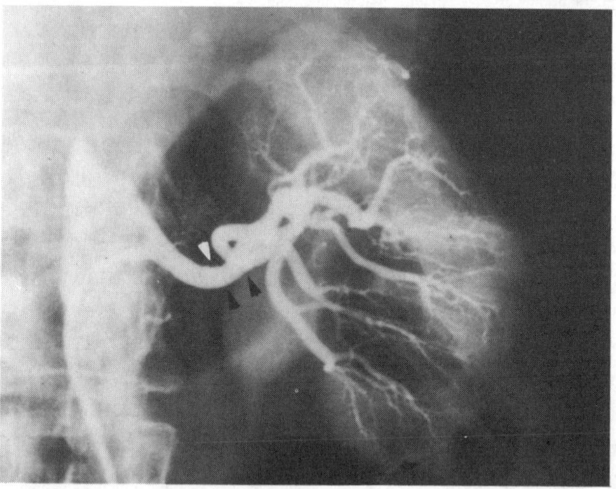

B

Figure 17-27 **A** Fibrous dysplasia of both renal arteries (same patient as Figure 17-26). Note: 1) obvious beaded appearance in distal two thirds of right renal artery, 2) no obvious involvement of the left renal artery by fibrous dysplastic process, 3) abdominal aorta relatively free of atherosclerotic signs, 4) tortuosity of the abdominal aorta and its iliac branches, most probably secondary to chronic hypertension. **B** Selective arteriogram of left renal artery reveals subtle changes of fibrous dysplasia in its distal one-third (arrowheads).

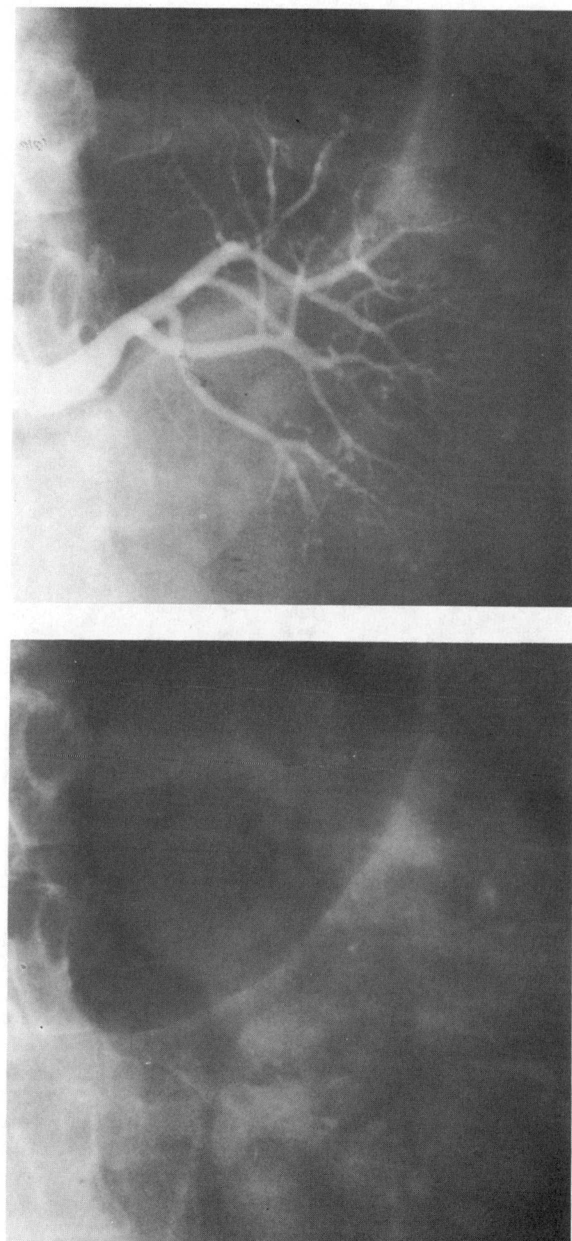

Figure 17-28 **A** Polyarteritis nodosa—left kidney. Note: aneurysms of varying sizes characteristically located at branching points of the interparenchymal arteries within the kidney. **B** Parenchymal phase of selective arteriogram, showing pooling of contrast within aneurysms. (Images courtesy of Dr Christos A. Athanasoulis, Boston, MA.)

branches, and the pulmonary arteries. It can produce stenosis, occlusion, dilatation, or aneurysm. It most commonly affects young women, but also occurs in men.[49] Though its etiology is not clear, most investigators believe it to be due to an autoimmune disorder.[50-52] Pathologically, all three layers of the arterial wall may be involved in a mononuclear cell inflammatory process. Destruction of the elastic fibers of the media results in aneurysmal and intimal proliferation, and fibrosis leads to luminal stenosis. Vessel occlusion is usually secondary to thrombus. There may also be extensive periaortic adhesions.

Angiographically, the findings in Takayasu's arteritis include: occlusive disease, stenotic lesions, aneurysmal changes, or any combination (Figure 17-29).

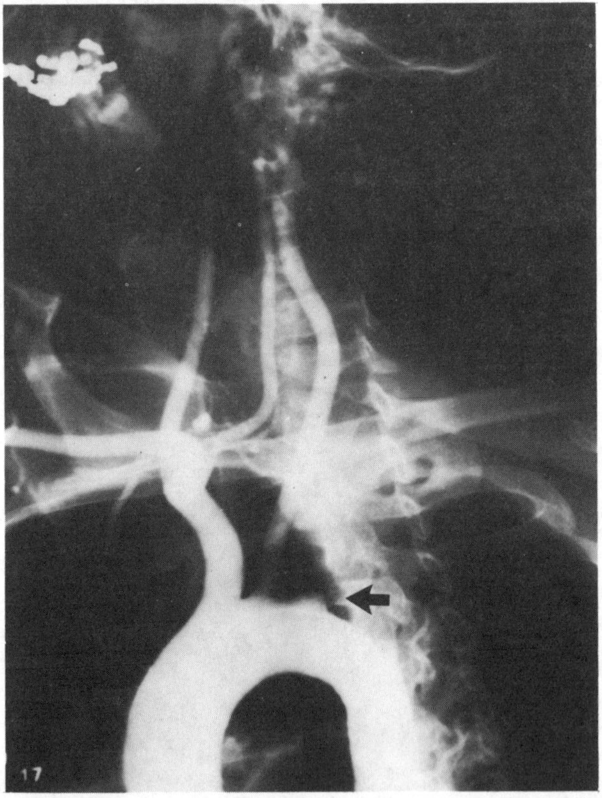

Figure 17-29 **A** Takayasu's arteritis (24-year-old male). Note: thoracic aortogram shows occlusion of left subclavian artery (arrow). **B** Takayasu's arteritis (same patient). **C** Takayasu's arteritis (same patient). Note: totally occluded right renal artery and stenosis of left renal artery in its proximal part (arrow). The aorta and its branches are free of any other disease, which would be atypical if this were primarily atherosclerotic disease.

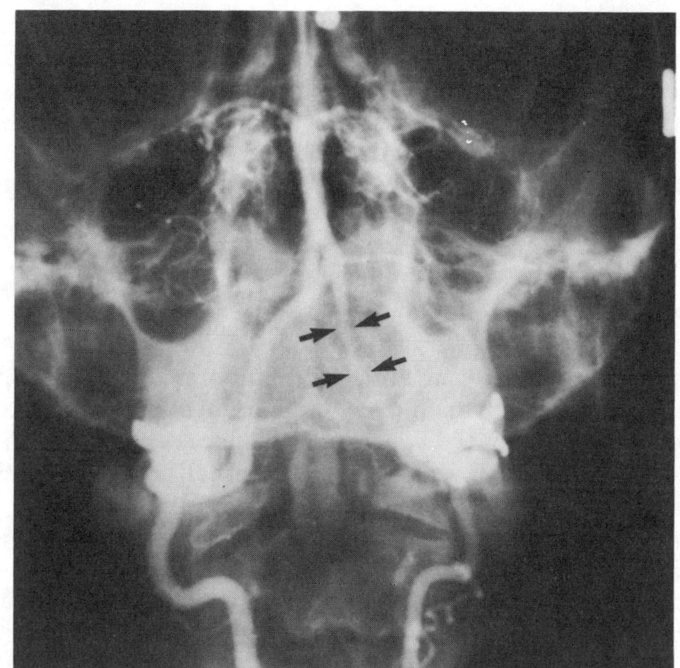
B

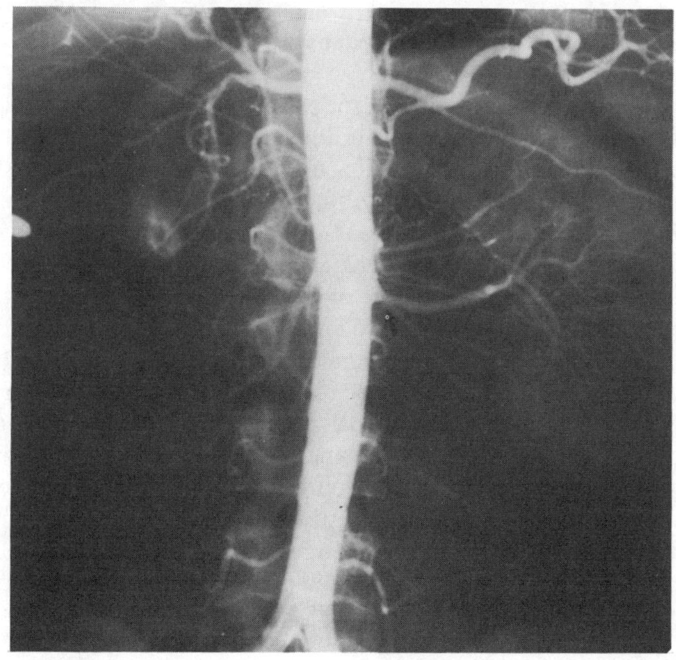
C

Takayasu's arteritis may superficially resemble atherosclerosis; but the latter is infrequent in nondiabetic, premenopausal women and often involves the iliac and femoral arteries. Furthermore, ischemic necrosis of the extremities has not been reported in Takayasu's arteritis. This is probably explained by the abundant collateral circulation usually present in patients afflicted with this disease, especially the younger ones.

TEMPORAL ARTERITIS

Temporal or cranial arteritis is an inflammation of arteries in elderly persons (usually men). Any large or medium sized artery may be involved, including the superficial temporal artery. The distribution and histopathology of the lesions in giant cell arteritis resemble the pathology of Takayasu's disease. In Takayasu's, however, the lesions tend to be more common in the thoracic aorta, its carotid and subclavian branches, and begin early in life, particularly in women during the second and third decades. Angiographically, the lesions of giant cell arteritis are similar to those of Takayasu's arteritis (Figure 17-30). Hence, the diagnosis of temporal arteritis can be definitely made only by arterial biopsy.

Thrombotic and Embolic Diseases

Thrombosis and embolic episodes in the arterial system are best defined through angiographic studies. Angiography can identify the site and extent of thrombosis and/or embolus formation (Figure 17-31).

Angiographically, fresh thrombus formation is suggested if a filling defect is identified within a vessel. The defect will usually have well-defined margins, which are distinct within the column of contrast (Figure 17-31C). The distinctness of the margins is secondary to adjacent contrast being radiographed in a tangential plane. If the x-ray exposure is not in a tangential plane to the thrombus and contrast, the filling defect's margins may not be sharply defined. Other sources for the filling defect, such as unopacified blood from a collateral or contributing vessel, air, or some normal vascular structure, should be looked for before diagnosing an acute thrombus. Filling defects secondary to unopacified blood usually appear as lucencies with ill-defined margins, which usually change configuration from one film to the next. Air bubbles are usually well circumscribed and not present on a repeat radiograph (Figure 17-32).

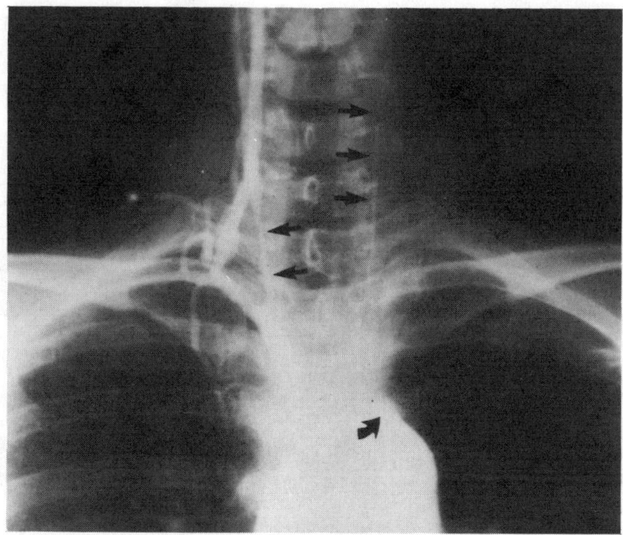

Figure 17-30 Seventy-two-year-old male with giant cell arteritis, biopsy proven. Note: 1) stenosed common carotid arteries (straight arrows), 2) totally occluded left subclavian artery (curved arrow), 3) the angiographic appearances of these lesions are very similar to those of Takayasu's arteritis.

Neoplasms of Blood Vessels

Though there are many tumor-like lesions, which arise in association with blood vessels, many lack the essential feature of true neoplasms, that is, continuous growth. For that reason, some authors have divided these lesions into two groups: true neoplasms, which may be either benign or malignant; and non-neoplastic, tumor-like lesions, which Albrecht called *hamartomas.*[53] He defined hamartomas as tumor-like malformations composed of tissues indigenous to the part, but lacking the growth potential of true neoplasms.[54] Using these criteria, hamartomas include: capillary hemangiomas, cavernous hemangiomas, and lymphangiomas. True neoplasms of blood vessels include: benign hemangioendotheliomas, hemangioblastomas, hemangiopericytomas, hemangiosarcomas, and Kaposi's sarcomas. It is not in the scope of this chapter to discuss these lesions in detail. Hence, it will suffice to say that angiography may be indicated to better describe the nature of tumor-like lesions and serve as a mapping procedure prior to surgical intervention. Figures 17-33 and 17-34 are examples of vascular neoplasms studied angiographically.

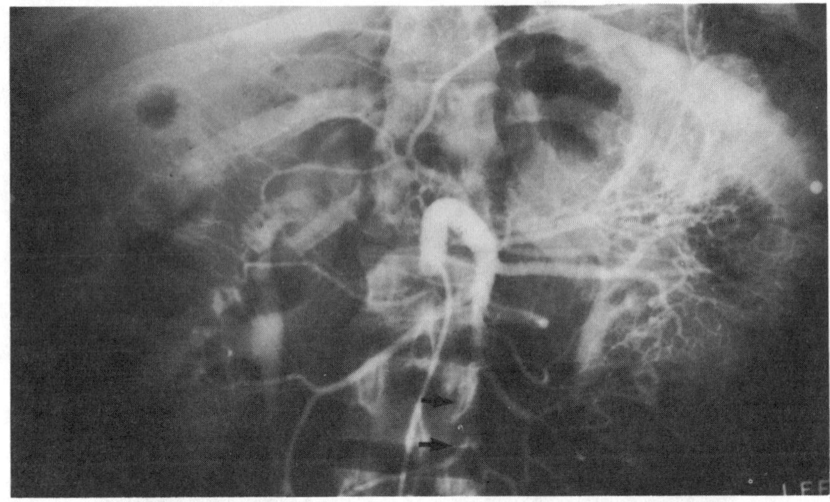

A

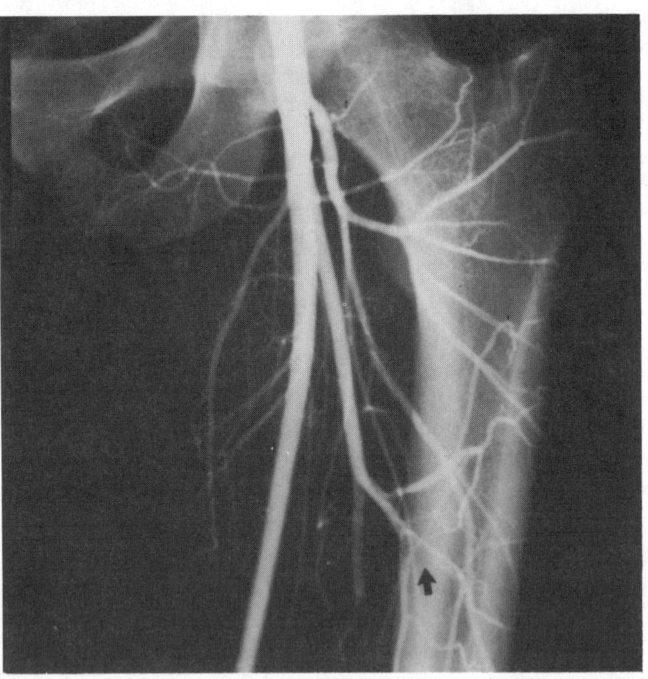

B

Figure 17-31 **A** Selective superior mesenteric arteriogram, showing occluded segment of its distal part (arrows). **B** Femoral arteriogram, showing fresh thrombi in profunda femoris branches (arrows). **C** Popliteal arteriogram, showing fresh thrombi in the common peroneal artery. **D** Left anterior oblique aortogram, revealing pseudoaneurysm (arrow), in patient postthoracic trauma. This pseudoaneurysm was thought to be the source of emboli.

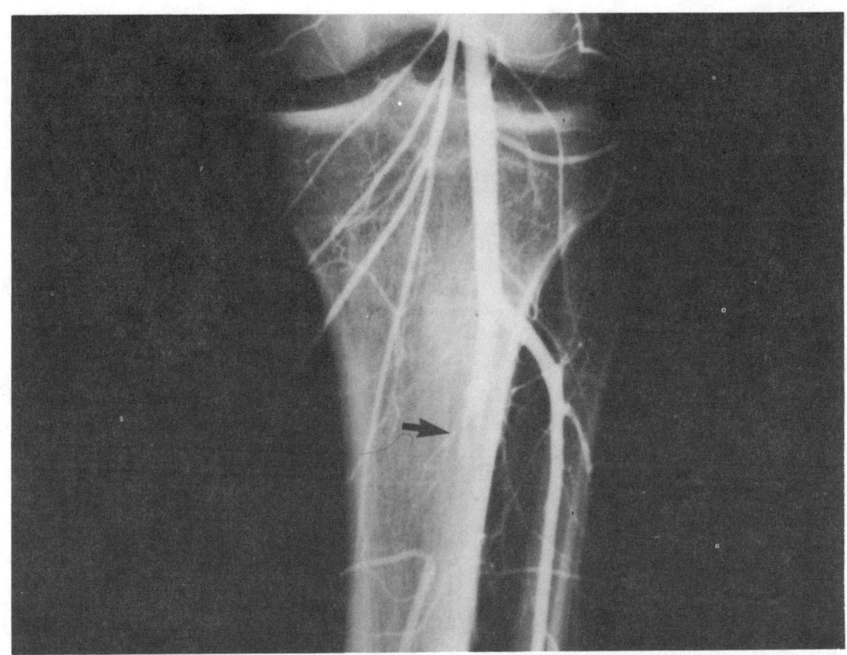

C

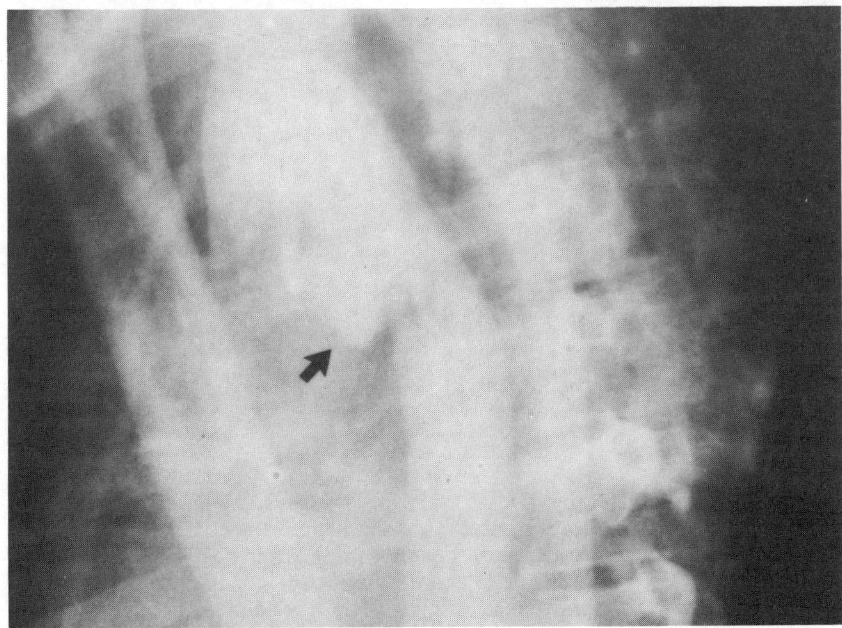

D

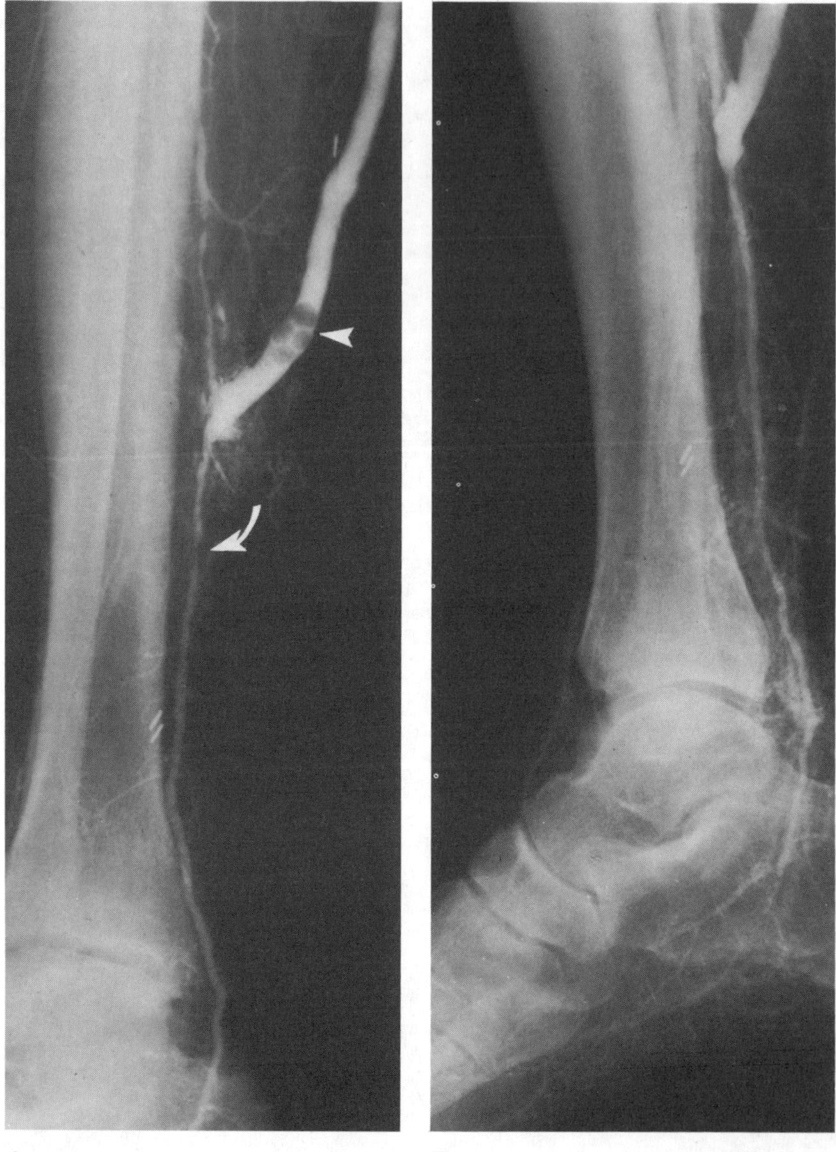

Figure 17-32 **A** Intraoperative arteriogram, postsaphenous vein graft to right posterior tibial artery. Note: 1) circumscribed lucencies, with sharply outlined margins within the vein graft, represent air, 2) stenosis in posterior tibial artery, approximately 1.5 cm distal to anastomotic site of vein graft (curved arrow). **B** Repeat intraoperative arteriogram. Lucent defects no longer present. Also, the stenosis within the posterior tibial artery was corrected by passing increasing sized probes (up to 6-french) through it.

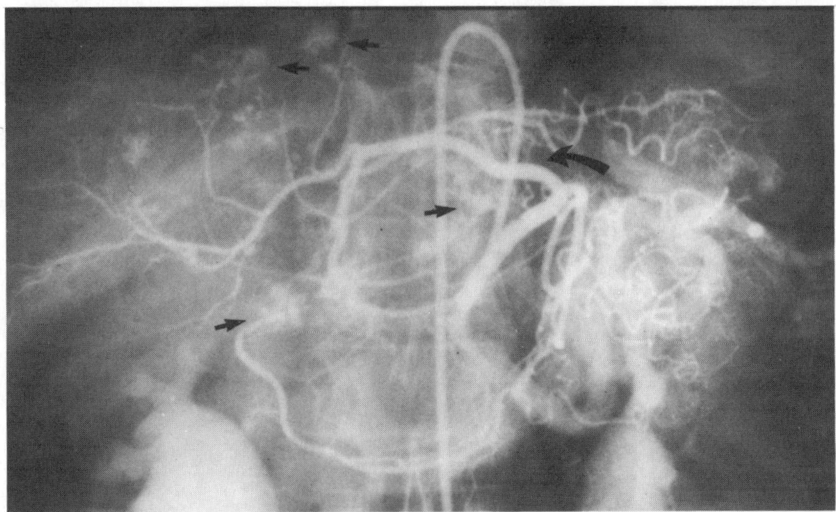

A

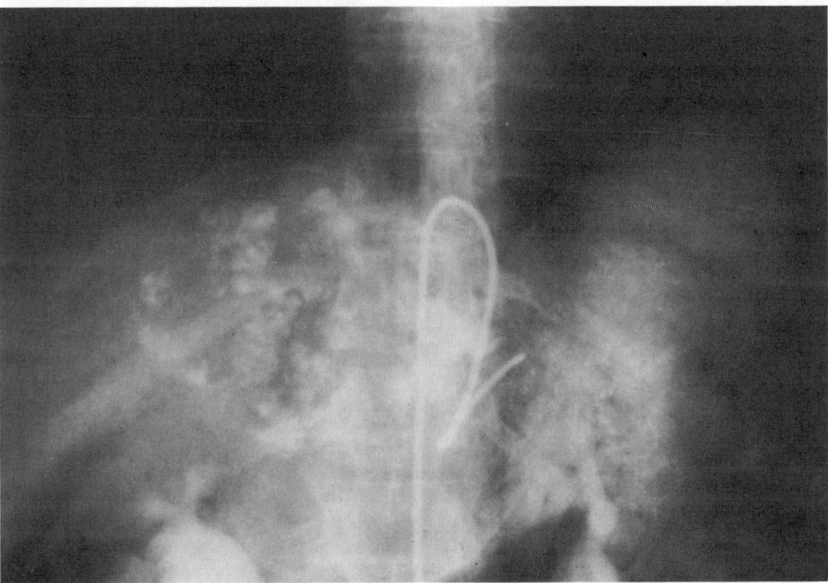

B

Figure 17-33 **A** Cavernous hemangioma in left lobe of liver. Selective left gastric arteriogram. Note: 1) left hepatic artery arises from left gastric artery (large curved arrow), 2) relatively large mass, with local blushing throughout (small arrows), 3) the blushing areas represent contrast pooling in vascular sinusoids and is characteristic of this tumor. **B** Late phase of arteriogram. Accentuates typical pooling of contrast in the sinusoids of the cavernous hemangioma.

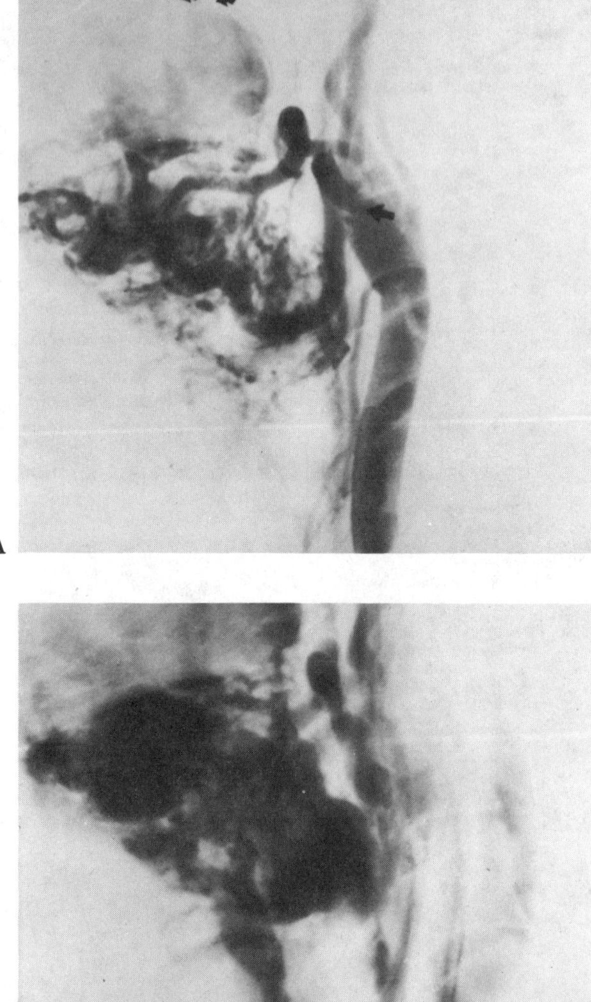

Figure 17-34 **A** Submandibular hemangiopericytoma metastatic to lung. Left common carotid arteriogram. Note: 1) large vascular submandibular mass pushing the left carotid arteries posterior, 2) huge lingular artery feeding the mass (large arrow), 3) early filling of a huge venous structure (curved arrows). **B** Venous phase of carotid arteriogram. Shows generous venous drainage into the left thyroid (curved arrow) and left jugular (straight arrow) veins.

Thoracic Outlet Syndrome

Patients having occlusions or narrowings in their subclavian artery secondary to chronic external trauma are said to have thoracic outlet syndrome. The source of trauma varies from congenital anomalies, such as cervical ribs, variations in head and neck anatomy, to acquired conditions such as callous formation on the clavicle secondary to fracture, muscle hypertrophy secondary to exercise, or repeated trauma from carrying heavy objects on the shoulder.[55] The thoracic outlet syndrome may be due to damage and/or compression of a nerve, vein, artery, or any combination of these three structures within the supraclavicular space. Angiography is helpful in confirming the etiology. The patient's upper extremity should be filmed in the position that produces the most symptoms, when compression of the vessel is thought to be the cause of his ischemia.[56] Figure 17-35 is an arteriogram of a young female with compression of the subclavian artery secondary to hypertrophy of the scalenus anticus muscle.

Thromboangiitis Obliterans (Buerger's Disease)

The etiology of this disease is unknown. It was first described by Dr Leo Buerger, an American surgeon, in 1908.[57] The disease affects relatively young men only, and they are usually excessive cigarette smokers. Symptoms usually occur in early adult life and present as claudication when exercising. The claudication subsides rapidly with rest. However, as the disease process worsens, pain and gangrene of the extremities may occur. The disease usually affects the arteries of the leg below the knee, that is, the popliteal arteries, and extends downward to involve their branches and small digital vessels with skip areas in between. The veins in the lower extremities are also involved. Buerger's disease may involve the arm arteries and, rarely, the cerebral, coronary, or mesenteric arteries. At one time, it was estimated that one in 6000 men in this country had Buerger's disease,[58] but it has become rare in the Western world. Opinions differ as to whether Buerger's disease is a single specific entity. Some people believe that Buerger's disease is an exaggerated form of atherosclerotic thrombo-occlusive disease,[59] and that it may have been overdiagnosed in the past.

Histologically, the affected vessels may show areas with early inflammatory changes with an abundance of neutrophiles, lymphocytes, macrophages, and a few giant cells dominating the latter phase. Later, endothelial cell proliferation and thrombosis within the lumen of the vessel occur. The thrombus becomes organized, leaving a characteris-

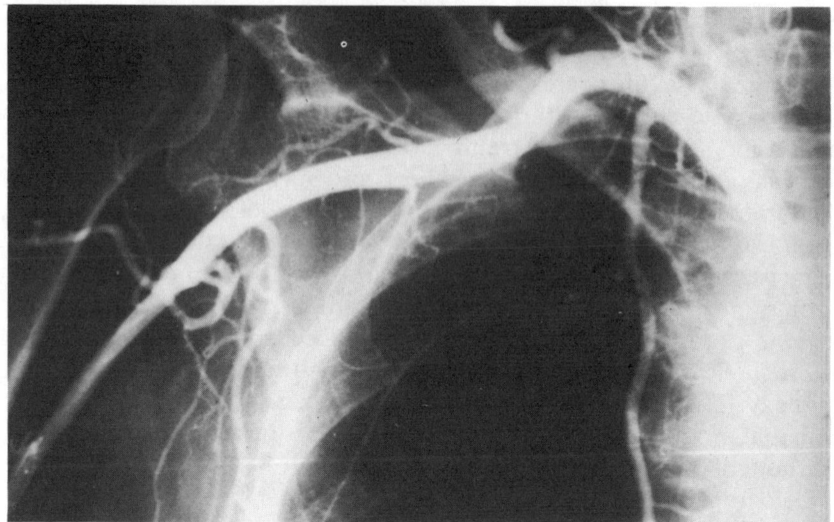

A

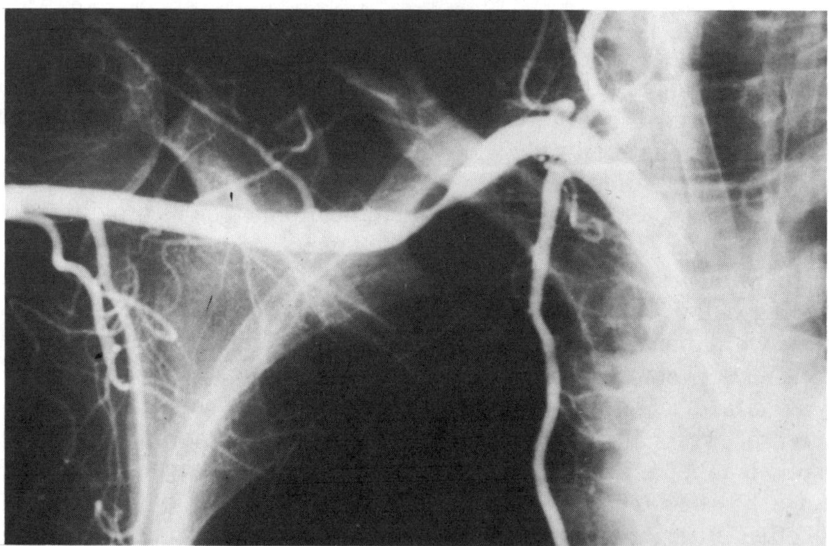

B

Figure 17-35 **A** Twenty-five-year-old female gymnast, experiencing numbness and tingling in the right finger tips, after several minutes of constant elevation of the right arm. Note: 1) selective right subclavian arteriogram with patient's arm by her side, 2) normal right subclavian artery. **B** Thoracic outlet syndrome. Repeat right subclavian arteriogram, with right arm raised to height. Note: severe narrowing of subclavian artery where one would expect it to leave the scalenus triangle.

tically cord-like segment of vessel and a highly convoluted, but well-preserved, internal elastic lamina. The preservation of the internal elastic lamina is a distinguishing histological feature of Buerger's disease from that of conventional atherosclerotic process.[59] Angiographically, one sees a relatively normal peripheral arterial tree down to the level of the popliteal arteries, after which one can expect stenoses and abrupt occlusions of the popliteal arteries and their branches to the feet (Figure 17-36).

Acquired Arteriovenous Fistuli

Arteriovenous fistuli, secondary to trauma, are fairly common and may occur anywhere. They may be small, causing no symptoms, or large enough to produce cardiac failure.[60–62] Hemodynamically, they cause left-to-right shunting which, if significant, increases cardiac output and pulse pressure. Tachycardia also ocurs. Plain radiographs of the chest, in symptomatic patients, usually show cardiomegaly and pulmonary-vascular engorgement. In the extremities, plain radiographs may show soft tissue swelling secondary to edema and occasional pulmonary osteoarthropathy of the affected limb. Calcifications in veins are the so-called *varicose aneurysms* and may be seen in chronic cases.[60,61] Angiographically, one looks for early opacification of a vein, after injecting contrast on the arterial side to make the diagnosis of arteriovenous fistula. More often than not, the exact site of the fistula can be shown angiographically. Both artery and vein are enlarged; however, the vein is commonly larger than the artery. Figures 17-37 and 17-38 are examples of iatrogenic traumatic fistuli.

Percutaneous Transluminal Angioplasty (PTA)

Percutaneous transluminal angioplasty (PTA) is rapidly becoming an adjuvant and/or alternative technique to surgery in correcting peripheral vascular problems secondary to atherosclerosis. The technique was first reported in this country by Dotter and Judkins in 1964.[63] The success of the procedure, however, had to await the invention of a catheter, with a balloon at its end, and with the appropriate physical characteristics (ie, with enough tensile strength to withstand several atmospheres of pressure without rupture, and which would take the shape of a blood vessel when inflated[64,65] (Figure 17-39). Under fluoroscopic control, a catheter with a deflated balloon (near or at its tip), is placed into a stenosed or occluded vessel (after passage of a guidewire). The balloon is inflated to about four atmospheres for at

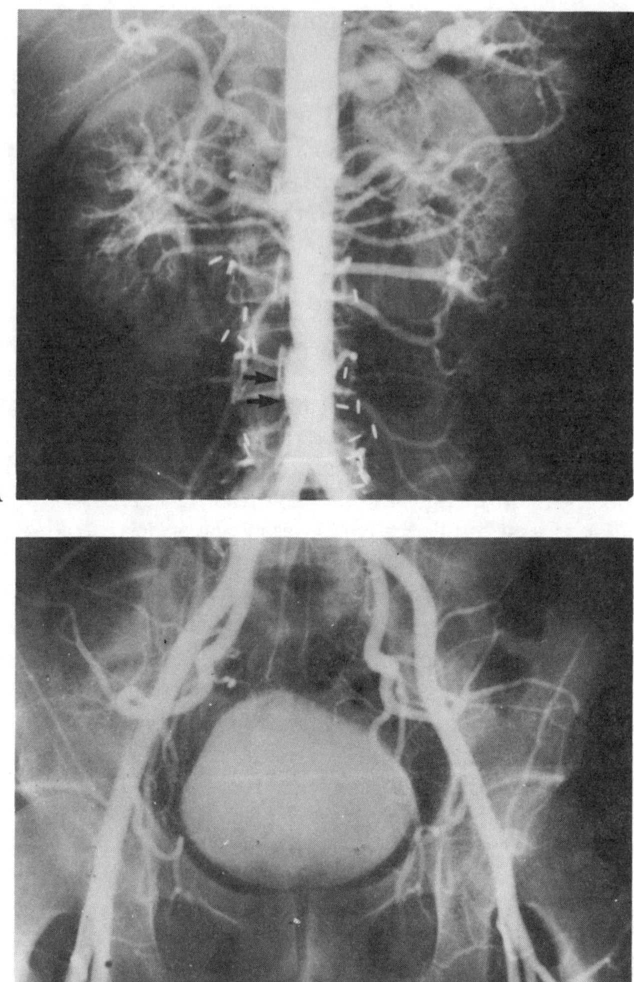

Figure 17-36 **A** Buerger's disease. Forty-two-year-old male (heavy smoker, with impending gangrene of both feet. Note: 1) abdominal aortogram, revealing mild atherosclerotic changes just above its bifurcation (arrow); otherwise, it is unremarkable. 2) Metallic clips from bilateral lumbar sympathectomies. **B** Buerger's disease. Note: normal pelvic arteries. **C** Buerger's disease. Note: both superifical femoral arteries are normal. **D** Buerger's disease. Note: 1) essentially normal-appearing right popliteal artery, 2) mild stenosing lesion in left popliteal artery (arrows), 3) occlusion of all three popliteal artery branches to the foot (circular arrows). **E** Buerger's disease. Note: 1) occlusion of all three right popliteal artery branches just above the ankle, 2) abrupt occlusion in right posterior tibial artery, with poor distal collateral formation (arrow). A similar abrupt occlusion, with poor distal collaterals, can be seen in the left anterior tibial artery (curved arrow), 3) these angiographic findings are typical of Buerger's disease, but not diagnostic.

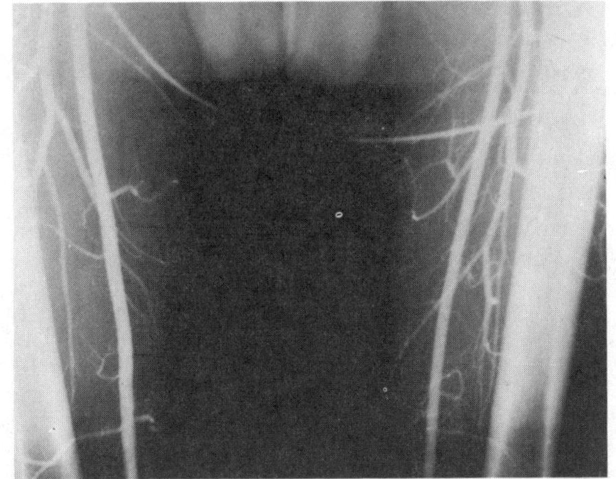

C

D

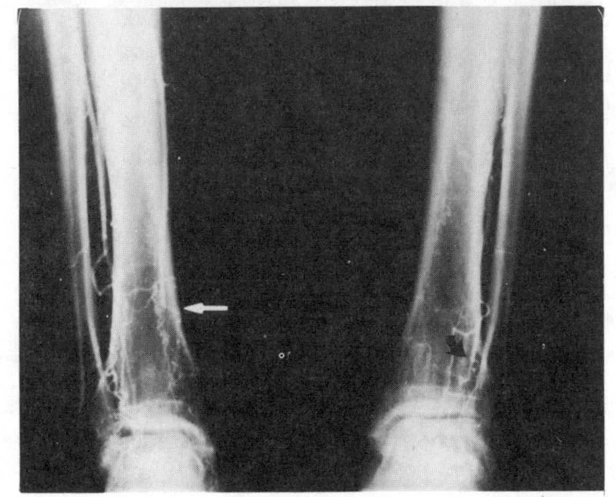

E

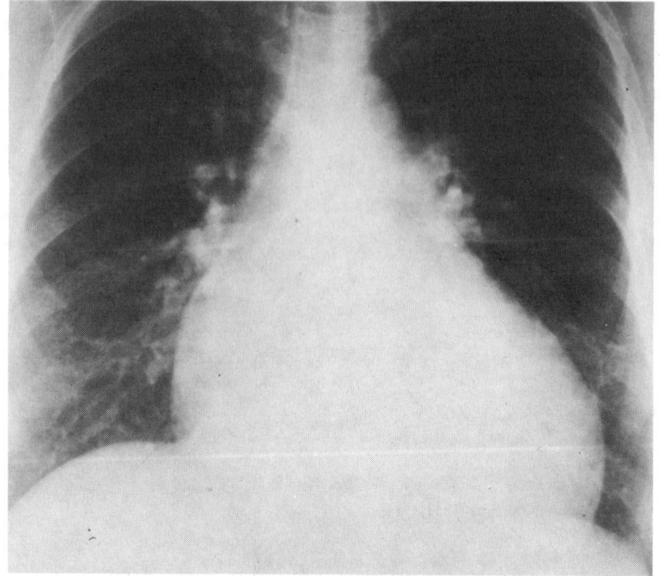

A

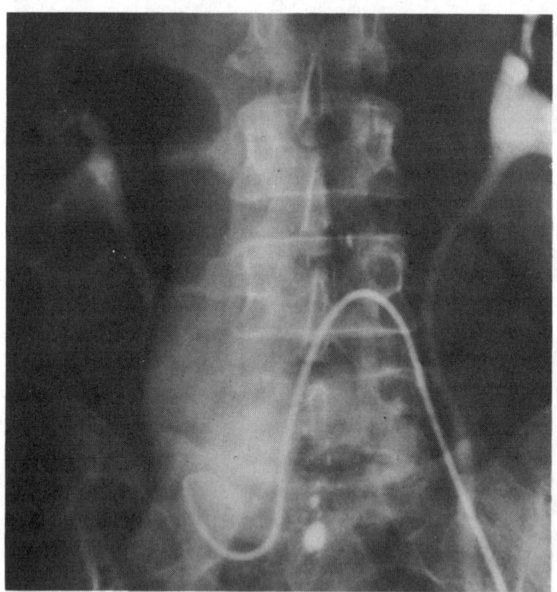

B

Figure 17-37 **A** Acquired arteriovenous fistuli. Thirty-six-year-old female with episodes of congestive heart failure one year post back surgery for a ruptured disk. Note: 1) posterior anterior chest film, 2) cardiomegaly, 3) pulmonary vessel plethora. **B** Arteriovenous fistuli. Note: 1) catheter tip placed into the fistuli via the right common iliac artery, 2) enlarged inferior vena cava, 3) residual pantopaque from past myelogram.

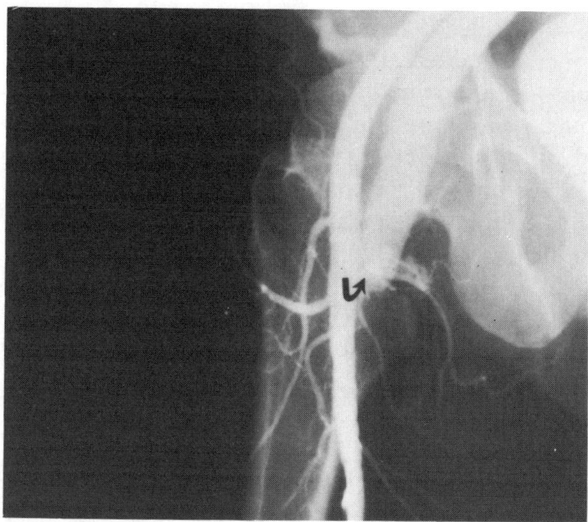

Figure 17-38 Acquired arteriovenous fistuli. Patient had a previous cardiac catheterization, using the common femoral artery approach. Note: 1) right superficial femoral arteriogram from a contralateral catheterization, 2) early opacification of femoral vein, 3) origin of fistūli (arrow) suggests a low femoral artery puncture was performed at the time of cardiac catheterization.

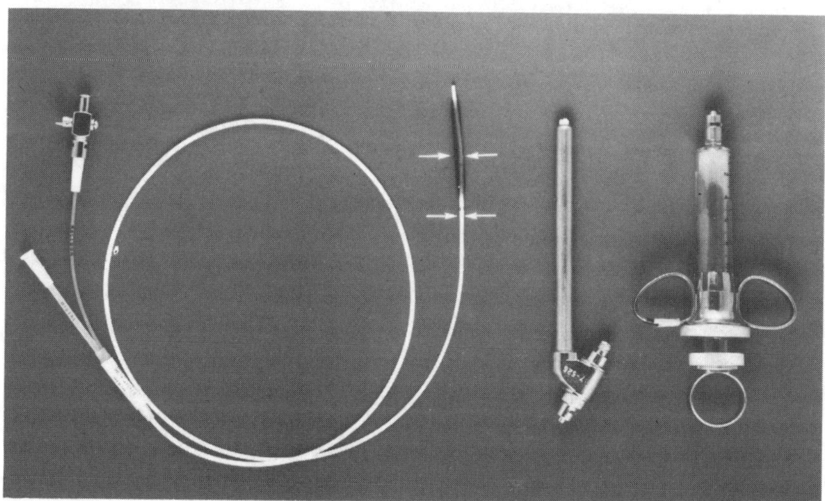

Figure 17-39 Percutaneous transluminal angioplasty equipment (from left to right). Note: 1) a balloon dilatation catheter (7-french catheter with 5 mm balloon), used to dilate stenoses in vessels with sizes similar to the superficial femoral or renal arteries. Balloon has an oblong shape, 2) pressure gauge, to control inflation pressure, 3) syringe, to inflate balloon with. Dilute contrast is used to inflate the balloon in order to better monitor its expansion and deflation.

least one minute; the balloon may be deflated and inflated several times to its recommended atmospheric pressure, depending upon the circumstances. The occlusion or stenosis is thus opened. At this writing, thousands of atherosclerotic narrowings and occlusions have been treated successfully using this method in essentially every major artery within the human body.[66-75]

Specific contraindications are: 1) atherosclerotic lesions of blood vessels with direct flow to the brain; 2) recanalization or dilatation of an artery at the point of origin of an essential and principal collateral that cannot be sacrificed; 3) a long segmental occlusion (ie, greater than 10 cm long). This is not an absolute contraindication, but is a less favorable situation; and 4) intraluminal calcification, which indicates total occlusion by calcified plaque.

The mechanism for increasing the lumen size of a stenosed or occluded vessel secondary to balloon dilatation is not fully understood. However, published data suggests that a controlled injury to the intimal and medial portions of the vascular wall, at the site of stenosis or occlusions, allows for immediate local expansion.[76,77] If the arterial pressure is sufficient to maintain adequate blood flow at the site of controlled injury, the healing process will serve to fix the expanded area and, in many instances, further increase the interluminal diameter of the vessel through retraction of the media and intima.[76,77] One of the authors states that desquamation and redispersion of the plaque elements sometimes occur.[77]

Major complications leading to surgical intervention have occurred in less than one percent of patients having this procedure performed (excluding the coronaries).[64] No reported deaths have occurred. Published data regarding long-term patency in iliac arteries compare favorably with surgery.[64,65] With regard to long-term patency in other arteries versus surgical repair or bypass procedures, no published data are available primarily due to the newness of the procedure. However, preliminary results have been very encouraging.[64] At present, no clear guidelines have been established as to when to employ the PTA procedure in treating stenotic or occlusive vascular lesions. The decision to use PTA in correcting vascular stenoses and/or occlusions should be a joint one on the part of the referring physician, angiographer, and vascular surgeon. Figures 17-40 and 17-41 illustrate atherosclerotic lesions that were corrected using PTA.

Digital Fluoroscopy

Recent technical advances have given the angiographer hope of becoming less invasive in his approach to diagnostic problems. A new

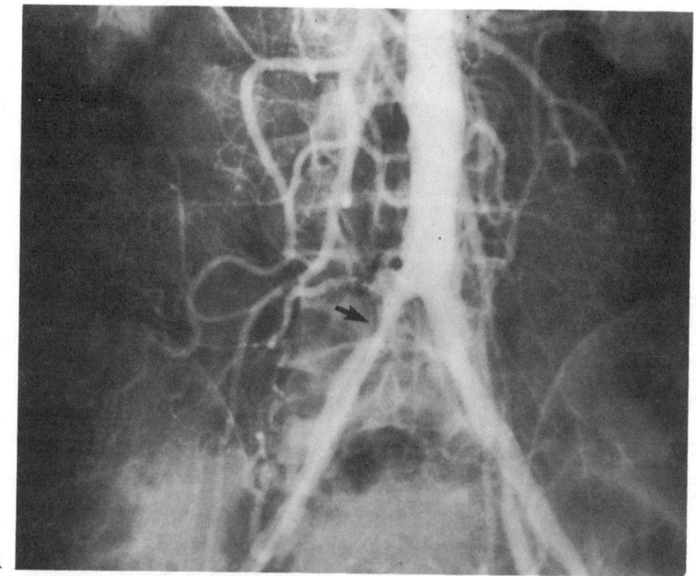

A

B

Figure 17-40 **A** Abdominal aortogram in 54-year-old male, with right buttock, thigh and calf claudication when exercising. Note: 1) stenosis in right common iliac artery (arrow), 2) there was a 25 mm Hg resting gradient across the stenosis. **B** Arteriogram postpercutaneous transluminal angioplasty. Shows minimal residual narrowing in right common iliac artery. No gradient across the area of residual narrowing was present at rest or postreactive hyperemia testing.

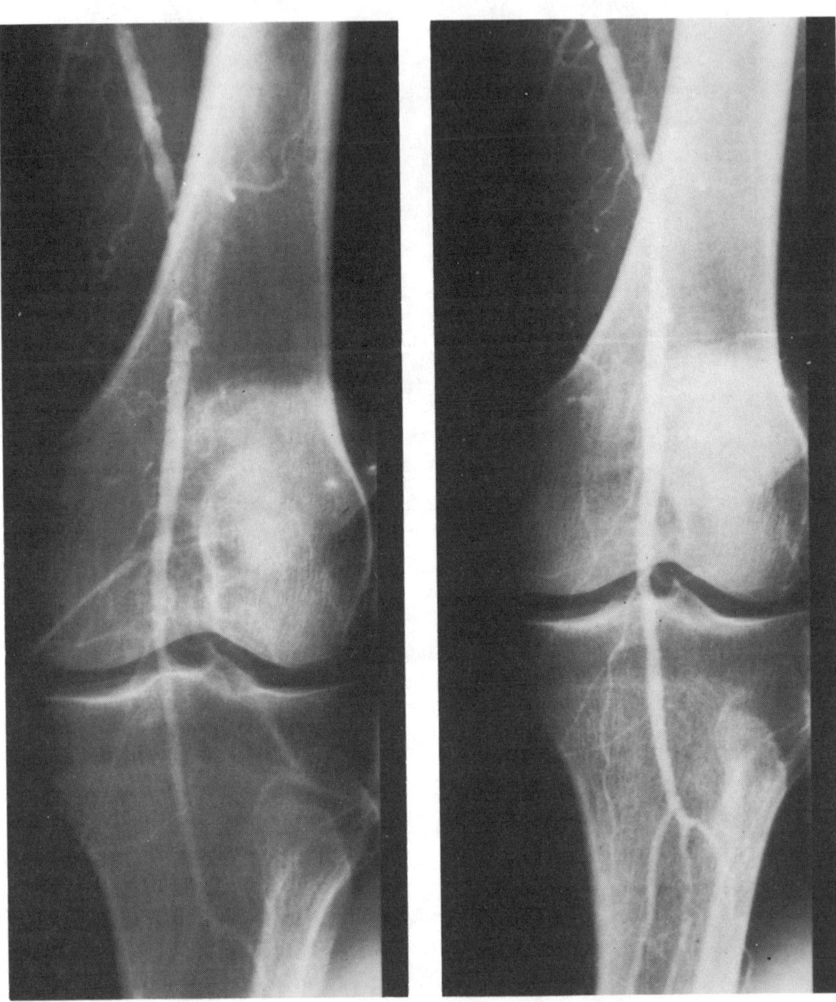

Figure 17-41 **A** Left superficial femoral artery occlusion in a 84-year-old male with impending gangrene of the left foot and severe cardiac disease. **B** Re-establishment of the left superficial femoral artery lumen post percutaneous transluminal angioplasty of this vessel, using a 7-french catheter with a 5 mm dilatation balloon. The patient's foot recovered and he was without pain when ambulating.

system, currently referred to as *computerized fluoroscopy,* allows digital subtraction angiography after bolus injection of contrast agent via an antecubital vein.[78,79] Though the technique has been described in the past,[80,81] only now has it begun to be considered as a clinically useful diagnostic tool. All computerized fluoroscopic units to date consist of some form of a specially designed computer system, integrated with a fluoroscopic and radiographic apparatus for digitalization, manipulation, and display of data. The images of blood vessels are enhanced using low-dose contrast and subtraction techniques which, in effect, result in the removal of unwanted background images. This is done

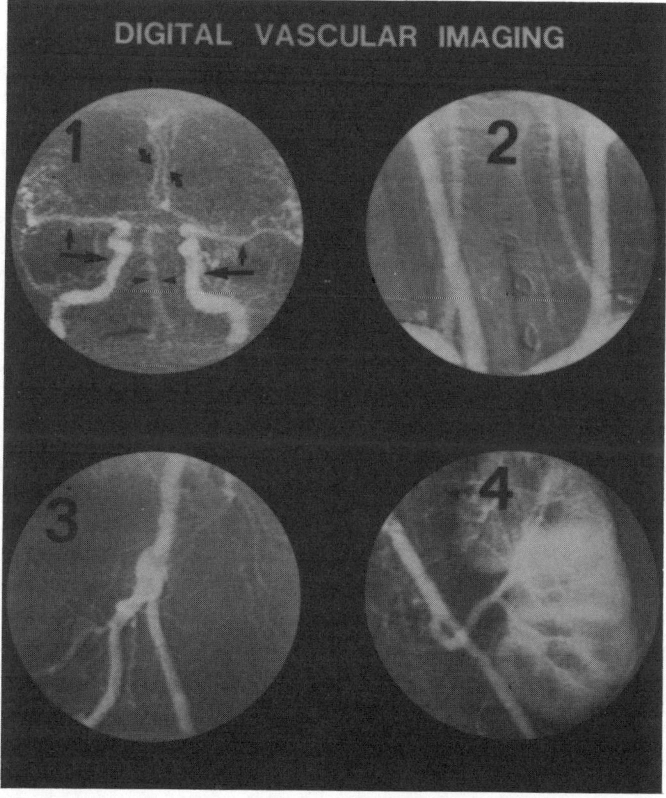

Figure 17-42 Digital vascular imaging. 1) Image of the cerebral arteries in the anterior-posterior plane. Note: both carotids (large, straight arrows), middle cerebrals (small, straight arrows), anterior cerebrals (small, curved arrows), and the basilar artery (arrowheads) are well visualized. 2) Anterior-posterior view of both common carotid and vertebral arteries. 3) Anterior-posterior view of the right common femoral artery and its bifurcation into the profunda and superficial femoral branches. 4) Anterior-posterior view of a left transplanted renal artery and kidney. (Images courtesy of Philips Medical Systems, Inc.)

first by imaging the area to be studied without contrast, followed by an image of the area with contrast enhancement. The image taken without contrast enhancement is of the background. This background image is then subtracted from the image which includes the contrast-enhanced object (blood vessels) plus the background. The final image is one of the contrast-enhanced object without its background.

Preliminary reports have shown that, after bolus injection of contrast via an antecubital vein, images of the heart, carotid, thoracic, abdominal, and femoral arteries can be obtained with remarkable clarity, obviating the need for conventional angiography in many instances. The technique is simple, safe, inexpensive, and avoids puncture of an artery. It requires only an intravenous puncture (although more recently, use of a small catheter in the superior vena cava has been advocated); the potential problems of guidewire and catheter manipulations are eliminated. It also requires less time on the part of the technician, nurse, and angiographer to perform the study.

Early recognized disadvantages to the procedure are inability to do selective arteriography and problems of vessel overlap and patient motion, causing image degradation. These can be reduced to a minimum by performing the study in more than one projection and by the selection of patients who can control their breathing and body movements. Antiperistaltic agents, such as glucagon, have been used to minimize bowel motion in abdominal or mesenteric arteriography. No doubt, continued technical advances will at least minimize, if not completely resolve, these problems. Currently, the technique is being heralded as a screening procedure and, in many instances, as an alternative to angiography. Figure 17-42 shows examples of studies performed using the computerized fluoroscopic technique.

REFERENCES

1. Hessel SJ, Adams DF, Abrams HL. Complications of angiography. *Radiology* 138(2):273–281, 1981.

2. Mani RL, Eisenberg RL, McDonald EJ Jr, et al. Complications of catheter cerebral arteriography: Analysis of 5,000 procedures. I. Criteria and incidence. *Am J Roentgenol* 131:861–865, 1978.

3. Mani RL, Eisenberg RL. Complications of catheter cerebral arteriography: Analysis of 5,000 procedures. III. Assessment of arteries injected, contrast medium used, duration of procedure, and age of patient. *Am J Roentgenol* 131:871–874, 1978.

4. Steinberg I, Stein HL. Congenital arterial disease. *Semin Roentgenol* 5(3):213–227, 1970.

5. Ricketts RR, Finck E, Yellin AE. Management of major arteriovenous fistulas by arteriographic techniques. *Arch Surg* 113(10):1153–1159, 1978.

6. Gomes MMR, Bernatz PE. Arteriovenous fistulas: A review and ten-year experience at the Mayo Clinic. *Mayo Clin Proc* 45:81–102, 1970.

7. Holman E. The physiology of an arteriovenous fistula. *Arch Surg* 7:64–82, 1923.

8. Holman E. The anatomic and physiologic effects of an arteriovenous fistula. *Surgery* 8:362–382, 1940.

9. Holman E. Contributions to cardiovascular physiology obtained from clinical and experimental observations of abnormal arteriovenous communications. *J Cardiovasc Surg* 3:48–63, 1962.

10. Coleman CC Jr. Diagnosis and treatment of congenital arteriovenous fistulas of the head and neck. *Am J Surg* 126:557–565, 1973.

11. Nagasue N, Inokuchi K, Kobayashi M, et al. Hepatoportal arteriovenous fistula in primary carcinoma of the liver. *Surg Gynecol Obstet* 145:504–508, 1977.

12. Brinsfield DE, Shuford WH, Plauch WH Jr, et al. In Lindsay J JR, Hurst JW (eds). *The Aorta,* ed 1. New York, Grune and Stratton, Inc, 1979, pp 271–292.

13. Senning A, Johansson L. Coarctation of the abdominal aorta. *J Thorac Cardiovasc Surg* 40:517–523, 1960.

14. Becker AE, Becker MJ, Edwards JE. Anomalies associated with coarctation of the aorta: Particular reference to infancy. *Circulation* 41:1067–1075, 1970.

15. Jang GC, Brody WR, Dinsmore RE. Radiologic diagnosis of aortic disease. In Lindsay J Jr, Hurst JW (eds). *The Aorta,* ed 1. New York, Grune and Stratton, Inc, 1979, pp 334–337.

16. Roberts WC. The aorta: Its acquired diseases and their consequences as viewed from a morphologic perspective. In Lindsay J Jr, Hurst JW (eds). *The Aorta,* ed 1. New York, Grune and Stratton, Inc, 1979, pp 56–67.

17. Jang GC, Brody WR, Dinsmore RE. Radiologic diagnosis of aortic disease. In Lindsay J Jr, Hurst JW (eds). *The Aorta,* ed 1. New York, Grune and Stratton, Inc, 1979, p 308.

18. Blakemore AH, Voorhees AB. Aneurysm of the aorta: A review of 365 cases. *Angiology* 5:209–231, 1954.

19. Blakemore AH. The clinical behavior of arteriosclerotic aneurysm of the abdominal aorta: A rational surgical therapy. *Ann Surg* 126:195–207, 1947.

20. Crane C. Arteriosclerotic aneurysm of the abdominal aorta. Some pathological and clinical correlations. *N Engl J Med* 253:954–961, 1955.

21. Ferguson MJ, Arden MJ. Gastrointestinal hemorrhage secondary to rupture of aorta. A review of four duodenal and three esophageal cases. *Arch Intern Med* 117:133–140, 1966.

22. Steinberg I, Dotter C, Peabody G, et al. The angiographic diagnosis of syphilitic aortitis. *Am J Roentgenol* 62:655-660, 1949.

23. Smith WG, Leonard JC. The radiological features of syphilitic aortic incompetence. *Br Heart J* 21:162–166, 1959.

24. Segal J, Harvey WP, Hufnagel C. The clinical study of one hundred cases of severe aortic insufficiency. *Am J Med* 21:200–210, 1956.

25. Kampmier RH. Saccular aneurysm of the thoracic aorta: A clinical study of 633 cases. *Ann Intern Med* 12:624–651, 1938.

26. Wagenvoort CA, Neufeld HN, Edwards JE. Cardiovascular system in Marfan's syndrome and in idiopathic dilatation of the ascending aorta. *Am J Cardiol* 9:496–507, 1962.

27. Chapman DW, Beazley HL, Peterson PK, et al. Annuloaortic ectasia with cystic medial necrosis. Diagnosis and surgical treatment. *Am J Cardiol* 16:679–687, 1965.

28 Whittaker SRF, Sheehan JD. Dissecting aortic aneurysm in Marfan's syndrome. *Lancet* 2:791–792, 1954.

29. Jang GC, Brody WR, Dinsmore RE. Radiologic diagnosis of aortic disease. In Lindsay J Jr, Hurst JW (eds). *The Aorta,* ed 1. New York, Grune and Stratton, Inc, 1979, p 316.

30. Anagnostopoulos CE. *Acute Aortic Dissections.* Baltimore, Baltimore University Park Press, 1975, p 70ff.

31. Daily PO, Trueblood HW, Stinson EG, et al. Management of acute aortic dissections. *Ann Thorac Surg* 10:237–247, 1970.

32. Debakey ME, Beall AC Jr, Cooley DA, et al. Dissecting aneurysms of the aorta. *Surg Clin North Am* 46(4):1045–1055, 1966.

33. Crawford ST. Blood and lymphatic vessels. In Anderson WAD, Krisene JW (eds). *Pathology,* ed 7. St. Louis, The CV Mosby Co, 1977, p 909.

34. Roberts WC. The hypertensive diseases. Evidence that systemic hypertension is a greater risk factor to the development of other cardiovascular diseases than previously suspected. *Am J Med* 59:523–532, 1975.

35. Himmet D, Richardson IW, Mohan OI. Seat belt aorta: Acute dissection and thrombosis of the abdominal aorta. *Surgery* 95(3):263–267, 1979.

36. Beckman CB, Geha AS, Hammond GL, et al. Results and complications of intraaortic balloon counterpulsation. *Ann Thorac Surg* 24(6):550–559, 1977.

37. McCabe JC, Abel RM, Subramanian VA, et al. Complications of intraaortic balloon insertion and counterpulsation. *Circulation* 57(4):769–773, 1978.

38. Jang GC, Brody WR, Dinsmore RE. Radiologic diagnosis of aortic disease. In Lindsay J Jr, Hurst JW (eds). *The Aorta,* ed 1. New York, Grune and Stratton, Inc, 1979, p 324.

39. Parmley LF, Mattingly TW, Manion WC, et al. Nonpenetrating traumatic injury of the aorta. *Circulation* 17:1086–1101, 1958.

40. Eller JL, Ziter FM Jr. Avulsion of the innominate artery from the aortic arch. An evaluation of roentgenographic findings. *Radiology* 94:75–78, 1970.

41. Himmet D, Richardson IW, Mohan OI. Seat belt aorta: Acute dissection and thrombosis of the abdominal aorta. *Surgery* 95(3):263–267, 1979.

42. Kincaid OW, Davis GD, Hallerman FJ, et al. Fibromuscular dysplasia of the renal arteries: Arteriographic features, classification, and observations on natural history of the disease. *Am J Roentgenol* 104(2):271–282, 1968.

43. Mannik M, Gilliland BC. Vasculitis. In Isselbacher KJ, Adams RD, Braunwald E, et al (eds). *Harrison's Principles of Internal Medicine,* ed 9. New York, McGraw-Hill Book Co, 1980, pp 351–355.

44. Zeek OM. Periarteritis nodosa and other forms of necrotizing angiitis. *N Engl J Med* 248(18):764–772, 1953.

45. Clark E, Kaplan B. Endocardial arterial and other mesenchymal alterations associated with serum disease in man. *Arch Pathol* 24:458–475, 1937.

46. Levo Y, Gorevic PD, Kassab HJ, et al. Association between hepatitis B virus and essential mixed cryoglobulinemia. *N Engl J Med* 296(26):1501–1504, 1977.

47. Fisher RG, Graham DY, Granmayeh M, et al. Polyarteritis nodosa and hepatitis B surface antigen: Role of angiography in diagnosis. *Am J Roentgenol* 129:77–81, 1977.

48. Chumbley LC, Harrison EG Jr, DeRemee RA. Allergic granulomatosis and angiitis (Churg-Strauss syndrome): Report and analysis of 30 cases. *Mayo Clin Proc* 52:477–484, August 1977.

49. Hachiya J. Current concepts of Takayasu's arteritis. *Semin Roentgenol* 5(3):245–259, 1970.

50. Makao K, Ikeda M, Kimata S. Takayasu's arteritis: Clinical report of eighty-four cases and immunological studies of seven cases. *Circulation* 35:1141–1155, 1967.

51. Paloheimo JA. Obstructive arteritis of Takayasu's type: Clinical roentgenological and laboratory studies of 36 patients. *Acta Med Scand Suppl* 468:7, 1965.

52. Riehl J-L, Brown WJ. Takayasu's arteritis: An autoimmune disease. *Arch Neurol* 12:92–97, 1965.

53. Crawford ST. Blood and lymphatic vessels. In Anderson WAD, Kissane JM (eds). *Pathology,* ed 7. St. Louis, The CV Mosby Co, 1977, pp 917–923.

54. Willis RA. *Pathology of Tumours,* ed 4. London, Butterworth and Company, 1967, p 718.

55. Imparato AM, Spencer FC. Peripheral arterial disease. In Schwartz SI, Shiris GT, Spencer FC, et al (eds). *Principles of Surgery,* ed 3. New York, McGraw-Hill Book Co, 1979, p 947.

56. Lang EK. Arteriography of thoracic outlet syndrome. In Abrams HL (ed). *Angiography,* ed 2. Boston, Little, Brown and Company, 1971, pp 691–692.

57. Buerger L. Thrombo-angiitis obliterans: A study of the vascular lesions leading to presenile spontaneous gangrene. *Am J Med Sci* 136:567–580, 1908.

58. Allen EV, Barker NW, Hines E. *Peripheral Vascular Disease,* ed 3. Philadelphia, WB Saunders Company, 1962.

59. Crawford ST. Blood and lymphatic vessels. In Anderson WAD, Kissane JM (eds). *Pathology.* St. Louis, The CV Mosby Company, 1977, p 904.

60. Bell D, Cockshott WP. Angiography of traumatic arteriovenous fistulae. *Clin Radiol* 16(3):241–247, 1965.

61. Lore L, Braun T. Arteriography of peripheral vascular trauma. *Am J Roentgenol* 102(2):431–440, 1968.

62. Staple TW, Friedenberg MJ. Ilio-iliac arteriovenous fistula following intervertebral disc surgery. *Clin Radiol* 16(3):248–250, 1965.

63. Dotter CT, Judkins MP. Transluminal treatment of arteriosclerotic obstruction. Description of a new technic and a preliminary report of its application. *Circulation* 30:654–670, 1964.

64. Gruntzig A. *Die perkutane transluminale rekanalisation chronisher arterienverschlusse mit einer neven dilatationionstechnik.* Baden-Baden, Gerhard Witzstrock, 1977. English translation by Wipfelder R, Kumpe D, 1979.

65. Gruntzig A, Kumpe DA. Technique of percutaneous transluminal angioplasty with the Gruntzig balloon catheter. *Am J Roentgenol* 132:547–552, 1979.

66. Waltman AC. Percutaneous transluminal angioplasty: Iliac and deep femoral arteries. *Am J Roentgenol* 135:921–926, 1980.

67. Greenfield AJ. Femoral, popliteal, and tibial arteries: Percutaneous transluminal angioplasty. *Am J Roentgenol* 135:927–935, 1980.

68. Motarjeme A, Keifer JW, Zuska AJ. Percutaneous transluminal angioplasty of the iliac arteries: 66 experiences. *Am J Roentgenol* 135:937–944, 1980.

69. Sprayregen S, Sniderman KW, Sos TA, et al. Popliteal artery branches: Percutaneous transluminal angioplasty. *Am J Roentgenol* 135:945–950, 1980.

70. Block PC. Percutaneous transluminal coronary angioplasty. *Am J Roentgenol* 135:955–959, 1980.

71. Schwarten DE. Transluminal angioplasty of renal artery stenosis. *Am J Roentgenol* 135:969–974, 1980.

72. Saddekni S, Sniderman KW, Hilton S, et al. Percutaneous transluminal angioplasty of nonatherosclerotic lesions. *Am J Roentgenol* 135:975–982, 1980.

73. Novelline RA. Percutaneous transluminal angioplasty: Newer applications. *Am J Roentgenol* 135:983–988, 1980.

74. Cope C. Balloon dilatation of closed mesocaval shunts. *Am J Roentgenol* 135:989–993, 1980.

75. Bachman DM, Kim RM. Transluminal dilatation for subclavian steal syndrome. *Am J Roentgenol* 135:955–996, 1980.

76. Casteneda-Zuniga WR, Formanek A, Tadavarthy M, et al. The mechanism of balloon angioplasty. *Radiology* 135:565–571, 1980.

77. Block PC, Fallon JT, Elmer D. Experimental angioplasty: Lessons from the laboratory. *Am J Roentgenol* 135:907–912, 1980.

78. Crummy AB, Strother CM, Sackett JF, et al. Computerized fluoroscopy: Digital subtraction for intravenous angiocardiography and arteriography. *Am J Roentgenol* 135:1131–1140, 1980.

79. Ovitt TW, Christenson PC, Fisher HD III, et al. Intravenous angiography using digital video subtraction: X-ray imaging system. *Am J Roentgenol* 135:1141–1144, 1980.

80. Bernstein ER, Greenspan RH, Loken MK. Intravenous abdominal aortography. A preliminary report. *Surgery* 44:29–535, 1958.

81. Steinberg I, Finby N, Evans JR. A safe and practical intravenous method for abdominal aortography, peripheral arteriograhy and cerebral angiography. *Am J Roentgenol* 82:758–772, 1959.

18 Overview of Vascular Surgery

Anthony M. Imparato

In this overview of vascular surgery as it has developed during this century, the emphasis will be upon arterial surgery, since the great progress in this part of the discipline has overshadowed the early attempts to affect the course of venous diseases. Furthermore, emphasis will be on arterial diseases as opposed to arterial trauma. Although to many it has meant restoring arteries to *normalcy,* either functionally or morphologically, its essence is twofold: to deal with ischemia resulting from arterial occlusion or interruption, and to correct abnormalities of the blood vessel wall that threaten its integrity and may lead to rupture and exsanguinating hemorrhage. The basic surgical maneuvers aim at restoring the arterial surface or substituting a nonthrombogenic, nonembolizing conduit for an occluded, narrowed, or dilated thrombogenic one.

The early development of the art, leading to its present state, has been due to a number of advances: technical-surgical, diagnostic, and ideational. Amongst the technical-surgical have been the development of relatively simple techniques for anastomosing blood vessels and the introduction of acceptable arterial substitutes. The basic diagnostic innovation of arteriography permitted the study of vascular pathologic conditions in vivo, leading to an understanding and accurate planning of arterial reconstructive procedures. Because of early successes in arterial reconstructions, large numbers of patients were operated on and their courses followed, leading to the present refinements of more precise patient selection, based upon clinical stages of disease and the ability to influence its course favorably. The durability of vascular reconstructive procedures can now be weighed against the risks of surgical intervention, factors that vary widely from one part of the body to another and with the pathologic process involved.

The most recent proliferation of *noninvasive* diagnostic techniques, which permit arterial imaging and arterial pressure, pulse wave, and velocity determinations, has added much needed refinement to diagnosis and has proven to be of value in follow-up. The use of the computer in radiology, which permits image intensification, promises to be a most dramatic innovation. It not only results in excellent studies of soft tissues of the body, but more recently with the introduction of computerized fluoroscopic image intensification following intravenous injection of small amounts of contrast medium, it promises to eliminate the discomfort and risks of intraarterial angiography.

Surgery for Ischemia

Although there had been sporadic attempts to deal with either damaged or diseased arteries prior to the twentieth century (Matas and Murphy having dealt with aneurysms),[1] a major landmark in the development of vascular surgery was the pioneering work of Carrel and Guthrie (1906),[2] who over a period of years developed many of the techniques of vascular anastomosis still in use today. Substitution of a vein for an artery was reintroduced by Kunlin.[3] The work of Blalock, Gross and Crafoord[4–6] in the 1940s, resulted in the successful treatment of tetralogy of Fallot, patent ductus arteriosus, and coarctation of the thoracic aorta. Thereafter, interest in vascular problems increased markedly.

The general surgical management of arterial occlusive diseases differs somewhat from the management of aneurysms and will be dealt with separately. There are five general ways to deal with ischemia due to interference with arterial blood supply:

1. Replace or bypass the occluded or narrowed artery with an arterial substitute,

2. Reopen the occluded or narrowed artery by endarterectomy or embolectomy/thrombectomy,
3. Reopen the occluded or narrowed artery by transluminal dilatation,
4. Develop or promote collateral circulation, or
5. Remove the ischemic tissue or organ if possible.

ARTERIAL REPLACEMENT

Graft Materials

Although it has been known since the early part of this century that a vein placed in an arterial location will function well and become *arterialized* (meaning that its wall generally thickens), there has been an intensive search for an ideal arterial substitute,[7] stimulated by the first report of Blakemore and Voorhees that Vinyon-N cloth, fashioned as a tube, remained patent when used as an arterial substitute. Various modifications have evolved since then and included investigation of different inert plastic substances, including nylon, polyvinyl sponge, Teflon, Dacron, and lastly Goretex. Fabrication of these has been either as woven, knitted, or extruded fabric with variable surface characteristics, ranging from crimped to filamentous to relatively smooth. The variations in materials and methods of construction have been spurred by the realization that in humans a true neoendothialized neointima does not develop in any of the plastic substitutes; rather, the prostheses become coated on their vascular surfaces with compacted fibrin and varying degrees of cellular invasion occur.[8]

The knitted prostheses, being more porous, have the advantage of becoming firmly anchored, and incorporated into the body structure through the invasion of the porous wall by fibroblasts. They remain relatively nonthrombogenic, providing satisfactory long-term patency rates in vessels as large as the aorta, iliac, and common femoral arteries, where autologous tissue substitutes are not available, but faring less well in smaller vessels. They suffer from the minor disadvantage of requiring preclotting prior to use, and of leaking blood through their interstices when anticoagulants are used in the early postoperative period. A more serious disadvantage is their susceptibilityto immediate and even progressive dilatation.[9] This may destroy their nonthrombogenic properties, resulting in the accumulation of laminated gelatinous thrombus and reocclusion. The introduction of changes in the blood/plastic interphase by making the prosthesis filamentous is an attempt to maintain nonthrombogenicity by promoting a more cellular neointima. Whether this modification is significant and will overcome the thrombogenicity introduced by progressive dilatation is not as apparent yet. Another major disadvantage, shared by all artificial plastic prostheses, is their susceptibility to infection.

Although they have been employed in large numbers in arteries smaller than the common femoral, it is generally agreed that late patency rates of knitted prostheses are not comparable to those obtained by autologous venous substitutes of similar caliber. Indeed, the reversed autologous saphenous vein graft has become the standard for comparision of results of all other small arterial replacements.[10]

Woven prostheses, being relatively nonporous, require no preclotting and can be employed when postoperative anticoagulants need to be given or when intraoperative coagulopathy is anticipated, as, in operations for ruptured aneurysms. They do not appear to be subject to dilatation. Their major disadvantages are that they are more difficult for the surgeon to handle and they develop a fibrinous neointima, which is only loosely attached to the graft, becoming firmly anchored by fibrous invasion only at suture lines. There have been sporadic reports of embolization of detached neointima from woven prostheses. Although woven Teflon enjoyed a vogue 15 years ago, Dacron has now replaced it and is available either knitted or woven. It is crimped, permitting longitudinal stretching of the graft for easy placement.

A recent development in graft constuction has been the introduction of polytetrafluoroethylene (PTE) (Goretex)[11] which is extruded, resulting in a randomized distribution of fibers rather than in orderly arrangements, ie, weaves and knits. The resultant graft grossly appears to be smooth. It is relatively nonexpandable and nonstretchable longitudinally. It can be constructed in various sizes, ranging from aorta to small vessels the size of the tibials. It is now undergoing intensive investigation in clinical situations. There have been varying degrees of success in small arterial replacements, reports varying from superior to autologous tissue to no better than any other plastic arterial substitute of equal caliber. Goretex suffers from the disadvantages of: 1) being relatively untried in terms of long-term (five-year) results, 2) of requiring early reoperation for thrombectomy for, as yet, not fully explained reasons to maintain long-term patency, and 3) of acting as a foreign body in the presence of infection. Its future is unpredictable.

Other substitutes for smaller arteries have been introduced during the past two decades, some the products of great ingenuity. The umbilical vein biograft, obtained from human placenta, is a case in point.[12] Fixed in glutaraldehyde (a fixative used for preparation of specimens for electron microscopy), which accurately preserves the architecture of the vein, it is a nonliving graft with a relatively nonthrombogenic surface but subject to dilatation since it has no arterial contractile properties. It, therefore, requires reinforcement with an externally applied net of plastic to prevent aneurysm formation. It, too, becomes lined with a fibrinous, relatively acellular neointima. It is now undergoing active clinical trials in the *small* vessel location with as yet uncertain results when compared to autologous vein.

The utilization of homologous grafts, both arterial and venous, has undergone cyclic popularity. Homologous arteries harvested from cadavers and lyophilized were the first to be used in large numbers between 1955 and 1965. They suffered from problems of availability, marked variations in quality control starting with nonuniform harvesting techniques, and exhibited both early failures due to autolysis with rupture and late failures due to marked degenerative changes, including aneurysm formation and calcification. The major advantages of ease of handling and accurate diameter replacement were therefore lost.[13]

Noteworthy, however, has been the realization that the technique of preparation of the homologous vein prior to implantation may play a major role in the manner in which it is perceived by the body. Freshly harvested veins appear to be least well tolerated. Lyophilization may introduce the tendency for degenerative changes while supercooling in a liquid medium may yield the most favorable results by destroying antigenicity while preserving the integrity of vein structure. Nevertheless, homograft veins appear to be frequently perceived as nonliving structures acting as inert fibrous tubes that may become invaded with fibrous tissue. In spite of occasional enthusiastic reports regarding their usefulness, they have not achieved universal appeal.[14]

Replacement Techniques

There are three different ways to achieve arterial replacement:

1) Resection of thrombosed arteries and interposition of prostheses,
2) Employment of the bypass principle in which an arterial replacement is anastomosed to an open artery above and to one below the artery to be replaced, or
3) Employing an *extra-anatomical* route in which a prosthesis is anastomosed proximally to a distant artery, ie, the subclavian, and distally to an artery beyond the obstructed segment, ie, the femoral artery. The possible combinations based upon this principle are almost limitless.

Of the currently popular arterial substitutes for both large and small vessel replacement, namely knitted and woven Dacron, Goretex, umbilical vein and autologous vein, all share some common properties. If the grafts dilate inappropriately, the nonthrombogenic properties are lost and gelatinous thrombus forms, which may lead to eventual closure. Suture lines are particularly vulnerable to thrombus deposition and when technical imperfections occur, they are subject to immediate or early closure. When lesser amounts of thrombus are deposited at suture lines, organization of this by fibrous tissue may result in fibrous stenosis and eventual closure. No arterial substitute exactly reproduces the compliance of native normal arteries and, therefore, the arteries in contact with the arterial substitutes are subjected to abnormal flow patterns, which may predispose to intimal proliferation and eventual closure.[15,16]

An unfortunate property shared by all artificial plastic prostheses is their previously mentioned susceptibility to infection and the inability of the body to limit or eradicate such infection, which spreads along the adventitional or outer surface of prostheses creating limb-threatening and life-threatening situations. Ordinarily, if infection occurs in the area of a plastic prosthesis, the prosthesis must be removed in order to control the infection and prevent life-threatening breakdown of arterial anastomotic suture lines with exsanguinating hemorrhage. Since a new prosthesis cannot be brought through infected tissues, extraanatomical pathways, if available, must be used to prevent distal ischemia. Surgical ingenuity has made it possible to cope successfully with a number of such complications.[17,18]

The introduction of microsurgical techniques, which involves the use of magnification of varying degrees during the performance of vascular anastomoses, the use of very fine suture material and appropriately scaled instruments, has permitted access to arteries as small as 1 to 2 mm in the limbs, kidneys, and brain.[19]

ENDARTERECTOMY

Endarterectomy, literally the cutting out of the inner wall of an artery, is universally employed in some areas, occasionally or infrequently in others, and never in some for chronic arterial occlusions or stenoses. There appears to be a universal distrust of the procedure, since it is commonly thought that blood exposed to the deeper layers of the arterial wall clots and that the endothelium is necessary to maintain a nonthrombogenic surface. Early reports of the healing of endarterectomized arteries suggested that thrombus deposition occurred universally and that the neointima, which formed, developed through the fibrous organization of thrombus.[20] Our own experiments indicate that this may not necessarily be so. Indeed, when thrombus deposition occurs unevenly, healing may occur due to organization of thrombus. When thrombus deposition does not occur, healing occurs through the deposition of white blood cells in monolayers on the endarterectomized surface, and neointima forms through the transformation of exposed smooth muscle cells in the arterial wall which transform to participate in the regeneration of an appropriately thin neointima lined with neoendothelial cells.[21] The endarterectomized arterial wall indeed may be nonthrombogenic, a property that is lost only when certain abnormalities of flow occur, ie, from leaving behind intimal or smooth muscle flaps and threads. Unimpeded flow helps to maintain the nonthrombogenic properties of the endarterectomized arterial wall. It is apparent, therefore, that endarterectomy is not necessarily followed by thrombosis.

The results of endarterectomy in the carotid location universally are accepted as excellent. Immediate closure is due to technical imperfections, and late closures occur relatively infrequently (1% to 4%). Our experiments suggest that the late proliferative reactions (hypertrophied neointima) are the result of *abnormal* flow, the precise characteristics of which are not clear. The late results of endarterectomy in the aortoiliac segment, too, are accepted as being outstanding. In the femoral-popliteal location, there are reports of early and late results being identical to results employing autologous veins.[22] Endarterectomy of arteries smaller than the proximal tibials, including the coronaries, is not as favorable. In part, this may be due to technical-surgical factors and in part related to velocity of flow in these smaller arteries.

The disadvantages of endarterectomy procedures basically are related to technique. Especially where long segments are involved, ie, in the aortofemoral location or in the femoral-popliteal location, a high degree of expertise is needed. The procedures tend to be more time-consuming and costly of blood and, thus, not suitable for high risk patients.

A major advantage is the minimal amount of foreign material used. Indeed, only the suture material can be considered a foreign body, and so the risk of infection, an ever present hazard with plastic prostheses, is decreased. These procedures permit conservation of major venous structures, ie, the greater saphenous vein for use in other areas such as the coronary site where no universally acceptable arterial substitute exists except for the internal mammary artery. For vessels down to and including the caliber of the proximal third of the tibial arteries, the results appear to be equal to those obtained by employing autologous vein.[23]

Techniques

Endarterectomy usually is performed in open fashion in those areas where the length to be cleared is short, no more than 5 or 10 cm, and particularly is useful in the carotid, common femoral, and profunda femoris locations. Where longer segments require disobliteration, ie, in the aortoiliac, common femoral and the femoral popliteal locations, arterial strippers are used.

An ingenious technique with limited applicability is *gas* endarterectomy.[24] This technique cannot be used to perform endarterectomy procedures in the limbs of diabetic patients who have a particularly adherent and friable type of medial calcification of the media. Carbon dioxide gas under pressure is injected through a needle into the arterial wall. The gas finds the path of least resistance, which usually is through the media, deep to atherosclerotic plaques. This effectively may free up the atherosclerotic intima. It was the hope of the originators that the gas would travel the entire length of the atherosclerotic involvement, the dissection stopping at normal intima, which is ordinarily quite adherent and difficult to separate. This appears to have been somewhat successful in the coronary arteries and perhaps in the carotids, but in the extremities such completely normal intima is rarely encountered, and particular surgical maneuvers are required to limit the dissection by the gas. Specially designed spatulae are available for insertion into the arterial lumen to help complete the endarterectomy. On occasion, however, the use of such spatulae has resulted in total disruption of the arterial wall. Although appealing in concept, this technique has not achieved universal popularity, in part because of the failure of the technique to live up to the hope that it would permit precise end points in the endarterectomy, and in part because of its ineffectiveness for use in diabetic leg arteries.

The *gas* procedure does not appear to save time for the experienced surgeon, since most of the time required for successful long endarterectomy procedures is spent not in the actual disobliteration but rather in the reconstructive phases. The risk of arterial wall disruption by the gas spatulae has constituted a major objection since, in our hands, the ring strippers do not suffer from the above disadvantages. The ring strippers also are quite successfully employed in diabetic patients.

EMBOLECTOMY/THROMBECTOMY

The occurrence of acute limb ischemia, resulting from embolization of large thrombi (usually from the heart), produces major technical-surgical problems due to the propagation of stasis clot distal to the site of lodgment of emboli. It is the propagation of such clot that usually results in progressively severe ischemia since its propagation blocks collateral channels. Such clot almost universally is encountered distal to emboli. Techniques for extracting the emboli have been relatively simple, but until the advent of the Fogarty balloon catheter,[25] disobliteration of the distal arterial system posed extremely difficult problems. With the catheter, it is possible to reopen the distal system down to the level of dorsal pedal arteries by passage of such balloon catheters through small arteriotomy incisions. The procedure succeeds provided propagation of clot into secondary branches has not occurred. A simple embolectomy/thrombectomy procedure fails, too, in the presence of a combination of chronic occlusive atherosclerotic disease and acute embolic occlusions, unless it is realized that such combinations exist and appropriate bypass or angioplastic reconstruction is performed in conjunction with the embolectomy/thrombectomy procedure.

TRANSLUMINAL ANGIOPLASTY

The concept of dilating atherosclerotic arteries transluminally was first popularized by Dotter,[26] who employed progressive catheter dilatation of both occluded and stenotic vessels in the aortoiliac and femoral popliteal segments. Gruntzig[27] adopted the balloon catheter technique, which consists of insertion of a catheter with a balloon at its distal end into the atherosclerotic lumen. The balloon is inflated to compact both thrombus and atherosclerotic debris. It then is possible to reopen either a short segment of occlusion or to dilate a soft stenotic segment provided it is not severely calcified. The earliest attempts, and to date perhaps the most successful, have been the dilatation of stenotic segments of iliac arteries, with lesser success in the femoral popliteal location. Notable success has been achieved, too, in the dilatation of stenotic renal arteries due to either atherosclerosis or arterial dysplasia, the dilatation of coronary arteries both preoperatively and intraoperatively, and the dilatation of stenotic arterial bypass grafts.[28-30]

The procedure offers a relatively nonstressful technique for restoring flow in carefully selected situations. Hemodynamically significant short lesions of the iliac system can be dilated significantly prior to operative procedures on the femoral popliteal or tibial arterial system, thereby decreasing the magnitude of the open procedure for lower extremity revascularization. Short segmental occlusions of 5 cm or less, or stenoses of the femoral-popliteal system if hemodynamically significant, can be dilated to avoid major open intervention in some patients. Approximately 10% of patients who present for limb salvage revascularization procedures have lesions that are amenable to transluminal angioplasty. In 10% to 15% of patients treated in this manner, immediate operative intervention becomes necessary because of extensive thrombosis following balloon angioplasty. Embolization of atheromatous debris probably occurs universally following balloon dilatation, but to date no serious consequences have been described.

The exquisite susceptibility of the brain to atheroemboli has precluded the widespread use of the technique for carotid artery dilatation, although the anatomical distribution of the atherosclerotic plaque in that location would appear to offer an ideal situation for such maneuvers. The plaques are rarely longer than 2 to 3 cm in length, and the distal intima in the internal carotid artery is normal. On the other hand, the smooth surface characteristics of the stenotic renal artery afflicted with arterial dysplasia, including fibromuscular hyperplasia, make it an ideal situation for balloon angioplasty. The long-term results of this technique have not yet been observed, and it is in danger of being overused. A major danger now exists because of the relative simplicity of the technique. There has been an unfortunate tendency to attempt balloon angioplasty in patients with mild extremity ischemia who do not need any surgery, thus exposing them to unnecessary risks. It will probably be a discredit to the technique if it is so indiscriminately employed. The technique will undoubtedly find its place in the armamentarium needed to cope with ischemic conditions, and will prove to be a major advance provided it is employed with the discretion that has become the hallmark of the thoughtful vascular surgeon.

PROMOTION OF COLLATERAL CIRCULATION (SYMPATHECTOMY)

Sympathectomy for the relief of extremity ischemia, upper and lower, has never achieved a respectable or recognizable position in the surgeon's armamentarium.[31] It is admitted by most that some patients experience dramatic improvement following lumbar sympathectomy, while many exhibit transient or no improvement, there being no reliable technique to help in patient selection. Numerous attempts to test for residual sympathetic function preoperatively, and then demonstrate the ability to block such function, have given poor correlation with surgical results. The most recent attempt to correlate the pressure readings obtained with the aid of Doppler devices applied to the pedal arteries has made it possible to identify a small group in whom the chance of response is virtually zero. It has not improved, however, the prediction ratio to any appreciable extent in those who have some pressure in the pedal vessels.

IDEATIONAL ADVANCES

A number of important concepts have developed during the past three decades of intensive vascular surgical activity that reflect the growing understanding of the proper management of ischemic syndromes.

Limb

In the management of ischemic conditions of the limbs, perhaps the most important concept developed has been the need to conserve the patient's vascular resources. Where it was considered advisable to operate on all patients with chronic arterial occlusions, even with mild symptoms, it now is apparent that surgical intervention is only mandatory in patients whose ischemia is limb or life threatening, since those with minor degrees of ischemia, (ie, experienced by most claudicators) fare quite well without surgery. Surgical revascularization procedures in the limbs may remain functional for relatively short periods of time. With graft failure, not only might the patient's most useful surgical replacement, the saphenous or brachial vein, have been used up, but ischemia may be worse because of propagation of thrombus into the most distal vessels. Paradoxically, limb salvage rates in patients who have arterial reconstructions for threatened limb loss usually exceed late patency rates, attesting to the continued elaboration of the collateral circulation. When limb infection is controlled with the aid of a revascularization procedure, a stage of compensated ischemia may be restored and the limb preserved. These observations led to a change in the surgical population subjected to limb revascularization procedures so that the majority now are those requiring salvage procedures.

In patients with acute ischemic states, realization that the differential diagnosis between cardioembolization and in situ thrombosis is essential for proper successful surgical management promises to improve the results of therapy. Simple embolectomy/thrombectomy procedures in patients with embolic occlusion superimposed upon chronic arterial occlusion, or for acute in situ thrombosis, often are not adequate. This realization led to the appreciation of the importance of the role of intraoperative angiographic studies when combinations of embolectomy/thromboectomy and angioplastic or bypass procedure may be required. It is clear now also that some patients with acute arterial occlusion should be treated with large doses of heparin so long as improvement occurs.[32] As collateral circulation enlarges appropriately, informative angiographic studies can be performed to more accurately assess the true condition of the arterial system and permit more precise surgical intervention, if indicated by the persistence of residual ischemia. Angiographic studies in patients with acute arterial occlusions are frequently misleading because of failure of vessels distal to sites of acute occlusions to opacify even when mechanically patent. This nonsurgical approach to acute ischemia, however, requires close hourly follow-up and precise knowledge of what constitutes worsening or improvement of ischemia.

The recognition of low flow states due to cardiac pump failure in patients with otherwise compensated chronic arterial occlusions, resulting in focal ischmia distal to such chronic occlusions, is best managed by improving cardiac function. This is a major ideational advance that has avoided unnecessary or unusually hazardous operations in critically ill patients. Indeed, in the presence of such impaired flow due to poor cardiac function, the failure rate of either otherwise successful disobliterative or bypass procedures is inordinately high.

Atheroembolization of limbs (*purple toe* syndrome), formerly thought to be due to emboli from plaques in the suprarenal aorta and usually accompanied by embolization to the kidneys, is now recognized to be probably more frequently due to embolization from relatively easily accessible arteries, ie, the infrarenal aorta, the iliacs, and even the femorals for the lower extremities, and subclavian for the upper extremities. These arterial sources of emboli are approached surgically with ease, and the sources of emboli usually can be removed by endarterectomy. The classic situation, of course, occurs in embolization from the carotid bifurcation.[33]

Realization of the importance of major arterial occlusions (macroangiopathy) in the diabetic, as opposed to microangiopathy and the added role of the susceptibility to burrowing necrotizing infections in producing limb- and life-threatening situations, has led to successful limb salvage procedures through combinations of surgical debridement and major arterial reconstructions. The early fears that microangiopathy would preclude successful revascularization by arterial reconstruction, or even control of the necrotizing infections, have not been realized. In the presence of open major arteries, such infections can be debrided radically and healing can be expected. In those with occluded major arteries, the debridement usually requires the addition of a major vascular reconstruction. Microangiopathy does not appear to play a significant role in the outcome.

Cerebral Circulation

The major ideational advances in the management of ischemic brain syndromes have been the realization that ischemic strokes are caused by lesions in the extracranial carotid arteries, and that transient symptoms and cerebral infarcts are often the result of embolization of either atheromatous debris or platelet fibrin particles to the intracranial arteries. These facts were amply uncovered by the National Cooperative Stroke Study.[34] This study further emphasized the role of safe surgical technique as a major factor in favorably altering the natural course of ischemic brain disease. Those most severely afflicted with multiple arterial lesions, after successful operative procedures, appeared to enjoy the greatest protection from future stroke. This study also emphasized the futility of attempting to revascularize a brain that had sustained an acute infarct, emphasizing the prophylactic nature of the surgical procedures. This is a concept quite at variance with what has been learned for the management of ischemic extremities.[35,36]

The mechanism of brain stem ischemia in vertebrobasilar arterial insufficiency is probably inadequate flow rather than embolization. This is attested to by the observation that correction of hemodynamically significant carotid lesions frequently relieves vertebrobasilar symptoms. Furthermore, we observed that the only patients upon whom vertebral arterial reconstructions was necessary for the relief of symptoms were those with severe, bilateral flow-impeding lesions of their vertebrals who were not relieved by carotid repair.[37] Unilateral vertebral angioplasty has been effective in these cases. Low flow in the vertebrals usually is due to ostial stenosis from subclavian lesions.

The study of carotid plaque morphology provided insights into the nature of the atherosclerotic process as it occurs in those vessels. The common denominator in all lesions is intimal fibrous thickening with variable secondary changes, including: intramural hemorrhage, intramural atheromatous debris, ulceration, thrombosis even in the absence of marked stenosis or ulceration, and finally exuberant hypertrophy of the intima due simply to fibrous proliferation and leading to critical flow-impeding stenosis. A most important change occurring in approximately 50% of symptomatic patients, is plaque hemorrhage, which often leads to ulceration and embolization.[38]

The pathologic findings in the asymptomatic contralateral carotid artery frequently are identical with those in the symptomatic one.These suggest that although the intimal fibrous plaque may be an almost universal finding in the late adult population, the occurrence of secondary changes is dependent upon specific factors in particular patients, which determine the type of evolutionary changes that may occur. This is quite at variance with the traditional concept that the atherosclerotic plaque, in its development from inception to eventual thrombosis, follows a stereotyped course, each plaque going through sequential stages and finally resulting in either thrombosis or sufficient interference with circulation to produce ischemia. Perhaps it is important, therefore, to know the precise details of pathologic changes in particular patients to permit understanding of the factors that result in these specific secondary changes. It then might be possible to achieve specific therapeutic regimens for specific groups of patients based upon specific pathology.

Renal Circulation

Stenotic lesions of the kidney arteries, though once aggressively treated surgically, now are less frequently treated in this manner, partly because of the relatively poor results achieved in patients with atherosclerotic lesions. Surgical results appear to be inversely related to the severity of the atherosclerotic process in arteries not directly related to the renal arteries. Surgical mortality experienced in renal arterial revascularization procedures occurs predominantly in the atherosclerotic population.[39] For patients with arterial dysplasias of various types, the availability of numerous drugs effective in controlling hypertension has raised the question of whether surgical therapy is preferable to medical therapy in terms of long-term survival. The answer is not clear. The basic data available refer predominantly to the effect of the surgical procedure upon arterial hypertension. Control of hypertension, by implication, is thought to improve survival, but the superiority of surgical over medical therapy is not apparent. On the other hand, renal arterial reconstructive procedures for salvage of renal function are performed most aggressively, even in patients in whom small kidneys are found distal to totally occluded renal arteries.[40] Various microsurgical techniques and bench procedures,[41] which permit the kidney to be cooled, temporarily removed from the body to permit precise arterial reconstruction into smaller branches, and reimplanted at the iliac level, have helped in such salvage operations. Surprisingly, previously thought functionless kidneys in two of our patients resumed function and sustained life for many years.

Mesenteric Circulation

Ischemic conditions of the bowel continue to pose difficult problems of diagnosis and therapy. The most significant advances have been the earlier and more frequent use of angiographic studies in patients with acute and chronic ischemic bowel problems. Attempts at pharmacologic relief of acute ischemic states have been successful. This can be achieved through the fluoroscopic control of catheters advanced into appropriate vessels, and infusion of vascular smooth muscle relaxants.[42] Revascularization procedures for acute ischemic bowel syndromes have not achieved the success of arterial reconstructions in other areas, in part owing to the difficulties of establishing diagnoses before intestinal infarction occurs. On the other hand, studies of the arterial circulation in patients with incapacitating abdominal symptoms, not otherwise diagnosed by more conventional studies, have led to the proliferation of a number of successful techniques for relieving such chronic ischemia through the use of either bypass or endarterectomy procedures.[43]

EVALUATION OF PATIENTS WITH CEREBROVASCULAR INSUFFICIENCY

Selection of Patients for Study as Prospective Surgical Candidates

Lesions in carotid arterial bifurcations appear to expose patients to the greatest risks of stroke. Their nature is illustrated by the patients who have transient ischemic attacks (TIA). Episodes of TIA, either of the monocular or cerebral hemispheric type, denote a risk of future stroke that is estimated to be approximately 10% to 15% per year, being greatest in the first two years following the attack. Indeed, there are series which report that from one fourth to one third of all patients who experience such episodes will ultimately sustain major strokes. It also is apparent that approximately three fourths of all patients who sustain a major stroke have had a prior warning transient ischemic episode.[44] Consequently, although there is some evidence from the Canadian antiplatelet study[45] that males who experience transient episodes and receive aspirin have a diminution in their transient attack frequency and perhaps a decreased incidence of stroke in the ensuing years, all patients who experience TIA's, men and women, are studied. The definitive study performed is angiography. Although there are some data to suggest that the deleterious effects of carotid plaques increase as they become hemodynamically significant, it is not possible to predict the details of the pathologic changes in the plaque either from hemodynamic studies or from angiographic studies. Other patients with transient symptoms referable to the cerebral hemispheres or the brain stem, including patients with unexplained syncopal episodes, may require cerebral angiographic studies after nonvascular causes have been ruled out.

A second problem group is made up of patients who are totally asymptomatic. They either present with bruits over the carotid bifurcations that are clearly separable from aortic murmurs, or are referred for evaluation because noninvasive procedures, ie, oculoplethysmography or imaging, have suggested hemodynamically significant carotid lesions are present. In these, a decision regarding the need for angiography must be made. Based upon a number of observations suggesting that the significance of lesions in terms of future cerebral ischemic damage increases proportionately to the degree of stenosis, noninvasive pressure studies have become a major determinant in deciding whether to subject such patients to cerebral angiography.

Selection of Patients for Carotid Surgery

The selection of patients for surgery is determined by: the neurologic status of each patient, the radiographic appearance of the lesions, evaluation of systemic conditions that may be apparent in determining life expectancy, and the ability of each patient to withstand surgical procedures. Where a cerebral hemisphere appears to have been completely destroyed, as manifested by dense unresolving hemiplegia, surgical intervention cannot be expected to change the condition of the patient. If, however, areas of the brain have been spared (such as occur with monoparesis or hemiparesis of the dominant cerebral hemisphere in which the speech area was unaffected, and the syndrome occurred appropriate to a stenotic carotid artery), surgical intervention then might be expected to protect the remaining portion of the partially infarcted hemisphere.

The radiographic appearance of the lesion is evaluated in terms of its ability to interfere with flow and ability to discharge emboli. A 50% or greater diametric luminal narrowing and/or an irregular surface of the filling defect are the criteria for operability. A second lesion in the intracranial portion of the carotid artery, which produces marked stenosis in the range of 70% to 90%, is considered a contraindication to surgical intervention in the carotid bifurcation. Relief of the more proximal stenosis cannot be expected to increase total cerebral blood flow. Total occlusion of the internal carotid artery could result from surgical procedures proximal to a markedly stenotic carotid siphon. Since areas of recent cerebral infarction may hemorrhage after blood flow is restored, preoperative CAT scans are performed to detect infarcts in patients with flow-impeding lesions. When infarcts are found, surgical intervention for flow-impeding lesions is postponed for four weeks. Intervention for nonhemodynamically significant lesions, which have been the source of emboli, usually does not need to be delayed.

Operations are avoided for total occlusion of the internal carotid artery. Propagated thrombus from the bifurcation to the siphon makes disobliteration impossible by current techniques. Simple coiling or tortuosity of the internal carotid artery, unless symptoms can clearly be attributable to such kinks, do not require operation.

In a patient with bilateral carotid stenoses, a decision must be made regarding surgical intervention as a secondary procedure on the side opposite the symptomatic artery. In our own patient population, a second operation is performed on the asymptomatic contralateral carotid artery when the asymptomatic artery demonstrates flow-impeding stenoses greater than 50% to 70%, or when the symptomatic artery contains intramural hemorrhage, intramural atheromatous debris, ulceration of the intimal surface, or intraluminal thrombosis. Our own retrospective study revealed that the pathologic changes at the carotid bifurcation are frequently bilaterally symmetrical and a patient exhibiting hemorrhage in one carotid artery is apt to have a hemorrhage in the other asymptomatic one. A patient with a smooth fibrotic plaque on one side is apt to have a similar type of plaque on the other.

Operations upon the external carotid artery have now become important in this day of extracranial-intracranial bypass procedures. Patients who have persistent symptoms referable to the cerebral hemisphere, distal to a totally occluded internal carotid artery, and who have a stenotic external carotid artery, are subjected to restoration of the lumen of the external carotid artery. This permits extracranial-intracranial bypass procedures, usually from the superificial temporal branch of the external carotid artery.[46]

Other Cerebrovascular Surgery

Operations upon the vertebral artery origins are undertaken in patients with persistent basivertebral arterial symptoms in the absence of carotid stenosis. Only those with bilateral vertebral arterial involvement are chosen for surgical intervention, and the procedure in our own series invariably was a unilateral vertebral operative procedure.

Patients with subclavian steal syndromes can be treated with simple bypass procedures to restore blood pressure in the involved arm. Lesions of the innominate artery rarely require surgical intervention but, on occasion, have been responsible for symptoms either because of total occlusion or embolization from ulcerated plaques. More frequently, total occlusion of either common carotid artery requires a surgical intervention.

Those patients with isolated total occlusion of an internal carotid artery and persistent symptoms referable to a cerebral hemisphere, distal to the occlusion, are considered to be candidates for extracranial-intracranial bypass procedures.

SURGERY FOR CEREBROVASCULAR INSUFFICIENCY

The essence of surgical procedures performed for cerebral vascular insufficiency syndromes involves either restoration of normal hemodynamics or removal of one or more lesions suspected of being the source of cerebral emboli. The surgical maneuvers required to achieve these aims are fairly well standardized. Endarterectomy procedures universally are accepted for carotid bifurcation lesions, while all other lesions usually are treated by either bypass or some variation of an angioplastic procedure to restore appropriate lumen size. The controversial aspects of surgical intervention deal with anesthetic management during carotid procedures and the selection of patients who have various types of strokes in evolution.

Carotid Bifurcation Lesions

Clamping of the carotid artery represents a significant risk to the patient during endarterectomy. Various maneuvers have been tried to protect the brain from becoming ischemic during the period of carotid clamping. These include: the successful use of temporary inlying plastic shunts inserted at the time of carotid clamping and removed just prior to completion of the surgical procedure, and unsuccessful attempts to increase total and regional cerebral blood flow by alterations of intracerebral resistance, employing carbon dioxide inhalations and carbonic anhydrase inhibitors, ie, acetazolamide. These latter measures fail, since the nonischemic area of the brain responds by vasodilatation and competes for cerebral blood with the ischemic areas. General body hypothermia also has been used, but it is unwieldy and difficult to manage. Barbiturates offer a protective effect in animals, but are precluded in humans because of depression of cardiac function.

Various monitoring techniques have been used intraoperatively. The electroencephalogram may indicate ischemia, and monitoring of flow specifically by carotid stump pressures can predict the likelihood of ischemia. Both techniques are unreliable, however, and because of this, our own series was performed in conscious patients under cervical block anesthesia. Symptoms of ischemia appear within 8 to 30 seconds of carotid clamping in only 4% of our patients. Those who exhibited ischemia were managed with temporary carotid shunts. In spite of the lack of uniformity in management during this most critical phase of surgical reconstruction, a number of experienced carotid vascular surgeons have reported comparable surgical results. Neurological complication rates have been in the range of 1% to 3%.

The carotid bifurcation is exposed, care being exercised to avoid the occurrence of embolization from the carotid bulb by occluding the internal carotid artery prior to completion of the dissection. The artery is opened through a longitudinal arteriotomy, extending from the distal common carotid to the proximal internal carotid artery. The plaque rarely extends beyond the proximal 1 to 2 cm of the internal carotid artery, the intima beyond presenting a perfectly normal thin, glossy appearance. The endarterectomy plane ordinarily is developed easily and the plaque removed from the common, internal and external carotid arteries. The distal site of intimal transection is inspected carefully to be sure there are no irregularities that might attract platelets and form thrombi. When such are encountered, they are sutured with tacking sutures. The arteriotomies then are closed, either primarily with fine sutures or by the use of autologous venous patches. Some groups employ artificial plastic roof patches. A routine is employed to again protect the brain from embolization during the critical phase of restoration of flow to the brain. The internal carotid artery is flushed into the carotid bulb, and then reclamped. Flow is restored to the external carotid artery before finally reopening the internal carotid artery.

During the postoperative period, if the carotid baroreceptor nerves found between the internal and external carotid arteries have been carefully preserved, patients can be expected to exhibit hypotension, which is then easily managed by the use of mild, intravenously administered vasopressors. If the carotid baroreceptor nerves have been damaged, or if hypercarbia occurs in the postoperative period, hypertension can be expected to occur and can be extremely dangerous as it may lead to intracranial hemorrhage.

In addition to hypertension or hypotension, the postoperative course of such patients occasionally is complicated by the occurrence of either frank myocardial infarction or EKG changes leading to the suspicion of infarction. Such events are carefully evaluated and appropriately treated.

The most serious direct surgical complications encountered are: occasional hemorrhage into the wound, which then requires immediate surgical evacuation, and the occurrence of a frank neurologic deficit, either transient or unremitting. Neurologic deficits occur from inadequate cerebral protection during carotid clamping, thrombosis of the repaired vessel, or embolization from the operative site. When the event occurs in the recovery room, the patient is taken immediately to the operating room where the neck wound is opened and an angiographic study is performed. The arteriotomy is reopened when a filling defect is found or when total occlusion of the vessel has occurred. When the neurologic syndromes occur later in the early postoperative period, the patient is usually taken to the radiographic suite for a complete angiographic survey of the operated vessel and reoperation is guided by the findings. Totally reoccluded vessels are reopened and clots at the operative site in the vessel lumen are removed to prevent reembolization. Fortunately, such events are rare among experienced carotid surgeons, occurring in less than 1.5% of patients in our series.

The patients are given antiplatelet therapy in the postoperative period to minimize thrombus deposition at the operative site. Our laboratory animal studies indicate that healing at the endarterectomy site perhaps may be accelerated and occur earlier if thrombus deposition at the site can be avoided. Long-term antiplatelet therapy is also prescribed in the hopes of protecting these patients from having other vascular disorders. When a second procedure is to be performed on the contralateral asymptomatic carotid artery, it usually is performed one week later. When hypoglossal nerve or recurrent laryngeal nerve palsies occur, operative procedures are postponed until recovery of either the vocal cord or the tongue has occurred, since bilateral palsies interfere with respiratory exchange. The patients are followed closely for the rest of their lives, and yearly oculoplethysmography is performed.

The Vertebral Artery

Since most surgically accessible vertebral arterial stenotic lesions result from atherosclerotic plaques in the subclavian arteries, which rarely extend beyond the proximal 2 to 3 mm of the vertebral, surgical correction of the larger of paired stenotic arteries can be achieved in two ways. The vertebral artery can be transected prior to its entrance into the foramina transversaria with reanastomosis of the distal cut end to the side of the carotid artery. Alternatively, vertebral angioplasty can be performed by placing a vein patch over the stenotic vertebral-subclavian junction and shortening the reduplicated vertebral by an internal plication procedure when such kink is present. The procedures can be performed under either general anesthesia or cervical block anesthesia. Clamping of the vertebral artery universally has been tolerated regardless of the combination of lesions in the carotids and contralateral vertebral. No brain complications resulted in our series from vertebral arterial reconstructions. The incision is in the supraclavicular area with preservation of the phrenic nerve and division of the anterior scalene muscle to permit access to the subclavian-vertebral junction.

The major postoperative problems have been related to peripheral nerve palsies, which included: Horner's syndrome usually of a mild degree, paralysis of the ipsilateral diaphragm due to temporary damage to the phrenic nerve, and on the right side, partial vocal cord paralysis due to trauma to the right recurrent laryngeal nerve.

Total Occlusion of the Common Carotid Artery

Total occlusion of the common carotid artery, either right or left, although infrequently encountered, requires restoration. The internal and external carotid arteries usually remain patent and communicate with each other in spite of the total common carotid occlusion. Restoration of flow into the carotid bifurcation, therefore, almost always is possible. This can be achieved by a bypass procedure from the ipsilateral subclavian artery to the carotid bifurcation where a routine endarterectomy ordinarily is required also. On the right side, endarterectomy of the common carotid artery frequently is possible without resorting to thoracotomy. On the left side, where thoracotomy would be needed to disobliterate the origin of the left common carotid artery from the aortic arch, left subclavian to left common carotid bulb bypass procedures are favored.

Surgical exposure of the common carotid artery is obtained in a fashion similar to exposure of the carotid bifurcation with extension of the incision downward to the head of the clavicle. When subclavian bypass is required, the lower end of the incision is curved laterally to proceed parallel to the clavicle. The subclavian artery is exposed by dividing the anterior scalene muscle.

The Innominate Artery

Innominate arterial lesions that require surgical correction appear relatively infrequently. Satisfactory and direct correction of lesions of this vessel usually are performed best by entering the mediastinum through midsternotomy incisions, exposing the ascending thoracic aorta and performing a bypass procedure with artificial plastic prostheses to the right common carotid artery. When the lesion to be dealt with in the innominate artery is the source of emboli, then that vessel, as well, requires interruption to exclude the site of origin of the emboli from the cerebral circulation. Endarterectomy procedures have been performed on the innominate aortic junction, but these are difficult technically because controlling the thoracic aorta without interrupting the left common carotid artery is inconvenient. Endarterectomy, therefore, is avoided.

Subclavian Steal Syndrome

Since the subclavian steal syndrome results from occlusion of one subclavian artery proximal to the vertebral origin, and since thoracotomy is best avoided, two satisfactory bypass techniques have been developed for its correction. The least troublesome for the patient is the axillo-axillary bypass graft with a plastic prosthesis, usually of the knitted Dacron type, anastomosed to each axillary artery in the infraclavicular region. The two small incisions require communication through a subcutaneous tunnel across the anterior chest, through which the plastic prosthesis is passed.

The second procedure available, which requires a somewhat more extensive dissection but which permits the use of autologous tissue in the form of saphenous vein, is the ipsilateral carotid to subclavian bypass performed through a curvilinear supraclavicular incision. We prefer axillo-axillary shunting because of its simplicity and high rate of success.

The Temporary Carotid Shunt

Regardless of the combination of extracranial and intracranial arterial lesions found in symptomatic patients on the operative angiogram, only 4% of conscious patients in whom carotid clamping is performed develop signs of cerebral ischemia. These appear rapidly within 8 to 30 seconds of carotid clamping and recovery is equally prompt upon removal of the clamps. Approximately 90% of those who develop such signs of ischemia do so only when the internal carotid artery is clamped, clamping of the common carotid artery being well tolerated. Based upon these observations, the insertion of the temporary carotid shunt during carotid bifurcation endarterectomy is performed only in these selected patients. The technique involves placing the shunt in the common carotid artery while the internal and external remain patent to each other, and the patient remains neurologically intact. It requires a relatively short period of ischemia to then clamp the internal and external and insert the shunt into the internal carotid artery.

Although a number of techniques have been proposed to improve the tolerance to carotid clamping, the only effective technique other than shunt insertion has been the artificial elevation of the arterial systolic blood pressure. This may convert a patient from intolerant, to clamping, to tolerant, but at the expense of an eightfold increase in postoperative myocardial infarctions in patients who have a previous history of heart disease.

RESULTS OF CEREBROVASCULAR SURGERY

Although the results of carotid surgery have been debated since the earliest reports, it is generally agreed upon by surgeons and neurologists alike that, if a surgical neurologic complication rate between 1% and 3% is achieved, the natural course of ischemic brain disease is favorably altered, decreasing the incidence of transient ischemic attacks and most important, the incidence of future strokes. In the Joint Study of Extracranial Arterial Occlusion, it was further noted that patients with bilateral carotid involvement who survived the operative procedure had the most dramatic benefits. Here, too, the key to success was a low operative complication rate, achieved by some groups but not others. Our own series of now over 1000 carotid procedures confirmed the cooperative study findings. The series comprised all patients with carotid lesions (since 1962) and included the patients who, during the early portion of the series, were operated on during the acute stroke phase. Patients operated on with amaurosis fugax as the only finding sustained a 1.5% stroke rate; those with hemispheric TIAs had a 2.5% stroke rate, and those with acute strokes without alteration of sensorium sustained a 4% stroke rate. Asymptomatic patients, to date, have a 0% operative stroke rate.

In the majority of cases, these strokes were minor, and the patients had good recovery of function. Operations for acute strokes with altered consciousness resulted in a 50% mortality. The major determinant of postoperative neurologic complications in our series, therefore, was the neurologic status of the patient. Although the combination of lesions of the extracranial vessels determined the tolerance to carotid clamping in conscious patients, this appeared to play no major role in the postoperative stroke rate in our series of patients operated on under local anesthesia.

As yet unresolved is the problem of strokes in evolution or the *stuttering stroke.* Some groups continue to advocate an aggressive attitude, recommending surgical intervention during the progression phase. Although some dramatic results are achieved (progression coming to a halt following operation, dramatic improvement occurring in others), it is not yet apparent that this can be achieved with a sufficiently low complication rate to warrant general application. It has been suggested that careful control of hypertension in the postoperative period will decrease the incidence of postoperative intracerebral hemorrhage, which accounts for a large number of the postoperative strokes in this group. Such blood pressure control may not prevent postoperative cerebral edema, which we have noted in this group.

Acute myocardial infarctions occurred in 2.5% of our patients. The most serious infarcts occurred in patients in whom artificial elevation of blood pressure was employed during the carotid clamping phase. Artificial elevation of blood pressures above the patient's resting blood pressure is no longer employed.

Operations on stenotic carotid arteries opposite totally occluded vessels were performed with a high degree of safety in our series, the complication rate in the distribution of the asymptomatic contralateral carotid approaching zero. This procedure appears to improve favorably the future stroke rate.

Data for lesions other than carotids are less well documented. Our own series of over 65 patients with vertebral operations (followed for over 15 years) suggests that syncopal episodes, ataxia, and vertigo can be relieved by vertebral procedures in carefully selected patients. The late stroke rate is remarkably low in this group with the most severe and widespread arterial involvement, and is less than 1% per patient year during the 14-year follow-up. An unanswered question is whether sudden, otherwise unexplained deaths are prevented by vertebral arterial procedures.

The efficacy of other operative procedures, ie, axillo-axillary bypass, innominate bypass, and common carotid procedures, have only been tested with reference to relief of symptoms, which seems to be quite safisfactory in this group of patients with hemodynamically significant and otherwise nontreatable involvement.

Another major unresolved problem concerns the coincidence of carotid occlusive disease in patients who are to undergo coronary arterial procedures or surgical procedures unrelated to the cerebral circulation. In three recently reported series in which patients with carotid bruits were identified prior to surgical intervention in unrelated areas, stroke-prone patients were not identified by their bruit, since strokes occur predominantly in patients without bruit.[47] Screening procedures involving basically noninvasive techniques, ie, oculoplethysmography and carotid imaging, which often can be performed preoperatively, may help to solve the problem of identification of stroke-prone patients. When carotid disease is present in patients who are to be subjected to coronary artery procedures, various schemes have been tried, including staged operations on one system or the other as well as simultaneous operations. At present, it appears that the system, which seems to be most threatening on the basis of symptoms and angiographic findings, should receive priority attention. In patients with severe symptomatic carotid and left mainstem coronary artery disease, the most favorable approach at present appears to be the performance of both operative procedures at the same session, performing the carotid procedure first and proceeding directly to the coronary operation.

CHRONIC LOWER EXTREMITY ISCHEMIA

Selection of Patients for Surgery

One of the major ideational concepts, which evolved from treatment of patients with lower extremity ischemia, is that treatment should be determined and directed at correction or prevention of ischemia and not merely at restoring flow through or around occluded blood vessels. This in part developed from the realization that surgical procedures for arterial occlusions are not curative, and that arterial occlusions of the lower extremities symptomatically respond quite well to measures that promote the development of collateral circulation. Thus, unless a patient afflicted with intermittent claudication is seriously incapacitated so that employment is threatened or life style is inordinately changed, treatment consists of total cessation of smoking and participation in an active walking program, either outdoors or indoors on a treadmill, up to two miles per day, stopping to rest each time claudication appears. Follow-up is performed at several-month intervals to reassess the circulatory status of the limb and provide encouragement to continue in the exercise program. The follow-up of ambulatory patients who have stopped smoking reveals approximately two-thirds achieve either marked improvement or at least tolerable stability so that they can function and not wish to consider surgical intervention. The remaining one third is made up of those patients who absolutely cannot tolerate the claudication or whose ischemia progresses to the point of either frank gangrene or threatened limb loss. The incidence of gangrene is approximately 2% per year. Indeed, many of those who develop gangrene would be considered inoperable since they have extensive occlusions of the tibial and pedal arteries, making bypass procedures impossible.[48]

Claudicators who are subjected to operative intervention are those whose symptoms become worse in spite of therapy, or those in whom ischemic changes appear in the skin. One must be quite wary of operating on the patient who persists in smoking since operative results may be short-lived. One must also be wary of operating on the nonexerciser or the patient with disabling angina pectoris. The general condition of the patient warrants major consideration before subjecting one to the rather major operative procedures required for the relief of symptoms. It is also important to have the patient realize that, on occasion, an operative procedure for a condition as mild as intermittent claudication may lead to loss of either limb or life.

Patients with ischemic rest pain, ischemic ulcers, or frank gangrene are seriously considered for operative intervention. If the gangrene is localized to a toe, is dry and nonpainful, the patient may be treated without a revascularization procedure depending on his course. If the gangrene is spreading to the foot, then revascularization for limb salvage becomes a major consideration.

Ischemic ulcers frequently can be treated conservatively with bedrest, massive doses of antibiotics, and local care to the sites of ulceration. If granulation tissue appears in these ulcers, then the likelihood of healing without revascularization is good. If the base of the ischemic ulcer remains gray and has a purulent exudate, then healing is unlikely without additional blood supply.

Under general anesthesia, diabetic patients with necrotizing infections of the feet require radical debridement, with removal of all of the necrotic infected tissue. If the major arteries are open, this procedure should suffice for granulations to grow in the wound, which will permit the application of skin grafts. If, however, the major arterial supply is blocked, then shortly after the debridement, surgical intervention becomes necessary to insure healing.

Sexual impotence is rarely a primary indication for a revascularization procedure. The results are unpredictable although sometimes quite dramatic. Prior to accepting a patient for a revascularization procedure for this symptom, there is a careful discussion regarding alternative methods for managing the problem, namely the use of penile prostheses. Most patients when they understand that operations for sexual impotence can be major and life threatening, are satisfied to eliminate that symptom as a major consideration for a surgical procedure.

The general condition of the patient, including age, heart, lungs, kidneys and the presence or absence of hypertension and diabetes mellitus, are evaluated before accepting a patient for possible surgical intervention.

Only after it has been decided that the patient requires an operative procedure is the decision made to perform angiographic studies. The angiograms performed require visualization of the aortoiliac, femoral, popliteal, and tibial arteries, usually at least to the level of the ankles when the operation is performed for other than gangrene or necrotizing infection. When a limb salvage procedure is indicated, visualization of the terminal portions of the tibial arteries, including the pedal arches, is mandatory to permit planning a predictable revascularization procedure. In the absence of a pedal arch, revascularization of the toes and foot is not accomplished satisfactorily.

Surgical Techniques

Regardless of the degree of ischemia in the extremities, the operative procedure performed is determined by the levels of occlusion. Most claudicators who require surgical intervention have occlusions of either the aortoiliac system or the femoral-popliteal system, and can be treated by disobliteration of the aortoiliac system into the profunda femoris or of the femoral popliteal system to above the knee. Patients who require limb salvage procedures usually, though not invariably, require reconstructions into the distal popliteal artery, to the proximal tibial arteries, or to the arteries on the dorsum of the foot. The preoperative angiographic studies are the key to success in these extended procedures. It is imperative that the inflow and outflow vessels be completely opacified and visualized. Frequently, special techniques are required to opacify the distal tibial and pedal arteries. The reaction to ischemia induced by application of a blood pressure cuff to the calf, inflating it to above arterial pressure level for a period of 3 to 5 minutes, and releasing it immediately prior to the injection of the angiographic bolus will assist in this. On occasion, a direct puncture into the femoral artery with injection of the contrast media in the direction of flow is useful. On other occasions, the angiographic visualization, under general anesthesia, obtained in the angiographic suite is amplified by intraoperative angiograms. Care must be taken to limit the amount of contrast medium administered. Especially in diabetics, renal function may be severely impaired following the angiographic study or may even result in renal shutdown if the studies are repeated too frequently.

Aortoiliac Surgery

When the aortoiliac system is totally occluded, bypass either directly from the aorta to the iliac or common femoral segment, endarterectomy over the same segment, or an extraanatomical bypass using the axillary artery in the infraclavicular area as the inflow vessel and the common femoral as the outflow vessel results in marked improvement in the ischemia provided the common femoral artery communicates with a widely patent profunda femoris artery. This is true even in the presence of an occluded superficial femoral artery. When there are stenotic or occlusive lesions of the proximal profunda femoris artery, these usually can be corrected by endarterectomy and patch angioplasty. It is essential, however, to establish the hemodynamic significance of these aortoiliac lesions since correction of lesser degrees of stenosis, if not producing marked pressure gradients, will not improve distal ischemia. Lesser degrees of stenosis or short segments of occlusion can be dealt with by balloon catheter transluminal angioplasty.

The specific operative procedure selected, of the three described, depends upon the age and condition of the patient. The aortoiliac femoral endarterectomy procedures, though somewhat more difficult to perform requiring greater expertise, appear to be more durable and are employed in young patients (usually under the age of 60). The aortofemoral bypass procedures and the extraanatomical bypasses are performed in patients less tolerant to major surgical interventions.

Results of bypass for severe aortoiliac occlusion are quite good. Claudication can be relieved almost entirely in at least 90% to 95% of the patients, and ischemic skin lesions can be made to heal in 50% to 70% of the patients by progressing no lower than the profunda femoris artery. The remainder of patients with ischemic skin lesions require more distal reconstructions. It can be expected that 80% to 90% of these reconstructions will be open five to ten years postoperatively. There is, however, a high attrition rate from deaths from coronary arterial disease.

Femoral Popliteal Surgery

Patients who have lesions in the femoral popliteal segment, regardless of the degree of ischemia, can be improved by performing bypass procedures across occlusions of the superficial femoral artery, employing preferably autologous saphenous vein. When feasible, depending upon the experience of the surgeon, long, semiclosed endarterectomy can be used. Least desirable is the employment of one of a number of artificial prostheses, which range from Dacron to Goretex to tanned umbilical vein. The reconstructive procedures in the femoral-popliteal segment are most successful when there is at least one vessel beyond the popliteal artery reaching the ankle. This so-called one vessel run-off should comprise either the anterior or posterior tibial artery in marked preference to only a peroneal artery. Under such conditions, the immediate patency rate is approximately 95% and by the life table cumulative patency, there is a 50% to 70% survival-patency rate at five years. Occasional patients are made worse when the reconstructed segment reoccludes at a later date. On occasion, late reocclusion is followed by loss of limb in those unfortunate patients in whom the outflow tract has either become severely involved with atherosclerosis, or in whom thrombus has propagated into those vessels and has become nonextractable. Those patients who have their procedures performed for limb salvage, however, exhibit a limb salvage rate that is greater than the late patency rate.

Tibial-Pedal Arterial Reconstructions

When the occlusive process in the arterial system extends beyond the distal popliteal artery into the tibial vessels, surgical intervention for intermittent claudication becomes too risky. Reconstructions in the tibial arteries then are reserved for patients who require limb salvage procedures. Precise angiographic survey is essential to perform predictable reconstructions. The predictability of the reconstruction is essential since, upon failure of a reconstruction into the tibial arteries, there may be extension of the thrombotic process so that the knee joint may have to be sacrificed at subsequent amputation.

Combinations of endarterectomy and autologous venous bypasses can be performed to the upper third of the calf with immediate and late patency rates comparable to those obtained for the femoral popliteal segment. For patients with occlusions of tibial arteries in the calf, the persistence of vessels suitable for bypass at the level of the malleoli or the dorsum of the foot permits bypass procedures to these vessels, again using either autologous vein or a plastic artificial prosthesis. The patency rates are approximately 85% immediately, and the durability is approximately one half that of the more proximal reconstructions. Nevertheless, limb salvage is approximately five times greater than graft patency at ten years. This is very prominent among diabetics who may come to amputation not because of progression of ischemia but because of the superimposition of infection, which then causes decompensation of the circulation. Once the bypass procedure is performed and the infection is controlled, they revert to a state of compensation that may last for many years provided that care is taken to protect the feet from trauma and infection.

There is a small but definite group of patients who can be treated by revascularization in the absence of any major arterial run-off from the popliteal artery. This so-called bypass into a blind popliteal segment again usually is performed only for limb salvage. It requires considerable experience to predict from the angiographic study which patient can be successfully treated. Basically, description of the blind popliteal segment is that it resembles a pine tree with many branches.

A word of caution is offered regarding the peroneal artery as an outflow vessel. It ordinarily ends at the level of the malleoli in two small branches. This type of peroneal artery is unsuitable as an outflow vessel. If, however, it communicates with the remains of the dorsalis pedis or posterior tibial at the ankle and fills the pedal arch, then it works quite well as an outflow vessel and can be employed for revascularization.

RENOVASCULAR HYPERTENSION

Selection of Patients for Operation

The patients whom we have subjected to renal arteriography were selected from a relatively large population of hypertensive patients who, because of refractoriness to therapy or because of young age, were considered candidates for surgical intervention. Those having renal arterial lesions were then evaluated specifically in terms of the possibility of obtaining long-term results from correction of the renal arterial stenoses. In our series, multiple confirmatory tests have been performed through the years, but no one test alone has been reliable in predicting the outcome of the operation. Our criteria at present rest upon the finding of 50% or more stenosis of the diameter of at least one renal artery, and one positive confirmatory test, be it an excretory urogram, a positive split renal function study, or a positive renal venous renin assay. This combination constitutes an indication for surgical intervention.[49]

The criteria for a positive split renal function test are: a reduction of urine volume of 50%, and a reduction in urine sodium concentration of at least 15%, or an increase of urinary creatinine concentration of at least 15% from the involved kidney. If a Stamey test is to be performed, the criteria for positive test are a 66% decrease in urine volume and a 100% greater para-aminohippurate concentration on the involved side.[50]

A positive rapid-sequence excretory urogram is based upon the finding of a unilateral delay of opacification of the involved kidney, a decrease in renal length of 1.5 cm on the involved side, and unilateral decreased concentration of the medium on the early films on the involved side, with unilateral hyperconcentration on the late films. This can be intensified further by rehydrating the patient and producing a washout of the contrast medium from the normal kidney.

The renal venous renin assay has been helpful when available. The basic criterion is a 1.5 renin ratio when comparing renin levels from the involved and uninvolved kidneys. Renin determinations through the years were particularly troublesome until it was learned what the various factors were that may influence them. The currently available chemical determinations are more reliable. Posture plays a role in determination of renin levels and it is advisable to have the patient upright prior to the test. Sodium restriction before pretesting is important, and restriction of antihypertensive drugs such as propranolol, reserpine, and methyldopa is critical. The renin determination should be performed prior to the angiographic study. The adminstration of hydralazine may accentuate the renin difference between the two kidneys.[51]

Preoperative Preparation

The preparation of the patient preoperatively is aimed at preventing cardiovascular collapse during the administration of general anesthetics in patients who may be on potent antihypertensive medication such as rauwolfia drugs, which should be discontinued approximately two weeks prior to the operative procedure. When antihypertensive therapy is mandatory because of the severity of hypertension, methyldopa, a relatively short-acting agent that does not deplete the nerve endings of norepinephrine stores, may be employed. Indeed, because of the ability to control blood pressure easily on a hospital regimen, it is not unusual for us to admit the patients several days prior to the surgical intervention to permit stabilization of blood pressure at closer to normal levels.

There should be a two or three day lapse between the performance of angiographic studies and split function studies, during which time creatinine clearance studies should be performed to be certain that renal damage has not been accentuated by the diagnostic studies.

Operative Treatment

Two groups of patients then would be suitable for renal arterial reconstruction for relief of hypertension. One group constitutes those with arterial dysplasias of various sorts involving the major renal arteries, either unilaterally or bilaterally. The decision to repair one or both arteries simultaneously is a difficult one. Assessment is made preoperatively in our clinic and occasionally confirmed by the measurement of pressure gradients across the areas of stenosis intraoperatively in instances in which a second artery may be involved whose significance is not readily apparent. The operative procedures for the arterial dysplasias for the most part involve performance of bypass grafting usually with autologous tissue, either autologous vein or autologous artery. The autologous artery, which is employed often, is the hypogastric artery. It suffers from having atherosclerotic changes within its wall relatively early, even in young patients. As a consequence, Wylie et al[52] have suggested employing the external iliac artery, which is then replaced with a plastic prosthesis.

The bypass material in some clinics is made of plastic, either Dacron or Goretex. We have had very little experience with plastic prostheses in this location and have avoided their use in young patients.

Variations of the bypass principle have been employed in dealing with renal arterial dysplasia and include transection of the renal artery at the site of poststenotic dilatation and reimplantation into another site on the aorta. Patch graft angioplasties have been useful in the management of the single mural hypoplastic type of lesion.

Where the arterial dysplastic lesion extends into branch arteries, two techniques have been employed, both of which are satisfactory. The first was proposed by Fry and Baker and involves transluminal dilatation of the branch lesions with olive-tip dilators.[53] The second technique is the so-called *bench* technique. In this procedure, the kidney is removed from its bed by transecting the artery and vein but leaving the ureter intact, and perfused with ice cold normal saline or lactate Ringer's irrigation. Angioplastic repairs of the branch lesions then are performed, and the renal artery and renal vein are reimplanted in the pelvis to the iliac vessels. This has avoided the need for nephrectomy for branch lesions.

The other group of patients, those with atherosclerotic stenosis or occlusion of renal arteries, have often required complex operative procedures of the aorta, iliac, and renal arteries as well. In those patients with atherosclerotic plaque confined to the origin of the renal arteries, a transaortic endarterectomy has been found most useful. This can be performed by clamping the aorta above and below the renal arteries, making an arteriotomy at the level of the origins of the renal arteries and performing transluminal endarterectomy of the aorta and of both renal arteries. This has been found more satisfactory than various types of localized endarterectomies performed by incising the renal artery and aorta transversely. The bypass principle also has been employed in patients with renovascular hypertension due to atherosclerosis, and here either autologous vein or plastic prostheses have been employed.

Postoperative Management

The postoperative management of these patients is critical. Most have a diuresis following successful renal arterial repair. In some it may be massive, resulting in severe electrolyte disturbances requiring accurate replacement.

Severe hypotension may occur and has been observed on the operating table. This poses problems in differential diagnosis between hypovolemic shock and exaggerated response to correction of renal arterial stenosis, which may require vasopressors. Blood volume determinations, cardiac output determinations, and careful fluid balance studies will help in making the differential diagnosis.

Severe hypertension can occur in the postoperative period and is not an uncommon problem. It may be due to fluid overload, to hypothermia with peripheral vasoconstriction, or to unknown causes. Nevertheless, it may require intensive therapy. When hypertension becomes overwhelming, one must presume the arterial reconstruction has thrombosed, and then diagnostic studies, ie, excretory urograms, radioactive renograms, or even renal angiographic studies, may be necessary.

Varying degrees of renal failure can be expected in the postoperative period, especially if both renal arteries have been operated on.

Especially in patients in the atherosclerotic age group, congestive heart failure and frank pulmonary edema may supervene during the early postoperative period. In these patients, the Swan-Ganz catheter may be of value following the hemodynamic changes that occur rapidly at this time.[54]

Results of Surgery

Obviously, the operative results should be evaluated in terms of blood pressure response and patient survival. It is imperative to separate the two major groups of patients, namely the atherosclerotic from those with arterial dysplasias. The term *cure* is rather loosely used by some groups. It is said by some that adults with documented diastolic hypertension who have a diastolic blood pressure of less than 90 mm Hg three months after surgical treatment may be considered cured. On the other hand, we have seen patients, in whom the blood pressure response occurs gradually over a period of several months, achieve a long-term result over a period of many years. We have also seen patients with perfectly satisfactory blood pressures for three or more months postoperatively then develop a reexacerbation of their hypertension, with no apparent explanation obtained on the basis of repeat renal arteriography.

It is difficult to compare results from group to group because of the differences in the criteria of cure. As an example, Foster[55] considers normotension at the end of three months as a cure, while we have taken one year after surgery as the time for evaluation. Consequently, in the atherosclerotic group, cures range from 53% for Foster, 32% for Fry, to 25% for Imparato, and improvement occurred in 36% for Foster, 56% for Fry, and 40% for Imparato. The failure rate is 11% for Foster, 12% for Fry, and 35% for Imparato. In the cooperative study, the cured-improved rate was 63% while the failure rate was 37%. It is of interest to note the deaths that were incident to surgical intervention, which varied from 5% to 6.6%, occurred in the atherosclerotic age group. Indeed, when multiple operative procedures are added to what may be required to repair renal arterial lesions, the operative mortality in this group may be as high as 10%.

In the arterial dysplasia group, the results are more uniform and more encouraging. Here the cure rates are 72% for Foster, 55% for Fry, and 54% for Imparato, while the improvement group, consisting of a decrease in diastolic pressure of 20 mm Hg, is reported as 24% for Foster, 40% for Fry, and 40% for Imparato. The failure rate is 4% for Foster, 5% for Fry, and 6% for Imparato. The reported combined cured–improved rates are 80% for the cooperative study with a 20% failure rate, and 96% for Wylie with a 4% failure rate.[56]

A number of attempts have been made to refine the selection of patients in the atherosclerotic group for repair of renal arterial lesions. In terms of the response of hypertension, it is apparent that the more extensive the atherosclerotic process in the systemic arterial system of the patient, the less dramatic is the blood pressure response after repair of renal arterial lesions.

As a consequence of the less favorable results of surgical therapy in patients in the atherosclerotic age group, we have adopted a highly selective approach to these patients with renal arterial stenoses, and will subject to surgical intervention only those patients who have accelerated hypertension unresponsive to therapy, or who have evidence of renal failure with marked bilateral renal arterial stenoses or total occlusion. We have three patients who had revascularization of kidneys, distal to occluded renal arteries. All three are surviving on these single, formerly contracted kidneys. Two of the patients have been normotensive, one for 15 years and the other for five years. Incidental renal arterial lesions encountered during abdominal aortic aneurysm operations or aortoiliac reconstructive procedures for other reasons are not routinely repaired.

Those patients with arterial dysplastic lesions in the young age groups are operated on when the procedure is a primary one and one not previously attempted. When previous attempts at renal arterial reconstructions fail, then surgical intervention is performed for threatened thrombosis of the renal arteries only.

Transluminal Renal Artery Angioplasty

Isolated renal artery stenoses are now being subjected to transluminal catheter angioplasty. In some, the results are quite dramatic. It is impossible at the present time to judge the efficacy or durability of the procedure and, more importantly, to evaluate the long-term complications that might be anticipated, ie, microembolization.

INTESTINAL ISCHEMIA

As with other organ systems, ischemia of the intestine may occur acutely, producing characteristic symptoms, or it may occur gradually over long periods of time. The arterial blood supply of the bowel is well branched with numerous communications among the major intestinal arteries, including the coeliac axis, the superior mesenteric, the inferior mesenteric, and the hypogastric arteries by way of the hemorrhoidal. As in other organ systems, slowly developing arterial occlusion is relatively well tolerated while acute occlusion associated with propagating stasis clot is not. For each type of occlusion, the mechanisms and therapy differ.

Acute Bowel Ischemia

Acute bowel ischemia, resulting most often from acute occlusion of the superior mesenteric artery and less often from low flow states, may produce a characteristic syndrome of acute onset of abdominal pain associated with tenderness, vomiting, diarrhea of watery or bloody stool, pronounced leukocytosis, acidosis, and very early in its course, vascular collapse. Fever may not occur at the outset but appears as infarction of the intestine progresses. Bowel necrosis and perforation soon ensue, resulting in the picture of generalized peritonitis and sepsis.

Not infrequently, this syndrome occurs in a patient who has recently sustained an acute myocardial infarct, or in an atrial fibrillator with or without mitral stenosis. Less often, the syndrome occurs in patients in the atherosclerotic age group who have ostial stenosis of the superior mesenteric artery due to atherosclerosis, which then progresses to complete occlusion. On other occasions, it occurs in cardiac patients with low flow syndromes. There may be other manifestations of decreased peripheral arterial flow, ie, mottling of the skin of the extremities, low or absent urine output, and other signs of forward failure.

Its precise management depends upon making an accurate differential diagnosis between occlusive and nonocclusive intestinal ischemia and among a number of other entities that may produce the characteristic picture of the acute surgical abdomen (ie, acute cholecystitis, acute diverticulitis, acute pancreatitis, and perforation of peptic ulcer, conditions that usually demand immediate or at least early surgical intervention). If the surgeon is not convinced the diagnosis is due to causes other than mesenteric arterial occlusion, then the only technique that permits accurate diagnosis is the angiographic study. This is performed usually through the introduction of a catheter into the femoral artery, passed under fluoroscopic control into the abdominal aorta where it is possible to perform selective opacification of each of the mesenteric vessels. The value of this technique is twofold: 1) it permits the diagnosis of nonocclusive mesenteric ischemia, which on occasion can be treated successfully by the infusion of vasodilating drugs, ie, papaverine, isoproterenol, or tolazoline hydrochloride, thereby avoiding surgical intervention in a certain number of acutely ill patients, and 2) it permits the accurate diagnosis of the occlusive mesenteric vascular conditions that demand immediate surgical intervention.[57]

Reported mortality rates from acute intestinal infarction vary from 50% to close to 100%. Until 1957, when Shaw and Rutledge[58] reported the first successful superior mesenteric artery embolectomy not requiring associated bowel resection, the only surgical procedure considered in these patients was bowel resection. Often, the extent of bowel necrosis is such that resection is either so shocking that death ensues or that so much bowel needs resection that life is not possible thereafter. In recognizing that revascularization might be possible, acute diagnosis is mandatory. The mainstay of such accurate diagnosis is the angiographic study.

Once the abdomen is opened, the surgeon then must decide whether to perform a bypass procedure from either the aorta to one of the major mesenteric arteries or its branches, or from a distant uninvolved artery to a mesenteric vessel. After revascularization, once considered irrevocably damaged ischemic areas may rapidly improve. It is essential, however, following revascularization procedures and the removal of any residually ischemic bowel, to reexplore the patients at 24- to 36-hour intervals to be certain that minute areas of ischemia, which may go on to perforation, are not evident. Indeed reexploration, in our experience, should be repeated until no more infarcted bowel is evident. Although mortality rates are very high, a few patients can be salvaged.

Chronic Visceral Arterial Occlusion

Chronic occlusion of mesenteric arteries, because of the rich collateral circulation enjoyed by the intraabdominal organs, requires multiple vessel occlusions before symptoms will appear. Some patients may remain asymptomatic. When the syndrome of chronic intestinal ischemia appears, it is recognizable from the characteristic appearance of generalized cramping abdominal pain, which comes on soon after eating, lasts as long as three hours, and may be associated with a sense of distension or bloating. The pain then disappears only to return again upon the ingestion of food. This is in the picture of intestinal angina. It leads to a reluctance on the part of the patient to eat, resulting in the avoidance of food and weight loss, though without evidence of other malaise. A malabsorption syndrome, manifest by foamy stools, high in fat and protein content, leads to additional weight loss. In approximately one third of the patients who present with intestinal infarction, it is possible to obtain a history of preceding intestinal angina.

Physical findings are variable and may be related to the presence of generalized arteriosclerosis with a more specific finding of a bruit heard in the upper midabdomen.

The syndrome produced must be differentiated from other commonly occurring intraabdominal pathologic entities. The diagnosis often is made by exclusion of such entities by the routine workup. Specific diagnosis can only be made by the use of the angiographic technique. The diagnostic arteriograms usually show stenosis or complete occlusion of multiple mesenteric arteries including the coeliac, superior mesenteric, inferior mesenteric, and often the hypogastric. Characteristically, the sites of stenosis or occlusion are close to the origins of those vessels from the aorta. There may be poststenotic dilatations of those vessels. There may be a markedly enlarged marginal artery, which fills from the inferior mesenteric artery to compensate for a collapsed superior mesenteric.

Surgical intervention is advised not only to correct the symptoms of intestinal angina but also in the hopes of preventing the progression to intestinal infarction.

Two basic techniques are available for correction of chronic intestinal ischemia. Transaortic endarterectomy has been popularized by Stoney,[59] and consists of: approaching the abdominal aorta through a retroperitoneal, thoracoabdominal incision, controlling the aorta and its major branches in the upper abdomen, opening the aorta posteriorly, and performing endarterectomy procedures of the aortomesenteric vessels. The mesenteric vessels, coeliac and superior mesenteric, are very close to each other and the procedure can be performed with relatively short aortic occlusion times. The other approach is through bypass procedures; the aorta and mesenteric vessels are exposed transperitoneally and bypass grafts are placed from the aorta to either the superior mesenteric or coeliac axis artery or branches.

The results of operative procedures for chronic intestinal ischemia cannot be easily analyzed statistically since major series are few. In general, when diagnosis and differential diagnosis have been performed carefully, intestinal ischemia can be relieved by appropriate revascularization. In the interpretation of results, however, dilution occurs because of the frequent finding of associated conditions, ie, gall stones, unsuspected pancreatitis, undiagnosed peptic ulcers or tumors of the gastrointestinal tract. It is not clear either, that intestinal infarction can be prevented. It is apparent that a number of patients with symptoms of chronic intestinal ischemia have ischemia of other end organs (ie, heart, brain, and extremities), further hampering the statistical evaluation of results.

Mesenteric Venous Occlusion

Mesenteric venous occlusion may produce a clinical syndrome similar to that which occurs with acute arterial occlusion, but with the added feature of large amounts of fluid in the bowel wall and peritoneal cavity, leading to rapid abdominal distension and shock. The condition is rarely diagnosed preoperatively. The definitive treatment is surgical since without operation, mortality approaches 100%. The surgical treatment consists of removal of thrombi from the major venous structures, resection of necrotic bowel, and aggressive treatment with angicoagulants and second-look operations.

The results depend upon the extent of the venous occlusive process, the ability to institute and continue anticoagulant therapy, and the ability to remove relatively short segments of necrotic bowel.[60]

SURGERY FOR VASOSPASTIC DISORDERS

For some years, upper dorsal and lower cervical sympathectomy was considered to be a specific therapy for Raynaud's phenomenon. Greater experience has demonstrated that only 50% of patients subjected to sympathectomy will show any improvement and in some, the improvement is short-lived.

When sympathectomy is to be performed, the surgeon has at least four surgical techniques available to him. Originally it was performed through a posterior approach, which includes exposing the sympathetic chain by resecting short segments of the second and third ribs posteriorly, and extrapleural dissection to isolate the sympathetic chain. This approach now has few proponents. The supraclavicular approach, in which the incision is made in the base of the neck, does not permit easy access to the third dorsal ganglion of the chain, which is considered important in achieving a satisfactory result. This approach also invariably results in a Horner's syndrome. A third method, providing access to the midportions of the dorsal sympathetic chain as well as to the lower half of the stellate ganglion, is the transthoracic approach. This involves opening the hemithorax in the third or fourth intercostal space. More recently, the transaxillary approach has been popularized and is performed through a short incision in the axilla followed by resection of the first, second, or third rib. It can be combined with the transaxillary resection of the first rib to achieve thoracic outlet decompression as well, where such is indicated.

The nonsurgical treatment of Raynaud's phenomenon has permitted medical control of significant segments of the patient population. At present, in the selection of patients for sympathectomy, it is desirable to exhaust medical therapy first, which includes the use of vasodilating drugs and intraarterial reserpine, reserving surgical intervention only for those patients who suffer repeated breakdown of skin or whose symptoms become incapacitating.[61,62]

THORACIC OUTLET COMPRESSION SYNDROMES

Until the advent of the transaxillary approach to the thoracic outlet popularized by Roos,[63] it was not possible to observe clearly the compression mechanisms involving the subclavian artery and vein, and brachial plexus in the living patient. The transaxillary approach allows dissection of all the components of the thoracic outlet and clear delineation of any pathologic abnormalities in the area.

Anatomy

The subclavian artery leaves the thorax, passes over the first rib posterior to the anterior scalene muscle, and then enters the axilla under cover of the pectoralis minor muscle tendon. The more posteriorly located cords of the brachial plexus, separated from the artery medially by the scalenus medius muscle, leave the cervical foramina, pass over the first rib, and enter the axilla. They too pass under the pectoralis minor muscle. Directly posterior to the plexus on the curvilinear line formed by the first rib is the posterior scalene muscle, and importantly, as viewed from the transaxillary approach, the plexus is nestled in the convexity of the posterior angle of the first rib. The subclavian vein, on the other hand, lies anterior and medial to the anterior scalene muscle, subject to compression in the angle between the clavicle and the first rib. Various muscle slips traverse this area, including slips of the sternocleidomastoid muscle. When a cervical rib is present, a bony or ligamentous structure in continuity with the anterior end of the cervical rib passes under the brachial plexus to attach to the first rib. This acts as a compressing mechanism of the lower portion of the brachial plexus.

Compression of one or more of the three major structures may occur either singly or in combination. The brachial plexus and subclavian artery are more likely to share a compressing mechanism from unusual bands or slips of posterior and middle scalene muscles. The subclavian vein is more apt to be compressed alone by the peculiarities of the anatomy at the costoclavicular and costosternal junctions. It is easy to visualize how hyperabduction could produce compression under the pectoralis minor muscle.

Syndromes

Compression of the neural structures, resulting in pain, paresthesias and numbness (most pronounced along the distribution of the C8–T-1 nerve root distributions), and more rarely muscular weakness, paralysis, or muscle atrophy, may occur independently of all other symptoms. It was anticipated that careful electrical studies of the motor and sensory nerves of the plexus would provide unequivocal diagnostic evidence of the presence of thoracic outlet compression of the plexus. This has not proven to be completely true. Although electromyography and ulnar nerve conduction velocities measured across the thoracic outlet would appear to be the ideal diagnostic modalities upon which to rest the diagnosis, there are false positive and false negative tests. It becomes an extremely difficult matter to select patients who predictably will be improved by the surgical procedure. In selecting such patients, it is necessary to rule out conditions of the cervical spine and peripheral portions of the ulnar and median nerves at their distal sites of compression. Carpal tunnel syndromes as well as ulnar nerve injuries at the medial aspect of the elbow must be ruled out.

The vascular disorders associated with thoracic outlet compression may be either vasospastic, producing classical Raynaud's phenomenon, or occlusive, resulting in stenosis with embolization or total occlusion of the subclavian artery under the anterior scalene muscle.

As a third alternative, the subclavian artery may be aneurysmal just distal to the lateral border of the anterior scalene muscle, producing either a pulsatile supraclavicular or infraclavicular mass or embolization to the upper extremity. Pathology in the area of the thoracic outlet can be suspected from the presence of a unilateral Raynaud's phenomenon, from the appearance of focal ischemia of the digits or hand, characteristic of atheroembolization, or from the appearance of claudicatory symptoms involving the upper extremity associated with diminished or missing wrist pulse.

Venous compression can be suspected from the incidence of recurrent cyanosis of the hand on exertion. A pattern of collateral veins on the ipsilateral chest wall or shoulder may appear. Often, the unilateral elevation of venous pressure of the hand can be determined by simple simultaneous elevation of both upper extremities until the level is reached at which venous collapse occurs. On occasion, the presenting manifestation occurs as a result of acute total occlusion of the subclavian vein, producing the characteristic picture of sudden onset of pain, swelling, cyanosis, and dilated veins of the chest wall. This usually follows some type of exertion involving that extremity, ie, bowling or ironing clothes.

Surgical Treatment

Surgical treatment of thoracic outlet compression depends upon the presenting clinical manifestations and, therefore, upon the structures being compressed. For compression of the arterial system, it further depends upon the specific symptoms produced, the degree of ischemia present, and the mechanism by which ischemia is occurring.

Intermittent claudication of the upper extremities associated with subclavian arterial thrombosis frequently can be treated without surgical intervention, relying upon an active exercise program to promote the development of collateral circulation. The chronically thrombosed artery is not apt to discharge emboli and if the ischemia, which is maximal at the time of occlusion, has been tolerated, no additional treatment of the artery or of the thoracic outlet may be required. When, however, either acute occlusion of the artery is encountered or embolization from the aneurysmal or atherosclerotic compressed subclavian artery has occurred, emergency surgical intervention may be necessary to deal with limb-threatening ischemia. The operative intervention requires disobliteration of occluded arteries in the arm and forearm through arteriotomies of the distal brachial artery and passage of balloon catheters into the major ulnar and radial branches to extract emboli and thrombus. It requires decompression of the thoracic outlet, as well, usually by the transaxillary route, to permit removal of the first rib and division of the scalene muscles. Reconstruction of the subclavian artery is performed then through a supraclavicular approach, either to restore an occluded artery or refurbish an artery that is the source of emboli. Replacement usually is effected with a segment of autologous vein, often taken from the groin. Plastic prostheses are avoided in this group of relatively young patients to obviate having to deal with anastomotic false aneurysms later.[64]

In some rare instances in which typical and severe Raynaud's phenomenon occurs in association with thoracic outlet compression, transaxillary resection of the first and cervical ribs is followed immediately by an upper dorsal sympathectomy performed through the same axillary incision, removing the sympathetic ganglia from the dorsal third to the lower half of the stellate ganglion.

Decompression of the brachial plexus requires careful division of all of the scalene muscle attachments to the first rib, paying particular attention to removal of the posterior portion of the first rib, and its periosteum. If periosteum is left, there may be regrowth of rib. It becomes apparent from this surgical approach when decompression is complete. The neural structures can be seen to drop free of any bony or ligamentous compression from beneath. To achieve this requires division of the entire insertion of the posterior scalene muscle to the first rib. Cervical ribs, when present, can be removed through the same incision.

Decompression of the venous structures in the thoracic outlet has posed more complex problems than arterial or neural release. In approximately one half of our patients, transaxillary resection of the first rib did not permit satisfactory decompression of the vein. Second operative procedures were needed to remove the medial half of the clavicle to achieve complete venous decompression. There have been associated abnormalities, which have been detected through the combined transaxillary and transclavicular approach, including abnormal relationships between the phrenic nerve and the subclavian vein (the nerve markedly compressing the vein), and venous webs at the junction of the subclavian and internal jugular veins. The latter has required opening of the vein, excision of such webs, and venoplasty with patches of autologous vein taken from the groin. Sometimes fibrous and tendinous bends compress the vein anteriorly, mandating a combined posterior transaxillary and supraclavicular approach to thoroughly decompress the system.

Results of Surgery

The results of thoracic outlet decompression of neurovascular structures vary with the structures affected. The most satisfactory and predictable results are obtained in instances in which there has been embolization from either a compressed or aneurysmally dilated subclavian artery. In such instances, it is possible to achieve satisfactory revascularization of the upper extremity and remove the site of pathology as well as prevent its recurrence.

With venous compression, results have been less satisfactory. Approximately two thirds of the patients have satisfactory decompression of the venous system with relief of symptoms, when operative intervention is carried out before total occlusion of the vein occurs. It is necessary to perform intraoperative angiographic studies following the decompression of the venous system to be certain that additional compressing structures and especially intraluminal webs are not present. When complete occlusion of the vein is encountered, it is treated nonsurgically with anticoagulants and antiedema measures, which result in satisfactory function.

Decompression of the brachial plexus is the most difficult to evaluate and cope with. In approximately one half of the patients, the results are dramatic. Pain, paresthesia, and muscle weakness all abate. In the other 50%, although improvement occurs, many annoying symptoms often persist. In some, these can be ameliorated by decompression of the carpal tunnel and, occasionally, by transplantation of the ulnar nerve at the elbow. On other occasions, additional treatment of the cervical spine is required to relieve possibly minor compressions of the nerve roots. On still other occasions, a complete change of occupation is required. There is no question that thoracic outlet decompression of the brachial plexus can provide marked improvement. The difficulty is in the proper selection of patients, there being no totally reliable method for excluding patients who are apt not to have a good response to the operative procedure. On rare occasions, the brachial plexus neuropathy may be aggravated by the surgical procedure, which may produce other peripheral neuropathies as well, such as that of the long thoracic nerve of Bell with winging of the scapula or of the intercostobrachial nerve, which results in numbness of the inner aspect of the upper arm.

ANEURYSMAL DISEASE

Aneurysms, in general, produce symptoms either by expansion and compression of neighboring organs, by the formation of intraluminal thrombus and embolization of portions of this thrombus or by rupture. Since the advent of suitable arterial substitutes, surgical conduits, invariably of plastic material for the larger arteries and frequently autologous vein for the smaller, have been employed often.

ABDOMINAL AORTIC ANEURYSMS

Abdominal aortic aneurysms, which characteristically originate 1 to 2 cm below the level of the renal arteries, are the most commonly encountered, are found frequently in association with other evidence of atherosclerotic disease involving the brain, heart, kidneys, limbs, or bowel, and may present with a large variety of manifestations. At present, most aneurysms that come to the vascular surgeon's attention are discovered incident to either physical examination for unrelated symptoms, or abdominal or back x-ray studies for bowel, urinary tract or musculoskeletal symptoms. Those patients presenting with the syndrome of impending rupture, characterized by the presence of an abdominal aortic aneurysm and abdominal or back symptoms otherwise undiagnosed, are fewer in number than they were a decade ago, since aneurysms are now being found earlier and, therefore, are smaller in size. On rare occasions, the presenting manifestation is gastrointestinal hemorrhage due to the formation of an aortoenteric fistula.

Any symptom complex of the gastrointestinal tract, the urinary tract, or even of distal circulatory obstruction, can be produced by abdominal aortic aneurysms. The incidence of embolic occlusion of distal arteries is not clearly known since routine angiographic studies are not performed of the lower extremity vessels in patients with aneurysms. Nevertheless, there are patients whose presenting symptoms may be ischemic, referred to the extremities, and ranging from intermittent claudication to more severe ischemia with acute onset of impending limb gangrene. On occasion, a *blue toe* syndrome will result from an aneurysm.

Although most abdominal aneurysms can be felt on physical examination and the experienced observer can arrive at a rather accurate estimate of the transverse diameter of the vessel, ultrasonic studies and computerized axial tomography are of invaluable assistance in estimating the true diameter of the outer wall of the abdominal aorta. Because the incidence of rupture appears to increase markedly when aneurysms exceed a 5 to 6 cm transverse diameter, this fact is relied upon heavily in selecting patients for operation. Although rupture can occur in aneurysms smaller than 5 cm, in our experience it appears to happen rather infrequently and does not justify an aggressive attitude towards all patients with small aneurysms.

Preoperative Evaluation

Since the incidence of rupture of clinically significant aneurysms appears to be approximately 50% within a three-year follow-up, and since the curve of survival of operated patients is definitely improved over the curve of rupture, the attitude towards surgical correction of abdominal aneurysms is rather aggressive.[65,66] The patients who will be advised not to undergo immediate surgical intervention are those who have:

1) Asymptomatic aneurysms which are well under the 5 cm range,
2) Markedly impaired renal function with creatinine clearances of less than 15 or 20 ml per minute,
3) Uncorrectable cerebrovascular insufficiency states,
4) Advanced coronary arterial disease with much muscle destruction, or
5) Inoperable or terminal cancers.

Even octogenarians are considered for surgical intervention.

Because of the age group of the patients involved and the frequent association of unrelated intraabdominal conditions, preparations are made for performing other intraabdominal surgical procedures in addition to the procedure for abdominal aneurysm when gallstones, previously diagnosed gastrointestinal malignancies or urinary tract malignancies are encountered. Frequently, it is necessary to repair large inguinal hernias to prevent postoperative intestinal obstruction. This is easily accomplished transperitoneally through the abdominal incision.

When clinically significant abdominal aortic aneurysms are encountered during operations for nonemergency conditions or when abdominal aortic aneurysm is diagnosed at the time of workup for an unrelated condition, usually the abdominal aortic aneurysm takes precedence over other intraabdominal or intrathoracic conditions since rupture may occur unexpectedly. In the presence of unrelated intraabdominal conditions, it is possible to perform the operative procedure on the aneurysm, cover the prosthesis with neighboring structures including the old aneurysm wall, left colon mesentery, or greater omentum, and then proceed with the secondary procedure.

Surgical Procedure

The operation for infrarenal abdominal aortic aneurysm has reached a high stage of development. Because the only arteries uninvolved by aneurysmal disease in the abdomen below an abdominal aortic aneurysm are the proximal external iliac and proximal hypogastric arteries, this fact is made use of in our technique for applying vascular clamps. Our routine is to clamp the external iliac and hypogastric arteries before clamping the infrarenal abdominal aorta. We open the aneurysm then, evacuate it of thrombus and atheromatous debris and usually interpose a knitted (or sometimes a woven) Dacron prosthesis between the transected end of the infrarenal aorta and the transected ends of the distal common iliac arteries. The endarterectomized aneurysm wall then is sutured around the graft.

This approach avoids the problem of embolization to lower extremity vessels, which may be brought about by application of clamps to common iliac arteries that frequently have marked degeneration within their walls, in spite of the fact that there may not be marked dilatation of the circumference of the vessel. The maneuver also permits the flushing of the prosthesis into the hypogastric arteries before restoring flow to the external iliacs. There is a gradual restoration of circulation to the lower half of the body following the removal of the aortic clamps, which helps not only in avoiding distal embolization but also in avoiding declamping shock. The aneurysm prosthesis then is isolated from the peritoneal cavity by being wrapped with the old aneurysm wall.

Recovery from the operative procedure usually is uneventful. The major complications are cardiac and pulmonary. There may be transient intestinal obstruction, which almost invariably is correctable through intestinal intubation with a mercury-weighted suction tube, such as a Cantor tube.

Results of Operation

Operative intervention electively performed for abdominal aortic aneurysms, excluding only patients with the most serious unrelated organ involvement and including octogenarians, can be performed with 5% or less operative mortality. On the other hand, when operative intervention is performed for frank rupture, mortality rates of up to 80% to 90% can be anticipated depending upon the promptness with which patients are brought to the hospital and the degree of shock experienced prior to the surgical procedure. Operations for impending rupture, which not infrequently must be performed at odd hours without complete evaluation, carry a somewhat higher mortality than elective procedures.

The long-term results of abdominal aortic aneurysm operations are excellent. Survival curves are improved. These patients are subject to atherosclerotic problems in other areas. Indeed, patients who have prior history of cerebral vascular insufficiency or who are found to have neck bruits or altered carotid artery pressures on oculoplethysmography, may be subjected to cerebral angiographic studies and possibly surgical intervention on their carotid arteries prior to elective abdominal aortic aneurysm operations. Those with severe angina pectoris as part of their preoperative evaluation may have coronary angiographic studies performed and, on rare occasions, may require simultaneous operative intervention on the coronary arterial system and the abdominal aortic aneurysm.

In late follow up, one must search for aneurysms that might appear at a later date in either the femoral or popliteal areas, or at sites of anastomosis to the plastic prosthesis, the so-called anastomotic junctional aneurysms.

Suprarenal Abdominal Aortic Aneurysms

Suprarenal abdominal aortic aneurysms involving the major visceral arteries, namely the coeliac axis and superior mesenteric arteries as well as the renals, occur in less than 5% of patients with abdominal aortic aneurysms and carry the additional operative risk entailed in transplantation of the mesenteric and renal vessels to the prosthesis. In addition, the spinal cord blood supply may originate from a portion of the lower thoracic aorta, which may require exclusion in order to permit the placement of the prosthesis, thereby resulting in postoperative paraplegia. To minimize the risk of paraplegia, certain precautions are taken, such as preserving the back wall of the lower thoracic aorta and incorporating it into the prosthesis, and similarly, transplanting the major intraabdominal vessels as a unit attached to a segment of aortic wall. Even with meticulous technique, however, operative mortality is still considerably higher than it is for the infrarenal abdominal aortic aneurysm. The risk of paraplegia has been a reason for a number of patients to refuse to undergo operative intervention. Another reason for refusal has been the inability to provide a documented series of patients who have experienced rupture of the suprarenal abdominal aortic aneurysm, thereby making it impossible to supply specific numbers regarding the relative risks of nonoperative and operative intervention. On the other hand, those patients who become so acutely uncomfortable from the expansion of the suprarenal aneurysm usually are quite happy to accept the risks in the hopes of getting rid of the symptoms and prolonging life.

The operative procedure usually requires thoracoabdominal incision with the technique described by Crawford[67] for excising a segment of the wall of the aneurysm containing the origins of the renal arteries and the mesenteric arteries to permit transplantation to the prosthesis as a unit. The suggestion of Connolly, that the lower intercostal artery origins be preserved and transplanted to the prosthesis, is worthwhile.[68]

POPLITEAL ANEURYSMS

Popliteal aneurysms may appear prior to the discovery of an abdominal aortic aneurysm, may be found at the time that an abdominal aortic aneurysm is discovered, or may appear some years after successful surgical treatment of an infrarenal abdominal aortic aneurysm. The major hazard is the development of ischemia of the lower extremity. Two or three decades ago, popliteal aneurysms measured 8 to 10 cm in diameter when they appeared for surgical treatment. At the present time, most popliteal aneurysms are encountered while they are still 2 to 4 cm in diameter.

This aneurysm is particularly dangerous since severe ischemia of the extremity may occur, either through propagation of clot or embolization, or thrombosis of the aneurysms. It is for this reason that popliteal aneurysms, when encountered, are usually considered for surgical therapy. Angiographic studies are performed and operative intervention usually consists of bypassing the aneurysms with popliteal-reverse autologous venous grafts. On occasion, when the vessels are unusually large, the substitute conduit may consist of a plastic prosthesis, ie, knitted Dacron or Goretex. When aneurysms are large and fill the popliteal space, it may be necessary to decompress the popliteal fossa by opening the aneurysm, evacuating it of thrombus, and suturing back bleeding geniculate arteries.

The results of elective operative intervention for popliteal aneurysms are excellent. This is in contrast to operations for either thrombosed aneurysms or aneurysms that already have reduced distal flow by embolization. In such instances, the aneurysm can be removed but ischemia may not be relieved. Fortunately, a considerable number of patients with ischemia due to popliteal aneurysms can be improved by the performance of lumbar sympathectomy in conjunction with exclusion of the aneurysms.[69,70]

VISCERAL ANEURYSMS

Splenic Artery Aneurysms

Splenic artery aneurysms are notable for their rarity, the difficulty of diagnosing their presence prior to rupture, and the fact that they are prone to rupture in pregnant women. They are best treated by operative intervention since rupture of the aneurysms carries an extremely high mortality rate. In part, this may be due to failure to uncover the presence of the aneurysm during exploration for massive intraabdominal bleeding. Diagnosis can be suspected when ring-like calcifications are found in the upper quadrants of the abdomen. Angiographic studies should be performed to confirm their presence.[71,72]

Hepatic Artery Aneurysms

Hepatic artery aneurysms are quite rare. The author has encountered only three in the past 25 years. They may present as a pulsatile upper abdominal mass, and mimic hydrops of the gallbladder or even empyema. Occasionally, a hepatic artery aneurysm can rupture into the portal vein producing the picture of portal hypertension with bleeding esophageal varices. Surgery is always indicated for this lesion after preoperative angiography. An isolated aneurysm of a hepatic artery can be replaced with a venous autograft, but hepatic artery ligation may sometimes be necessary to control life-threatening hemorrhage.[73,74]

In one instance in which intraabdominal bleeding due to a ruptured hepatic artery aneurysm resulted in successful replacement of the hepatic artery with a venous autograft, death ensued days later from rupture of intrahepatic arteries through the capsule of the liver from unrecognized intrahepatic aneurysmal disease.

Mesenteric Artery Aneurysms

Superior mesenteric artery aneurysms are extremely rare. They have been encountered in our experience usually during a workup for unexplained abdominal symptoms or incident to angiographic studies for totally unrelated conditions. There are no large series of reported cases to help determine the prognosis. When encountered in symptomatic patients, they should be replaced with autologous venous grafts.

Renal Artery Aneurysms

Aneurysms of the renal artery usually are diagnosed incidental to angiographic study for either renal vascular hypertension or for totally unrelated conditions. On occasion, the presence of the aneurysm is suspected when a concentric ring of calcium is found. Multiple aneurysms of the renal artery can occur in association with fibromuscular hyperplasia of that vessel. It is said that rupture of renal artery aneurysms occurs rarely when there is concentric calcification. On the other hand, the rupture rate for uncalcified lesions is extremely high.

When aneurysms are encountered incident to workup of hypertension, operative intervention is indicated. At present, it is possible to preserve the kidneys in most patients with even branch aneurysms by dividing the major renal vessels, leaving the ureter intact, cooling the kidney with iced lactate Ringer's irrigation, and performing an autologous graft with the kidney on the abdominal wall. Following the correction of the aneurysmal problem, the renal artery and vein are reimplanted into the iliac vessels.[75,76]

CAROTID ARTERY ANEURYSMS

Carotid artery aneurysms occur infrequently. They usually present as pulsating neck masses with or without pain. On occasion, the pulsating mass will appear in the oropharynx. They must be differentiated from tortuous common carotid or subclavian arteries in the base of the neck that are innocuous, from carotid body tumors at the carotid bifurcation, and from metastatic lymph nodes that may lie upon the carotid artery.[77,78]

The definite diagnostic technique is carotid angiography. When the aneurysm involves the distal common carotid or the carotid bifurcation, replacement with autologous vein can be relatively easily performed, taking the usual precautions to monitor the brain and institute protective measures when necessary. On the other hand, when the aneurysm involves the internal carotid artery, filling the space between the angle of the mandible and the mastoid process, surgical exposure may be quite difficult and challenging. It may be necessary to place a distal occluding clamp on the internal carotid artery close to the base of the skull. This involves: division of the digastric muscle, division of the styloid process, sometimes detachment of the insertion of the sternocleidomastoid muscle into the mastoid process, and the considerable hazard of trauma to the hypoglossal, glossopharyngeal, facial, and vagus nerves. Nevertheless, surgery is indicated because aneurysms tend to enlarge, can be the origin of emboli, and can rupture.

In the management of these patients, we have elected to perform the operative procedures under local anesthesia whenever possible. This permits test clamping of the carotids, which when tolerated, requires no indwelling shunt to protect the brain during the surgical procedure, rendering it technically easier. When test clamping is not tolerated, then an indwelling shunt is utilized, rendering the surgical procedure more difficult. For extremely large aneurysms that may require very extensive dissection, general anesthesia may be necessary to complete the operation. However, it is used only after deciding upon subsequent proper course that insures protection of the brain from ischemia. There was no operative mortality in our series.

REFERENCES

1. Matas R. Endoaneurysmorrhapy, *Surg Gynecol Obstet* 30:456, 1920.
2. Carrel A. Technique and remote results of vascular anastomoses. *Surg Gynecol Obstet* 14:246, 1912.
3. Kunlin J. Le Traitement de l'arterite obliterante par la greffe veineuse. *Arch Mal Coeur* 42:371, 1946.
4. Blalock A. Operative closure of the patent ductus arteriosus. *Surg Gynecol Obstet* 82:113, 1946.
5. Gross RE, Hubbard JP. Surgical ligation of patent ductus arteriosus. *JAMA* 112:729, 1939.
6. Crafoord C, Nylin G. congenital coarctation of aorta and its surgical treatment. *J Thorac Surg* 14:347, 1945.
7. Voorhees AB, Jaretski A III, Blakemore AH.The use of tubes constructed from Vinyon "N" cloth in bridging arterial defects, *Ann Surg* 135:332, 1952.
8. Sauvage LR, Berger K, Nakagawa Y, et al. An external velour surface for porous arterial prostheses. *Surgery* 70:940, 1971.
9. Kim GE, Imparato AM, Nathan I, et al. Dilation of synthetic grafts and junctional aneurysms. *Arch Surg* 114:1296, 1979.
10. Baird RJ. Management options for the occluded superficial femoral artery. *Surgery* 1, 1981.
11. Veith FJ, Moss CM, Fell SC. Comparison of extended polytetrafluoroethylene and autologous saphenous vein grafts in high risk arterial reconstructions for limb salvage. *Surg Gynecol Obstet* 147:749, 1978.
12. Dardik H, Ibrahim IM, Sprayregen S, et al. Clinical experience with modified human umbilical cord vein for arterial bypass. *Surgery* 79:618, 1976.
13. Harris PD, Kovalik AT, Marks JA, et al. Factors modifying aortic homograft structure and function. *Surgery* 63:45, 1968.
14. Perloff LJ, Reckard CR, Rowlands DT Jr, et al. The venous homograft: An immunological question. *Surgery* 72:961, 1972.
15. Imparato AM, Bracco A, Kim GE, et al. Intimal and neointimal fibrous proliferation causing failure of arterial reconstructions. *Surgery* 72:1007, 1972.
16. Nathan IM, Imparato AM. Vibration analysis in experimental models of atherosclerosis. *Bull NY Acad Med* 53:849, 1977.
17. Blaisdell FW, Hall AD. Axillary-femoral artery bypass for lower extremity ischemia. *Surgery* 54:563, 1963.
18. Guida PM, Moore SW. Obturator bypass techniques. *Surg Gynecol Obstet* 128:1307, 1969.
19. Smith JW. Microsurgery: Review of the literature and discussion of microtechnique. *Plast Reconstr Surg* 37:227, 1966.
20. Sabiston DC, Smith GW, Talbert JJ. Evaluation of experimental endarterectomy in vessels of different caliber. *Surg Gynecol Obstet* 110:563, 1960.

21. Imparato AM, Baumann G. Healing patterns in endarterectomized arteries (in preparation).

22. Imparato AM, Bracco A, Kim GE. Comparisons of three techniques for femoral popliteal arterial reconstructions. *Ann Surg* 117:375, 1973.

23. Imparato AM, Kim GE, Madayag M, et al. The results of tibial artery reconstruction procedures. *Surg Gynecol Obstet* 138:33, 1974.

24. Sobel S, Kaplitt MJ, Reingold M, et al. Gas endarterectomy. *Surgery* 59:517, 1966.

25. Fogarty TJ, Cranley JJ, Krause RJ, et al. A method for extraction of arterial emboli and thrombi. *Surg Gynecol Obstet* 116:241, 1963.

26. Dotter CP, Judkins MP. Transluminal treatment of arteriosclerotic obstruction: Description of a new technique and a preliminary report of its application. *Circulation* 30:654, 1964.

27. Gruntzig A, Kumpe DA. Technique of percutaneous transluminal angioplasty with a Gruntzig balloon catheter. *Am J Roentgenol* 132:547, 1979.

28. Gruntzig AR, Senning A, Siegenthaler W. Non-operative dilatation of coronary artery stenosis: Percutaneous transluminal coronary angioplasty. *N Engl J Med* 301:61, 1979.

29. Millan VG, Mast WE, Madias NE. Non-surgical treatment of severe hypertension due to renal artery intimal fibroplasia by percutaneous transluminal angioplasty. *N Engl J Med* 300:1371, 1979.

30. Freiman DB, Ring EJ, Oleaga JA, et al. Transluminal angioplasty of the iliac, femoral, and popliteal arteries. *Radiology* 132:285, 1979.

31. Imparato AM. Lumbar sympathectomy: Role in the treatment of lower extremity occlusive arterial disease. *Surg Clin North Am* 59:719, 1979.

32. Blaisdell FW. In vivo assessment of anticoagulation. *Surgery* 82:827, 1977.

33. Fisher ER, Hellstrom HR, Myers JD. Disseminated atheromatous emboli. *Ann J Med* 29:176, 1960.

34. Bauer RB, Meyer JS, Fields WS, et al. Progress report of control of long term survival in patients with and without operation. Joint study of extracranial arterial occlusion as a cause of stroke. *JAMA* 208:509, 1969.

35. Blaisdell WF, Clauss RH, Galbraith GJ, et al. A review of surgical considerations. Joint study of extracranial arterial occlusion as a cause of stroke. *JAMA* 209:1889, 1969.

36. Fields WS, Maslneikov V, Meyer JS, et al. Progress report of prognosis following surgery or nonsurgical treatment for transient cerebral ischemic attacks and cervical carotid lesions. Joint study of extracranial arterial occlusions as a cause of stroke. *JAMA* 211:1993, 1970.

37. Imparato AM, Riles TS, Kim EG, et al. Vertebral artery reconstruction. *Stroke* 12:125, 1981.

38. Imparato AM, Riles TS, Gorstein F. The carotid bifurcation plaque: Pathologic findings associated with cerebral ischemia. *Stroke* 10:238, 1979.

39. Foster JH. Surgically correctable hypertension. In Schwartz S (ed): *Principles of Surgery,* ed 3. New York, McGraw-Hill, 1979, p 1011.

40. Morris GC Jr, DeBakey ME, Crawford ES, et al. Late results of surgical treatment for renovascular hypertension. *Surg Gynecol Obstet* 122:1255, 1966.

41. Opa K, Mori S, Awane Y, et al. Ex situ repair of renal artery for renovascular hypertension. *Arch Surg* 94:370, 1967.

42. Boley SJ, Schwartz SS. Colonic ischemia: Reversible ischemia lesions. In *Vascular Disorders of the Intestine.* New York, Appleton-Century-Crofts. 1971.

43. Connolly JE, Kwaan JHM. Prophylactic revascularization of the gut. *Ann Surg* 190:514, 1979.

44. Fields WS, North RR, Hass WK, et al. Organization of study and survey of patient population. Joint study of extracranial arterial occlusion as a cause of stroke. *JAMA* 203:955, 1968.

45. Canadian Cooperative Study Group. A randomized trial of aspirin and sulfinpyrazone in threatened stroke. *N Engl J Med* 299:53, 1978.

46. Lazar ML, Clark K. Microsurgical cerebral revascularization. Concepts and practice. *Surg Neurol* 1:355, 1973.

47. Riles TS, Lieberman A, Koppelman I, et al. Bruit, stenosis and symptoms: Interrelationships in carotid artery disease. *Arch Surg* 116:218, 1981.

48. Imparato AM, Kim GE, Davidson T, et al. Intermittent claudication: Its natural course. *Surgery* 78:795, 1975.

49. Dean RH. Indications for operative management of renovascular hypertension. *JSC Med Assoc* 73:523, 1977.

50. Stamey TA. Renovascular hypertension-1965. *Am J Med* 38:829, 1965.

51. Pettinger WA, Mitchell HC. Renin release, saralasin and a vasodilator-beta blocker drug interaction in man. *N Engl J Med* 292;1214, 1975.

52. Wylie EJ, Perloff D, Stoney RJ. Autogenous tissue revascularization techniques in surgery for renovascular hypertension. *Ann Surg* 170:416, 1969.

53. Fry WJ, Brink BE, Thompson NW. New techniques in the treatment of extensive fibromuscular disease involving the renal arteries. *Surgery* 68:959, 1970.

54. Ganz W, Swan HJC. Measurement of blood flow by thermal dilution. *Am J Cardiol* 29:241, 1972.

55. Foster JH, Dean RH, Pinkerton JA, et al. Ten years experience with surgical management of renovascular hypertension. *Ann Surg* 177:755, 1973.

56. Genest J, Boucher R, Rojo-Ortega JM, et al. Renovascular hypertension. In Genest J, Loiw E, Kuchel O (eds): *Hypertension.* New York, McGraw-Hill Book Co, 1977, p 815.

57. Boley SJ, Brandt LJ, Veith FJ. Ischemic disorders of the intestines. *Curr Probl Surg* 15, 1978.

58. Shaw RS, Rutledge RH. Superior mesenteric artery embolectomy in the treatment of massive mesenteric infarction. *N Engl J Med* 257: 595, 1957.

59. Stoney RJ, Ehrenfeld WK, Wylie EJ. Revascularization methods in chronic visceral ischemia caused by atherosclerosis. *Ann Surg* 186:468, 1977.

60. Anane-Safah JC, Blair E, Reckler S. Primary mesenteric venous occlusive disease. *Surg Gynecol Obstet* 141:740, 1975.

61. Willerson JT, Decker JL. Raynaud's disease and phenomenon, a medical approach. *Am Heart J* 82:572, 1971.

62. Gifford RW Jr, Hines EA Jr, Craig WMcK. Sympathectomy for Raynaud's phenomenon: Follow-up study of 70 women with Raynaud's disease and 54 women with secondary Raynaud's phenomenon. *Circulation* 17:5, 1958.

63. Roos DB, Owens JC. Thoracic outlet syndrome. *Arch Surg* 93:71, 1966.

64. Kim GE, Imparato AM, Crowley GJ, et al. Arterial embolization of the upper extremity associated with thoracic outlet syndrome. *Vasc Surg* 12:85, 1978.

65. Estes JE Jr. Abdominal aortic aneurysm: A study of 102 cases. *Circulation* 2:258, 1950.

66. Szilagyi DE, Elliot JP, Smith RF. Clinic fate of the patient with asymp-

tomatic abdominal aortic aneurysm and unfit for surgical therapy. *Arch Surg* 104:600, 1972.

67. Crawford ES, Cho GC, Roehm JO. Thoracoabdominal aortic aneurysms involving celiac, superior mesenteric and renal arteries. In Bergan JJ, Yao JST (eds): *Surgery of the Aorta and Its Body Branches.* New York, Grune and Stratton Inc., 1979, p 148.

68. Wakabayashi A, Connolly JE. Prevention of paraplegia associated with resection of extensive thoracic aneurysms. *Arch Surg* 111:1186, 1976.

69. Alpert J. Aneurysms of the popliteal artery . *J Med Soc NJ* 67:791, 1970.

70. Edmunds LH, Darling RC, Linton RR. Surgical management of popliteal aneurysm. *Circulation* 32:517, 1965.

71. Bedford D, Lodge B. Aneurysm of the splenic artery. *Gut* 1:312, 1960.

72. Owens JC, Coffey RJ. Aneurysm of the splenic artery including a report of 6 additional cases. *Int Abstr Surg* 97:313, 1953.

73. Arujan S, Cahaw E, Greene FL, et al. Successful treatment of hepatic artery aneurysm with erosion into the common duct. *Ann Surg* 182:169, 1975.

74. Guida PM, Moore SW. Aneurysm of the hepatic artery. Report of 5 cases with brief review of previously reported cases. *Surgery* 60:229, 1966.

75. Cerny JC, Chang C, Fry WJ. Renal artery aneurysms. *Arch Surg* 96:653, 1968.

76. Poutasse EF. Renal artery aneurysm: Report of 12 cases, 2 treated by excision of the aneurysm and repair of renal artery. *J Urol* 77:697, 1957.

77. Kianouri M. Extracranial carotid aneurysms. *Ann Surg* 165:152, 1967.

78. Sanoudos GM, Ramp J, Imparato AM. Internal carotid aneurysms. *Am Surg* 39:118, 1973.

19 Podiatric Care in the Diabetic or Ischemic Foot

Robert B. Rakow
Gary S. Saphire

PODIATRY AND PERIPHERAL ARTERIAL INSUFFICIENCY

In no area of medicine are vigilance and preventive care more important than in the treatment of ischemic feet. The great majority of patients with peripheral arterial disease have adequate pedal blood flow under normal metabolic conditions, but many cannot increase blood flow to meet increased oxygen demand. Most amputations performed each year could be avoided through better foot care.

Patient education is the primary method of preventing complications of arterial insufficiency. The physician or podiatrist must take the time to explain certain simple rules of foot care to every patient with diabetes mellitus or absent pedal pulses. These include:

1. Avoidance of thermal trauma; anything applied to the foot should be neither hot nor cold,

2. Avoidance of physical trauma by wearing comfortable, well-fitting shoes and not walking bare-footed,
3. Regular podiatric care for toenails and hyperkeratotic lesions, and
4. Daily foot inspection.

The last item is particularly important for diabetics who often have significant sensory impairment due to neuropathy. Many such diabetics are also visually impaired and require the help of a family member for adequate foot inspection. Any break in the skin, rash, or evidence of skin irritation should prompt a visit to the physician or podiatrist.

THE ROUTINE PODIATRIC VISIT

Often, a well-meaning family member tries to care for a diabetic's feet with catastrophic results. Therefore, it must be stressed to both the patient and his family that their participation in foot care should be limited to daily inspections of the patient's feet and his foot gear, along with strict adherence to a daily pedal hygiene regimen. Nail care, reduction of corns and calluses, and the treatment of other pedal lesions should be restricted to a competent podiatrist. The patient must be trained to contact his podiatrist or physician at the first signs of pedal trouble so that proper treatment can be initiated promptly and further problems thereby obviated (Figure 19-1).

A diabetic patient should be seen by his podiatrist several times a year. At these routine visits, a complete examination of the lower extremities should be made. The skin should be inspected for ulcers, fissures, and infections or macerations. Close attention should be paid to the skin of the webspaces, as these are frequent sites of dermatophytosis and moniliasis in the diabetic. Hyperkeratotic areas should be thoroughly inspected since they are symptoms of abnormal pressure points which are subject to ulceration and gangrenous degeneration. Particular attention should be paid to clavi through which petechiae or hematoma are visible because intradermal hemorrhage is a sign of excessive shearing or point pressure which will most certainly lead to ulceration, infections, and gangrene if left untreated.

The nails should be inspected for incurvation, impingement of the ungual labia, subungual caseation, and trophic changes. Pedal pulses should be palpated and recorded at each visit. Vibratory sensation, light touch, sharp/dull discrimination, and deep tendon reflexes should also be tested and recorded.

The nails should then be prepared with a mild antiseptic solution

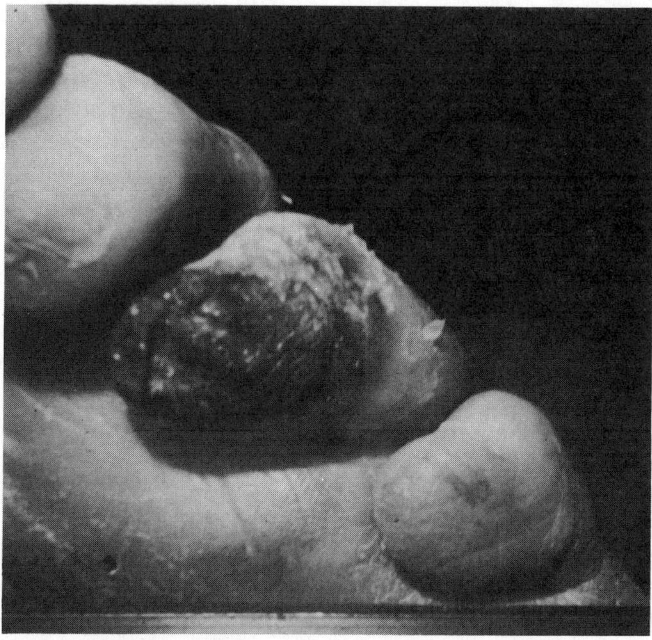

Figure 19-1 Gangrene of the distal aspect of the fourth toe caused by the patient's attempt at self care.

such as phenol 2% and trimmed straight across. Treatment of diseased nails will be discussed later in this chapter. Hyperkeratotic lesions should also be prepared with a 2% solution of phenol and debrided with the utmost care, using a sterile scalpel which is of the proper design for the lesion. After the nails and calluses have been reduced, a mild antiseptic solution such as thimerosal should be applied to the areas which have been treated. Thick callus should be aseptically debrided at least once a month. Protective felt pads may then be applied to shield the lesions from the causative pressures.

It is also very important to look for dermatophytosis between the toes. A very large proportion of patients with diabetes mellitus and peripheral arterial disease have at least some minimal evidence of interdigital fungal infection, although very few are symptomatic. In most cases, one sees only mild desquamation, mainly between the fourth and fifth toes. However, this harmless-looking lesion can progress to small, shallow ulcers through which bacteria can penetrate. The resulting cellulitis can lead to gangrene if blood flow is marginal. It is important to treat early lesions of dermatophytosis with a topical antifungal agent and advise the patient to dry the skin between the toes after bathing.

Dryness of the skin, notably in the heel region, is the cause of heel fissures. The patient must be advised about the application of an emollient ointment. Diabetic patients must be alerted to the importance of proper foot gear in cold as well as in warm weather. Exposure to extreme temperatures, whether cold or hot, should be avoided at all costs. The feet of these patients must never be exposed to direct sunlight, or to direct or indirect heat and cold.

CORNS AND CALLUSES (CLAVI)

Corns and calluses are basically traumatic keratoses. A corn is an elevated nodular lesion, often conical in shape, and commonly found on the dorsal aspect of the fifth toe. It is almost always over a bony prominence. An x-ray often shows a bony spur or phalangeal malalignment under the corn. A callus is a flatter area of hyperkeratosis, most often seen on the plantar surface. These lesions are merely symptoms of an underlying disease process. Normal skin responds to intermittent pressure or shearing forces by hypertrophy. This epidermal hypertrophy in turn increases the pressure on the basal cells, which again respond in kind. The cycle continues until the intermittent pressure becomes constant which, in turn, causes atrophy and ulceration by depriving the skin of an adequate blood supply.

It is beyond the scope of this chapter to discuss the pathomechanics of the foot in great detail, but a few points should be made. The inherent imbalances and instabilities of the foot are, for the most part, responsible for hyperkeratotic lesions; the type of shoe is not the primary source of such lesions. The most common biomechanical fault which causes both dorsal and plantar lesions is a rearfoot (subtalar) varus which makes the entire forefoot unstable and therefore vulnerable. This subtalar varus renders the foot a mobile adaptor during the phase of gait when it should optimally function as a rigid lever. More simply stated, the foot is pronating when it should be supinating at the subtalar joint. This abnormal pronatory force is ultimately responsible for bunions, hammertoes, and plantar-flexed metalarsals which present themselves as the prominences and pressure points of the foot where clavi tylomata are most likely to form.

In caring for corns and calluses, one should not cut them too deeply, especially if foot circulation is impaired. After removal of the cornified layer, steps are taken to inhibit further growth of the keratosis. This is accomplished by proper padding. A U-shaped pad, placed behind a corn, is often effective in dispersing pressure. Molded shoes may also be helpful. In severe cases, calluses are treated with various shoe inserts and inlays.

LATERAL TOENAIL PROBLEMS

Abnormal toenail growth is usually of no consequence to normal individuals, but can easily lead to infection and gangrene in patients with peripheral arterial insufficiency. The lateral borders of toenails may begin to burrow into the underlying skin for a variety of reasons including poor gait, malformed phalanges, osteoarthritis, subungual osteomas and chondromas, and poorly fitting shoes.

Lateral nail problems have been divided into three categories: onychocryptosis (ingrown nail), incurved (inverted) nail, and hypertrophic ungual labium.[1] All of these nail disorders represent a spectrum of progressive, pathologic changes. In an incurved nail, the lateral arc of the plate is exaggerated on one or both sides. Symptoms include pain on digital pressure and walking, but most patients, especially those with diabetic neuropathy, are asymptomatic. This problem can usually be prevented by trimming nails straight across so that the corners of the nail extend beyond the skin line. Shoes and socks must not be too tight. Treatment consists of removal of callus from the sharp margin and packing of the nail groove until the edge of the nail grows out beyond the skin line.

Onychocryptosis is a less common but more serious stage of nail deformity. In one series, it was found in 16% of normal individuals.[2] It is often a complication of incorrect trimming. If the nail is not cut straight across, a lateral sliver of an incurved nail can penetrate into subungual tissue, opening a track for infection.

Once the lesion is infected, it must be treated with vigor. It should be cultured immediately. If the area is already draining, warm saline soaks may be prescribed to promote drainage. The nail border which precipitated the problem must be removed with as little trauma as possible to the already compromised tissue. If there is no drainage and the area is fluctuant, incision and drainage must be performed immediately and followed by saline soaks.

When dealing with patients with diabetes or peripheral arterial disease, the physician is in a dilemma. If he does not incise and drain the infected, ingrown nail, the infection is likely to spread and produce more tissue damage. However, if the procedure is performed, the trauma of the surgery may occasionally precipitate gangrenous changes. Nevertheless, the physician has no choice but to drain the suppurative lesion.

It must be stressed that at no time and under no circumstance should a local anesthetic be injected into such an ischemic foot or toe. The trauma of the needle puncture alone may well be enough to cause necrosis and ulceration of the surrounding tissue, while introduction of exogenous fluid to a closed space (the toe) will increase the pressure in the fascial compartment, thereby increasing the interstitial pressure and impeding the capillary perfusion of the already ischemic area. In such cases we prefer to carry out the procedure under intravenous sedation, spinal anesthesia, or general anesthesia so as not to further compromise an already poor host.

Since host defenses are poor because of systemic problems, the infection must be treated with systemic antibiotics. Although the results of the culture and sensitivity tests may not be available for 72 hours, the patient should be immediately started on antibiotic therapy. The physician can choose a drug prudently if he is aware of the organisms which are most often cultured from similar infections.

A retrospective study of the cultures of 100 secondarily infected ingrown toenails treated by the authors revealed that 83% were caused by *Staphylococcus aureus* (Table 19-1). Since *Staphylococcus aureus* is a beta-lactamase producer, common sense dictates that one use a semisynthetic penicillin which will not be inactivated by the penicillinase. It is our practice to start such cases on oxicillin 500 mg po, qid pending the results of culture and sensitivity. However, if the patient has a past history of penicillin allergy, we prescribe either tetracycline or erythromycin in similar doses and intervals. We choose them as substitutes because about 90% of *Staphylococcus aureus* strains will be susceptible to either drug.

Table 19-1
Results of Cultures Taken of Secondarily Infected Toenails

Organism Cultured	No. (%)
Staphylococcus aureus	82 (82)
Enterococcus	5 (5)
Proteus	3 (3)
S. epidermidis	8 (8)
E. coli	1 (1)
P. aeruginosa	1 (1)
Total	100

The third disorder of the laternal nail, hypertrophic ungualabium, results from chronic inflammatory changes related to an ingrown or incurved nail. The lateral edges of the nail enlarge and thicken. In extreme cases, these hypertrophied edges may override the toenail plate. Surgical removal of this debris is sometimes necessary when the edges become inflamed.

THICKENED AND DYSTROPHIC NAILS

Figure 19-2 is a sketch of a normal nail. Many patients have thickening of the undersurface of the toenail plates (onychogryposis), which can be seen protruding under the free edge. This thickening occurs as a trophic change in elderly people and those with diabetes or arterial insufficiency, but it can also result from trauma, psoriasis, eczema and, onychomycosis. Whatever the cause, it is important to treat this lesion if it is marked. Unattended, it may become a sharp, heavy mass that puts undue pressure on the underlying skin and leads to secondary bacterial infection and subungual ulceration and gangrene (Figure 19-3).

Onychomycosis

Onychomycosis is an infection of the nail caused by a dermatophyte or yeast. The dermatophytes which are commonly responsible for ungual infections are *Trichophyton rubrum, Trichophyton gypseum,* and *Trichophyton mentagrophytes. Candida albicans* is the only yeast which has been demonstrated to infect the nails.

Clinically, the mycotic nail caused by *Tricophyton* will initially present as scaling along the ungual labia with an accumulation of caseous debris along the nail folds. As the disease progresses, the entire nail plate will become thickened, yellowed, and lusterless, with a copious

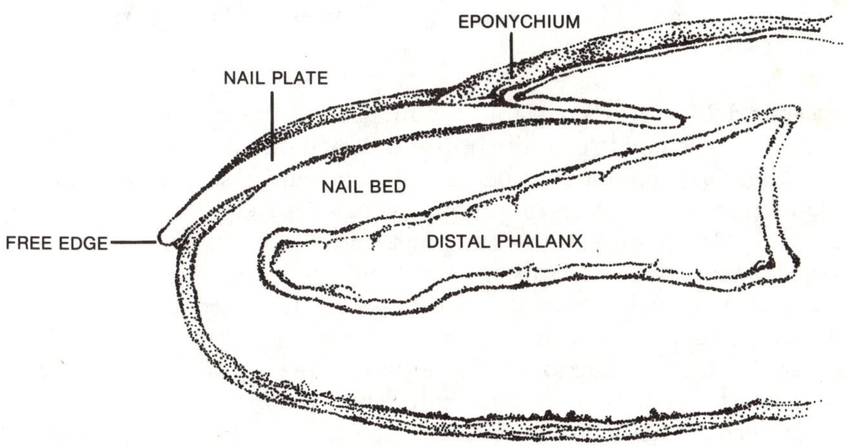

Figure 19-2 Sagittal section through second toe demonstrating the anatomy of the nail.

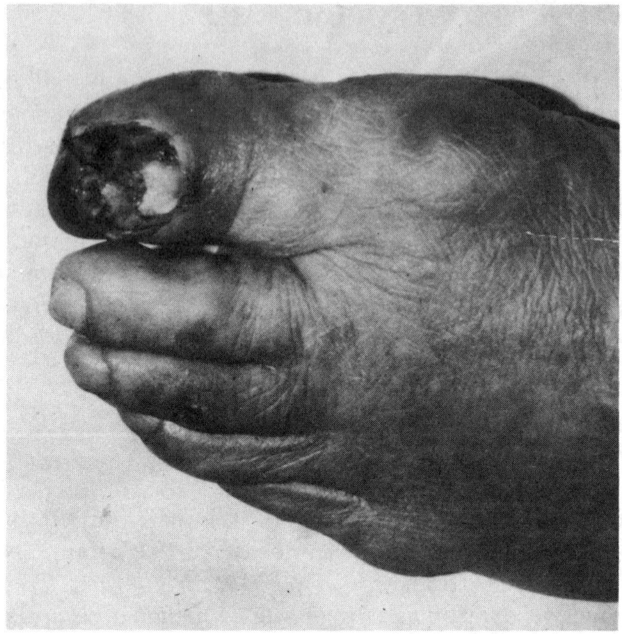

Figure 19-3 Subungual ulceration discovered on debridement of a mycotic hallux nail. The patient had absent pedal pulses, absent vibratory sensation to 15 cm below the tibial tuberosity, diminished deep tendon reflexes, and absence of proprioception. Although the patient suffered severe ischemic changes under the thickened nail plate, he was unaware of anything more than the increase in the thickness of the great toenail since the peripheral neuropathy of diabetes rendered his foot anesthetic. A second ulcer was found upon debridement of the clavus, which overlies the third proximal interphalangeal joint.

caseous debris clearly visiable subungually at the free edge. The nail plate will be noted to be quite brittle and easily fractured (Figure 19-4).

Monilial infections of the nail present with a soft, yellowed nail plate. A creamy white to yellow exudate is frequently noted subungually. In most cases the nail plate undergoes spontaneous lysis to reveal a subungual ulceration.

These mycotic infections must be differentiated from psoriatic nails, lichen planus, and tropic onychogryposis. The physician can make a definitive diagnosis by identifying spores and hyphae or budding yeast on a potassium hydroxide preparation.

Alternate methods of identification are: 1) use of the periodic acid-Schiff stain, and 2) inoculation of a DTM agar test plate with material obtained from the nail plate and subungually.

Once a definitive diagnosis of onychomycosis is made, treatment can be accomplished in several ways. The nail may be treated either medically or surgically. If the patient has no signs of cutaneous ischemia, the nail may be avulsed and the root resected by sharp dissection, or the root may be destroyed chemically. If the patient has circulatory impairment, the problem must be managed medically.

The medical treatment of onychomycosis consists of electromechanical debridement of the thickened nail plate with a high speed dental burr. Extreme caution must be employed during the debridement since the friction of the cutting action of the burr is apt to build up a great deal of heat which might easily induce thermal gangrene in the patient with impaired circulation or altered sensation. The debridement is repeated every four to six weeks. In conjunction with the local care, the patient is given a prescription for a topical antifungal agent to apply to the nail plate and folds twice a day. If the patient has no history of penicillin allergy, a regimen of oral griseofulvin is started after a baseline hemogram has been obtained. The patient must be made to understand from the outset that he will not note any results from the griseofulvin for a minimum of four to six months. He must also be made aware that good medical practice dictates that a blood count be done every month during therapy, since agranulocytosis or leukopenia is a well-documented side effect of the drug.

TREATMENT OF FOOT ULCERATION AND GANGRENE

The two major factors in the development of foot ulcers and gangrene are insufficient blood flow and trauma. The latter may be

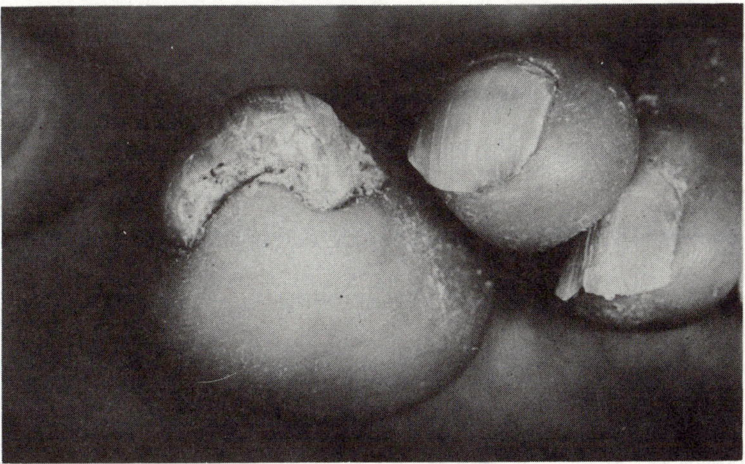

Figure 19-4 Characteristic changes of onychomycosis. Note the thickening of the nail plate, its lusterless appearance, and the caseous subungual debris.

thermal or physical in nature, and occur acutely or insidiously over a long period of time. Diabetic patients with peripheral neuropathy are often subject to repeated injury without being aware of it. Ill-fitting shoes, for example, can cause gradual erosion of skin in the instep area, and a hot bath or electric heating pad may produce painless blistering and ulceration. An even more surreptitious form of trauma occurs with ingrown toenails.

Infection also plays a role, sometimes as the primary factor and often as a complication of ulceration and gangrene. Diabetic patients are particularly susceptible to a rapidly spreading infection of the surface of these lesions and secondary cellulitis. Infection leads to tissue necrosis, not only by direct damage but also by an increase in the metabolic rate and oxygen demands of already hypoxic cells.

Because of loss of subtle reflexes, patients with severe diabetic neuropathy are at risk for traumatic ulceration even during normal walking and standing. Undue pressure on the plantar aspect of the foot produces a painless, neurotrophic ulcer (Figure 19-5). This lesion generally occurs in areas of thick callus under the metatarsals, but sometimes on the lateral aspects of the first and fifth metatarsophalangeal joints and on the distal aspects of the digits. These ulcers heal quickly when the source of trauma (pressure on standing) is relieved, but can easily recur when the patient again becomes ambulatory.

At the other end of the ischemia-trauma spectrum, severe arterial insufficiency may cause pure tissue infarction, which carries a worse prognosis than a traumatic lesion in a foot with milder arterial disease (Figure 19-6). However, even this type of gangrene can be arrested. If the lesion is well-demarcated, it can eventually slough off, and healing of healthy tissue around its borders can slowly take place.

The clinician must apply a few general principles in treating and preventing skin breakdown. These include:

1. Removal of all pressure on the lesion, which often requires complete rest,
2. Culture and sensitivity of the base of the ulcer,
3. Systemic antibiotics for any cellulitis surrounding the lesion,
4. Cautious debridement of devitalized tissue, and
5. Local medications and body temperature soaks as indicated.

One must be careful not to immobilize the patient longer than necessary because muscle atrophy and contractures may result from prolonged disuse of a limb. It is also important to protect major pressure points (heel and malleoli) from continuous pressure by the

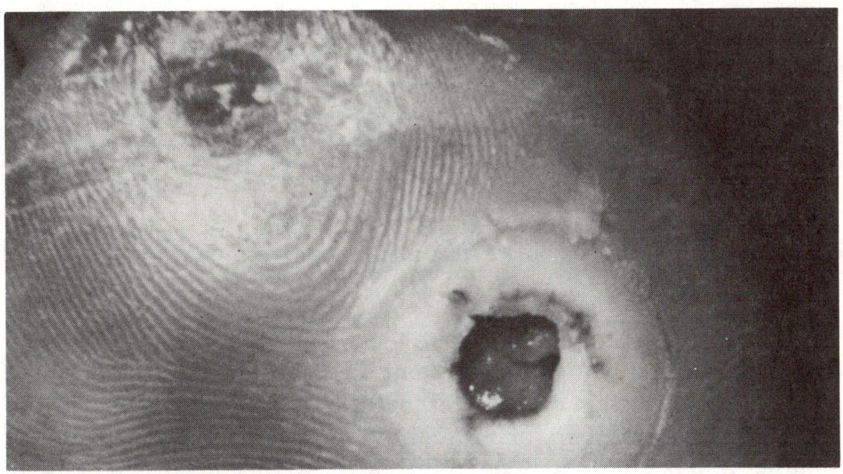

Figure 19-5 Mal perforans over the plantar aspect of the first metatarsal head.

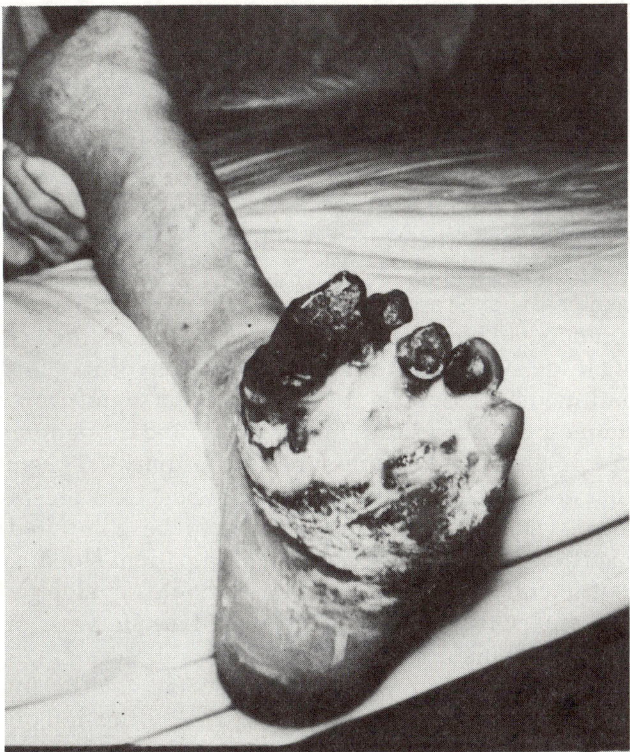

Figure 19-6 Dry gangrene of the toes with spread of necrosis onto the dorsum and plantar apsect of the foot.

mattress if the patient is at bed rest. Cushioned heel pads are useful, and pillows can be utilized to suspend the foot and ankle away from the mattress. Patients with dry gangrene can be ambulatory when the lesion has become well demarcated. Ulcerated lesions must be protected from pressure, even after healing has begun, in order to prevent recurrence.

Shoe Modifications and Relief of Pressure

Shoes must be modified to take the weight off the ulcerated area. The goal is to relieve completely any pressure on the lesion, while distributing the weight over the rest of the foot. If even weight distribution is not accomplished, one is merely trading one pressure point for another, and is quite likely to end up with two lesions instead of one. Throughout this discussion, one should bear in mind that these techniques can be applied to pressure points which have not as yet broken down, thereby preventing possible limb-threatening lesions.

The number of shoe modifications, latex shields, and inlays which can be fabricated is limited only by the physician's ingenuity and creativity. We shall therefore discuss and illustrate the basic types of appliances and modifications so as to allow the individual physician to expand upon these elementary forms.

Gangrenous lesions occurring either on the dorsum of the toes or their distal aspects can be easily managed. One can simply remove the toebox from the shoe, thereby preventing any pressure which might come to bear on the lesion.

Bauman et al[3] have reported an extensive study of plantar pressure in the trophic foot. They have shown that continuous pressure of only slight magnitude is enough to deprive the tissue of its blood supply. If this continuous pressure is maintained for a significant length of time, ischemic necrosis occurs. Kosiak[4] and Lindan[5] demonstrated in animal experiments that this pressure need be only 0.08 kg/cm^2. If we assume that total ischemia is produced when external pressure is greater than systolic blood pressure, it can be computed that 0.2 kg/cm^2 is sufficient to produce necrosis. If a patient stood completely still for a sufficiently long period of time, he could develop gangrene on the plantar aspect of the foot. This would occur with or without diabetes or arterial insufficiency.

Lesions which occur on the plantar surface of the foot can be treated either by shoe modifications or by the fabrication of a molded orthotic device which the patient can slip into his shoe. These devices can be made from many different types of material, generally divided into three classes: 1) rigid 2) semirigid, and 3) flexible (Table 19-2). We

Table 19-2
Materials Commonly Used in the Production of Orthotic Devices for Foot Correction

Rigid materials
Stainless steel
Rohadur
Fiberglass
Semirigid materials
Ortholon
Celastic
Flexible materials
Plastizote
Felt latex
Spenco
P.P.T.
Leather rubber butter

prefer to utilize the semirigid and flexible types to accommodate the lesions of the compromised foot because they are more easily modified to equalize the pathomechanical forces in the ischemic, diabetic or geriatric foot. We reserve the rigid type of device for the treatment of the younger, non-compromised patient who presents with a purely biomechanical problem.

The orthotic device which we use most often for the treatment of a plantar lesion is the dynamically fabricated Plastizote inlay. It is constructed as follows: A piece of ¼ inch Plastizote is cut to fit the contour of the shoe as an innersole. A medial flange is allowed to remain along the longitudinal arch. The form is then placed in the shoe and the patient is allowed to walk on the device for several days. At the next visit the inlays are examined. The points of maximal pressure are visualized as thinning or compression of the Plastizote. One must build up the undersurface of the device surrounding the areas of increased pressure. The build-up can be made from felt, cork, or Plastizote. The top of the orthotic device is then covered with a layer of leather or some other suitable fabric so as to prolong its useful life. The inlay is examined periodically to ascertain if any new pressure points have developed. Modifications are made accordingly.

Lesions which occur on the medial aspect of the first metatarsal head or on the lateral aspect of the fifth metatarsal head can be accommodated either by a shoe modification or by the fabrication of a latex shield (Figure 19-7). The shoe modification is easily accomplished by removing the entire toebox as is done for dorsal and distal, digital lesions. The shield is made from a plaster model of the foot or toe. We have found the shoe modification to be more easily and quickly accomplished.

Gangrenous lesions which occur around the heel are most easily treated with a posterior shoe modification (Figure 19-8). This alteration cannot be carried out in the office, but must be done by a shoemaker since it requires a build-up of the shank area of the shoe as well as the sole. One must be certain that the cut edge of the shoe has been adequately beveled and cushioned to avoid one area of pressure being traded for another.

Medication and Dressings

Local measures include the use of topical antibiotics, proteolytic enzymes, and a variety of other substances. Kanof[6] has reported preliminary studies with gold leaf, but this therapy has not proven to be helpful. Many other substances have been suggested, including powdered dextrose, salicylic acid, and vitamins, but they have not proved to be useful. When an ulcerated lesion is exudative, heavy ointment may block drainage and cause maceration. In such cases, lukewarm water or saline soaks may be most useful.

The antiseptic properties of the halogens have been known for years. However, methods of application were found wanting until Collens et al[7] published a method for the release of nascent, volatile iodine. This method of treatment is as satisfactory today as it was when the paper was published in 1962. Briefly, the solution is prepared by dissolving 0.5 gm of potassium iodide in 100 ml of water to which 0.5

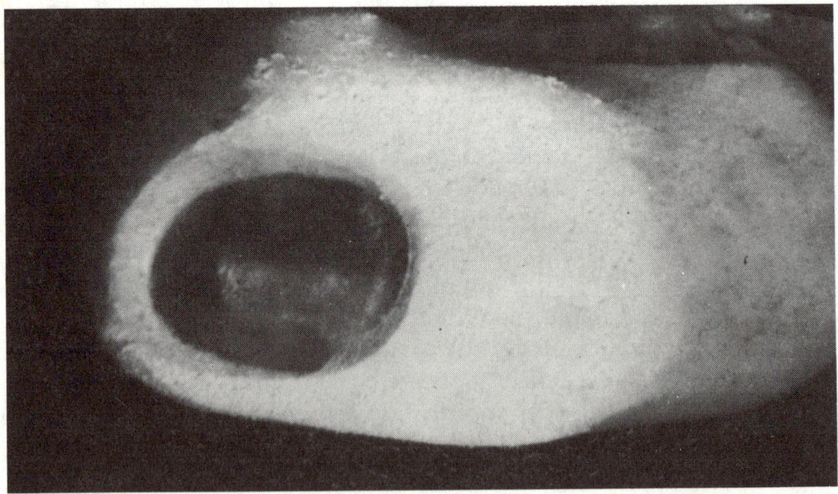

Figure 19-7 Latex shield to protect the lateral aspect of the fifth metatarsal head.

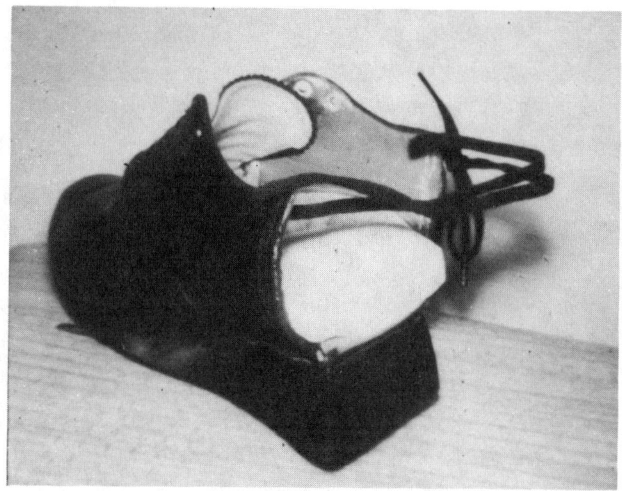

Figure 19-8 Shoe modification to accommodate heel lesion.

gm of iodine crystals is added. Approximately 0.4 gm of the iodine goes into solution, producing a supersaturated solution with crystal iodine and liberating a free triiodide complex (I_3^-). This unstable compound provides a rapid and continuous release of free, nascent iodine. The solution can be used in any of several ways and in a combination of dressings. Sinus tracts may be loosely packed and the iodine solution placed directly on the drain (Figures 19-9, 19-10). The triiodide solution may be applied directly into the slough or it may be placed upon a sterile gauze pad which is then sandwiched between two dry sterile gauze pads and incorporated into one dressing.

The use of Debrisan beads can be helpful. These hydrophilic beads absorb fluid and are helpful in drying out exudative wounds so that granulation can proceed. Proteolytic enzymes are often helpful in chemical debridement of necrotic and fibrinous material at the base of some nonpurulent ulcers. By application of these enzymes after soaking the lesion in body temperature water, one may often avoid the trauma of physical debridement of adherent material. Two useful agents are collagenase and sutilains (a product of *B. subtilis*). The latter must be applied at least three times per day to be fully effective.

RADIOLOGY OF THE DIABETIC FOOT

Radiographic changes encountered most frequently in the diabetic foot are: 1) Mönckeberg's medial calcinosis (Figure 19-11), 2) diabetic osteopathy (Figure 19-12), 3) Charcot's joint (neurotrophic arthrop-

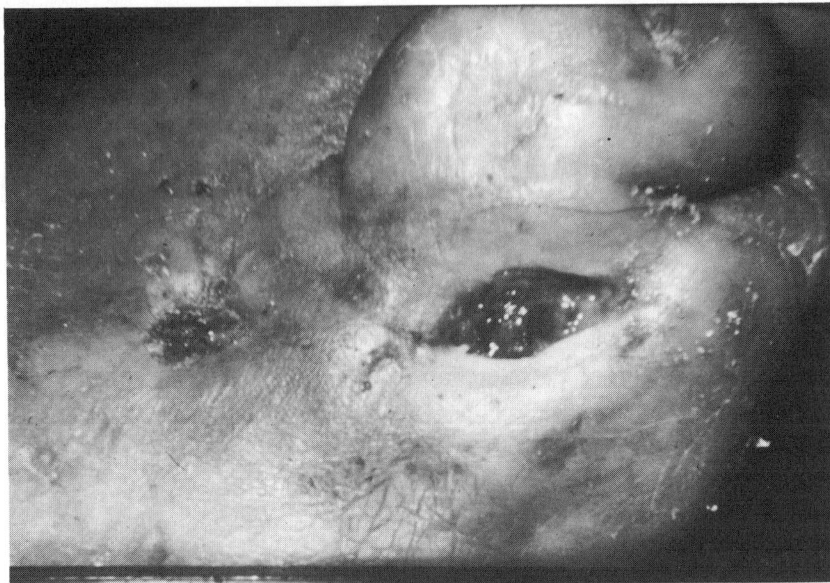

Figure 19-9 Communicating ulcers on the dorsum of the ischemic and anesthetic foot of a 72-year-old, insulin-dependent diabetic.

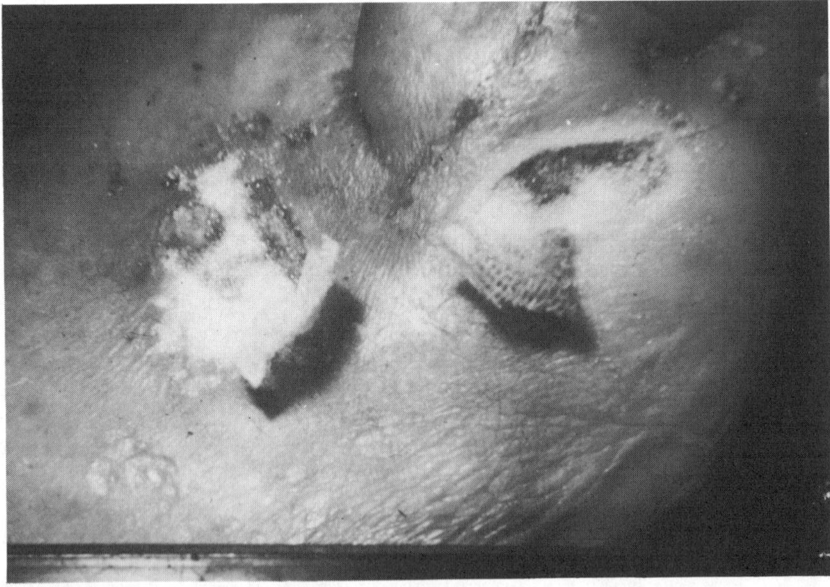

Figure 19-10 Same patient as in Figure 19-9 with through-and-through iodoform gauze drain in place.

athy); 4) generalized osteopenia (Figure 19-12), and 5) osteomyelitis (Figure 19-11, 19-13).

Since the radiographic changes of a Charcot's joint or diabetic osteopathy can easily be mistaken for those of osteomyelitis, it is imperative to correlate the clinical manifestations with x-ray findings before deciding on therapy. Osteomyelitis is almost always of the direct expansion type, preceded by a penetrating wound or a long-standing ulcer, whereas diabetic osteopathy and changes in a Charcot's joint can occur beneath an intact skin (Figure 19-14). Nevertheless, a trophic ulcer may overlie foot ulcers. To differentiate osteomyelitis from the concurrent existence of diabetic osteoarthropathy and a trophic ulcer, one must carefully examine the ulcer to be certain that there are no sinus tracts therein. If a sinus tract is found, a sterile probe may be gently introduced to ascertain if the tract has reached the bone. X-ray studies may be performed with the instrument in place to obtain a hard copy of the actual depth of the tract. If the sinus does in fact penetrate to the bone, it is safe to assume that the radiographic process is truly that of osteomyelitis.

If the exact etiology of a lesion cannot be determined by the correlation of clinical and radiographic findings, it may become necessary to per-

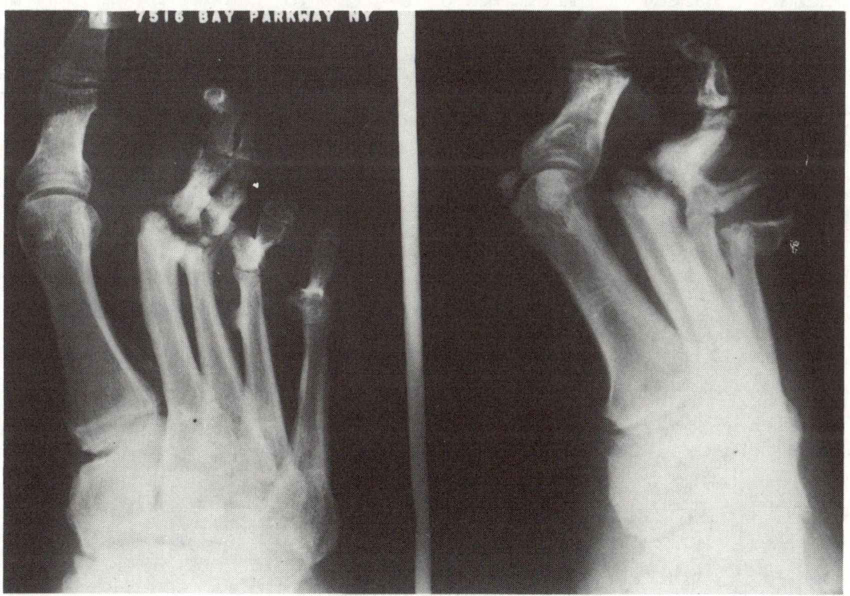

Figure 19-11 The above radiographs demonstrate: 1) Mönckeberg's medial calcinosis of the dorsalis pedis artery, 2) Diabetic osteopathy as evidenced by the resorption of the fourth and fifth distal phalanges, 3) Osteomyelitis of the fourth metatarsal head. This lesion was clearly exposed through a 2-cm ulcer on the plantar surface of the foot.

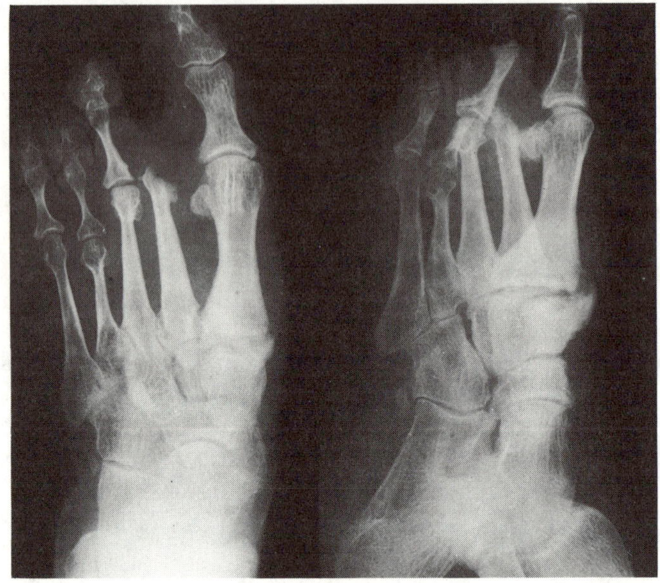

Figure 19-12 These films demonstrate the marked osteoporosis commonly seen in the diabetic foot. The second digit was disarticulated six months before because of chronic osteomyelitis.

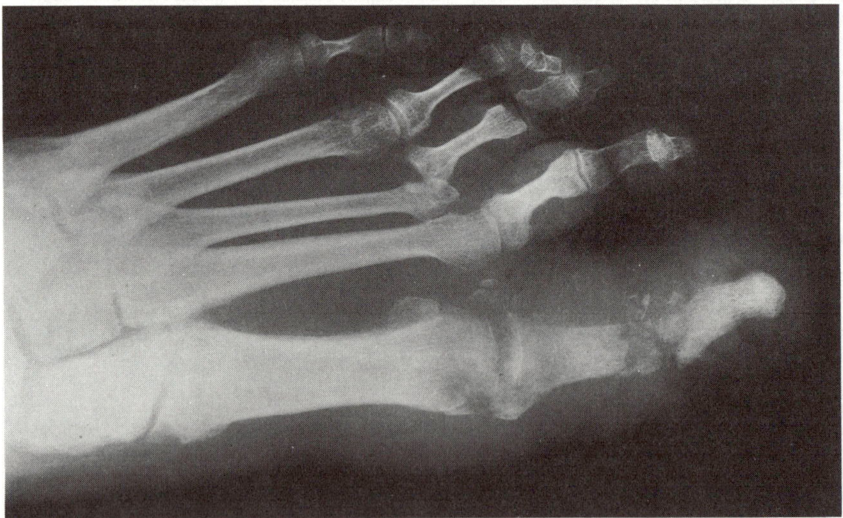

Figure 19-13 Note the destructive changes around the interphalangeal joint of the hallux. A soft tissue defect can be easily visualized at the same level in that toe. Histologic examination of bone retrieved from the sinus tract confirmed the diagnosis of osteomyelitis.

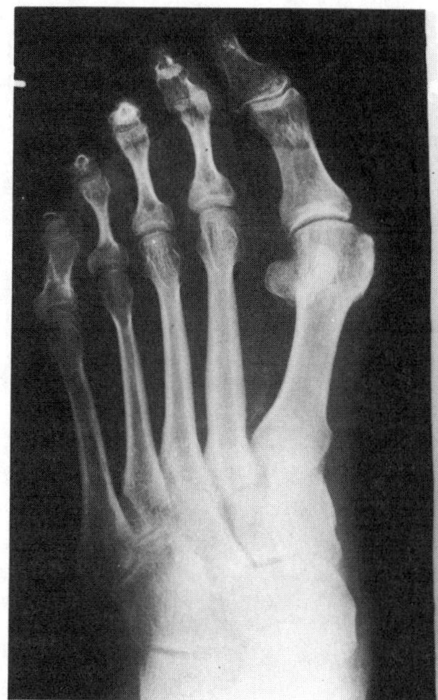
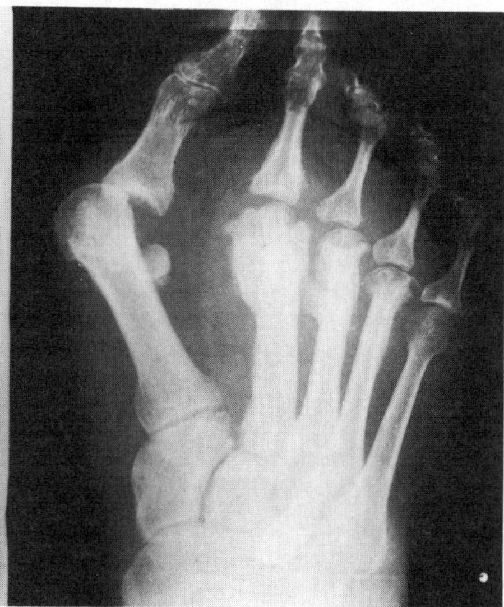

Figure 19-14 The left foot appears to be within normal limits, except for the calcification of the dorsalis pedis artery. The contralateral foot exhibits marked soft tissue swelling, dislocation of the first metatarsophalangeal joint, and Charcot's joint changes in the second, third, and fourth metatarsophalangeal joints.

form a bone scan to elucidate the nature of the osseous changes. Osteomyelitic changes will be clearly visualized on the scan early in the course of the disease. Dibos and Wagner[8] have reported that osteomyelitis can be detected on scan as early as 24 hours after the inflammatory reaction has begun, whereas the radiographic signs of osteomyelitis may not appear for 10 to 14 days after the onset of the infection.

REFERENCES

1. Frost L. Root resection for incurvated nail. *J Natl Assoc Chirop* 40:19, (Mar) 1950.
2. Krausz CE. A nail survey of 4,600 patients. *J Natl Assoc Chirop* 40:11 (May) 1950.
3. Bauman JH, Brand PW. Measurement of pressure between foot and shoe. *Lancet* 1:629, 1963.
4. Kosiak M. Etiology of decubitus ulcers. *Arch Phys Med Rehabil* 42:19, 1961.
5. Lindan O. Etiology of decubitus ulcers. *Arch Phys Med Rehabil* 42:774, 1961.

6. Kanof NM. Gold leaf in the treatment of cutaneous ulcers. *J Invest Derm* 43:441, 1964.

7. Collens WS, Vlahos E, Dobkin GN, et al. Conservative management of gangrene in the diabetic patient. *JAMA* 181:692, 1962.

8. Dibos P, Wagner H. *Atlas of Nuclear Medicine, Bone V.* Philadelphia, WB Saunders, 1978, p 65.

INDEX